SPINAL INSTRUMENTATION

SPINAL INSTRUMENTATION

Editors

HOWARD S. AN, MD

Assistant Professor
Director of Reconstructive Spine Surgery
Department of Orthopaedic Surgery
The Medical College of Wisconsin
Milwaukee, Wisconsin

Jerome M. Cotler, MD

Professor and Vice Chairman
Department of Orthopaedic Surgery
Thomas Jefferson University
Philadelphia, Pennsylvania

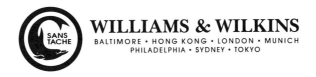

WILLIAMS & WILKINS
BALTIMORE · HONG KONG · LONDON · MUNICH
PHILADELPHIA · SYDNEY · TOKYO

Editor: Timothy H. Grayson
Managing Editor: Marjorie Kidd Keating
Copy Editor: Judith F. Minkove
Designer: Karen S. Klinedinst
Illustration Planner: Ray Lowman
Production Coordinator: Susan S. Vaupel
Cover Designer: Dan Pfisterer

Copyright © 1992
Williams & Wilkins
428 East Preston Street
Baltimore, Maryland   21202,   USA

Printed in the United States of America

Library of Congress Cataloging in Publication Data

Spinal instrumentation / editors, Howard S. An, Jerome M. Cotler.
    p.   cm.
  Includes bibliographical references and index.
  ISBN 0-683-00127-2
  1. Spine—Surgery.   2. Orthopedic implants.   I. An, Howard S.
II. Cotler, Jerome M.
  [DNLM: 1. Orthopedic Fixation Devices.   2. Spinal Fusion—
instrumentation.   3. Spine—abnormalities.   4. Spine—surgery.   WE
725 S7572]
RD768.S6534   1992
617.3′75059—dc20
DNLM/DLC
for Library of Congress   91-30654
                                       CIP

92 93 94 95 96
1 2 3 4 5 6 7 8 9 10

THIS BOOK IS DEDICATED TO
OUR WIVES, SUE AND FLORENCE

FOREWORD

What is the current state-of-the-art in spinal instrumentation? The editors have assembled a veritable "Who's Who" of recognized authorities to answer that question. Within this volume the reader will find the numerous techniques currently available to the spinal surgeon to deal with spinal instabilities ranging from unusual tumors, to more common traumatic conditions, to the most common problems that may accompany spinal degeneration.

How has spinal surgery progressed to this level of sophistication? In the overall scope of human endeavor, the history is short. Most spinal surgeons believe that Hadra (3) was the first surgeon to attempt spinal stabilization, an operation he undertook in a baby with wiring of C6–C7. In fact, Wiltse (8) attributes the first operation to B.F. Wilkins (7), whose case report is reminiscent of *The Wizard of Oz*. He describes a pregnant mother, who in the 8th month of pregnancy was struck by a table, propelled by a severe tornado! A day later she was delivered of a child with a peculiar "bunch in the back."

According to Wiltse, Dr. Wilkins observed this unusual mass, performed his operation when the child was 6 days old, reduced a dislocation of T12 on L1, and stabilized his reduction with carbolized silver sutures passed around the pedicles. Not only is the case study an extraordinary tribute to surgical courage, but it antedates the current popularity of the pedicle as a site of fixation by almost 100 years.

How have we progressed over that century? Clearly, the surgeon now has a formidable armamentarium of devices to treat spinal instability. This book describes highly sophisticated techniques applicable to all spinal levels, as well as multiple pathologies. The reader will be shown how clinical problems can be attacked by the anterior, posterior, or combined approach using many different devices. Because the author of the chapter usually has been the inventor of the device, the individual chapters have the benefit of the authors' large experience.

How should we select a particular operation for the particular patient who presents in our emergency rooms or clinical practice? With each patient, the surgeon faces numerous dilemmas. What is the basic pathology? Is instability really present? Is the desired instrumentation available? Do I have a team who knows how to use the instrumentation? In fact, do I have the requisite skill and experience to perform the operation? For many of us, these are thorny problems.

First, the definition of instability, particularly in nontraumatic conditions affecting the spine remains uncertain when rigorous clinical and radiologic criteria are employed. For example, the CT scan allowed spinal surgeons to differentiate potentially unstable burst fractures from the more common stable compression fracture (1,2,4). Ten years later, we have learned that patients with burst fractures, treated conservatively, appear to function well without stabilization. In fact, remodeling of the compromised spinal canal occurs over time (6).

Even more difficult are the clinical decisions that accompany the surgical treatment of patients with "degenerative instability." Clinical criteria are uncertain, imaging studies often equivocal or subject to significant measurement errors, and clinical results are less than satisfactory, as measured by the relief of pain and return to function.

Similarly, the highly sophisticated techniques are accompanied by a "steep learning curve." For example, pedicle screw fixation is accompanied by a significant rate of screw misplacement, iatrogenic neurologic complications, and failed surgery. These realities have to be measured against the fact that pedicle fixation, as one form of spinal stabilization, offers the surgeon a degree of rigid fixation unavailable with any other technique.

Finally, it is almost axiomatic that the majority of patients who require spinal stabilization also require a biologic arthrodesis. Obviously, exceptions exist, such as the patient with metastatic spinal disease and impending paraplegia, for whom a composite of internal fixation and methylmethacrylate, is an appropriate alternative. However, the use of methylmethacrylate is accompanied by significant complications, particularly when the construct is from a posterior approach and placed under tension (5). For most patients with a normal life expectancy, the modest additional morbidity of the biologic arthrodesis balances well against the durability that bone grafting affords.

These brief thoughts are meant to provoke you, the reader. There is no question that the editors and their distinguished authors, present a current and comprehensive guide that Wilkins, even in the context of *The Wizard of Oz*, could hardly have envisioned. The utility of the volume is its completeness and the bringing together of a diverse and emerging literature. The ultimate test will be finding answers to these questions: "How well do our patients fare when these techniques are used? Would they have done as well by less complex surgical techniques or, in fact, would they have fared better with a nonoperative approach?"

John W. Frymoyer, M.D.
Interim Dean, College of Medicine
Professor of Orthopaedics
Director, McClure Musculoskeletal
   Research Center
Department of Orthopaedics and
   Rehabilitation
University of Vermont
Burlington, Vermont

REFERENCES

1. Denis F, Armstrong G: Compression fractures versus burst fractures in the lumbar and thoracic spine. J Bone Joint Surg (Br) 1981; 63:462.
2. Denis F: The three column spine and its significance in the classification of acute thoracolumbar spinal injuries. Spine 1983; 8:817–831.
3. Hadra BE: Wiring the spinous processes in Pott's disease. Trans Amer Orthop Assoc 1891; 4:206–210.
4. McAfee PC, Yuan HA, Fredrickson GE, et al: The value of computed tomography in thoracolumbar fractures. J Bone Joint Surg 1983; 64A:461–473.
5. McAfee PC, Bohlman HH, Ducker T, et al: Failure of stabilization of the spine with methylmethacrylate. A retrospective analysis of 24 cases. J Bone Joint Surg (Am) 1986; 68:1145–1157.
6. Weinstein JN, Collalto P, Lehmann TR: Thoracolumbar burst fractures treated conservatively: A long-term follow-up. Spine 1988; 13:33–38.
7. Wilkins BF: Separation of the vertebrae with protrustion of hernia between the same-operation-cure. St Louis Med Surg J 1888; 54:340-341.
8. Wiltse LL: The history of spinal disorders. In: Frymoyer JW, ed. The adult spine: principles and practice. New York: Raven Press. 1991; 3–41.

FOREWORD

Breakthroughs in spinal surgery have included methods to control bleeding and infection, and the invention of tools for the surgeon. Certainly, the development of x-ray techniques, including new computed imaging methods, led to quantum leaps in the understanding of spinal disorders. Ultimately, it became obvious to spine surgeons that external immobilization, in the form of braces or casts, may not be sufficient to stabilize the spine, or to immobilize it during the fusion process. Consequently, internal stabilization by spinal instrumentation was born.

The evolution of these techniques has been fitful. Tissue damage was caused immediately on their insertion, or subsequently, as the result of migration, metal fatigue, or infection. Some devices were inappropriately designed, and these soon became unavailable. Methods of fixation of instruments to the spine were, in many instances, insecure.

The last decade saw a rebirth of spinal instrumentation. Fueled by committed spinal surgeons whose knowledge of spine function was enhanced by research and subtler imaging techniques, new methods of spinal instrumentation have evolved. Instruments have been designed for specific purposes related to specific disease entities. The use of newer alloys has reduced the incidence of metal failure. Enhanced techniques allow instruments to be fixed to the spinous processes, lamina, pedicles, and, occasionally, to vertebral bodies. These new developments have proved successful in the correction of deformities. At the same time, surgeons can be more optimistic about the permanency of their procedures.

The authors of this book are leaders in the renaissance of spinal instrumentation. Each has combined innovative mechanical skills with the detailed study of spinal anatomy and an abiding concern for a cure. They are pioneers, however, and as such, only time can distinguish the durable from the transient. Readers who are spine surgeons are entrusted to make long-term comparisons of these devices. With that trust is an obligation to study and review surgical results.

Spinal surgeons who read this book are challenged to match the integrity of Drs. An and Cotler. Having this book on your shelf will serve as a reminder to value their expertise while charting your own success with the innovative techniques described on these pages.

Frederick A. Simeone, M.D.
Professor of Neurosurgery
University of Pennsylvania School of Medicine
Chief of Neurosurgery
Pennsylvania Hospital
Philadelphia, Pennsylvania

PREFACE

The recent flood of new spinal instrumentations stimulated the editors to compile an up-to-date book on this topic. There have been significant advancements in the field of spine fusion and instrumentation in the last few decades. The aim of this book is to provide insight into the field of spinal isntrumentation as well as to present basic information on surgical anatomy, fusion techniques, and surgical indications. Biomechanics, surgical techniques, clinical results, and complications of various old and new instrumentation systems are presented.

Spinal Instrumentation is written for spine surgeons (orthopaedists and neurosurgeons), general orthopaedic surgeons, spine fellows, and residents. The editors were extremely fortunate to assemble pioneers and experts of spine instrumentation from all over the world. Chapter 1 deals with the surgical anatomy, surgical techniques of spine fusion, general surgical indications, and potential complications. Chapter 2 focuses on the standard and new methods of posterior cervical fixation. Chapter 3 presents new methods of anterior plate-screw instrumentations of the cervical spine. Chapters 4–7 deal with established spinal instrumentations such as Harrington rod, Luque rod, and Wisconsin segmental fixation, describing not only the original methods but also various improved modifications. Chapters 8–20 give examples of the recent flood of new posterior spinal instrumentations, using hooks and pedicle screws. Each author has carefully presented the philosophy, surgical techniques, results, and complications of each system. Various anterior thoracolumbar systems are presented from chapters 21 to 25. Lastly, Chapter 26 serves as a summary chapter, discussing general principles of different surgical constructs in terms of indications and complications.

We would like to acknowledge our teachers, clinical and research colleagues, who were indirectly involved in the preparation of this project. It is impossible to mention all of them by name. We must mention Ann Louise Smith and Patricia Dybro for their dedicated assistance in editing and secretarial efforts. What really made this project possible was the individual contributor of each chapter, as this book would not exist without their contributions.

Howard S. An, M.D.
Jerome M. Cotler, M.D.

CONTRIBUTORS

TODD J. ALBERT, M.D.
Chief Resident
Department of Orthopaedic Surgery
Thomas Jefferson University
Philadelphia, Pennsylvania

HOWARD S. AN, M.D.
Assistant Professor
Director of Reconstructive Spine Surgery
Department of Orthopaedic Surgery
The Medical College of Wisconsin
Milwaukee, Wisconsin

**GORDON W. D. ARMSTRONG, M.D.,
F.R.C.S.(C)**
Professor of Orthopaedic Surgery
University of Ottawa
Former Chief of Orthopaedics
Ottawa Civic Hospital (Retired)
Ottawa, Ontario, Canada

MARC A. ASHER, M.D.
Professor of Orthopaedic Surgery
University of Kansas Medical Center
Kansas City, Kansas

RICHARD B. ASHMAN, Ph.D.
Assistant Professor
Department of Orthopaedics
University of Texas Southwestern Medical Center
Scientific Director of Research
Texas Scottish Rite Hospital
Dallas, Texas

RICHARD A. BALDERSTON, M.D.
Clinical Professor of Orthopaedics
Department of Orthopaedic Surgery
Jefferson Medical College
Philadelphia, Pennsylvania

Cpt. JAMES C. BAYLEY, M.D., M.C., U.S.A.R.
Assistant Professor of Orthopaedic Surgery
Department of Orthopaedic Surgery
Mayo Clinic
Rochester, Minnesota

J. ABBOTT BYRD III, M.D.
Assistant Clinical Professor
Department of Orthopaedic Surgery
Eastern Virginia Medical School
and Vann Orthopaedic Associates, P.C.
Norfolk, Virginia

WILLIAM L. CARSON, Ph.D.
Professor
Department of Mechanical and Aerospace Engineering
University of Missouri-Columbia
Columbia, Missouri

FRANCO P. CERABONA, M.D.
Clinical Assistant Professor
Department of Orthopedic Surgery
New York Medical College
Chief of Spine Service
St. Vincent's Hospital and Medical Center
New York, New York

DONALD CHOW, M.D., F.R.C.S.(C)
University of Ottawa
Staff Surgeon
Division of Orthopaedics
Ottawa Civic Hospital
Ottawa, Ontario, Canada

HOWARD B. COTLER, M.D.
Associate Professor
Division of Orthopaedic Surgery
The University of Texas Medical School
Medical Director
Texas Back Institute
Houston, Texas

JEROME M. COTLER, M.D.
Professor and Vice Chairman
Department of Orthopaedic Surgery
Thomas Jefferson University
Philadelphia, Pennsylvania

DENIS S. DRUMMOND, M.D.
Chairman
Division of Orthopaedic Surgery
University of Pennsylvania School of Medicine
Children's Hospital of Philadelphia
Philadelphia, Pennsylvania

CHARLES C. EDWARDS, M.D.
Professor of Orthopaedic Surgery
Director, Section of Spinal Surgery
University of Maryland Medical Center
Baltimore, Maryland

BRUCE E. FREDRICKSON, M.D.
Professor of Orthopedic Surgery
Department of Orthopedic Surgery
State University of New York Health Science Center
Syracuse, New York

STANLEY D. GERTZBEIN, M.D.
Associate Professor
Chief, Department of Research and
Orthopaedic Surgery
Texas Back Institute and University of Texas
Houston, Texas

MICHAEL H. HAAK, M.D.
Spine Fellow
Spine Injury Center
McGaw Medical Center of Northwestern University
Chicago, Illinois

MARK F. HAMBLY, M.D.
Wiltse Spine Institute
Long Beach, California

CHARLES F. HEINIG, M.D.
Ware Neck, Virginia
Orthopaedic Surgeon (Retired)
Miller Clinic
Charlotte, North Carolina

J. ANTHONY HERRING, M.D.
Professor
Department of Orthopaedics
University of Texas Southwetern Medical Center
Chief of Staff
Texas Scottish Rite Hospital
Dallas, Texas

CHARLES E. JOHNSTON II, M.D.
Assistant Professor
Department of Orthopaedics
University of Texas Southwestern Medical Center
Orthopaedic Surgeon
Texas Scottish Rite Hospital
Dallas, Texas

KIYOSHI KANEDA, M.D.
Professor and Chairman
Department of Orthopaedic Surgery
Hokkaido University School of Medicine
Sapporo, Hokkaido, Japan

JOHN P. KOSTUIK, M.D.
Chief, Spine Division
Department of Orthopaedic Surgery
The Johns Hopkins University School of Medicine
Baltimore, Maryland

MARTIN H. KRAG, M.D.
Associate Professor
Vermont Rehabilitation Engineering Center
for Low Back Pain
Department of Orthopaedics and Rehabilitation
University of Vermont
Burlington, Vermont

CLAUDE LAVILLE, M.D.
Assistant
Service de Chirurgie Orthopédique et Traumatologique
Centre Hospitalier Pitié-Salpétrière
Paris, France

RÉNÉ LOUIS, M.D.
Professor
Service d'Orthopédie Traumatologie et Chirurgie
Vertebrale
Hôpital de le Conception
Marseille, France

EDUARDO R. LUQUE, M.D.
Director General
Hospital "Dr. German Diaz Lombardo"
Mexico City, Mexico

CHRISTIAN MAZEL, M.D.
Assistant
Service de Chirurgie Orthopédique et Traumatologique
Centre Hospitalier Pitié-Salpétrière
Paris, France

PAUL R. MEYER, JR., M.D.
Professor
Department of Orthopaedic Surgery
Northwestern University Medical School
Director, Spine Injury Center
McGaw Medical Center of Northwestern University
Chicago, Illinois

PASQUALE X. MONTESANO, M.D.
Assistant Professor
Department of Orthopaedic Surgery
University of California, Davis Medical Center
Sacramento, California

JAMES W. OGILVIE, M.D.
Director, Division of Spinal Surgery
and Twin Cities Scoliosis-Spine Center
Department of Orthopaedic Surgery
University of Minnesota
Minneapolis, Minnesota

RICHARD D. PEEK, M.D.
Clinical Instructor of Orthopaedics
Department of Orthopaedics
University of California-Irvine
Irvine, California
Long Beach Memorial Medical Center
and Wiltse Spine Institute
Long Beach, California

ROLANDO M. PUNO, M.D.
Instructor
Department of Orthopaedic Surgery
University of Louisville
Staff Surgeon
Kenton D. Leatherman Spine Center
Louisville, Kentucky

RAYMOND ROY-CAMILLE, M.D.
Professeur de Chirurgie Orthopédique et
Traumatologique à la Faculté Pitie-Salpetriere
Université Pierr et Marie Curie à Paris
Chef, Service de Chirurgie Orthopédique
et Traumatologique
Centre Hospitalier Pitié-Salpétrière
Paris, France

JOSEPH J. RUSIN, M.D.
Assistant Professor
Department of Orthopaedic Surgery
Medical College of Ohio
Toledo, Ohio
Former Spine Fellow
Spine Injury Center
McGaw Medical Center of Northwestern University
Chicago, Illinois

RICK C. SASSO, M.D.
Chief Resident
Division of Orthopaedic Surgery
The University of Texas Medical School
Houston, Texas

J. MICHAEL SIMPSON, M.D.
Spine Fellow
Department of Orthopaedic Surgery
Thomas Jefferson University
Philadelphia, Pennsylvania

WALTER E. STRIPPGEN
Delta Design
Golden, Colorado

JOHN S. THALGOTT, M.D.
Clinical Instructor
Department of Orthopaedics
University of Nevada Medical Center
Las Vegas, Nevada

JOHN G. THOMETZ, M.D.
Assistant Professor,
The Medical College of Wisconsin
Director of Pediatric Orthopaedics
Children's Hospital of Wisconsin
Milwaukee, Wisconsin

ALEXANDER R. VACARRO, M.D.
Chief Resident
Department of Orthopaedic Surgery
Thomas Jefferson University
Philadelphia, Pennsylvania

PABLO VASQUEZ-SEOANE, M.D.
Instructor of Orthopaedics
The University of Texas Health Science Center
at San Antonio
San Antonio, Texas

LEON L. WILTSE, M.D.
Clinical Professor of Orthopaedic Surgery
Department of Orthopaedics
University of California-Irvine
Irvine, California
Long Beach Memorial Medical Center
and Wiltse Spine Institute
Long Beach, California

HANSEN A. YUAN, M.D.
Professor of Orthopedic Surgery
Department of Orthopedic Surgery
State University of New York Health Science Center
Syracuse, New York

CONTENTS

Surgical Exposure and Fusion Techniques of the Spine

Howard S. An

INTRODUCTION

Successful spinal instrumentation depends significantly on the techniques of surgical exposure and fusion. Meticulous exposure is essential in performing proper instrumentation and in achieving a solid spinal fusion. Many potential complications can be avoided with careful and meticulous surgical approaches to the spine. The precise technique of surgical exposure depends on the nature of the lesion, its location, and the extent of the pathology. In this chapter, operative techniques of surgical exposure and fusion of the cervical spine, thoracic spine, and lumbar spine will be discussed.

UPPER CERVICAL SPINE

The upper cervical spine can be approached either anteriorly or posteriorly, depending on the pathoanatomy of the lesion. Many posterior occipitocervical fusion techniques of the upper cervical spine have been described in the literature (42,74,78,102). Wertheim and Bohlman recently reported successful fusion of the occipitocervical spine in 13 patients, using triple wires and iliac grafts (102). Atlantoaxial stabilization and fusion can also be accomplished with wires and iliac bone graft in the majority of cases (13,40,43,88). Complications associated with posterior occipitocervical or atlantoaxial fusion may be devastating. Care is required during passage of the wires to prevent injury to the brainstem or spinal cord. We recommend the use of somatosensory evoked potential monitoring in myelopathic cases. Postoperative halo-vest external support is recommended in the majority of cases.

Posterior Occipitocervical Exposure and Fusion

A halo-vest is generally applied preoperatively. Anesthesia and intubation must be done cautiously; awake intuba-

tion using fiberoptic light is recommended in all unstable cases to minimize neck manipulation. If traction is not required and preoperative alignment is acceptable, surgery can be performed in the halo-vest on the routine operating table. If traction is required, or spinal realignment is necessary during the procedure, the halo ring should be attached to a traction device on the Stryker table. To facilitate the exposure of the occiput and the upper cervical spine, a halo ring with a posterior opening is recommended.

A reverse Trendelenburg position allows venous drainage and less bleeding during the procedure (Fig. 1.1). A midline incision is made from the external occipital protuberance to the spinous process of C2. Surgical dissection on the occiput and the ring of the atlas must be done in a gentle manner, as excess pressure may result in a fracture or slippage of the instrument. The ring of the atlas should not be dissected more than 1.5 cm laterally because the vertebral artery is at risk beyond this margin. One should avoid dissecting the foramen magnum from the inferior edge of the foramen to prevent uncontrollable venous bleeding. Wiring and other methods for stabilization will be discussed in the section on posterior cervical instrumentation.

Anterior Exposure to the Upper Cervical Spine

Anterior approaches to the upper part of the cervical spine include dislocation of the temporomandibular joint (77), osteotomy of the mandible (44), transoral approach (37), and anterior retropharyngeal approaches (29,67,106). Each procedure has advantages and disadvantages, and the surgeon should be thoroughly familiar with the anatomy and potential complications associated with the particular procedure before undertaking this formidable task.

DeAndrade and Macnab described an anteromedial retropharyngeal approach to the upper cervical spine, which

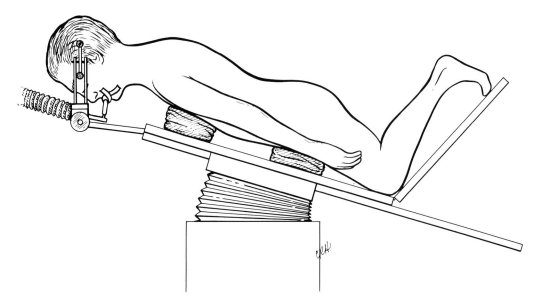

Figure 1.1. A reverse Trendelenburg position for posterior cervical spine surgery.

is an extension of Smith-Robinson approach to the lower cervical spine (29) (Fig. 1.2). The neck is hyperextended, and the chin is turned to the opposite side. The degree of neck hyperextension should be assessed preoperatively, as too much hyperextension may produce myelopathic signs and symptoms. A skin incision is made along the anterior aspect of the sternocleidomastoid muscle and curved toward the mastoid process. The platysma and the superficial layer of the deep cervical fascia are divided in the line of the incision to expose the anterior border of the sternocleidomastoid. Retract the sternocleidomastoid muscle anteriorly, and retract the carotid artery laterally. The superior thyroid artery and lingual vessels are ligated. The facial artery is identified at the upper portion of the incision, which helps to find the hypoglossal nerve adjacent to the digastric muscle. Careful retraction of this nerve is mandatory to avoid injury. The superior laryngeal nerve is in close proximity to the superior thyroid artery, and excessive retraction of this nerve causes hoarseness or inability to sing high notes. Stripping of the longus colli muscle exposes the anterior aspect of the upper cervical spine and basiocciput.

Another technique of retropharyngeal anterior exposure of the upper cervical spine has been described by McAfee and associates (67) (Fig. 1.3). A right-sided submandibular transverse incision and division of the platysma leads to the sternocleidomastoid muscle and its deep cervical fascia. The mandibular branch of the facial nerve should be identified with the aid of a nerve stimulator, and the retromandibular vein is ligated during the initial stage of dissection. The anterior border of the sternocleidomastoid muscle is mobilized. The submandibular

salivary gland and the jugular digastric lymph nodes are resected. Care should be taken to suture the duct in the salivary gland to prevent a salivary fistula. The digastric tendon is divided and tagged for later repair. The hypoglossal nerve is next identified and mobilized. In order to mobilize the carotid contents laterally, the carotid sheath is opened and arterial and venous branches are ligated. These include the superior thyroid artery and vein, lingual artery and vein, ascending pharyngeal artery and vein, and facial artery and vein, beginning inferiorly, progressing superiorly. The superior laryngeal nerve is also identified with the aid of a nerve stimulator and mobilized. The prevertebral fasciae are transected longitudinally to expose and dissect the longus colli muscles.

The anterolateral retropharyngeal approach described by Whitesides and Kelley also provides exposure of the upper cervical spine but not the basiocciput (106) (Fig. 1.4). This approach involves dissection anterior to the sternocleidomastoid but posterior to the carotid sheath. The skin incision is made from the mastoid along the anterior aspect of the sternocleidomastoid. The external jugular vein is ligated, and the greater auricular nerve is spared if possible. The sternocleidomastoid and splenius capitus muscles are detached from the mastoid, leaving a fascial edge for later repair. The spinal accessory nerve should be identified and protected. Retract the carotid contents along with hypoglossal nerve anteriorly, while retracting the sternocleidomastoid posteriorly. Blunt dissection leads to the transverse processes and anterior aspect of C1 to C3. Potential complications of this approach include injuries to the spinal accessory nerve, the sympathetic ganglion, and vertebral artery.

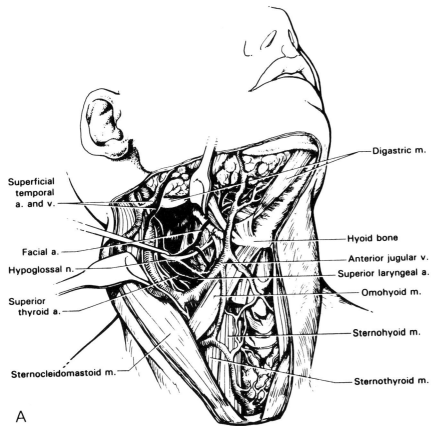

Superficial
temporal
a. and v.

Facial a.

Hypoglossal n.

Superior
thyroid a.

Sternocleidomastoid m.

Digastric m.

Hyoid bone

Anterior jugular v.

Superior laryngeal a.

Omohyoid m.

Sternohyoid m.

Sternothyroid m.

A

Figure 1.2. *A*, An anteromedial retropharyngeal approach to the upper cervical spine, described by DeAndrade and MacNab, which is an extension of Smith-Robinson approach to the lower cervical spine (From Cotler HB, Kaldis MG: Anatomy and surgical approaches of the spine. In: Cotler JM, Cotler HB, eds. Spinal Fusion. New York, Springer-Verlag, 1990; 102.) *B*, A cross-section of the upper cervical spine, showing the anteromedial approach. *C*, Anterior aspect of the upper cervical spine after stripping the longus collis muscle.

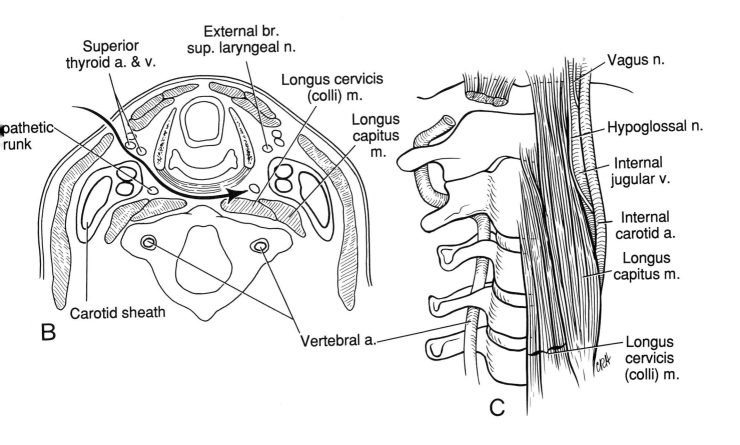

Superior
thyroid a. & v.

External br.
sup. laryngeal n.

Longus cervicis
(colli) m.

Longus
capitus
m.

pathetic
runk

Carotid sheath

Vertebral a.

B

Vagus n.

Hypoglossal n.

Internal
jugular v.

Internal
carotid a.

Longus
capitus m.

Longus
cervicis
(colli) m.

C

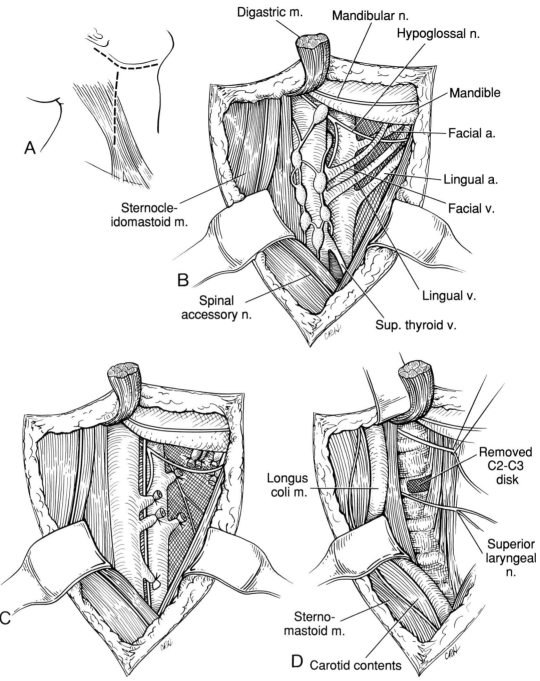

Figure 1.3. *A,* A right-sided submandibular transverse incision. *B,* The anterior border of the sternocleidomastoid muscle is mobilized, followed by division of the digastric tendon. The submandibular salivary gland and the jugular digastric lymph nodes are resected. The hypoglossal nerve is identified and mo-

bilized. *C,* The carotid sheath is opened and arterial and venous branches are ligated. *D,* The superior laryngeal nerve is also identified and protected. The prevertebral fasciae are transected longitudinally to expose and dissect the longus colli muscles.

Limited anterior exposure from the occiput to C2 may be achieved by the transoral technique of Fang and Ong (37) (Fig. 1.5). This involves splitting the soft palate and posterior pharyngeal wall, but it carries a high risk of infection (37). Fang and Ong reported six patients who

underwent anterior transoral approach to the upper cervical spine, and four had infections of the pharyngeal wall, including one patient who died of meningitis (37). The vertebral artery is also at risk of injury during transoral approach.

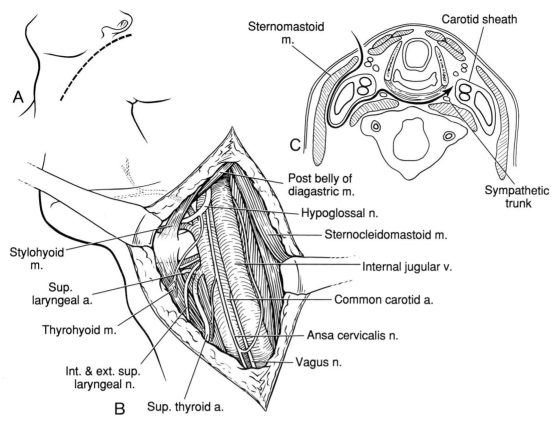

Figure 1.4. The anterolateral retropharyngeal approach described by Whitesides and Kelley. *A*, The skin incision is made from the mastoid along the anterior aspect of the sternocleidomastoid. *B*, The sternocleidomastoid and splenius capitus muscles are detached from the mastoid. *C*, Dissection is posterior to the carotid contents leading to the transverse processes and anterior aspect of C1-C3.

Potential complications associated with anterior operations of the upper cervical spine can be numerous. Proper positioning of the neck, fiberoptic nasotracheal awake intubation, and intraoperative monitoring of the spinal cord function are important measures to take in the prevention of spinal cord injury. Because dissection is intimately close to vital neural, vascular, and visceral structures, thorough knowledge of the anatomy and surgical experience are required to prevent injuries to these structures. Decompression of the spinal cord must be done adequately but not too laterally as to endanger the vertebral arteries. In the postoperative period, the patient should be intubated for 2 to 3 days until retropharyngeal edema subsides. Corticosteroids may decrease severe edema in the postoperative period. Airway obstruction and difficulty with swallowing due to retropharyngeal edema may require reintubation or tracheostomy.

LOWER CERVICAL SPINE

Surgical exposure and stabilization of the lower cervical spine can be approached anteriorly, posteriorly, or both ways, depending on pathoanatomic processes of the le-

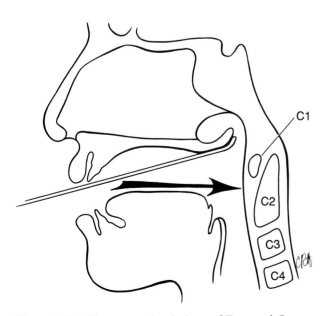

Figure 1.5. The transoral technique of Fang and Ong.

sion. If the spinous processes and lamina are intact, a standard triple wiring and fusion with bone graft is performed (12,68,71). If laminectomy has been performed, a lateral facet wiring, Luque rodding, or lateral mass plating can be performed. Decompressive laminectomy is infrequently indicated and is prone to progressive instability and late deformity, particularly in the younger individual (107). Use of methylmethacrylate for cervical stabilization is generally contraindicated, as only temporary benefit may be expected (31,66). In general, methylmethacrylate should be used only as an adjunctive material in patients with malignancy and short-term survival (66).

Posterior Exposure of the Lower Cervical Spine

Exposure of the posterior elements of the lower cervical spine is simple. Either Mayfield tongs or Gardner Wells tongs are used for positioning. A reverse Trendelenburg positioning allows venous drainage (Fig. 1.1). A midline incision is followed by subperiosteal dissection, exposing the spinous processes, lamina, and facet joints. One should expose only the levels to be fused, as creeping fusion extension is common. If cervical laminectomy is indicated, it should be done in a cautious manner. At the junction of the lamina and facet, a regular burr followed by a diamond burr is used to thin the cortices, and a small curette is used to finish the cut. To detect trauma to the spinal cord, somatosensory evoked potential monitoring should be used in myelopathic cases. Meticulous hemostasis is mandatory to prevent hematoma formation. Epidural hematoma may cause spinal cord compression or even death (63). Posterior stabilization of the cervical spine is a well-established procedure with a high success rate if done properly (12,71). Facet fusion or lateral mass plating can be done if laminectomy has been performed (18,34,79,100). The details of these procedures will be discussed under posterior cervical instrumentation.

Anterior Exposure of the Lower Cervical Spine

The anterior approach to the lower cervical spine has been well described in the literature (77,78). Meticulous and careful surgical technique is again paramount in preventing complications associated with surgical exposure. The patient is placed in a supine and slight reverse Trendelenburg position to minimize venous pooling in the surgical area (Fig. 1.6). Traction is applied to the head using Gardner Wells tongs or halter device, and caudally directed traction to the shoulders is applied using adhesive tape. To minimize injury to the recurrent laryngeal nerve, the cervical spine is often approached from the left, particularly at the C6-T1 region. The right-handed sur-

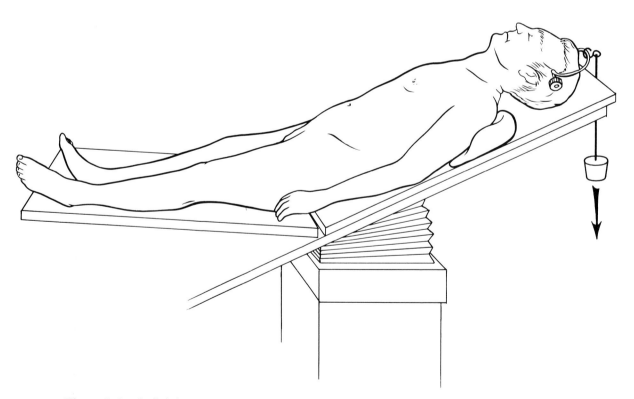

Figure 1.6. A slightly reverse Trendelenburg position for anterior approach to the cervical spine.

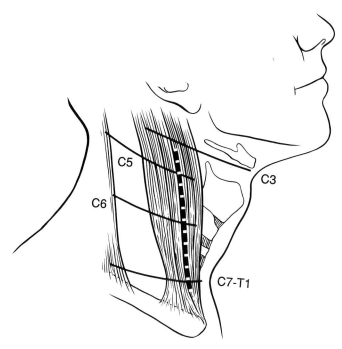

geon prefers the right-sided approach. On the right side, the recurrent laryngeal nerve may leave the carotid sheath at a higher level, and the surgeon must take caution during dissection, especially below C5. One should remember that the hyoid bone overlies the third vertebra, the thyroid cartilage overlies the C4-5 intervertebral disc space, and the cricoid ring at the C6 vertebra (Fig. 1.7). A useful alternative method involves measuring the distance from the clavicle to the appropriate level on a routine preoperative chest x-ray. A horizontal incision is used in the majority of cases, but a vertical incision anterior to the sternocleidomastoid may be necessary in cases where multiple levels need to be exposed. A transverse incision in line with the skin crease is made from the midline to the anterior aspect of the sternocleidomastoid muscle. The skin and subcutaneous tissue are undermined slightly, and division of the platysma muscle is completed. Retraction of the divided muscle exposes the sternocleidomastoid muscle laterally and strap muscles medially. The deep cervical fascia is divided between the sternocleidomastoid muscle and strap muscles, and blunt finger dissection is done through the pretracheal fascia along the medial border of the carotid sheath (Fig. 1.8). A self-

Figure 1.7. The hyoid bone overlies C3, the thyroid cartilage overlies C5, the cricoid ring at C6, and supraclavicular level for C7-T1 region.

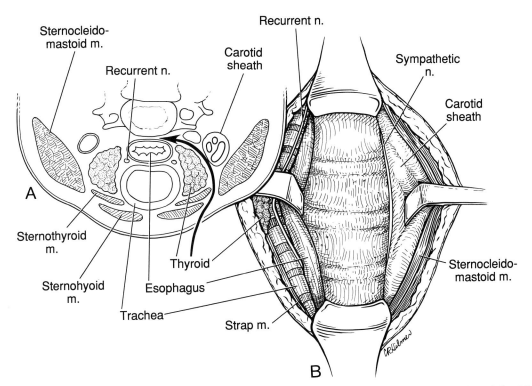

Figure 1.8. *Left*, Dissection is along the anterior aspect of the sternocleidomastoid muscle. The deep cervical fascia is divided between the sternocleidomastoid muscle and strap muscles, and blunt dissection is done through the pretracheal fascia while retracting the carotid contents laterally. *Right*, Division of the prevertebral fascia and dissection of longus colli lead to the vertebral bodies and the intervertebral discs.

retaining retractor is then positioned to expose the pre-vertebral fascia and longus colli muscles.

One must be careful not to enter the carotid sheath laterally to avoid injury to the carotid artery, internal jugular vein, or vagus nerve. Great caution should also be taken medially, as the strap muscles surround the thyroid gland, trachea, and esophagus. The surgical dissection should not enter the plane between the trachea and esophagus because the recurrent laryngeal nerve is at risk. A sharp self-retaining retractor should be avoided to prevent perforation of the esophagus medially. It is also important to check for the temporal arterial pulse when the retractor is spread. Prolonged occlusion of the carotid artery may cause brain ischemia and stroke. The superior thyroid artery is encountered above C4 and the inferior thyroid artery is seen below C6. These vessels should be identified and ligated as necessary. One should also be aware of the thoracic duct below C7 during the left-sided approach. Further dissection is performed by palpating the prominent disc margins ("hills") and concave anterior vertebral bodies ("valleys"). A bent 18-gauge needle is placed in the disc space, and a lateral radiograph is taken to confirm the correct level. The bent needle prevents inadvertent penetration to the spinal cord. To minimize bleeding and prevent injury to the sympathetic chain, the pretracheal fascia and the anterior longitudinal ligament must be divided in the midline and subperiosteal mobilization of the longus colli muscles completed. Also, take care not to dissect too far laterally, as the vertebral artery and nerve roots are in danger of injury.

This anteromedial approach to the cervical spine is utilized in the majority of cases. However, in special circumstances, lateral approaches described by Hodgson, Henry, and Verbiest may be used (47,52,53,96). Hodgson described an approach to the lower cervical area, dissecting posterior to the carotid sheath to expose the anterior and lateral aspect of the cervical spine (53). This approach avoids the thyroid vessel, vagus nerve, and superior laryngeal nerve. Verbiest modified the original approach for exposure of the vertebral artery by Henry: this involves dissecting anteriorly to the carotid sheath and exposing the vertebral artery and nerve roots posterior to the transverse processes (96). These lateral approaches may be better in cases where the lesion is localized laterally or if the vertebral artery must be exposed (Fig. 1.9).

Depending on the case, discectomy and interbody fusion at one or more levels or vertebrectomy with strut fusion are performed. The proper techniques of discectomy and fusion are crucial to successful outcomes. Neurologic consequences may be devastating, and bone graft complications are common. Proper lighting and loupe magnification of the surgical field are essential during discectomy. All of the disc material is removed, but the posterior longitudinal ligament is usually left alone. When the posterior longitudinal ligament is perforated by the offending disc material, further decompression should be performed up to the dural margin. Use of an operating microscope or loupe magnification and microsurgical instruments is important during dissection around the posterior longitudinal ligament and the dura.

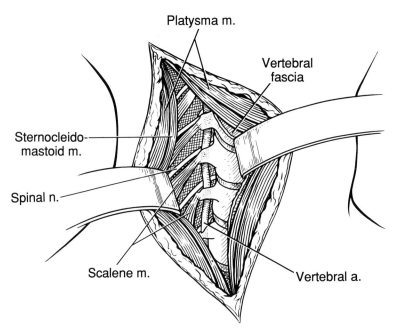

Figure 1.9. A lateral approach by Hogson.

A Smith-Robinson interbody fusion is found to be biomechanically superior compared with other counterparts (103,104). The graft should be about 8-9 mm in height or 2 mm greater in height than the degenerated disc space to obtain maximal compressive strength and to enlarge the neural foramina (17). Distraction of the intervertebral space can be achieved by skull traction and laminar spreader. Traction with the head halter or Gardner Wells tongs can also be effective. Graft extrusion can be avoided if the graft is countersunk 2 mm under the anterior cortical margin of the vertebral body (Fig. 1.10). Obviously, the graft should not be too deep, as posterior impingement of the spinal cord must be avoided. Exact measurement of width and depth of the bone graft slot should be made using a caliper or ruler in each case.

Vertebrectomy with strut grafting is frequently performed for patients with cervical spondylotic myelopathy, tumors or burst fractures (10,12). The iliac crest bone is adequate in most cases, but the fibula may be utilized in more than three level vertebrectomy cases (105). A power burr is used to remove bone down to the posterior longitudinal ligament (Fig. 1.11). A strut graft must be countersunk in order to prevent graft dislodgement. We have been satisfied with the slotted technique shown in Fig. 1.11. The bone graft is placed against the endplates to achieve greater stability and to prevent kyphosis and collapse (Fig. 1.7).

Potential complications associated with anterior exposure of lower cervical spine are numerous (Table 1.1). The most devastating complication is neurologic deterioration. Most spinal cord to nerve root injuries are as-sociated with technical mishaps. The first consideration is anesthesia and positioning. Awake intubation with the aid of a fiberoptic light is helpful to prevent excessive manipulation during intubation. Awake intubation and somatosensory evoked potential monitoring should be routine in all myelopathic cases. Utmost care should be taken when removing osteophytes and disc material in the lateral corner near the uncovertebral joint to avoid nerve root injury. If removal of the posterior longitudinal ligament or osteophytes is necessary because of perforating disc fragments or large osteophytes, great care should be taken. The depth of the graft should be measured carefully with the aid of magnification (the operative microscope). Gentle tapping is all that is necessary, and stability should be maintained by compressive force on the graft. If neurologic complications are discovered postoperatively, one should administer dexamethasone and take a lateral x-ray to determine the position of the bone graft. Computed tomography or magnetic resonance imaging may be valuable in determining hematoma or cord contusion. If hematoma or bone graft is suspected to be the culprit of postoperative myelopathy, expeditious reexploration is required.

Dysphagia after an anterior cervical surgery may be caused by postoperative edema, hemorrhage, denervation, or infection (100). If persistent dysphagia is present, barium swallow or endoscopy should be considered. Esophageal perforation is a rare but serious complication of anterior cervical spine fusion (6,50). It occurs in about 1 of 500 procedures (96). Sharp retractors must be avoided, and gentle handling of the medial soft structures is mandatory. Use of a nasogastric tube may be helpful in identifying the esophagus during surgery. If esophageal perforation is suspected during surgery, methylene blue can be injected for better visualization. The perforation is frequently not recognized until the patient develops an abscess, tracheosophageal fistula, or mediastinitis in the postoperative period. The usual treatment consists of intravenous antibiotics, nasogastric feeding, drainage, debridement, and repair. Early consultation with head and neck surgeons is recommended.

Minor hoarseness or sore throat after anterior cervical fusion may be due to edema or endotracheal intubation and occurs in nearly one-half of such patients. However, recurrent laryngeal nerve palsy may be the culprit of persistent hoarseness in a small number of patients (16). The incidence is about 1% (94), but one report was as high as 11% (46). The superior laryngeal nerve is a branch of the inferior ganglion of the vagus nerve and travels along with the superior thyroid artery to innervate the cricothyroid muscle. Damage to this nerve may result in hoarseness, but often produces symptoms such as easy

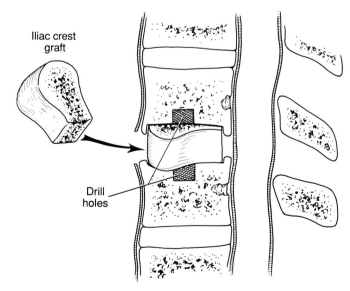

Figure 1.10. A diagram of interbody fusion using a tricortical iliac crest graft.

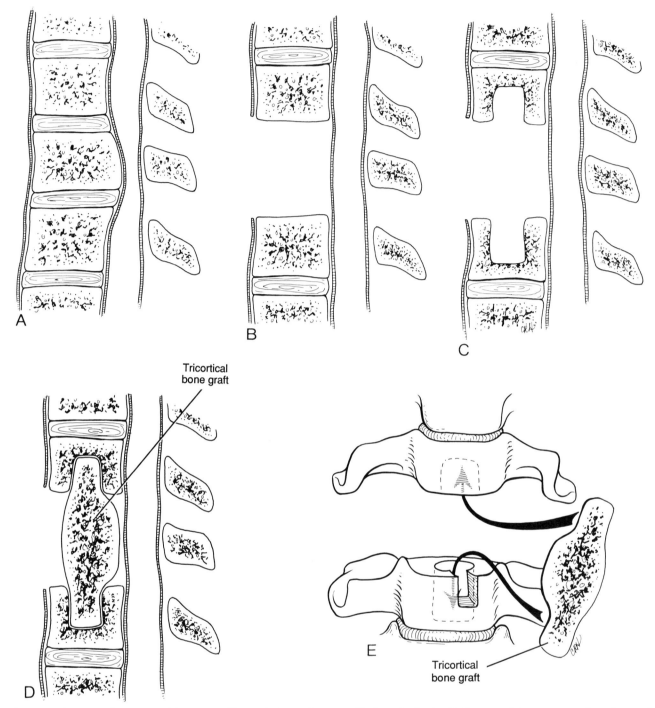

Figure 1.11.   Vertebrectomy with strut grafting technique. *A*, Anterior spinal cord compression. *B*, Vertebrectomy and discectomy above and below the body. *C*, Slot preparation above and below the body. *D*, Strut graft is countersunk against endplates. *E*, A window is made inferiorly in order to insert the strut graft.

fatiguing of the voice (16). The inferior laryngeal nerve is a recurrent branch of the vagus nerve which innervates all laryngeal muscles except the cricothyroid. On the left side, the recurrent laryngeal nerve loops under the arch of the aorta and is protected in the left tracheoesophageal groove. On the right side, the recurrent nerve travels around the subclavian artery, passing dorsomedially to the side of the trachea and esophagus. It is vulnerable as it passes from the subclavian artery to the right tracheoesophageal groove. The recurrent laryngeal nerve should be located when working from C6 downward. The best guideline to its location is the inferior thyroid

Table 1.1. Potential Complications of Anterior Cervical Fusion

Neural injury
   Spinal cord injury
   Nerve root damage
   Dural tear
Vascular injury
   Carotid artery
   Internal jugular vein
   Vertebral artery
Vocal cord damage (recurrent laryngeal nerve injury)
Esophageal perforation
Tracheal injury
Horner's syndrome
Thoracic duct injury
Pneumothorax
Bone graft complications
   Extrusion
   Collapse
   Nonunion
   Donor site complications
Infection
Wound problems (hematoma, drainage, dehiscence)

artery. The nerve usually enters the tracheoesophageal groove where the inferior thyroid artery enters the lower pole of the thyroid. It is also more common for the right inferior laryngeal nerve to be nonrecurrent where it travels directly from the vagus nerve and carotid sheath to the larynx. The incidence of nonrecurrent laryngeal nerve on the right side is reported as 1% (81). If hoarseness persists for more than 6 weeks following anterior cervical surgery, laryngoscopy should be done to evaluate the vocal cord and laryngeal muscles. Treatment of inferior laryngeal nerve should include waiting at least 6 months for spontaneous recovery of function to occur. Further treatment or surgery by the otolaryngologist may be necessary in persistent cases.

Injury to the sympathetic chain may result in a Horner's syndrome. The cervical sympathetic chain lies on the anterior surface of the longus colli muscles posterior to the carotid sheath. Subperiosteal dissection is important to prevent damage to these nerves. Horner's syndrome is usually temporary but may be permanent in some cases (56). The incidence of permanent Horner's syndrome is less than 1% (39). Ophthalmologic consultation may be needed for treatment of ptosis.

Serious bleeding complications following anterior cervical surgery is fortunately rare, but hematoma complication of the wound is relatively common up to a rate of 9% incidence reported in one series (86). Hematoma may complicate wound healing, but may rarely be responsible for airway obstruction or spinal cord compression (82). The patient's head should be elevated in the immediate postoperative period because the source of bleeding is frequently venous. Meticulous hemostasis and placement of a drain should be routine to prevent these complications. Arterial bleeding from either the superior or inferior thyroid artery can be prevented by careful identification and ligation during surgery. Great caution should be taken not to dissect too far laterally as the vertebral artery is in danger along with the nerve roots. Tears of the vertebral artery should be repaired by direct exposure of the vessel in the foramen rather than merely packing the bleeding site. Injuries to the carotid artery or internal jugular vein are exceedingly rare.

Airway obstruction after extubation may occur in the postoperative period. One must be certain that the patient can exchange air prior to extubation. In cases in which multiple vertebrectomy has been performed with retraction of soft tissues for a prolonged period of time, intubation should continue for a few days until retropharyngeal edema subsides. Corticosteroids may be used to decrease edema in these cases.

Complications associated with bone grafting and fusion are more common. Extrusion of graft usually occurs anteriorly away from the spinal cord and can be associated with dysphagia, tracheal obstruction, kyphotic deformity, or neurologic symptoms. The incidence is reported from 1 to 13%. As mentioned before, meticulous surgical technique is the key to prevention of these problems. Treatment may be observation or reoperation, depending on the situation. Graft collapse is another complication that may or may not require active treatment. The incidence of graft collapse appears to be slightly higher for allograft than autograft (14). If graft collapse results in a significant kyphosis, revision surgery may be required. The incidence of pseudarthrosis after anterior cervical fusion has been reported from 0 to 26%. Failure of fusion is reported to be greater using the dowel technique, whereas the keystone method described by Simmons had no cases of nonunion in one series (87). Multiple-level fusion has also been associated with a higher rate of nonunion compared with single-level fusion (103). Many are asymptomatic despite radiographic evidence of nonunion, and require no treatment (48,86). Those with symptomatic nonunions may benefit from prolonged immobilization or revision surgery. Posterior foraminotomy with posterior fusion is a good procedure following failed anterior cervical fusion for unilateral radiculopathy. Repeat anterior fusion may also be done in these cases with good success.

CERVICOTHORACIC JUNCTION

Surgical approaches to the upper thoracic vertebrae present a challenge to the spinal surgeon. Anterior exposure of the upper thoracic vertebrae may be accomplished through the low cervical, supraclavicular

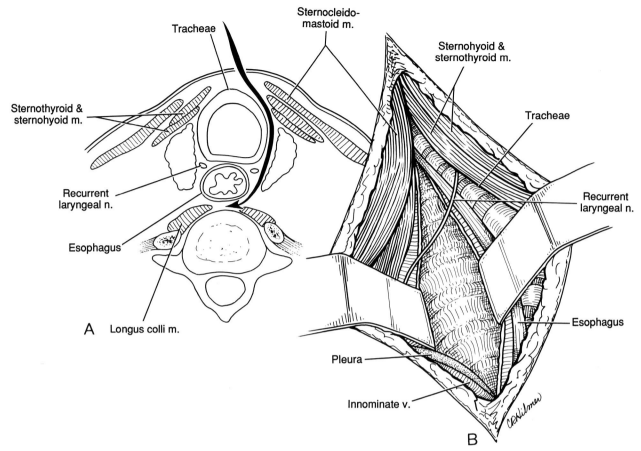

Figure 1.12. *A,* Low cervical approach, an extension of anteromedial approach to the low cervical spine. *B,* The recurrent laryngeal nerve muscle must be identified from the right-sided approach, whereas the thoracic duct may be injured from the left-sided approach.

approach, sternum-splitting approach, or transthoracic approach (2,8). Low cervical approach is an extension of the anteromedial approach to the lower cervical spine (26,38). An oblique cervical incision is made beginning 4 cm below the mastoid process extending to the sternoclavicular joint or horizontal incision at the base of the neck (Fig. 1.12). After division of the platysma muscle, the dissection is taken between the sternocleidomastoid muscle laterally and the esophagus and trachea medially to reach the spine. The inferior thyroid artery and vein are ligated. The recurrent laryngeal nerve muscle must be identified from the right-sided approach, whereas the thoracic duct must be spared from the left-sided approach.

The supraclavicular approach entails a transverse incision above the clavicle and a dissection posterior to the carotid sheath. After incision of the platysma muscle, division of the clavicular head of the sternocleidomastoid is done (58) (Fig. 1.13). The internal jugular and subclavian veins as well as the carotid artery must be protected from injury during division of the sternocleidomastoid muscle. After division of the sternocleidomastoid muscle, the fascia beneath is divided to release the omohyoid from its pulley. The subclavian artery and its branches, which include the thyrocervical trunk, suprascapular artery, and transcervical artery must be identified. The suprascapular artery, and transcervical arteries must be identified. The suprascapular and transcervical arteries should be ligated as necessary. The dome of the lung and the phrenic nerve are in close proximity to the scalenus anterior muscle. The phrenic nerve should be identified and retracted before division of the scalenus anterior muscle. The brachial plexus and supraclavicular nerves are more superficial at the lateral border of the scalenus anterior muscle.

Division of the scalenus anterior muscle exposes the Sibson's fascia in the floor of the wound, which covers the dome of the lung. Sibson's fascia is divided transversely using scissors, and the visceral pleura and lung should be retracted inferiorly. The trachea, the esopha-

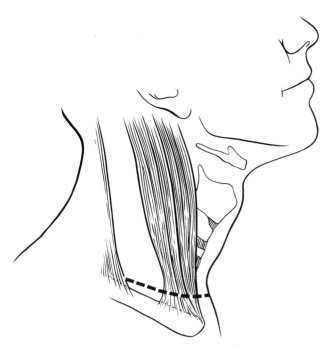

Figure 1.13. Supraclavicular approach entails a transverse incision above the clavicle and a dissection posterior to the carotid sheath, followed by release of the clavicular head of the sternocleidomastoid, omohyoid, and scalenus anterior.

gus, and the recurrent laryngeal nerve must be protected during medial retraction. The posterior thorax, stellate ganglion, and upper thoracic vertebral bodies are now visible looking from above downward through the thoracic inlet. The recurrent laryngeal nerve should be identified and protected. Likewise, the inferior thyroid artery and vertebral artery should be identified. The thoracic duct should be identified if approached from the left. If damaged, the thoracic duct should be doubly ligated both proximally and distally to prevent chylothorax.

The low cervical or supraclavicular approaches usually allow exposure of the lower cervical spine and the first and second thoracic vertebrae, but the distal extent of the exposure may be limited by the size and position of the anterior thorax. Additionally, obese or muscular patients with short necks would be poor candidates for these approaches due to limited distal extent of the exposure. Low cervical or supraclavicular approaches do not generally provide an extensile exposure of the upper thoracic spine. All the complications discussed in the anteromedial approach to the low cervical spine apply to these approaches, particularly the injury to the recurrent laryngeal nerve, the thoracic duct, the lung, or the great vessels.

Upper thoracic vertebrae may also be approached through a standard thoracotomy that enters the chest through the bed of the third rib, but access to the low cervical region is restricted by the scapula and remaining

ribs (60) (Fig. 1.14). Recently, Turner et al. described a surgical approach to the upper thoracic spine from T1 to T3 (95). The right-sided approach is preferred to avoid the left subclavian artery, which is more curved than the right brachiocephalic artery. The incision is medial and inferior to the scapula. The scapula is retracted laterally by dividing the trapezius, latissimus dorsi, rhomboids, and levator scapulae muscles. The posterior 7-10 cm of each of the 2nd, 3rd, 4th, and 5th ribs are removed. If T1 is involved, 2-3 cm of the first rib are also excised. Exposure of the vertebrae is made with an L-shape incision in the pleura and intercostal muscles. Potential complications of this approach may be restriction of scapular movement and paralysis of intercostal muscles due to the muscle-splitting aspects of this dissection. Turner and Webb recommend use of this approach in older patients and perhaps in patients with malignant conditions (95).

The sternum-splitting approach provides better access to the cervicothoracic junction from C4 to T4, particularly in the obese patient (19,52) (Fig. 1.15). The skin incision is made anterior to the left sternocleidomastoid muscle and extends along the midsternal area down to the xiphoid process. After division of the platysma muscle and superficial cervical fascia, blunt dissection is done between the laterally situated neurovascular bundle and medial visceral structures. The retrosternal adipose and thymus tissues are retracted from the manubrium. Median sternotomy should be performed carefully to prevent injury to the pleura. Sternohyoid, sternothyroid, and omohyoid muscles are identified and transected as necessary. The inferior thyroid artery is ligated and transected. Blunt dissection is performed from the cranial toward the caudal portion until the left brachiocephalic vein is exposed. This vein may be ligated and transected if necessary, but postoperative edema of the left upper extremity may be a problem.

Great caution should be taken to avoid injuries to the sympathetic nerves, the cupola of the pleura at the level of T1, the great vessels, and the thoracic duct, which passes into the left venous angle between the subclavian artery and the common carotid artery. Because there is a significant perioperative mortality associated with this approach, Sundaresan performs a less aggressive T-shaped incision on the anterior chest wall (Fig. 1.16) (92,93). Dissection is taken down to the level of the body manubrium and clavicle with ligation of the anterior jugular venous arch and medial supraclavicular nerves. The left-sided approach is preferred because the recurrent laryngeal nerve is less variable on the left and farther from the midline than the right. At the level of the manubrium and clavicle, the sternal and clavicular heads of the sternocleidomastoid muscle are detached and retracted. The

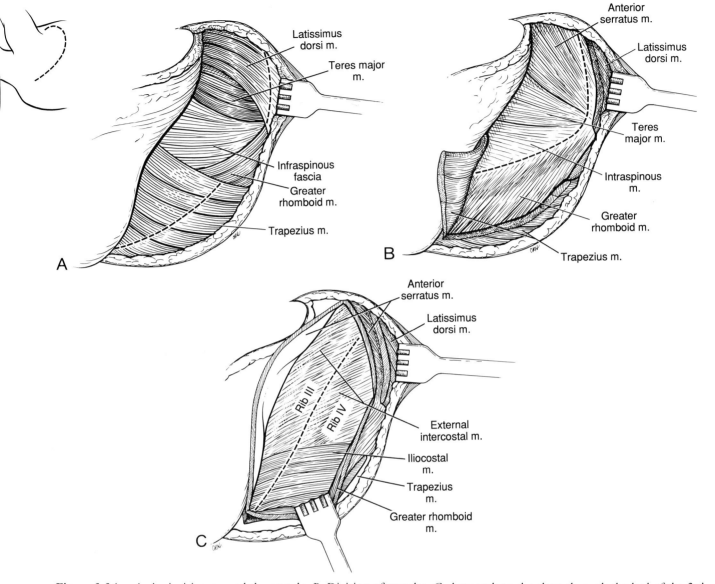

Figure 1.14. *A*, An incision around the scapula. *B*, Division of muscles. *C*, Approach to the chest through the bed of the 3rd rib.

strap muscles on the ipsilateral side of approach are similarly detached and retracted. After clearing the fatty and areolar tissues in the suprasternal space, the sternal origin of the pectoralis major is stripped laterally. The medial half of the clavicle is then stripped subperiosteally with removal of the medial third of the clavicle with a Gigli saw. A rectangular piece of the manubrium is removed along with its posterior periosteum. At this point, the exposed inferior thyroid vein, and if necessary, the innominate vein may be ligated. Dissection is then continued between the left carotid artery on the left and the

innominate artery, trachea, and esophagus on the right. Special attention must be given to protection of the thoracic duct and left recurrent laryngeal nerve. Sundaresan and associates used this approach on seven patients with tumorous involvement of the cervicothoracic junction (93). He noted one complication with this approach of a Steinman pin migration in a patient fused with methylmethacrylate filler.

Charles and associates used this approach on 10 patients with tuberculous or metastatic disease to the cervicothoracic junction. One death was noted in the

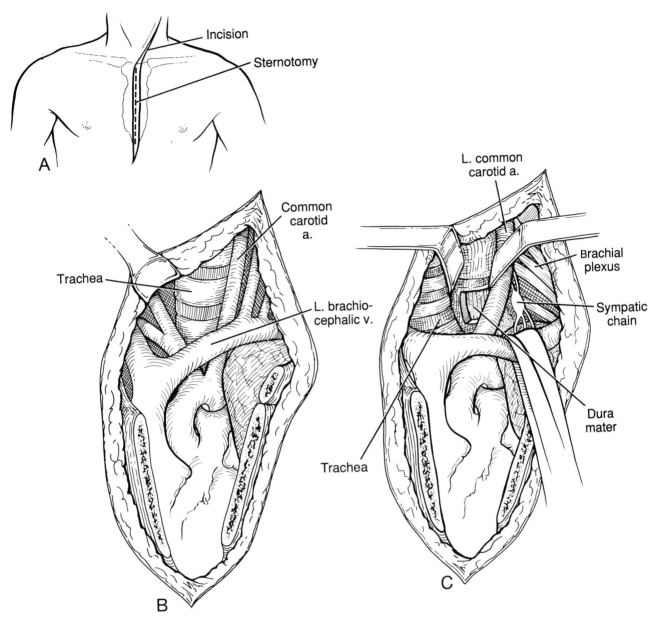

Figure 1.15. *A,* Sternum-splitting approach by an incision anterior to the left sternocleidomastoid muscle and extended along the midsternal area down to the xiphoid process. *B,* Blunt dissection between the carotid sheath and visceral structures proximally and median sternotomy distally. *C,* Following ligation and division of the inferior thyroid artery, the left common carotid artery and left brachiocephalic vein are retracted.

perioperative period due to respiratory failure in a patient with previous chronic obstructive pulmonary disease (20). No ipsilateral shoulder problems to the side of clavicular resection were found and all bone grafting matured to full fusion. One episode of early graft displacement without sequelae was recorded with an additional patient having temporary hoarseness. Recently, Kurz and Herkowitz presented a modified anterior approach to the cervicothoracic junction by removing the medial one-third of the clavicle (61). They reported no complications in four patients with tumors, but one patient had recurrence of tumor. A combined low cervical and transtho-

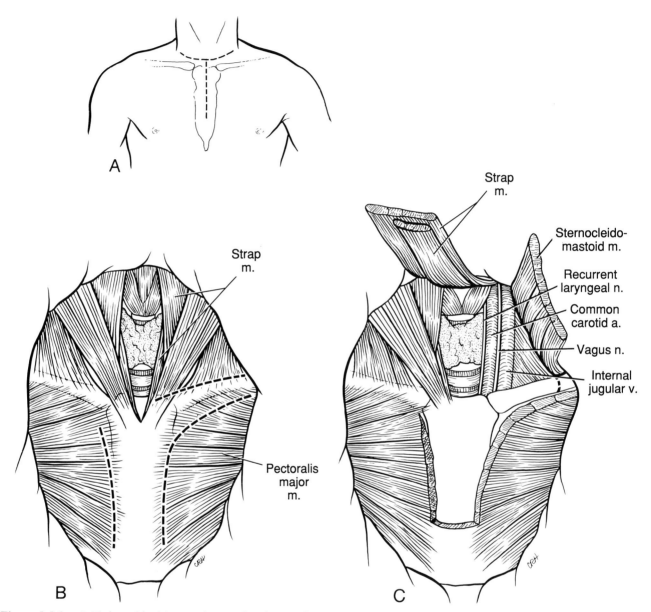

Figure 1.16. *A,* T-shaped incision on the anterior chest wall. *B,* Dissection is taken down to the level of the body manubrium and clavicle. *C,* The sternal and clavicular heads of the sternocleidomastoid muscle are detached and retracted. The strap muscles on the ipsilateral side of approach are similarly detached and retracted. *D,* The sternal origin of the pectoralis major is stripped laterally. The medial half of the clavicle is then stripped subperiosteally with removal of the medial third of the clavicle with a Gigli saw. A rectangular piece of the manubrium is removed along with its posterior periosteum. *E,* Dissection between the left carotid artery on the left and the innominate artery, trachea, and esophagus on the right. *F,* Self retaining retractor is in place.

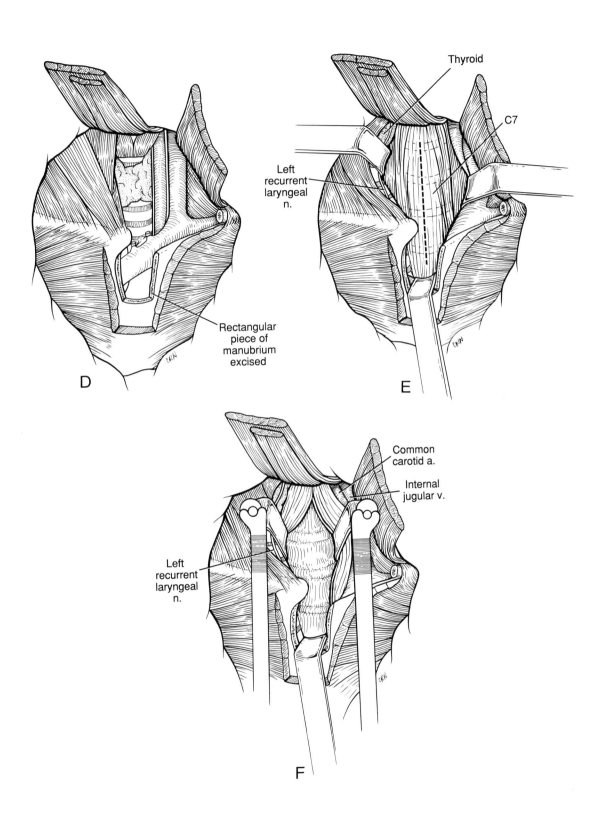

D

Rectangular
piece of
manubrium
excised

E

Thyroid

C7

Left
recurrent
laryngeal
n.

F

Common
carotid a.

Internal
jugular v.

Left
recurrent
laryngeal
n.

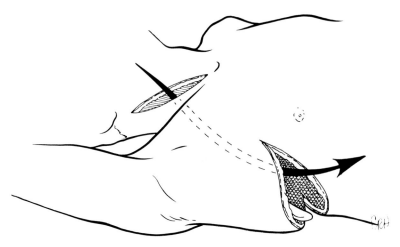

Figure 1.17.   A combined low cervical and transthoracic approach.

racic approach has also been described to gain greater access to the cervicothoracic junction in patients with severe kyphoscoliosis (70) (Fig. 1.17).

THORACIC AND THORACOLUMBAR SPINE

Posterior Approaches to the Thoracic and Thoracolumbar Spine

Posterior exposure of the thoracic and thoracolumbar spine is relatively simple, but meticulous techniques are required to achieve a successful fusion and to prevent complications.

The patient is usually positioned on the four-poster or Relton-Hall frame (Fig. 1.18). By adjusting all posters with regard to the patient's width and height, pressure points are evenly distributed on the chest and proximal thighs, while obtaining some reduction of the deformity. One must avoid pressure on the brachial plexus and ulnar nerves for obvious reasons. It is important that the abdomen is free of pressure to allow venous drainage of the lower extremities and to decrease blood loss during surgery. An increased blood loss due to pressure on the vascular system will only decrease the surgeon's vision at surgery and increase the complication rate from an excessive blood loss. Initial subperiosteal dissection is done with the Cobb elevator, exposing the spinous processes, lamina, facets, and the tips of the transverse processes. With a right-handed surgeon, the left wrist of the surgeon is always kept on the patient's body and firmly anchored on the instrument. Thus, the left upper extremity forms

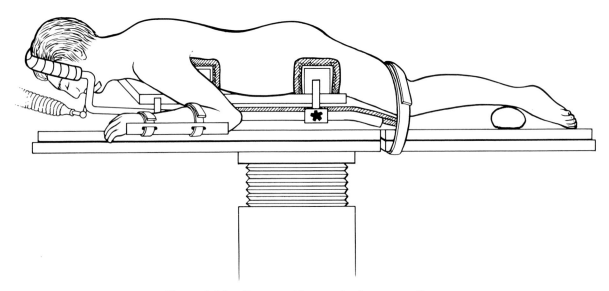

Figure 1.18.   Prone position on the four-poster frame.

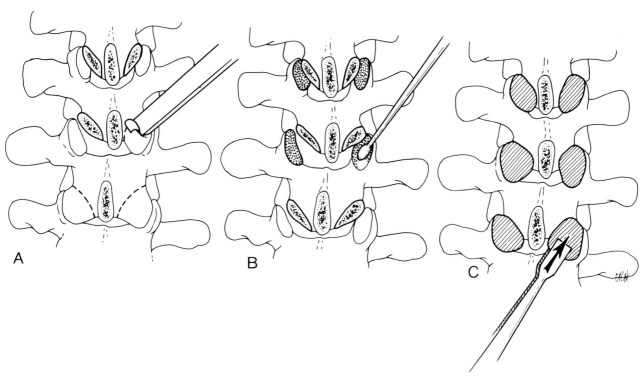

Figure 1.19. *A*, Partial excision of the inferior articular process. *B*, Removal of the articular cartilage. *C*, Packing of bone graft into the facet joint.

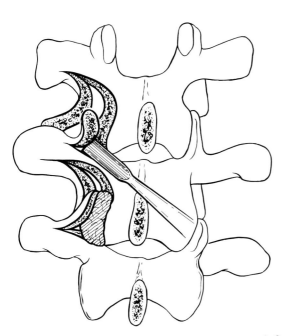

Figure 1.20. Decortication of the transverse process, inferior facet, and the lateral aspect of the superior facet.

a block to inadvertent penetration of the instrument anteriorly into the neural elements and provides much greater control of the instrument. Facet excision can be done with instruments such as osteotome, Lexcel rongeur or power burr (Fig. 1.19). Decortication should also be done meticulously using gouges, rougeur, or power burr (Fig. 1.20). Power instruments should again be held in both hands, resting both wrists or forearms on the patient to provide proprioceptive feedback to the surgeon and to minimize the risk of an unexpected wayward deviation of these instruments.

Occasionally, laminectomy may be indicated in intradural tumor surgery. Thoracic laminectomy should be done using a power burr because of minimal epidural space. Transpedicular approach is also useful for biopsy or decompression in the thoracic and thoracolumbar spine. Transpedicular biopsy or decompression requires a thorough knowledge of the anatomy of the thoracic pedicle. The thoracic pedicle is located by crossing a horizontal line at the midportion of the transverse process and a vertical line at the junction between the lamina and transverse process ("the valleys") (Fig. 1.21). A power burr is used to remove the outer cortex. A pin is placed to confirm the location of the pedicle with a roentgenogram. An angle-tipped curette can be used to remove

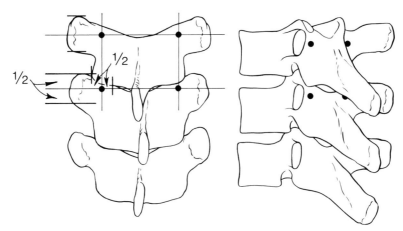

Figure 1.21. The thoracic pedicle is located by crossing a horizontal line at the midportion of the transverse process and a vertical line at the junction between the lamina and transverse process or midportion of the facet joint. This point is usually 1–2 mm below the facet joint.

tissues from the vertebral body. Decompression of the spinal cord can be done by excising the pedicle and by removing tissues from a posterolateral direction.

Another posterior approach to the anterior and lateral aspect of the thoracic vertebra is the posterolateral costotransversectomy technique (58) (Fig. 1.22). This approach is less extensive than a formal thoracotomy and may be preferred for lesions in the lateral aspect of the vertebral body, lesions that do not require a long strut graft, or patients who cannot tolerate a formal thoracotomy. The patient is placed halfway between a lateral decubitus and prone position with a pad in the axilla, and the upper arm is slightly extended and securely supported. A "C"-shape curved incision is made along the paraspinous muscles, spanning about four to five ribs. The middle part of the incision should be about 2.5 inches from the midline at the paraspinal depression. By undermining the skin and subcutaneous tissue, exposure of the par-

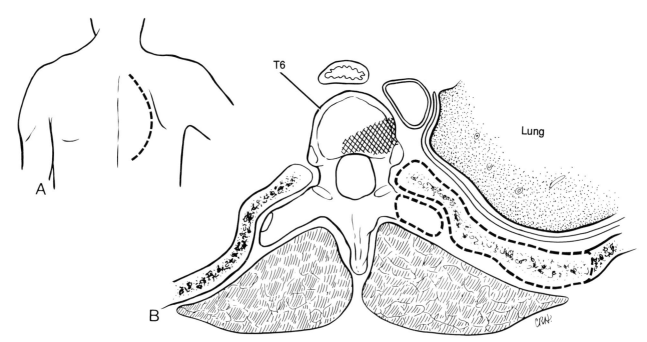

Figure 1.22. *A,* The posterolateral costotransversectomy incision. *B,* After division of the trapezius and latissimus dorsi muscles, the rib and transverse process are resected. The rib is exposed subperiosteally and excised approximately 3.5 inches lateral to the vertebra and disarticulated at the costovertebral junction. Retraction of the pleura will lead to the vertebrae.

aspinous muscles and posterior elements of the spine is completed. The trapezius and latissimus dorsi muscles are divided either longitudinally or transversely. The rib and transverse process are resected at one to four levels, depending on the extent of the lesion. The rib is exposed subperiosteally and excised approximately 3.5 inches lateral to the vertebra and disarticulated at the costovertebral junction. Careful retraction of the pleura will lead to the vertebrae. The pedicles, neural foramina, and spinal nerves should be identified. For neural decompression, the pedicles may be widened or excised to expose the dura. A strut bone graft may be applied if necessary.

Similarly, a posterolateral approach can be used to expose the anterolateral aspect of the vertebral body in the thoracolumbar region (11,62) (Fig. 1.23). The patient is placed in the lateral decubitus and rolled slightly toward the anterior side. A left- or right-sided approach can be done, depending on the pathoanatomy of the lesion. The skin incision may be in a C or J shape to expose the dorsolumbar fascia and latissimus dorsi fascia. These fascia are incised, and the erector spinae muscle group is retracted medially from the surface of the 11th and 12th ribs. These ribs are isolated subperiosteally and resected. The transverse processes of L1 and L2 may also be resected to gain exposure. The 12th or L1 nerve is identified and traced back to its foramen. The pedicle of the appropriate vertebra is resected using a Kerrison punch, and the dura is exposed laterally. Discectomy or vertebrectomy and fusion can then be performed.

Total spondylectomy through the posterolateral approach has been described for lesions that require en bloc excision (64,80,89,90). This operation is a formidable procedure and should be performed by those with prior experience.

Operative complications associated with posterolateral approaches of the thoracic and thoracolumbar spine may be spinal cord injury, dural tear, pneumothorax, bleeding, and fusion problems. Again, somatosensory evoked potential monitoring is recommended for scoliosis surgery or if decompression of the spinal cord is planned. Power drills, curettes or rongeurs should be used in a cautious manner, as neurovascular injury from use of these instruments may be devastating.

New instrumentation systems still require a meticulous fusion technique. A long-term good result depends primarily on achieving a solid arthrodesis. The incidence of pseudarthrosis may be decreasing with the current surgical devices, but it still remains a major problem in spinal fusion surgery. Although rigid instrumentations such as the Luque rod, Cotrel-Dubousset system, and transpedicular systems probably lower the incidence of pseudarthrosis, again, the meticulous fusion technique cannot be overlooked. Thorough decortication and facet excision are essential. Massive bone grafts from the iliac crest remain the gold standard. Allografts may be utilized for augmentation if the autogenous grafts are insufficient.

Pseudarthrosis occurs most commonly at areas of high stress such as the thoracolumbar junction or lumbar spine (9,69,72). Some argue that facet excision is not necessary in the thoracic spine (24), but meticulous decortication is necessary in all areas, particularly in the thoracolumbar and lumbar areas to decrease the incidence of pseudarthrosis. Adequate postoperative immobilization is also important to prevent pseudarthrosis and instrument failures (49). Inadequate spinal instrumentation or lack of postoperative support may contribute to the development of pseudarthrosis. Cigarette smoking has also been reported to be associated with pseudarthrosis (15). Electric stimulation may have a role in decreasing the overall rate of pseudarthrosis (32,59).

Anterior Approaches to the Thoracic and Thoracolumbar Spine

Exposure of the thoracic vertebral bodies is best accomplished by the anterior transthoracic approach (Fig. 1.24). A right-side of thoracotomy is preferred for the exposure of the upper thoracic spine to avoid the subclavian and carotid arteries in the left superior mediastinum. In the lower thoracic spine, a left-sided thoracotomy is preferred to avoid the liver. Because dissection is easier from above downward, the rib at the one or two upper levels should be removed, particularly if multiple levels are involved. For the thoracotomy approach, place the patient in the lateral decubitus position, moving the arm forward. Insertion of a double-branched endotracheal tube into the right and left mainstem bronchi is helpful to allow selective collapse of the lung. An axillary roll under the down arm is important in preventing compression of axillary neurovascular structures. The skin and subcutaneous tissues are opened from the lateral border of the paraspinous musculature to the sternocostal junction over the rib to be resected.

After the pleura is incised, exposure of the vertebral column is done by deflating the lung with a surgical laparotomy sponge. Remove the lap sponge periodically to prevent atelectasis. Exposure of the thoracolumbar junction is best achieved by a thoracoabdominal approach, which entails circumferential incision in the muscular portion of the diaphragm adjacent to the costal margin (Fig. 1.25). The key is to access the retroperitoneal space by splitting the costal cartilage after removal of the appropriate rib. The retroperitoneal space is identified by the light areolar tissue of fat, and blunt finger dissection is recommended. The peritoneum is bluntly dissected from the inferior surface of the diaphragm and

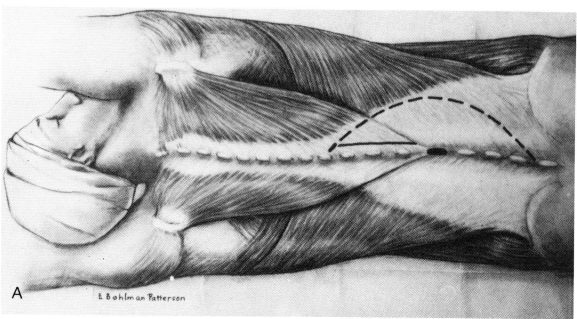

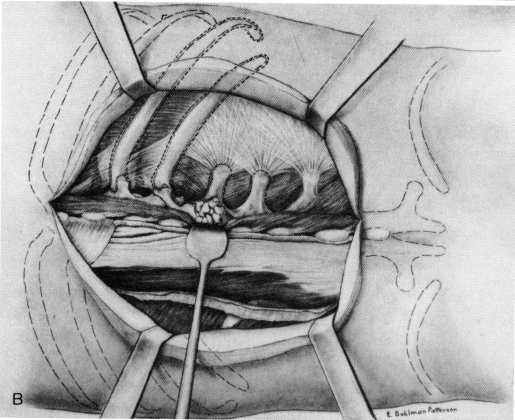

Figure 1.23. *A,* A posterolateral approach to the thoracolumbar spine. A skin incision is followed by incision of the dorsolumbar fascia and latissimus dorsi fascia. *B,* The erector spinae muscle group is retracted medially from the surface of the 11th and 12th ribs. The transverse processes of L1 and L2 may also be resected to gain exposure. The 12th or L1 nerve is identified and traced back to its foramen. The pedicle of the appropriate vertebra is resected to expose the dura laterally (From Bohlman HH, Ducker TB, Lucas JT: Spine and spinal cord injuries. In: Rothman RH, Simeone FA, eds. Spine. Philadelphia: WB Saunders, 1982;732).

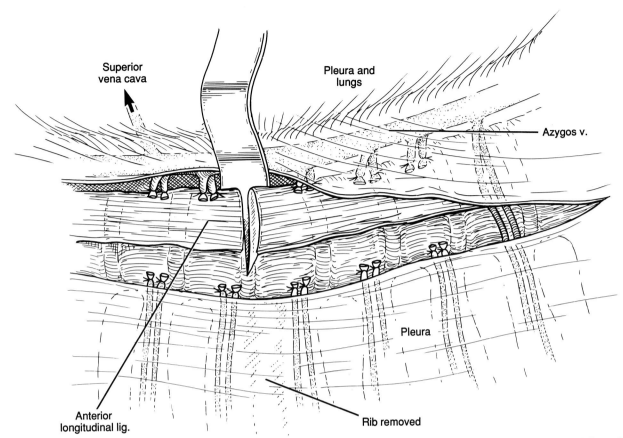

Figure 1.24. Transthoracic anterior approach to the thoracic spine. Ligation of the segmental artery and vein is followed by intervertebral disc excision.

swept medially off the psoas muscle. The diaphragm is detached about 2 cm from the periphery, and suture tags are placed in order to facilitate closure. In order to avoid disruption of the vascular anastomosis located at the intervertebral foramen, the segmental artery must be ligated at the midportion of the vertebral body. For exposure of T12-L1, the crus of the diaphragm is detached. The psoas muscle may also be reflected laterally for exposure.

After the spine is adequately exposed, removal of disc material is done for interbody fusion. All disc tissue must be removed to the posterior annulus and to the annulus on the opposite side. For scoliosis surgery, the vertebral endplates are removed to subchondral bleeding bone using a fine osteotome or angled curette. Minced rib can be used for the interbody fusion. Vertebrectomy for spinal cord decompression entails resecting the posterior one-third of the involved vertebrae down to the thecal sac. Resection of pedicles above and below the involved vertebrae facilitate the exposure of the spinal nerves and thecal sac.

A headlight, magnification loupe, and power burr are essential equipment during decompression. Strut fusion technique is performed by making a trough in the body of the cephalad vertebra up to the upper endplate and in the body of the caudad vertebra to the lower endplate (23,24) (Fig. 1.26). The iliac strut graft should extend from the upper endplate of the cephalad vertebra to the lower endplate of the caudad vertebra for maximum stability (Fig. 1.26). After insertion of the tricortical graft, the operating table is flexed back to the neutral position in order to lock the graft in place. There are numerous instrumentations that may be used to augment fixation anteriorly, and these are discussed elsewhere in this book.

Complications that may be associated with the anterior approach to the thoracic or thoracolumbar spine are numerous. Injury to the spinal cord is the most dreadful complication, which may be due to mechanical damage during removal of the intervertebral disc or vascular insult. Mechanical damage to the spinal cord is largely preventable with precise surgical techniques. Vascular insult to the spinal cord is rare if segmental vessels are ligated opposite the midportion of the vertebral body, allowing collateral vessels near the intervertebral foramen to supply blood to the spinal cord. The segmental artery on the left side around T10 should be preserved if at all possible, as this may be the major feeding artery to the spinal cord

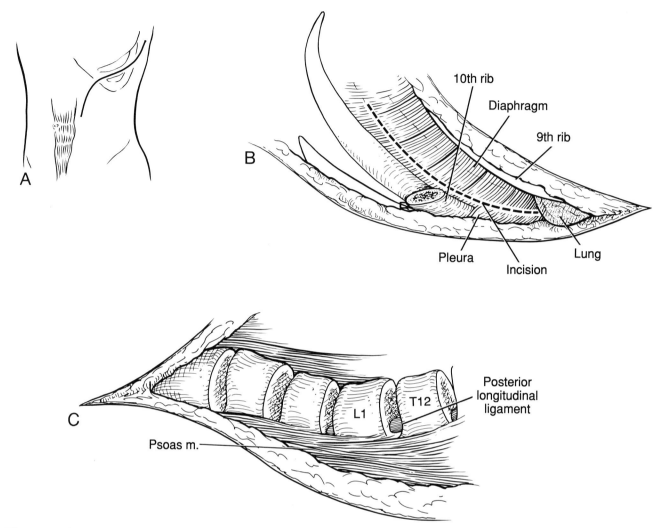

Figure 1.25. *A*, Incision for the exposure of the thoracolumbar junction. *B*, The retroperitoneal space is entered by splitting the costal cartilage of the 10th rib. Blunt dissection of the peritoneum from the inferior surface of the diaphragm is followed by detaching the diaphragm 2 cm from the attachment. *C*, Exposure of the anterolateral aspect of the spine is completed when segmental vessels are ligated and tied.

(30). In doubtful cases, clamping of the artery while observing the somatosensory evoked potentials should be done to prevent vascular compromise to the spinal cord (5). Preoperative angiography to identify the feeding vessel to the spinal cord is also helpful. If paraplegia is noted after surgery, x-rays should be taken to rule out penetration of the spinal canal by a bone graft or implant. Spinal cord contusion can be detected by magnetic resonance imaging.

The aorta or vena cava is at risk of injury during the anterior exposure of the thoracolumbar spine. Thorough familiarity of their anatomy is obviously important. Great caution should be taken when removing the annulus. To protect these vessels, an assistant should hold a malleable retractor between the vessels and the spinal column during disc removal. Late hemorrhage due to erosion, leakage, or false aneurysm formation of the vessel is known, but this complication is usually associated with prominent metal implants (33). Other complications that may be associated with the anterior exposure of the thoracic and lumbar spine are injury to the ureter (21,85), injury to the spleen (51), chylous leakage (22,35,84), sympathectomy effect, and other visceral damage (3).

LUMBAR SPINE AND SACRUM

Posterior Lumbar and Sacral Approach

A kneeling position lessens blood loss by reducing the intra-abdominal venous pressure (Fig. 1.27). A midline incision is made and subperiosteal dissection of the par-

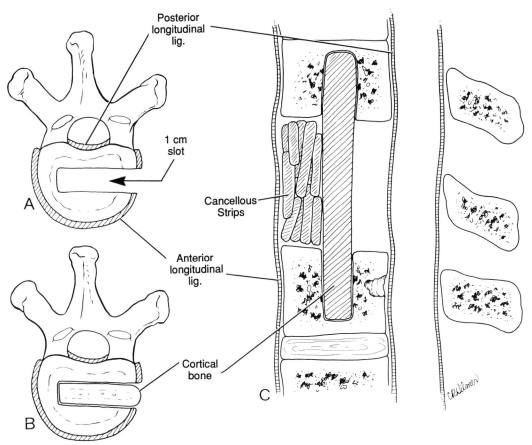

Figure 1.26. *A*, A slot for bone graft above and below the site of vertebrectomy. *B*, Tricortical bone graft in the slot. *C*, The bone graft spans from the upper endplate to the lower endplate for maximum stability.

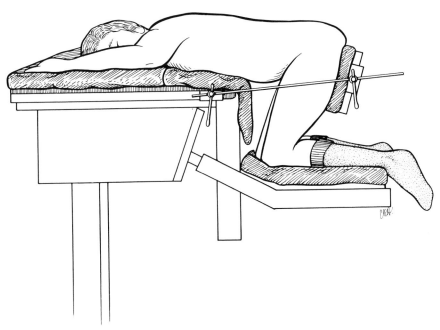

Figure 1.27. A kneeling position for lumbar surgery.

aspinous muscles is done, exposing the spinous process, lamina, facet joints, pars, and transverse processes. The inferior incision is curved in a J shape for the purpose of obtaining bone grafts from the posterior iliac crest. One must be careful not to destroy the facet capsule above the planned fusion site; degenerative changes or instability may develop later. At this time, laminectomy and foraminotomy are performed if necessary. The facet joints to be fused should be meticulously prepared by excising the cartilage from the joints and removing the cortical bone from the lateral portion of the superior articular process (Fig. 1.28). Decortication of the transverse process, the lateral gutter, and the sacral ala are performed carefully. Morselized bone from the iliac crest and/or allograft bone is placed in the prepared gutter. A hemovac drain is used routinely. Posterior lumbar interbody fusion is a technique that involves insertion of the bone grafts into the disc space by retracting the nerve roots. Great care must be taken to avoid damage to the nerve roots. Other possible complications associated with posterior lumbar interbody fusion may be anterior vessel damage

by penetrating the anterior annulus, posterior bone graft migration, perineural fibrosis, and pseudarthrosis.

The transpedicular approach is useful for biopsy, decompression, or stabilization with screws. Knowledge of pedicular anatomy in relation to neural structures is crucial. The pedicle entrance point is situated at the crossing of two lines (Fig. 1.29). The vertical line is the extension of the facet joint in line with the bony crest coming from the inferior articular facet. The horizontal line passes through the middle of the insertion of the transverse process, or 1 mm below the joint line. The sacral entrance point is at the lower point of the L5-S1 articulation. The nerve root is situated just medial and inferior to the pedicle as it exists into the intervertebral foramen. Therefore, one must avoid the area medial and inferior to the pedicle to prevent damage of the nerve root. A small rongeur or burr is used to decorticate the pedicle entrance. A Steinman pin with roentgenographic imaging can be used to confirm the location of the pedicle. A blunt instrument is advanced carefully through the pedicle into the vertebral body. The amount of medial an-

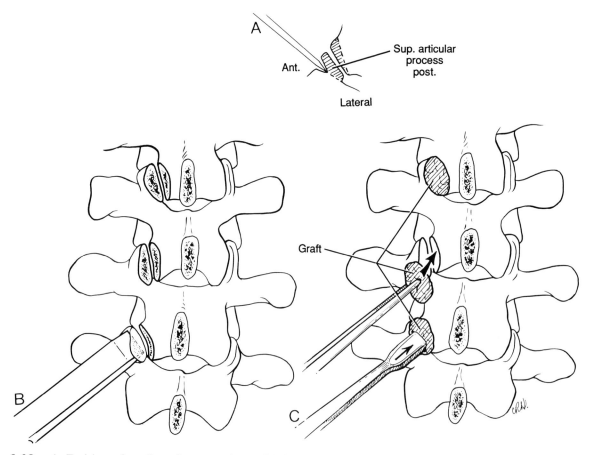

Figure 1.28. *A*, Excision of cartilage from superior and inferior articular facets. *B*, Lumbar facets are sagitally oriented. *C*, Packing of cancellous bone grafts to the facets.

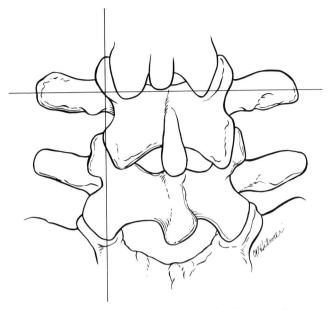

Figure 1.29. The pedicle entrance point is situated at the crossing of two lines. The vertical line is the extension of the facet joint in line with the bony crest coming from the inferior articular facet. The horizontal line passes through the middle of the insertion of the transverse process, or 1 mm below the joint line.

gulation varies, depending on the level. The medial direction of the pedicle is about 7° at L1 and L2, 8° at L3, 11° at L4, and 17° at L5 on the average (74). One should aim about 20° medially at S1. Depending on the cases, adjacent transverse process or lamina can be removed to better access the anterior vertebral body. Pedicle instrumentations are discussed in more detail in other chapters.

Posterior exposure of the sacrum and coccyx is done through a vertical midline incision. One must be careful to avoid dural tear in the midline, particularly in patients with occult spina bifida. Posterior sacral foramina are richly surrounded by venous structures and can be sources of significant bleeding. Subperiosteal dissection around the coccyx should be done carefully to avoid injury to the rectum anteriorly. Posterior laminectomy of the sacrum for exposures of the nerve roots along with anterior exposure of the sacrum may be necessary for resection of certain sacral tumors.

Potential complications of posterior lumbar spine surgery are many. These include neurologic deficits, dural tear, bleeding, pseudarthrosis, and instrument complications (4). Perforations of the dura may lead to neurologic impairment, pseudomeningocele formation, cerebrospinal fluid fistula, meningitis, or wound healing problems. Dural tears may occur during excision of the ligamentum flavum, but more commonly during manipulation of the dural sac to free adhesions, particularly in a stenotic canal. Gentle handling of the dural sac largely avoids this complication. Dural tears should be primarily closed using a 6:0 nonabsorbable suture in such a way as to avoid constriction of the cauda equina. A fascial or free fat graft may be used to augment the repair (36). The paraspinous muscle, overlying fascia, subcutaneous tissue and skin should be closed in multiple layers in a water-tight manner. Drains should be avoided.

The abdominal structures anterior to the intervertebral disc are at risk of damage if the anterior annulus is violated during disc removal (45,54), or if the pedicle screw penetrates the anterior cortex of the vertebral body, particularly the sacrum (1). The aorta bifurcates into the common iliac arteries at the L4-5 disc level. The right common iliac artery crosses the anterior surface of the L4-5 disc and fixes the left common iliac branch of the vena cava against the vertebral column. In addition to this vessel, the bowel and ureter are also in danger. The L5 nerve root courses anterior to the ala of the sacrum, and the pedicle screw should avoid this area. Great caution must be taken to avoid damage to these vital structures.

In addition to reducing venous bleeding and giving better exposure of the disc space, the kneeling position allows the intra-abdominal contents to fall anteriorly, away from the vertebral column. One should avoid overzealous attempts to remove the entire nucleus. Many patients with degenerative disc disease have fissuring of the annulus, and penetration of the annulus is possible if the surgeon pushes the instrument forward until resistance is met. The surgeon should always be aware of the depth of the instrument in the disc space. By maintaining contact with the vertebral endplates, the surgeon has better depth perception. The pituitary rongeur with a depth marking is helpful in avoiding excessively deep penetration. Preoperative lateral lumbar spine roentgenograms should also be reviewed carefully to measure the depth of the intervertebral disc space (41).

Many factors are involved in the pathogenesis of pseudarthrosis development. Patients who smoke cigarettes are at increased risk for pseudarthrosis (15), and those with previous failed fusion, grade III or IV spondylolisthesis or multiple level involvement do worse. As mentioned repeatedly, the key is the meticulous surgical technique and massive bone grafting in the prevention of pseudarthrosis. Adequate postoperative immobilization with a pantaloon cast or brace is also important if rigid internal fixation is not performed. With the advent of rigid internal fixation such as pedicle screw systems, the incidence of pseudarthrosis may decrease.

However, this device cannot replace the meticulous techniques of decortication and bone grafting, as Horowitch reported a 32% nonunion rate with the use of pedicle screw-plate system (55).

Anterior Lumbar and Sacral Approach

In the lower lumbar region, a standard retroperitoneal flank approach is used (Fig. 1.30). The patient is placed in the right lateral decubitus position. The incision extends from the midaxillary line to the edge of the rectus sheath. The level of the incision varies according to the level of the spine approached. Dissection is through the external oblique, internal oblique, and transversus abdominis muscles. The retroperitoneal space is entered laterally by identifying the retroperitoneal fat, taking care to avoid penetration of the peritoneum just lateral to the

rectus sheath. Blunt finger dissection anterior to the psoas muscle should lead to the spine. One should identify the genitofemoral nerve on the anterior surface of the psoas muscle, and the sympathetic chains medial to the muscle. Extreme caution must be used to avoid injuries to the ureter, which can be identified medially along the undersurface of the peritoneum, and the pulsating aorta, which is easily palpated. These structures are at risk with careless dissection. At the L4-L5 region, the iliolumbar vein should be identified and ligated to mobilize the great vessels. For the approach to L5-S1, the midline within the vascular bifurcation should be palpated by passing the finger over the left common iliac artery. The left common iliac vein is retracted to the left and cephalad, while the middle sacral vein and the superior hypogastric plexus are retracted to the right bluntly.

A transperitoneal approach through a vertical or trans-

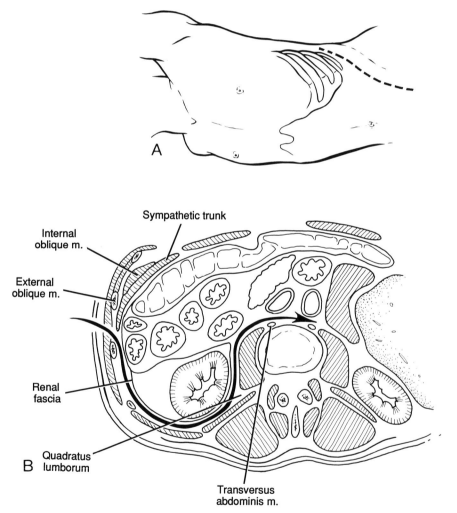

Figure 1.30. *A*, A standard retroperitoneal flank approach. The incision extends from the midaxillary line to the edge of the rectus sheath. *B*, Dissection is through the external oblique, internal oblique, and transversus abdominis muscles. The retroperitoneal space is entered laterally by identifying the retroperitoneal fat with blunt dissection anterior to the psoas muscle.

verse incision in the lower abdomen provides the best exposure to the lumbosacral junction (Fig. 1.31). The bowel contents are retracted, and the aortic bifurcation is palpated at the L4-L5 region. Infiltration of the tissue over the anterior surface of the sacral promontory may be done to elevate the peritoneum off the vascular structures (97,99). The posterior peritoneum is opened and the L5-S1 disc identified. The sacral artery runs down along the anterior aspect of the sacrum and is ligated for distal exposure. Great caution should be taken to protect the left iliac vein in the aortic bifurcation and to preserve the presacral plexus of parasympathetic nerves, which is important to sexual function. Exposure can be extended to the L4-L5 region by mobilizing the great vessels to

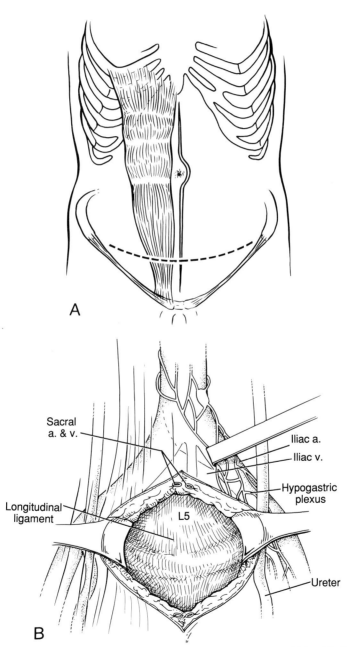

Figure 1.31. *A*, Transperitoneal approach through a vertical or transverse incision in the lower abdomen to expose the lumbosacral junction. *B*, The bowel contents are retracted, and the aortic bifurcation is palpated at L4-L5 region. Open the posterior peritoneum and identify the L5-S1 disc. The sacral artery runs down along the anterior aspect of the sacrum and is ligated for distal exposure. Careful retraction of the left iliac vein and the aortic bifurcation is done.

the right after ligating the L4-5 vessels. Take care not to injure the left ureter, which crosses the left common iliac vessels over the sacroiliac joint.

Anterior interbody fusion may be indicated in patients who have had failed surgery posteriorly due to pseudarthrosis or infection. Disc space infection may be another indication for this procedure. Although controversial, the results of anterior interbody fusion for mechanical and discogenic pain are at best equivocal. The techniques of anterior interbody fusion in the lumbar spine vary widely among different authors. Nonetheless, the technique should consist of meticulous excision of the entire disc material, preparation of the endplates to provide stability and vascularity, and tricortical plugs of autogenous iliac crests after disc space distraction (7,27,28,76,83,98).

Potential complications during anterior dissection along the lower lumbar spine and sacrum include hemorrhage from great vessel injury, retrograde ejaculation and sterility from superior hypogastric sympathetic plexus injury, ureteral injury, and bowel injury (3,85,99). Penile erection is predominantly under the parasympathetic system, and impotence is not anticipated after superior hypogastric sympathetic plexus injury, unless the patient also has advanced peripheral vascular disease (57).

REFERENCES

1. Abitbol JJ, Mirkovic, S, Steinmann J, et al: Anatomic considerations for sacral screw placement. Presented at the Annual Meeting of Scoliosis Research Society. Honolulu, Hawaii, September, 1990.
2. An HS, Vaccaro A, Cotler JM: Spinal disorders at the cervicothoracic junction. Presented at the Annual Cervical Spine Research Society, San Antonio, December, 1990.
3. An HS, Balderston RA: Complications in scoliosis, kyphosis, and spondylolisthesis surgery. In: Balderston RA, An HS, eds. Complications in spine surgery. Philadelphia: WB Saunders, 1991;5–40.
4. An HS, Booth RE, Rothman RH: Complications in lumbar disc disease and spinal stenosis surgery. In: Balderston RA, An HS, eds. Complications in spine surgery. Philadelphia: WB Saunders, 1991;61–78.
5. Apel DM, Marrero G, Goldie WD, et al: Avoiding paraplegia during anterior spinal surgery: The role of SSEP monitoring during temporary occlusion of segmental spinal arteries. Presented at the Annual Meeting of Scoliosis Research Society. Honolulu, Hawaii, September, 1990.
6. Balmaseda MT Jr, Pellioni DJ: Esophagocutaneous fistula in spinal cord injury: a complication of anterior cervical fusion. Arch Phys Med Rehabil 1985;66:783–784.
7. Barber B: Anterior lumbar interbody fusion: step-by-step procedures and pitfalls. In: White AH, Rothman RH, Ray CD, eds. Lumbar spine surgery. St. Louis: CV Mosby, 1987;368–382.
8. Bauer R, Kerschbaumer F, Poisel S: Operative approaches in orthopaedic surgery and traumatology. New York: Georg Thieme Verlag, 1987;13–16.
9. Bialik K, Piggott H: Pseudoarthrosis following treatment of idiopathic scoliosis by Harrington instrumentation and fusion without added bone. J Ped Orthop 1987;7:152–154.
10. Bohlman HH: Cervical spondylosis with moderate to severe myelopathy. Spine 1977;2:151–162.
11. Bohlman HH, Ducker TB, Lucas JT: Spine and spinal cord injuries. In: Rothman RH, Simeone FA, eds. The spine. (2nd ed.) Philadelphia: WB Saunders 1982;661–756.
12. Bohlman HH: Acute fractures and dislocations of the cervical spine: an analysis of 300 hospitalized patients and review of the literature. J Bone Joint Surg 1979;61A:1119–1142.
13. Brooks AL, Jenkins EB: Atlanto-axial arthrodesis by the wedge compression method. J Bone Joint Surg 1978;60A:279–284.
14. Brown MD, Malinin TI, Davis PB: A roentgenographic evaluation of frozen allografts versus autografts in anterior cervical spine fusions. Clin Orthop 1976;119:231–236.
15. Brown CW, Orme TJ, Richardson HD: The rate of pseudoarthrosis (surgical nonunion) in patients who are smokers and patients who are nonsmokers: a comparison study. Spine 1986;11:942–943.
16. Bulger RF, Rejowski JE, Beatty RA: Vocal cord paralysis associated with anterior cervical fusion: consideration for prevention and treatment. J Neurosurg 1985;62:657–661.
17. Burkus JK: Cervical disc disease. In Chapman M, ed. Operative orthopaedics. Philadelphia: JB Lippincott, 1988;2045–2054.
18. Callahan RA, Johnson RM, Margolis RN, et al: Cervical facet fusion for control of instability following laminectomy. J Bone Joint Surg 1977;59A:991–1002.
19. Cauchoix J, Binet J: Anterior surgical approaches to the spine. Ann R Coll Surg Eng 1957;27:237–243.
20. Charles R: Anterior approach to the upper thoracic vertebrae. J Bone Joint Surg 1989;71B:81–84.
21. Cleveland RH, Gilsanz V, Lebowitz RL, et al: Hydronephrosis from retroperitoneal fibrosis and anterior spinal fusion. J Bone Joint Surg 1978;60A:996.
22. Coletta AJ, Mayer PJ: Chylothorax: an unusual complication of anterior thoracic interbody spinal fusion. Spine 1982;7:46–49.
23. Cotler HB, Cotler JM, Stoloff A, et al: The use of autograft for vertebral body replacement of the thoracic and lumbar spine. Spine 1985;10:748–756.
24. Cotler HB, Kaldis MG: Anatomy and surgical approaches of the spine. In: Cotler JM, Cotler HB, eds. Spinal fusion. New York: Springer-Verlag, 1990;89–124.
25. Court-Brown CM, Stoll JE, Gertzbein SD: Thoracic facetectomy and bone grafting in the surgical treatment of adult idiopathic scoliosis. Spine 1987;12:992–995.
26. Crenshaw AH: Campbell's operative orthopaedics. 7th ed. St. Louis: CV Mosby, 1987;3094–3095.
27. Crock HV: Observations on the management of failed spinal operations. J Bone Joint Surg 1976;58B:193.
28. Crock HV: Anterior lumbar interbody fusion: indications for its use and notes on surgical technique. Clin Orthop 1982;165:157.
29. DeAndrade JR, Macnab I: Anterior occipitocervical fusion using an extra-pharyngeal exposure. J Bone Joint Surg 1969;51A:1621–1626.
30. Dommisse GF: The blood supply of the spinal cord. J Bone Joint Surg 1974;56B:225.
31. Dunn EJ, Anas PP: Tumors of the cervical spine. In: Evarts, CM, ed. Surgery of the musculoskeletal system. New York: Churchill Livingstone, 1983;4:175–189.
32. Dwyer AF: Direct current stimulation in spinal fusion. Med J Aust. 1974;1:73.

33. Dwyer AP: A fatal complication of paravertebral infection and traumatic aneurysm following Dwyer instrumentation. Proc Austral Orthop Assoc. J Bone Joint Surg 1979;61B:239.

34. Ebraheim NA, An HS, Jackson WT, et al: Internal fixation of the unstable cervical spine using posterior Roy-Camille plates: preliminary report. J Orthop Trauma 1989;3:23–28.

35. Eisenstein S, O'Brien JP: Chylothorax: A complication of Dwyer's anterior instrumentation. Brit J Surg 1977;64:339–341.

36. Eismont FJ, Wiesel SW, Rothman RH: The treatment of dural tears associated with spinal surgery. J Bone Joint Surg 1981;63A:1132.

37. Fang HSY, Ong GB: Direct anterior approach to the upper cervical spine. J Bone Joint Surg 1962;44:1588.

38. Fielding JW, Stillwell WT: Anterior cervical approach to the upper thoracic spine. A case report. Spine 1976;1:158–161.

39. Flynn TB: Neurologic complications of anterior cervical interbody fusion. Spine 1982;7:536–539.

40. Gallie WE: Fractures and dislocations of the cervical spine. Am J Surg 1939;46:495–499.

41. Gower DJ, Culp P, Ball M: Lateral lumbar spine roentgenograms: potential role in complications of lumbar disc surgery. Surg Neurol 1987;27:316–318.

42. Grantham SA, Dick HM, Thompson RC, Stinchfield FE: Occipitocervical arthrodesis. Clin Orthop 1969;65:118.

43. Griswold DM, Albright JA, Schiffman E, et al: Atlanto-axial fusion for instability. J Bone Joint Surg 1978;60A:285–292.

44. Hall JE, Denis F, Murray J: Exposure of the upper cervical spine for spinal decompression. J Bone Joint Surg 1977;59A:121–123.

45. Harbison SP: Major vascular complications of intervertebral disc surgery. Ann Surg 1954;140:342.

46. Heeneman, H: Vocal cord paralysis following approaches to the anterior cervical spine. Laryngoscope 1973;83:17–21.

47. Henry AK: Extensile exposure. Baltimore: Williams & Wilkins, 1959;53–72.

48. Herkowitz HN: A comparison of anterior cervical fusion, cervical laminectomy, and cervical laminoplasty for the surgical management of multiple level spondylotic radiculopathy. Spine 1988;13:774–780.

49. Herndon WA, Sullivan JA, Yngve DA, et al: Segmental spinal instrumentation with sublaminar wires. A critical appraisal. J Bone Joint Surg 1987;69:851–859.

50. Hilgenberg AD, Grillo HC: Acquired nonmalignant tracheoesophageal fistula. J Thorac Cardiovasc Surg 1983;85:492–498.

51. Hodge WA, DeWald RL: Splenic injury complicating the anterior thoracoabdominal surgical approach for scoliosis. J Bone Joint Surg 1983;65A:396–397.

52. Hodgson AR, Stock FE, Fang HSY, et al: Anterior spinal fusion: the operative approach and pathologic findings in 412 patients with Pott's disease of the spine. Br J Surg 1960;48:172–178.

53. Hodgson AR: An approach to the cervical spine (C3-7). Clin Orthop 1965;39:129.

54. Holscher EC: Vascular and visceral injuries during lumbar disc surgery. J Bone Joint Surg 1968;50A:383–393.

55. Horowitch A, Peek RD, Thomas JC, et al: The Wiltse pedicle screw fixation system. Early clinical results. Spine 1989;14:461–467.

56. Horwitz NH, Rizzoli HV: Postoperative complications in neurosurgical practice, recognition, prevention, management. Baltimore: Williams & Wilkins, 1988;30–98.

57. Johnson RM, McGuire EJ: Urogenital complications of anterior approaches to the lumbar spine. Clin Orthop 1981;154:114–118.

58. Johnson RM, Southwick WO: Surgical approaches to the spine. In: Rothman RH, Simeone FA, eds. The spine. Philadelphia: WB Saunders, 1982;67–188.

59. Kane WJ: Posterior arthrodesis of the thoracolumbosacral spine. In: Chapman MW, ed. Operative orthopaedics. Philadelphia: JB Lippincott 1988;1957–1964.

60. Kirkaldy-Willis WH, Allen PBR, Rostrup O, et al: Surgical approaches to the anterior elements of the spine: indications and techniques. Can J Surg 1966;9:294–308.

61. Kurz LT, Herkowitz HH: Modified anterior approach to the cervico-thoracic junction. Presented at the 18th annual meeting of Cervical Spine Research Society. San Antonio, Texas, November 1990.

62. Larson SJ, Holst RA, Hemmy DC, et al: Lateral extracavity approach to traumatic lesions of the thoracic and lumbar spine. J Neurosurg 1976;45:628–637.

63. Lesoin F, Bouasakao N, Clarisse J, et al: Results of surgical treatment of radiculomyelopathy caused by cervical arthrosis based on 1000 operations. Surg Neurol 1985;23:350–355.

64. Lesoin F, Rousseaux M, Lozes G, et al: Posterolateral approach to tumours of the dorsolumbar spine. Acta-Neurochir (Wien) 1986;81:40–44.

65. Light TR, Wagner FC, Johnson RM, et al: Correction of spinal instability and recovery of neurologic loss following cervical vertebral body replacement. Spine 1980;5:392–394.

66. McAfee PC, Bohlman HH, Ducker T, et al: Failure of stabilization of the spine with methylmethacrylate: a retrospective analysis of twenty-four cases. J Bone Joint Surg 1986;68A:1145–1157.

67. McAfee PC, Bohlman HH, Riley LH, et al: The anterior retropharyngeal approach to the upper part of the cervical spine. J Bone and Joint Surg 1987;69A:1371–1383.

68. McAfee PC, Bohlman HH, Wilson WL: The triple wire fixation technique for stabilization of acute cervical fracture-dislocations: a biomechanical analysis. Orthop Trans 1985;9:142.

69. McMaster MJ: Anterior and posterior instrumentation and fusion of thoracolumbar scoliosis due to myelomeningocele. J Bone Joint Surg 1987;69B:20–25.

70. Micheli JJ, Hood RW: Anterior exposure of the cervicothoracic spine using a combined cervical and thoracic approach. J Bone Joint Surg 1983;65A:992–997.

71. Meyer PR Jr: Surgical stabilization of the cervical spine. In: Meyer PR, ed. Surgery of spine trauma. New York: Churchill Livingstone, 1989;397–524.

72. Moe JH: Complications of scoliosis treatment. Clin Orthop 1967;53:21–30.

73. Moore CA, Cohen A: Combined arterial venous and urethral injuries complicating disc surgery. Am J Surg 1968;115:574.

74. Newman P, Sweetnam R: Occipito-cervical fusion. J Bone Joint Surg 1969;51B:423–431.

75. Olsewski JM, Simmons EH, Kallen FC, et al: Morphometry of the lumbar spine: anatomical perspectives related to transpedicular fixation. J Bone Joint Surg 1990;72A:541–549.

76. Raney FL: The Raney technique of anterior interbody fusion. In: White AH, Rothman RH, Ray CD, eds. Lumbar spine surgery. St. Louis: CV Mosby, 1987;403–407.

77. Riley LH Jr: Surgical approaches to the anterior structures of the cervical spine. Clin Orthop 1973;91:16–20.

78. Robinson RA, Southwick WO: Surgical approaches to the cervical spine. In: AAOS: Instructional Course Lectures. Vol XVII, St. Louis: CV Mosby, 1960;299–330.

79. Roy-Camille R, Saillant G, Mazel C: Internal fixation of the unstable cervical spine by a posterior osteosynthesis with plates and screws. In: The cervical spine (Sherk HH, ed.), Philadelphia: JB Lippincott, 1989;390–421.

80. Roy-Camille R, Mazel C, Saillant G, et al: Treatment of malignant tumors of the spine with posterior instrumentation. In: Sudaresan N, Schmidek HH, Schiller AL, et al, eds. Tumors of the spine. Philadelphia, WB Saunders, 1990;473–487.

81. Sanders G, Uyeda RY, and Karlan MS: Nonrecurrent inferior laryngeal nerves and their association with a recurrent branch. Am J Surg 1983;146:501–503.

82. Sang UH, Wilson CB: Postoperative epidural hematoma as a complication of anterior cervical discectomy. J Neurosurg 1978;49:288–291.

83. Selby DK, Henderson RJ, Blumenthal S, et al: Anterior lumbar fusion. In: White AH, Rothman RH, Ray CD: Lumbar spine surgery. St. Louis: CV Mosby, 1987; 383–402.

84. Shen YS, Cheung CY: Chylous leakage after arthrodesis using the anterior approach to the spine. Report of two cases. J Bone Joint Surg 1989;71A:1250–1251.

85. Silber I, McMaster W: Retroperitoneal fibrosis with hydronephrosis as a complication of the Dwyer procedure. J Pediatr Surg 1977;12:255.

86. Simeone FA, Rothman RH: Cervical disc disease. In: Rothman RH, Simeone FA, eds. The spine. Philadelphia: WB Saunders, 1982;440–499.

87. Simmons EH, Bhalla SK: Anterior cervical discectomy and fusion. A clinical and biomechanical study with eight-year follow-up. J Bone Joint Surg 1969;51B:225–232.

88. Simmons EH: Surgery of the spine in rheumatoid arthritis and ankylosing spondylitis. In: Evarts CM, ed. Surgery of the muscoloskeletal system. vol. 2. New York: Churchill Livingstone, 1983;85.

89. Stener B: Total spondylectomy in chondrosarcoma arising from the seventh thoracic vertebra. J Bone Joint Surg 1971; 53AB:288–295.

90. Stener B, Johnson OE: Complete removal of three vertebrae for giant cell tumor. J Bone Joint Surg 1971;53B:278–287.

91. Stener B, Gunterberg B: High amputation of the sacrum for extirpation of tumors. Spine 1978;3:351–366.

92. Sundaresan N, Shah J, Foley KM, et al: An anterior surgical approach to the upper thoracic vertebrae. J Neurosurg 1984;61:686–690.

93. Sundaresan N, Shah J, Feghali JG: A transsternal approach to the upper thoracic vertebrae. Amer J Surg 1984;148:473–477.

94. Tew JM Jr, Mayfield FH: Surgery of the anterior cervical spine: Preventions of complications. In: Dunsker SB, ed. Cervical spondylosis. New York: Raven Press, 1981;191–208.

95. Turner PL, Webb JK: A surgical approach to the upper thoracic spine. J Bone Joint Surg 1987;69B:542–544.

96. Verbiest H: Antero-lateral operations for fractures and dislocations in the middle and lower parts of the cervical spine. J Bone Joint Surg 1969;51A:1489–1530.

97. Watkins RG: Surgical approaches to the spine. New York: Springer-Verlag, 1983.

98. Watkins RG: Results of anterior interbody fusion. In: White AH, Rothman RH, Ray CD, eds. Lumbar spine surgery. St. Louis: CV Mosby, 1987;408–432.

99. Watkins RG: Cervical, thoracic and lumbar complications—anterior approach. In: Garfin SR, ed. Complications of spine surgery. Baltimore: Williams & Wilkins, 1989;211–247.

100. Weidner A: Internal fixation with metal plates and screws. In: Sherk HH, et al., ed. The cervical spine, Philadelphia: JB Lippincott, 1989;404–421.

101. Welsh LW, Welsh JJ, Chinnici JC: Dysphagia due to cervical spine surgery. Ann Otol Rhinol Laryngol 1987;96:112–115.

102. Wertheim SB, Bohlman HH: Occipitocervical fusion. J Bone Joint Surg 1987;69A:833–836.

103. White AA III, Southwick WO, DePonte RJ, et al: Relief of pain by anterior cervical fusion for spondylosis—a report of sixty-five patients. J Bone Joint Surg 1973;55A:525–534.

104. White AA III, Jupiter J, Southwick WO, et al: An experimental study of the immediate load bearing of three surgical constructions for anterior spine fusions. Clin Orthop 1973;91:21–28.

105. Whitecloud TS, LaRocca H: Fibular strut graft in reconstructive surgery of the cervical spine. Spine 1976;1:33–43.

106. Whitesides TE Jr, Kelley RP: Lateral approach to the upper cervical spine for anterior fusion. South Med J 1966;59:879–883.

107. Yasuoka S, Peterson HA, MacCarty CS: Incidence of spinal column deformity after multilevel laminectomy in children and adults. J Neurosurg 1982;57:441–445.

Two

Posterior Instrumentation of the Cervical Spine

Howard S. An

INTRODUCTION

Wiring techniques of posterior cervical stabilization have been well described in the literature in the past, but other forms of stabilization have been presented recently. The advantages and disadvantages of each method are presented in this chapter, and various wiring methods and selected alternative techniques of posterior cervical fixation will be discussed. The indications, techniques, and potential complications of these techniques will be presented.

UPPER CERVICAL SPINE

The indications for posterior atlantoaxial stabilization may be traumatic atlantoaxial instabilities with rupture of the transverse ligament, the type II odontoid fractures with a high risk of nonunion as in old patients with a significant displacement, and late atlantoaxial instabilities due to Jefferson's fracture of C1 ring or odontoid nonunion. Atlantoaxial instabilities may also be caused by nontraumatic disorders such as rheumatoid arthritis, congenital anomalies, and metabolic problems. Anterior atlantoaxial subluxation is assessed radiographically by measuring the atlantodens interval. This is measured from the midposterior margin of the anterior ring of C1 to the anterior surface of the dens. A measurement of this difference of more than 3 mm in the adult or 4 mm in the child on flexion/extension views is accepted as being unstable or potentially unstable. In nontraumatic disorders, an atlantoaxial interval greater than 3 mm is not necessarily an indication for surgery. For example, in rheumatoid arthritis, indications for surgery include significant progressive neurologic deterioration, intractable pain, or severe instability (>9 mm). Many patients with an atlantoaxial interval greater than 3 mm due to nontraumatic disorders do well, as the disease process may be protracted and nonprogressive.

Posterior atlantoaxial arthrodesis may be performed using either the Gallie or Brooks technique (8,25,29,38). The Gallie technique is safer because the spinous process of C2 is utilized instead of the lamina of C2, but the Brooks technique provides additional rotational stability. The author recommends the Gallie technique in most flexion injuries. The Brooks technique, however, is preferred in extension injuries or if more rigid fixation is required (41,75). Autogenous iliac crest graft material is preferable, but allograft material can be supplemented in patients whose pelvic bone is too osteoporotic. Internal fixation without fusion is not recommended, as a higher failure rate would be expected (47). The fusion should extend to the occiput when the arch of C1 is deficient or when the patient exhibits superior migration of the odontoid in rheumatoid arthritis. The author recommends halo-vest external support in the postoperative period for the majority of patients to prevent failure of fusion or wire breakage.

Surgical Techniques

Posterior Atlantoaxial Arthrodesis A halo ring is applied just prior to surgery to maintain traction during the operation and to facilitate vest application after surgery. Preoperative halo traction may be helpful in cases where a significant deformity is present. If traction is not required, the patient can be fitted with a posteriorly opened halo ring and the vest preoperatively. A midline incision from the occiput to the third cervical vertebra is made. The tips of the spinous processes are exposed and subperiosteal dissection carried out along the lamina of C2 and the posterior arch of C1. All soft tissues are then carefully removed from the bony surfaces. The arch of C1 should not be exposed more than 1.5 cm from the midline in adults and 1 cm in children to avoid injury to the vertebral arteries. Great care must be taken not to fracture the posterior ring of C1 while dissecting the ligamentum flavum. Muscular insertions on the spinous

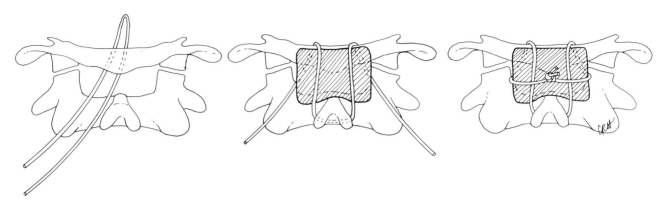

Figure 2.1. A modified Gallie technique using an H-shaped bone graft from the iliac crest contouring it to fit over the posterior arches of C1 and C2. A double U-shaped 18- or 20- gauge wire is passed under the arch of C1 from inferior to superior.

process of C2 should be preserved as much as possible to prevent the weakness or instability at C2-C3.

The C1-2 Gallie wiring with onlay bone graft is still used and is adequate for flexion types of instability. There are several techniques of wiring, and the author prefers a technique by Simmons, who advocates the use of a modified Gallie H-graft from the iliac crest contouring it to fit over the posterior arches of C1 and C2 (66). A doubled U-shaped 18- or 20-gauge wire is passed under the arch of C1 from inferior to superior. A bone block is taken from the posterior iliac crest and shaped to fit between C1 and C2 as well as the wires (Fig. 2.1). The loop of the wire goes over the bone block and the spinous process of C2. The ends of the wire are tightened around the graft between C1 and C2. The deep cancellous surfaces of the graft must be contoured to fit over the curved posterior surface of C1 and C2 so that the graft is in firm contact with the underlying vertebrae, immobilizing the involved segment. Additional cancellous bone chips are placed in defects to promote fusion.

In the Brooks type fusion, doubled-twisted 24-gauge wires are passed under the arch of C1 and then under the lamina of C2 (Figs. 2.2 and 2.3). Rectangular iliac crest bone grafts (1.25 cm × 3.5 cm) are harvested and beveled to fit in the interval between the arch of C1 and each lamina of the axis. The wires are then tightened, securing the graft in proper position.

Aprin and Harf recommend internal fixation of C1-C2 by passing two 18-gauge stainless wires beneath the posterior arch of the atlas and around a threaded Steinman pin that is drilled through the base of the spinous process of the axis (4). They reported excellent results in eight patients treated with this technique. Meyer's technique is a variation of the Brooks technique in that sublaminar wires are placed under C1 and C2, followed by fixing the bone grafts with the wires that threaded

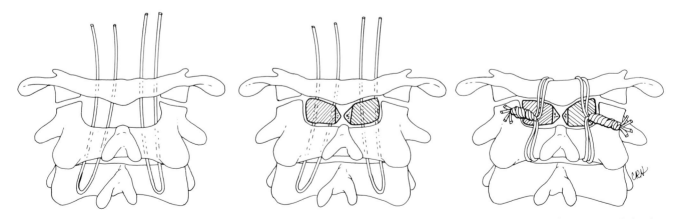

Figure 2.2. The Brooks type fusion with doubled-twisted 24-gauge wires that are passed under the arch of C1 and then under the lamina of C2. Rectangular iliac crest bone grafts are fitted in the interval between the arch of C1 and each lamina of the axis.

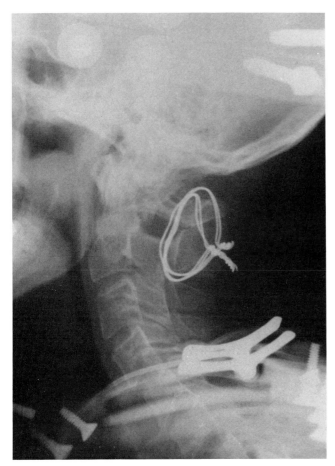

Figure 2.3. Lateral roentgenogram of a Brook wiring and fusion of C1-C2.

through holes in the grafts instead of wiring over the grafts (48). Fielding also described other variations of Gallie techniques for atlantoaxial stabilization (24). Triple-wire technique is another good method of stabilizing the upper cervical spine (73).

Posterior fusion may be reinforced with metal mesh or polymethylmethacrylate in selected patients with severe osteoporosis or malignancy to enhance stability (6,9,13,14,55). When stabilizing and fusing the upper cervical spine with wires, adequate external immobilization with a halo-vest should be carried out for approximately 12 weeks.

Although wiring and bone graft fixation methods give satisfactory stabilization in the majority of the cases, other forms of internal fixation have been reported in the literature in recent years. One method of posterior atlantoaxial arthrodesis utilizes an interlaminar clamp (16,34,49,70). This clamp may be used in selected cases where sublaminar wires would be difficult or dangerous to pass (Fig. 2.4). Potential problems with interlaminar

clamp fixation are implant slippage, difficulty with bone grafting, and pseudarthrosis. Another method of atlantoaxial fixation utilizes transarticular screws. Magerl described a transarticular screw technique for those who have deficient posterior arch of the atlas (44,72). This procedure provides a rigid fixation, but requires a meticulous surgical technique. A midline approach is used to expose the occiput to C3. Subperiosteal dissection is done on the cranial aspect of C2 to expose the C1-C2 facet joints bilaterally. Magerl recommends the use of K-wires to retract the soft tissues containing the greater occipital nerve and its accompanying venous plexus. The screws are inserted by entering C2 at the inferior aspect and exiting at the posterior aspect of upper articular process. The screws are placed through the facet joints into the lateral masses of C1 (Fig. 2.5). In a recent biomechanical study, this Magerl technique was found to be significantly stiffer in rotation than the Gallie wiring technique (50). Magerl recommends Gallie wiring and fusion in addition to transarticular screws in patients with an intact C1 ring (44,72). Recently, a technique of atlantoaxial stabilization using pediatric Cotrel-Dubousset rods and hooks has been reported (69).

Posterior Occipitocervical Fusion

Several techniques have been described. The author prefers the method described by Wertheim and Bohlman (Fig. 2.6) (74). A midline posterior approach is made, exposing the external occipital protuberance to the fourth cervical vertebra. Sharp subperiosteal dissection is completed, exposing the occiput and the cervical laminae. The external occipital protuberance is thick and represents the ideal location for passage of wires without having to go through both tables of the skull. A high-speed diamond burr is used to create a trough on both sides of the protuberance at a level 2 cm above the foramen magnum. A

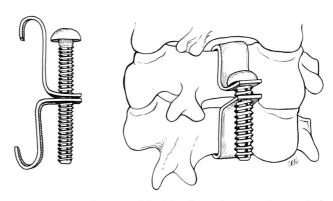

Figure 2.4. Diagram of Halifax clamp for posterior cervical fixation.

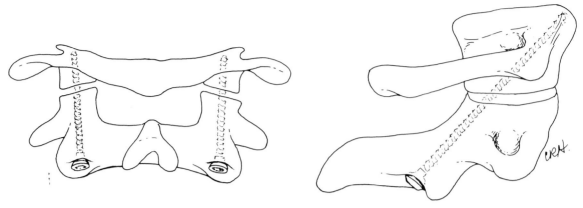

Figure 2.5. Magerl's technique of C1-C2 arthrodesis by screw fixation through the articular facets into the lateral masses of C1.

towel clip is then used to create a hole under the ridge. A second wire loop is passed around the arch of C1, and a third is passed through and around the base of the spinous process of C2. The posterior iliac crest is then exposed, and a large, thick, slightly curved graft of corticocancellous bone of appropriate width and length is obtained. The graft is then divided and three drill holes placed in each graft. The occiput is decorticated and the grafts anchored in place by the wires. Additional cancellous bone is then packed between the two grafts. Halo cast immobilization is required for 12 weeks.

Other wiring techniques of occipitocervical fusion have been described in the literature (28,33,48,57). Some authors utilize the occipital bone just above the occipitoatlantal space, and penetrate the opposite cortex to pass the

wires. Great care should be taken not to injure the dura or venous structures. The author prefers the technique in which a trough is created in the occipital protuberance for wire passage (28,74). Although isolated cases have been reported (53), occipitocervical arthrodesis with onlay grafts without internal fixation is generally not recommended. Without internal fixation, the patient may require prolonged bed rest, and a higher rate of pseudarthrosis is expected. This technique is acceptable in young children if patients are immobilized postoperatively with halo fixation (40).

Occipitocervical fusion can also be achieved by using Luque segmental instrumentation (7,35,56), or plate-screw fixation devices (23,32,60,61,69). Itoh and associates reported 13 rheumatoid patients who underwent

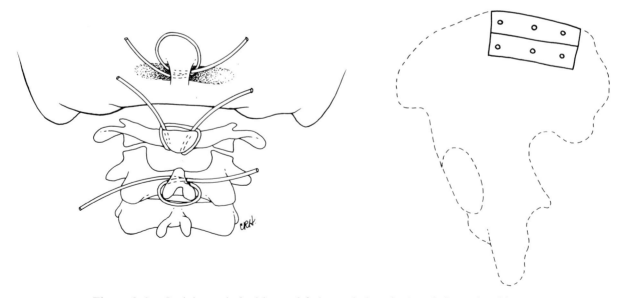

Figure 2.6. Occipitocervical wiring and fusion technique by Wertheim and Bohlman.

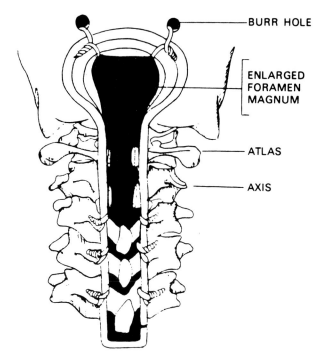

BURR HOLE

ENLARGED
FORAMEN
MAGNUM

ATLAS

AXIS

Figure 2.7. Ransford loop for occipitocervical fixation (From Ransford AO, Crockard HA, Pozo JL, et al: Craniocervical instability treated by contoured loop fixation. J Bone Joint Surg 1986;68B:173.

a posterior occipitocervical fusion reinforced by Luque's segmental spinal instrumentation (Fig. 2.7) (35). Twelve of 13 patients had union, and improvement of pain was observed in all patients. Ransford et al. also reported three patients with craniocervical instability treated by contoured loop fixation with good results (56). The author believes that this technique provides a better stability than wiring, but potential complications associated with sublaminar wiring prohibits its routine use. This sublaminar wiring technique may be advantageous in patients who require multiple-level fixation from the occiput to the lower cervical spine. At the risk of compromising stability, facet wires may be used instead of sublaminar wires in some cases.

Other authors recommend the use of screws onto the occiput (23,32,60,61,69). Roy-Camille devised an occipitocervical plate that is contoured to fit the occipito-cervical junction (60,61). Fidler presented three patients with metastasis who underwent plate-screw fixation on the occiput and sublaminar wire fixation on the upper cervical spine (23). This plate is screwed to the midline where the bone is thicker. A modified Cotrel-Dubousset system is also available for use in the occipitocervical spine. This system utilizes screws on to the occipital bone and hooks into the cervical spine (39). No clinical series are reported at this time. One can also use cement as an adjunctive fixation to enhance the stability of the construct. Recently, Stambough et al. described a technique of occipitocervical stabilization with bone cement in the osteoporotic spine (67).

Complications associated with posterior fusion of the upper cervical spine may be serious. Care is required during passage of the wires or application of the screws to prevent injury to the brain or spinal cord. We recommend the use of somatosensory evoked potential monitoring in high-risk procedures. Dissection on the ring of the atlas must be done in a gentle manner, as the direct pressure may result in fracture or slippage of an instrument. One should dissect laterally only approximately 1.5 cm to minimize risk to the vertebral artery. To prevent uncontrollable venous bleeding, one should avoid dissecting the foramen magnum from the inferior edge of the foramen. We recommend halo-vest immobilization after surgery to prevent failure of the surgical construct and to lessen the likelihood of pseudarthrosis.

LOWER CERVICAL SPINE

Posterior fusion of the lower cervical spine may be indicated in patients with traumatic instabilities, extensive laminectomies for neural decompression, or destruction of bony elements by neoplasm. The goals of the treatment include stabilization, maintenance of alignment, fusion, and early rehabilitation. There are numerous methods of posterior stabilization of the cervical spine (5,11,12, 16,17,22,27,34,43–45,51,54,59–61,64,65,68,70). Each has its advantages and disadvantages.

Wiring Procedures

Since Rogers initially described a method of cervical wiring and fusion (58), other techniques have been described in the literature (5,10,11,22,48,54,64,73). Wiring techniques are quite effective in preventing flexion but less effective in preventing extension or rotation. The author favors a triple-wire technique with interspinous process wires to compress bone grafts to lamina (Figs. 2.8,–2.9). This triple-wiring technique has been shown to be safe and effective, and biomechanically superior to many other constructs (5,45).

The patient should be in skull tong traction on the Stryker frame to maintain alignment. After preparation and draping of the patient, the skin and subcutaneous tissue are dissected down to the midline fascia. At this time, a lateral radiograph is taken to be certain of the level. Subperiosteal dissection is followed to expose the spinous processes, lamina, and facets, taking care to avoid dissecting beyond fusion sites to prevent creeping fusion extension. A 3- or 4-mm burr is used to drill a hole at

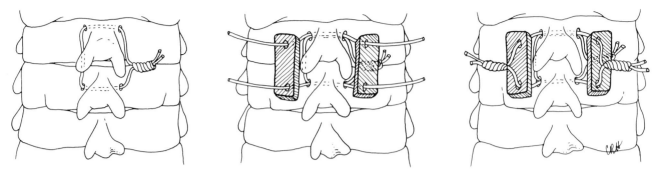

Figure 2.8. A triple-wire technique with interspinous process wires, compressing bone grafts to lamina.

the base of the spinous process on both sides at the spinolaminar junction. The drill hole site should be at the proximal aspect of the cephalad spinous process and at the distal aspect of the caudad spinous process. A towel clip is gently passed through the holes to create a tunnel for wires. A 20-gauge wire is then passed from one side to the other and tightened.

If more than one level is to be fused, the figure of 8 wiring is used to incorporate the middle spinous process in the wiring construct. If the middle spinous process or lamina are fractured, wiring should be avoided at this level. The second and third wires are passed through the cephalad and caudad holes in the base of the processes, respectively. Decortication of the lamina and facets is done carefully using a water-cooled power burr. Corticocancellous bone grafts of appropriate length are next taken from the outer table of the iliac crest. The bone grafts are drilled to make two holes and laid down on the lamina bilaterally. The wires are passed through the holes in the bone grafts and tightened. Additional can-

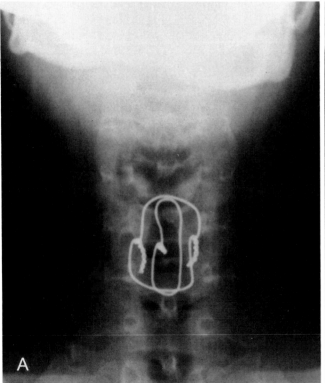

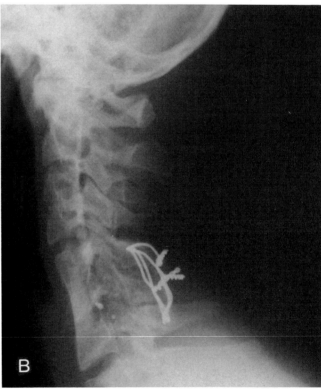

Figure 2.9. *A,* Anteroposterior view of triple-wiring. *B,* Lateral view of triple-wiring (anterior vertebrectomy and strut graft fusion is also shown).

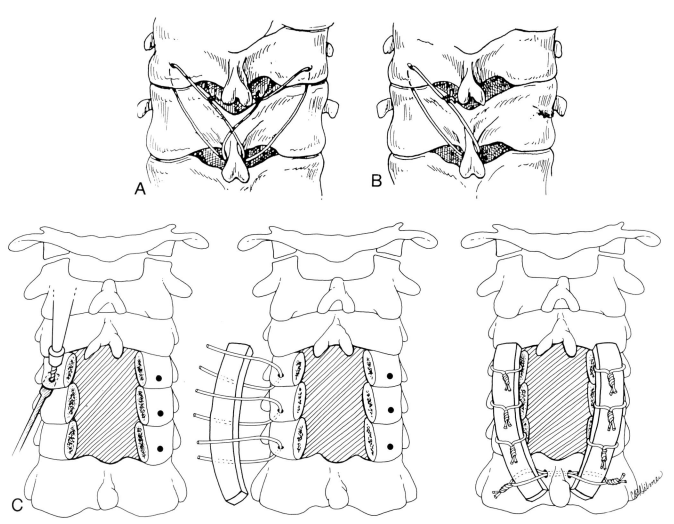

Figure 2.10. Facet wiring. *A*, Unilateral facet wiring. *B*, Bilateral facet wiring (From Wilber RG, Peters JG, Likavec MJ: Surgical techniques in cervical spine surgery. In: Errico TJ, Bauer RD, Waugh T, eds. Spinal trauma. Philadelphia: JB Lippincott, 1991). *C*, Facet wiring after laminectomy by Callahan. (Drilling is done on the inferior articular facets, and wires are passed at each level.) Bone grafts are then tied down on the facets (Modified from Callahan RA, Johnson RM, Margolis RN, et al: Cervical facet fusion for control of instability following laminectomy. J Bone Joint Surg 1977;59A:991–1002.)

cellous chips are laid on the exposed lamina or facets. The patient is usually kept in a cervicothoracic orthosis or halo-vest for 4-6 weeks, depending on the stability of the construct and compliance of the patient.

Facet fracture or subluxation can be managed with the oblique wiring technique or wire loop by passing the wire through the lateral mass (Fig. 2.10*A* and 2.10*B*) (10,22,76). If laminectomy has been performed, interfacet wiring and fusion can be applied (Fig. 2.10*C*) (11). The facet wire is passed by placing a small Penfield dissector into the facet joint, followed by making a 2-mm drill hole into the facet from superior to inferior. Twenty or 22-gauge wire is passed through this hole and looped around the inferior spinous process for one-level fusion, as in unilateral facet dislocation.

Facet wires may be extended to adjacent facets for multiple-level facet stabilization, as in postlaminectomy instability. The facet wires may be tied to bone grafts for fusion and also can be tied to rods to gain additional stability (26,51). Sublaminar fixation has also been described (Fig. 2.11) (76). The author does not recommend sublaminar fixation in the lower cervical spine because this technique is associated with a greater risk of neurologic injury. An alternative fixation is the "Dewar procedure," in which Kirschner wires are inserted through the bases of the spinous processes and secured with wire

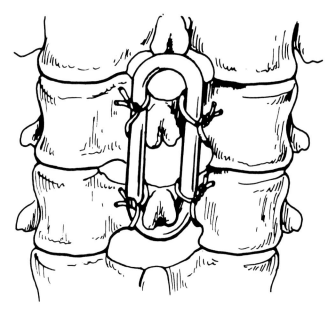

Figure 2.11. Luque loop fixation with sublaminar wires. (From Wilber RG, Peters JG, Likavec MJ: Surgical techniques in cervical spine surgery. In: Errico TJ, Bauer RD, Waugh T, eds. Spinal trauma. Philadelphia: JB Lippincott, 1991;155.)

in a loop fashion (Fig. 2.12) (17,59,65). Use of methylmethacrylate is generally discouraged due to high complication rates and early failures, except in special circumstances in which the bone is severely osteoporotic or the patient's life expectancy is short (19,45).

Complications associated with posterior interspinous wiring in the cervical spine are relatively infrequent. One must avoid unnecessary exposure of the cervical levels beyond fusion areas to prevent creeping fusions to adjacent vertebrae. Inadvertent penetration into the ligamentum flavum and the spinal canal can occur if one is not careful during subperiosteal dissection. Dural penetration can also occur during drilling or passing of the wires, if the holes are placed too close to the dura or with broken wires (20). The most common complication associated with the wiring procedure in the cervical spine is loss of fixation and subsequent recurrence of deformity. This complication is directly related to bone quality, the surgeon's technique, and postoperative external support. If a more rigid construct is accomplished, such as the triple-wiring and bone-block procedure, the patient can be managed with a cervicothoracic orthosis in the postoperative period. On the other hand, if the surgical construct is not quite stable, or if the patient's compliance is questionable, halo-vest should be used for postoperative external support.

Rigid Internal Fixation

Although the majority of patients with an instability of the cervical spine can be treated with wiring methods,

there are situations in which more rigid internal fixation is more beneficial. Most apparent are instances in which the spinous processes are absent or deficient, as in postlaminectomy cases and fractures of the spinous processes. Also, stable fixation of multiple levels is another advantage of other techniques such as rodding or plating. More rigid fixation is of greater benefit in patients with multilevel injuries or extensive neoplasm at multiple levels. Rigid fixation also allows for earlier mobilization of the patient with minimal postoperative external support, which may be paramount in the treatment of multiple trauma victims.

Numerous instrumentations of the cervical spine provide a greater stability. Harrington or Luque rods with wires have been used in the cervical spine (26,51). Pediatric Cotrel-Dubousset hooks can be used in the adult cervical spine for hook-rod fixation. The Halifax clamps have been mentioned before with regard to the upper cervical spine; this device utilizes the lamina, and provides good stability against flexion, but not against extension or rotation (16,34,49,70,75).

Posterior stabilization of the cervical spine using screws and plates was pioneered by Roy-Camille in Paris (Fig. 2.13A and 2.13B) (60,61). Louis utilizes a similar type of plate-screw fixation onto the lateral masses (42,52). Magerl devised a plate-screw system for the cervical spine, in which the inferior portion of the plate is a hook configuration, the so-called hook-plate (Fig. 2.14A–2.14E) (30,36,43,44). Recently, Anderson et al. presented 30

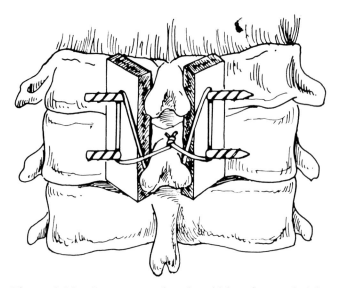

Figure 2.12. Dewar procedure in which a figure of eight wiring with Kirschner pins are secured on the spinous processes. (From Wilber RG, Peters JG, Likavec MJ: Surgical techniques in cervical spine surgery. In: Errico TJ, Bauer RD, Waugh T, eds. Spinal trauma. Philadelphia: JB Lippincott, 1991;154.)

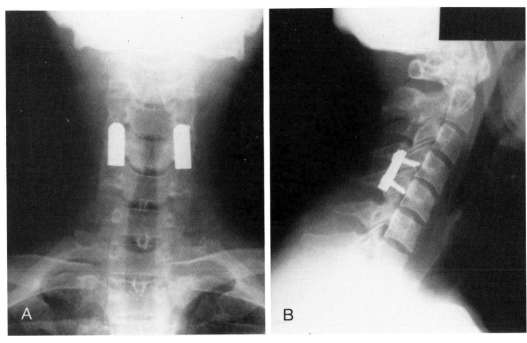

Figure 2.13. *A* and *B*, Roy-Camille plate-screw fixation on the lateral masses of the cervical spine in a patient with C4-C5 instability.

patients with unstable cervical spines, who had posterior arthrodesis with AO reconstruction plates (Fig. 2.15*A*–2.15*C*) (3). All had solid fusions with no neurologic or vascular complications. Three patients had screw loosening without clinical sequelae. Biomechanical strengths of these plates have been shown to be superior to posterior wiring, especially in extension and torsion (71). Clinical reports to date are also quite encouraging (3,15,18,21,37,63). These reports showed good correction of the deformity and maintenance of alignment until fusion. Although the author has not experienced any significant complications, potential problems associated with posterior plating with screws include injury of the vertebral artery or cervical nerve roots. Thorough familiarity of the articular pillar anatomy and surgical technique are important in the prevention of these complications.

A cadaveric study was done to find out potential dangers of posterior plate-screw osteosynthesis of the cervical spine (1). The vertebral artery and spinal cord were virtually free of danger with known techniques. The nerve root exits at the anterolateral portion of the superior facet, and the more medial angulation or the more cephalad angulation of the screw, the more likely it is to impinge on the nerve root. The ideal exit point of the drill was determined to be the juncture between the transverse process and the facet. The safest screw direction is determined to be about 30° lateral and 15° cephalad, starting

at 1 mm medial to the center of the lateral mass for C3 to C6 in avoiding both the nerve root and the facet joint (Fig. 2.16). The lateral mass is thin at the transitional C7 level, and lateral mass screw is potentially dangerous in disrupting the nerve root or the facet joint. Hook-plate design would be preferred at the C7 region. This cadaveric study allowed for measurement of the interfacet distances from the center of the lateral mass to the next lateral mass from C3 to C7. Results show that interfacet distances vary widely among different individuals, ranging from 9 mm to 16 mm with an average of 13 mm (Fig. 2.17).

A new plate design with oblong holes is necessary to better accommodate the differences of interfacet distances among different patients and different levels. The posterior plate-screw fixation of the cervical spine must be done with thorough knowledge of lateral mass anatomy. Bilateral exposure to the limits of the lateral masses is made. The center of the articular pillar is located and the cortex pierced with an awl or small burr at 1 mm medial to the center. As mentioned before, there are many techniques of drilling. Based on anatomical dissection to avoid potential injury to the nerve root, the pillar is drilled at 25–30° laterally and 15° cephalad for C3–C6, using a 2.5-mm drill bit. The drilling should be about 10–15° medially and 35° superiorly at C2 to avoid injury to the vertebral artery (Fig. 2.18). The opposite cortex is penetrated, using a drill with a stop guide. The drill hole is

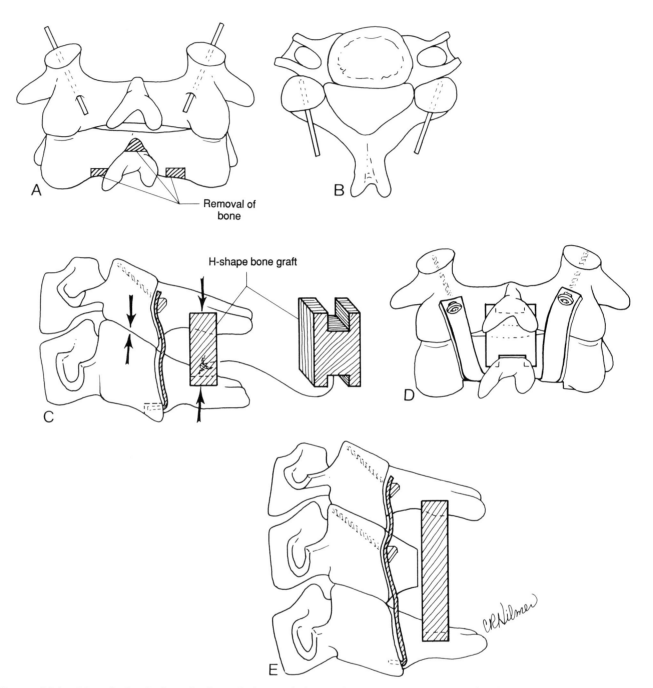

Figure 2.14. Magerl's hook-plate fixation of the cervical spine. *A*, Preparation of the inferior lamina for hook insertion. *B*, Lateral angulation of the screw at 25°. *C*, Superior screw angulation of the screw at 45° and H-shape bone graft between spinous processes. *D*, One-level stabilization of the cervical spine with hook-plate and bone graft. *E*, Two-level stabilization of the cervical spine with hook-plate and bone graft.

tapped with a 3.5-mm tap, and a contoured posterior cervical plate with a 3.5-mm diameter and appropriate length cortical screws are placed and secured.

In addition to Roy-Camille plates, other plates such as AO reconstruction plates, titanium plates, and Harm's posterior cervical plates are becoming available. The ti-

tanium device has an advantage of magnetic resonance imaging capability after implantation. The posterior elements adjacent to the plates are decorticated, and bone grafts are added. Complications associated with rigid posterior fixations of the cervical spine can be numerous. Devices such as Harrington or pediatric Cotrel-Dubous-

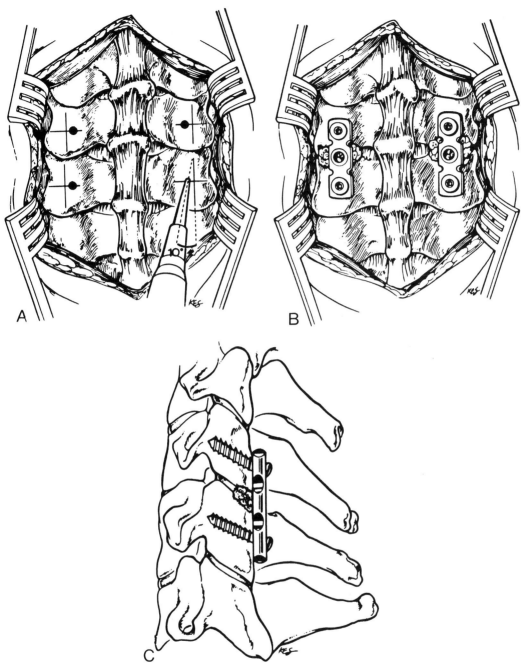

Figure 2.15. *A–C,* Posterior arthrodesis with AO reconstruction plates. Entry hole is 1 mm medial to the midpoint of the lateral mass, and the drill is directed 10° laterally and 30–40° cranially. (From Anderson PA, Henley MB, Grady MS, et al: Posterior cervical arthrodesis with AO reconstruction plates and bone graft. Spine 1991;16:S72–S79).

set hooks should be used cautiously, as hooks may impinge on the underlying dura, particularly if used bilaterally on the same level. Laminar hooks should be avoided in the injured level, where the spinal cord has been already compromised by edema or mechanical compression. Screw-plate fixation on the lateral mass may be complicated by injuries to the spinal cord, vertebral artery, or the nerve roots. Meticulous exposure of the lateral mass and strict adherence of surgical technique will prevent these complications. Implant loosening may occur if postoperative external support is ignored or pseuarthrosis results. If rigid fixation has been achieved,

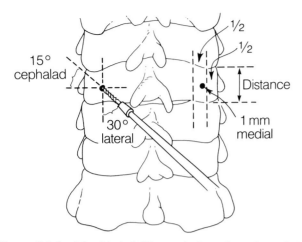

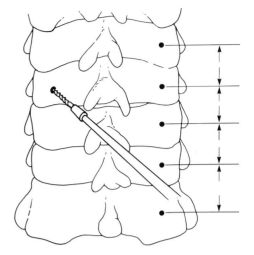

Figure 2.16. The ideal drilling technique for safety of the nerve root. The starting point is 1 mm medial to the center of the lateral mass, and the drill is directed 30° laterally and 15° cranially.

Figure 2.17. The average of interfacet distances is 13 mm, but ranges from 9 mm to 16 mm among different individuals.

halo-vest external immobilization is generally unnecessary, except in noncompliant patients.

CERVICOTHORACIC JUNCTION

Spinal disorders at the cervicothoracic junction may require stabilization due to trauma, tumors, infection, or postlaminectomy instability (2). Many lesions are located anteriorly and require anterior dissections through supraclavicular, transthoracic, or transsternal approaches. In selected cases, posterior fixation may be needed in addition to the anterior procedure. Posterior fixation is rather straightforward if laminae are intact. Triple-wiring with bone grafts, Luque rods with sublaminar wirings,

Harrington rods, or Cotrel-Dubousset rods with pediatric hooks may be used if laminae are intact.

If laminectomy has been performed, pedicles may be utilized even at C7, T1, or T2. The anatomy of the pedicles at this junction does not allow much room for error. A cadaveric study was done on the pedicles at the cervicothoracic junction (1). The pedicle entry point was 1 mm inferior to the midportion of facet joint for C7, T1, and T2 (Fig. 2.19). The medial angulation averaged 34° at C7, 31.8° at T1, and 26.5° at T2. The medial-lateral and superior-inferior outer pedicle diameters were 6.9 mm and 7.5 mm at C7, 8.5 mm and 9.5 mm at T1, and 7.5 mm and 10.7 mm at T2, respectively. The medial-lateral inner diameter averaged 5.18 mm, 6.4 mm, 5.5

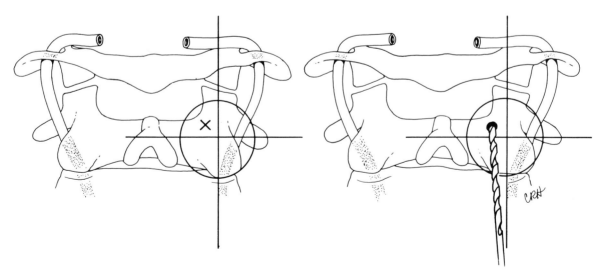

Figure 2.18. Drilling technique at C2 should be at 35° cranial and 10–15° medial angulation.

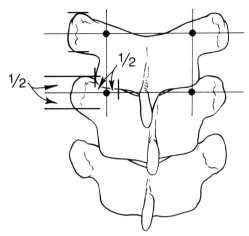

Figure 2.19. Entry point of the pedicle at the cervicothoracic junction. The pedicle is located by crossing a horizontal line at the midportion of the transverse processes and a vertical line at the lamina-transverse process junction or the midportion of the facet. This point is about 1-2 mm below the facet joint.

mm for C7, T1, and T2, respectively. The pedicle distances (from the entry point to the posterior vertebral body line) measured 9.1 mm, 9.9 mm, and 10.4 mm for respective levels (Fig. 2.20). The margins for error are small when using pedicle screws at these levels. If a pedicle screw must be used at C7, T1, and T2, precise knowledge of the entrance point, diameters, and 25–30° medial direction is required. The cervicothoracic region is a tran-

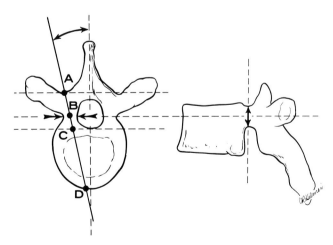

Figure 2.20. Morphometry of the pedicle at the cervicothoracic junction. *A,* Starting point. *B,* The middle or narrowest point of the pedicle. *C,* Posterior vertebral line. *D,* Anterior vertebral margin. Medial angulation should be about 25–30°. Superior-inferior diameter is relatively greater than medial-lateral diameter in the thoracic spine as compared with the lumbar spine.

sitional zone between mobile cervical and rigid thoracic spine, and injuries of laminectomy frequently cause significant instability. Internal fixation should be relatively rigid in this region, and postoperative immobilization should be done with a halo-vest in most cases.

In summary, posterior fixation of the cervical spine may be done by a simple and reliable triple-wiring method or other rigid fixation methods, depending on the pathoanatomic process of the lesion. One must be thoroughly familiar with the surgical anatomy, surgical techniques, and potential complications prior to using a particular method of stabilization of the cervical spine.

REFERENCES

1. An HS, Gordin R, Renner K: Anatomic consideration for plate-screw fixation of the cervical spine. Presented at the Cervical Spine Research Society, San Antonio, Nov. 1990.
2. An HS, Vaccaro A, Cotler JM: Spinal disorders at the cervicothoracic junction. Presented at the Cervical Spine Research Society, San Antonio, Nov. 1990.
3. Anderson PA, Henley MB, Grady MS, et al: Posterior cervical arthrodesis with AO reconstruction plates and bone graft. Spine 1991;16:S72–S79.
4. Aprin H, Harf R: Stabilization of atlantoaxial instability. Orthopaedics 1988;11:1687–1693.
5. Bohlman HH: Acute fractures and dislocations of the cervical spine: an analysis of 300 hospitalized patients and review of the literature. J Bone Joint Surg 1979;61A:1119–1142.
6. Brattstrom H, Granholm L: Atlanto-axial fusion in rheumatoid arthritis: a new method of fixation with wire and bone cement. Acta Orthop Scand 1976;47:619–628.
7. Bridwell K: Treatment of markedly displaced Hangman's fracture with a Luque rectangle and a posterior fusion in a 71-year-old man. Spine 1986;11:49–52.
8. Brooks AL, Jenkins EB: Atlanto-axial arthrodesis by the wedge compression method. J Bone Joint Surg 1978;60A:279–284.
9. Bryan WJ, Inglis AE, Sculco TP, et al: Methylmethacrylate stabilization for enhancement of posterior cervical arthrodesis in rheumatoid arthritis. J Bone Joint Surg 1982;64A:1045–1050.
10. Cahill DW, Bellegarrigue R, Ducker TB: Bilateral facet to spinous process fusion: a new technique for posterior spinal fusion after trauma. Neurosurgery 1983;13:1–4.
11. Callahan RA, Johnson RM, Margolis RN, et al: Cervical facet fusion for control of instability following laminectomy. J Bone Joint Surg 1977;59A:991–1002.
12. Capen D, Zigler J, Garland D: Surgical stabilization in cervical spine trauma. Contemp Orthop 1987;14:25–32.
13. Clark CR, Keggi KJ, Panjabi MM: Methylmethacrylate stabilization of the cervical spine. J Bone and Joint Surg 1984;66A:40–46.
14. Clark CR, Goetz DD, Menezes AH: Arthrodesis of the cervical spine in rheumatoid arthritis. J Bone Joint Surg 1990;71A:381–392.
15. Cooper PR: Posterior stabilization of the cervical spine using Roy-Camille plates: A North American experience. Trans Orthop 1988;12:43.
16. Cybulski GR, Stone JL, Crowell RM, et al: Use of Halifax interlaminar clamps for posterior C1-2 arthrodesis. Neurosurgery 1988;22:429–31.

17. Davey JR, Rorabeck CH, Bailey SI, et al: A technique of posterior fusion for instability of the cervical spine. Spine 1985;10:722–728.

18. Dominella G, Berlanda P, Bassi G: Posterior approach osteosynthesis of the lower cervical spine by the R. Roy-Camille technique. Ital J Orthop Traumat 1982;8:235–244.

19. Duff TA: Surgical stabilization of traumatic cervical spine dislocation using methylmethacrylate. J Neurosurg 1986;64:39.

20. Dunn V, Smoker WR, Menezes AH: Transdural herniation of the cervical spine cord as a complication of a broken fracture-fixation wire. Amer J Neurorad 1987;8:724–726.

21. Ebraheim NA, An HS, Jackson WT, et al: Internal fixation of the unstable cervical spine using posterior Roy-Camille plates: preliminary report. J Orthop Trauma 1989;3:23–28.

22. Edwards CC, Matz SO, Levine AM: The oblique wiring technique for rotational injuries of the cervical spine. Trans Orthop 1985;9:142.

23. Fidler MW: Pathological fractures of the cervical spine. J Bone Joint Surg 1985;67B:352–357.

24. Fielding JW, Hawkins RJ, Ratzan SA: Spine fusion for atlanto-axial instability. J Bone Joint Surg 1976;58A:400–407.

25. Gallie WE: Fractures and dislocations of the cervical spine. Am J Surg 1939;46:495–499.

26. Garfin SR, Moore MR, Marshall LF: A modified technique for cervical facet fusions. Clin Orthop 1988;230:149–153.

27. Glynn MK, Sheehan JM: Fusion of the cervical spine for instability. Clin Orthop 1983;179:97–101.

28. Grantham SA, Dick HM, Thompson RC, et al: Occipitocervical arthrodesis. Clin Orthop 1969;65:118–129.

29. Griswold DM, Albright JA, Schiffman E, et al: Atlanto-axial fusion for instability. 1978;60A:285–292.

30. Grob D, Magerl F: Dorsal spondylosis of the cervical spine using a hooked plate. Orthopaedics 1987;16:55–61.

31. Grob D, Magerl F: Surgical stabilization of C1 and C2 fractures. Orthopaedics 1987;16:46–54.

32. Grob D, Dvorak J, Panjabi M, et al: Posterior occipitocervical fusion. A preliminary report of a new technique. Spine 1991;16:S17–S24.

33. Hamblen DL: Occipito-cervical fusion. J Bone Joint Surg 1967;49B:33–45.

34. Holness RO, Huestis W, Howes WJ, et al: Posterior stabilization with an interlaminar clamp in cervical injuries: Technical note and review of the long term experience with the method. Neurosurgery 1984;14:318–322.

35. Itoh T, Tsuji H, Katoh Y, et al: Occipitocervical fusion reinforced by Luque's segmental spinal instrumentation for rheumatoid diseases. Spine 1988;13:1234–1238.

36. Jeanneret B, Magerl F, Halterward E, et al: Posterior stabilization of the cervical spine with hook plates. Spine 1991;16:S56–S63.

37. Karlstrom G, Olerud S: Internal fixation of fractures and dislocations in the cervical spine. Orthopaedics 1987;10:1549–1958.

38. Larsson S, Toolanen G: Posterior fusion for atlanto-axial subluxation in rheumatoid arthritis. Spine 1986;11:525–530.

39. Lesoin F, Autricque A, Jomin M: Use of C-D instrumentation for cranio-cervical junction osteosynthesis. 6th proceeding of the international congress on Cotrel-Dubousset instrumentation. Montpellier, France, Sauramps Medical, p. 249, 1989.

40. Letts M, Slutsky D: Occipitocervical arthrodesis in children. J Bone Joint Surg 1990;72A:1166–1170.

41. Lipson SJ: Cervical myelopathy and posterior atlanto-axial subluxation in patients with rheumatoid arthritis. J Bone Joint Surg 1985;67A:593–597.

42. Louis RP: Surgery of the spine. Berlin: Springer-Verlag, 1983;49–83.

43. Magerl F, Grob D, Seemann P: Stable dorsal fusion of the cervical spine (C2-T1) using hook plates. In: Kehr P, Weidner A, eds. Cervical spine I, Wien-New York: Springer-Verlag, 1987;217.

44. Magerl F, Seemann P: Stable posterior fusion of the atlas and axis by transarticular screw fixation. In: Kehr P, Weidner A, eds. Cervical spine I, Wien-New York: Springer-Verlag, 1987;322.

45. McAfee PC, Bohlman HH, Wilson WL: The triple wire fixation technique for stabilization of acute cervical fracture-dislocations: a biomechanical analysis. Trans Orthop 1985;9:142.

46. McAfee PC, Bohlman HH, Ducker T, et al: Failure of stabilization of the spine with methylmethacrylate: a retrospective analysis of twenty-four cases. J Bone Joint Surg 1986;68A:1145–1157.

47. McLaurin RL, Vernal R, Slamon JH: Treatment of fractures of the atlas and axis by wiring without fusion. J Neurosurg 1972;36:773–780.

48. Meyer PR Jr: Surgical stabilization of the cervical spine. In: Meyer PR, ed. Surgery of spine trauma. New York: Churchill Livingstone, 1989;397–524.

49. Mitsui H: A new operation for atlanto-axial arthrodesis. J Bone Joint Surg 1984;66B:422–425.

50. Montesano PX, Juach EC, Anderson PA, et al: Biomechanics of cervical spine internal fixation. Spine 1991;16:S10–S16.

51. Murphy MJ, Daniaux H, Southwick WO: Posterior cervical fusion with rigid internal fixation. Orthop Clin North Amer 1986;17:55–65.

52. Nazarian SM, Louis RP: Posterior internal fixation with screw plates in traumatic lesions of the cervical spine. Spine 1991;16:S64–S71.

53. Newman P, Sweetnam R: Occipito-cervical fusion. J Bone Joint Surg 1969;51B:423–431.

54. Oro JJ, Watts C: Sublaminar and epilaminar wire fusion: a new technique for posterior subluxation injuries of lower cervical spine. Trans Orthop 1985;9:142.

55. Ranawat CS, O'Leary P, Pellici P, et al: Cervical spine fusion in rheumatoid arthritis. J Bone Joint Surg 1979;61A:1003–1010.

56. Ransford AO, Crockard HA, Pozo JL, et al: Craniocervical instability treated by contoured loop fixation. J Bone Joint Surg 1986;68B:173–177.

57. Robinson RA, Southwick WO: Surgical approaches to the cervical spine. In the American Academy of Orthopaedic Surgeons: Instructional Course Lectures. Vol XVII, 1960; St. Louis: The CV Mosby.

58. Rogers WA: Fractures and dislocations of the cervical spine: An end-result study. J Bone Joint Surg 1957;39A:341.

59. Rorabeck CH, Rock MG, Hawkins RJ et al: Unilateral facet dislocation of the cervical spine. An analysis of the results of treatment in 26 patients. Spine 1987;12:23–27.

60. Roy-Camille R, Mazel C, Saillant G: Treatment of cervical spine injuries by a posterior osteosynthesis with plates and screws. In: Kehr P, Weidner A, eds. Cervical spine I, Wien-New York: Springer-Verlag, 1987;163.

61. Roy-Camille R, Saillant G, Mazel C: Internal fixation of the unstable cervical spine by a posterior osteosynthesis with plates and screws. In: Sherk HH, ed. The cervical spine. 2nd ed., Philadelphia: JB Lippincott, 1989;390–403.

62. Sakou T, Kawaida H, Morizono Y, et al: Occipitoatlantoaxial fusion utilizing a rectangular rod. Clin Orthop 1989;239:136–144.

63. Savini R, Parisini P, Cevellati S: The surgical treatment of late instability of flexion-rotation injuries in the lower cervical spine. Spine 1987;12:178–182.

64. Schlicke LH, Schulak DJ: Wiring of the cervical spinous process. Clin Orthop 1981;154:319–20.

65. Segal D, Whitelaw GP, Gumbs V, et al: Tension band fixation of acute cervical spine fractures. Clin Orthop 1981;159:211–222.

66. Simmons EH: Surgery of the spine in rheumatoid arthritis and ankylosing spondylitis. In: Evarts CM, ed. Surgery of the muscoloskeletal system. vol. 2. New York: Churchill Livingstone, 1983;85.

67. Stambough JL, Balderston RA, Grey S: Technique for occipito-cervical fusion in osteopenic patients. J Spin Dis 1990;3:404–407.

68. Stauffer ES: Wiring techniques of the posterior cervical spine for the treatment of trauma. Orthopaedics 1988;11:1543–1548.

69. Steib JP, Kehr P, Mitteau M: C1-C2 instrumentation with C-D pediatric material. 6th proceeding of the international congress on Cotrel-Dubousset instrumentation. Montpellier, France, Sauramps Medical, 1989;245.

70. Tucker HH: Technical report: Method of fixation of subluxed or dislocated cervical spine below C1-2. Can J Neurol Sci 1975;2:381–382.

71. Ulrich C, Woersdoerfer O, Kalff R, et al: Biomechanics of fixation systems to the cervical spine. Spine 1991;16:S4–S9.

72. Weidner A: Internal fixation with metal plates and screws. In: Sherk HH (ed.) The cervical spine, Philadelphia: JB Lippincott, 1989;404–421.

73. Weiland DJ, McAfee PC: Posterior cervical fusion with triple-wire strut graft technique: one hundred consecutive patients. J Spin Dis 1991;4:15–21.

74. Wertheim SB, Bohlman HH: Occipitocervical fusion. J Bone Joint Surg 1987;69A:833–836.

75. White AA, Panjab MM: Clinical biomechanics of the spine. Philadelphia: JB Lippincott, 1991.

76. Wilber RG, Peters JG, Likavec MJ: Surgical techniques in cervical spine surgery. In: Errico TJ, Bauer RD, Waugh T. Spinal trauma. Philadelphia: JB Lippincott, 1991;145–162.

THREE

PART ONE

Anterior Instrumentation of the Cervical Spine

Paul R. Meyer, Jr., Joseph J. Rusin, and Michael H. Haak

INTRODUCTION

Anterior cervical instrumentation techniques of the atlantoaxial and the lower cervical spines have their origins in the European literature.

In this chapter, the authors will discuss the historical development of anterior instrumentation of the atlantoaxial and lower cervical spine. The authors will present the current indications for surgery, illustrated surgical technique, and discuss results of anterior instrumentation of the cervical spine as currently practiced at the Midwest Regional Spinal Cord Injury Center Acute Care Unit located at Northwestern Memorial Hospital in Chicago, Illinois.

ANTERIOR INSTRUMENTATION OF THE LOWER CERVICAL SPINE

In the United States, the anterior approach to achieving fusion of the cervical spine has become an accepted and popular approach since first noted in the literature by Bailey and Badgley (1), Smith and Robinson (25), and Cloward (8). Although the technique of an anteriorly applied graft has been widely used in achieving fusions in degenerative conditions of the cervical spine, this technique, when applied to the acutely unstable cervical spine, has been plagued with complications (26,29). Reported complications include migration of the graft, creating instability with potential neurologic compromise of the cord, loss of angular correction, and failure to maintain the spine in a reduced position. Historically, these problems have required the augmentation of additional methods for immobilizing the cervical spine. These corrective measures have included prolonged recumbent traction, the use of a halo device, minerva cast, or additional posterior cervical surgical stabilization. These alternatives create less than ideal situations with regard to early patient mobilization and rehabilitation or multiple surgical procedures, particularly with the acute or debilitated patient.

It was in the European literature that the first reports of anterior metallic fixation of the cervical spine were described. In 1970, Orozco and Llovet (18) described the application of a stainless steel AO small fragment plate for anterior cervical osteosynthesis. In 1971, they improved the technique with the use of an H-shaped stainless steel plate, and, in 1975, used the current H and double-H AO stainless steel plate (Fig. 3.1.A). Senegas and Gauzere (24) described the use of similar H-shaped stainless steel AO plates in 1975.

One problem with stainless steel plates and screws is the artifacts that are produced in the postoperative CT or MRI. Recent reports in the literature have shown that good images can be obtained in the presence of titanium implants with both CT and MRI (11, 22). In 1986, Morscher et al. (16) reported on the use of a pure titanium anterior cervical plate and a hollow plasma-sprayed titanium screw that wedges into the screw holes of the plate. The head of the screw is cylindrical and has an expansile shoulder. The proximal end of the screw has a cross-cut for the insertion of an expansion screw that locks the screw shank into the cylindrical holes of the plate to give a solid connection with the plate (Fig. 3.1B, C, and D). The plate design allows for securing screws in the plate holes by means of a locking screw. The rigid plate-screw construct becomes a monocortically intrinsically stable implant, unlike the usual application of the stainless steel AO H-plate, which requires that the fixation screws pierce the dorsal cortex for bicortical purchase to prevent loosening. Without the need for dorsal cortex purchase, there is also a professed decreased risk of screw misplacement.

Since the first report, many articles have reported on

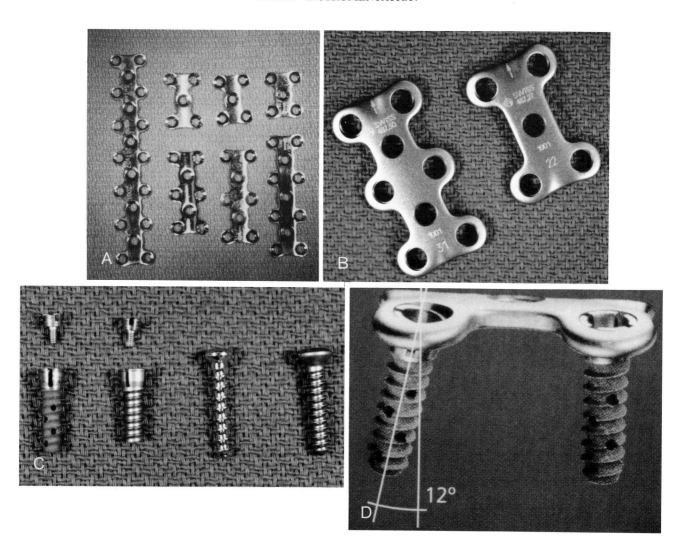

Figure 3.1. *A*, AO Orozco stainless steel cervical plate. This plate is available in various sizes from a small 5-hole plate to the large 20-hole plate in lengths from 23 mm to 133 mm. Screw hole placement varies from 16 mm to 21 mm in each of the various sizes. The plates can be cut and contoured. The standard AO stainless steel 3.5-mm screws may also be placed through the plate at angles up to 45° if needed. *B*, AO Morscher pure titanium cervical plate. This plate is available in 5- and 8-hole configurations with total length from 24 mm to 63 mm (15 intermediate sizes) and hole spacing from 16 mm to 55 mm (15 intermediate sizes). Screws lock into the plate with a fixed angle. The screw hole pair at one end of the plate is set at a 12° angle to facilitate insertion where the anatomical situation hinders a 90° approach. A standard 3.5-mm titanium screw is available for conventional bicortical technique. *C*, Screws (*left to right*) (*1*) 14-mm titanium cervical spine hollow perforated expansionhead screw 4 mm diameter; (*2*) 14-mm titanium cervical spine expansionhead screw 4 mm diameter. *Note*: in both of the expansionhead screws, the head of the screw is cylindrical and has an expansile shoulder. The proximal end of the screw has a cross-cut for the insertion of the expansion screw that locks the screw shank into the cylindrical holes of the plate; (*3*) 3.5-mm standard titanium screw; (*4*) 3.5-mm stainless screw with 2.7-mm head. *D*, Cut-away view showing AO Morscher titanium plate and hollow expansionhead screw configuration. The head of the screw is cylindrical and has an expansile shoulder. The proximal end of the screw has a cross-cut for insertion of an expansion screw that locks the screw shank into the cylindrical holes of the plate. The stability of this configuration depends on the unity between screw and plate for intrinsic stability with only unicortical purchase versus bicortical purchase with the Orozco system.

the use of an anterior plate and screw fixation in stabilizing the lower cervical spine in traumatic, degenerative, tumorous, and infectious processes (2,4,6,7,10,12,15, 16,19,20,28). These studies all stress the benefits of allowing simultaneous neural decompression and immediate stability provided by the use of the anterior plate fixation. These authors have, however, differed at times in their surgical technique, specific fixation device, and methods/duration of postoperative immobilization. Our own experiences and observations follow.

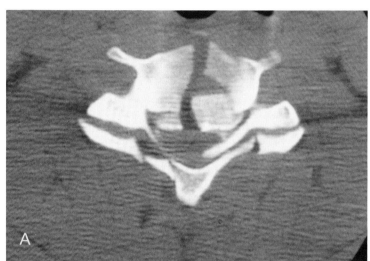
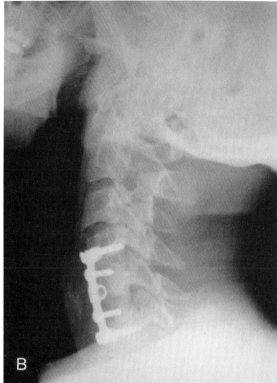

Figure 3.2. *A*, Preoperative CT demonstrating a grossly unstable three-column injury. Note the comminuted vertebral body fracture with fracture fragments in canal and associated laminar fracture. *B*, Four months postoperative lateral x-ray with solid fusion.

INDICATIONS FOR SURGERY

The indications of anterior plating may include:

- Excision of retropulsed vertebral body bone after trauma:
- Excision of intervertebral disc or vertebral body for cervical spondylosis;
- Anterior longitudinal ligament rupture with instability; and
- Evacuation of epidural abscess or tumor.

In acute cervical spine trauma treated at the Midwest Regional Spinal Cord Injury Center, five "injury patterns" were identified and treated with anterior management. The most common indication for anterior management observed in over half of the trauma patients was that of a grossly unstable "three-column" injury. While the Denis (9) and Holdsworth (13) classifications of the stable versus unstable spine injury were descriptive of injury to the thoracolumbar spine, the three-column theory may apply to the cervical spine. Instability is thought to exist when any two of the three columns are disrupted. The three-column injury is most often recognized by the pathognomonic triad of a vertebral body fracture with associated retrolisthesis of the involved vertebra on the next most inferior vertebra and associated bilaminar fracture. This particular injury pattern with gross instability and disruption of associated posterior structures clearly precludes the ability to manage this fracture from only the posterior approach. Adequate anterior vertebral body decompression, anatomic realignment, tricortical iliac crest grafting, and instrumentation with plate and screws provide a complete treatment in a single surgical approach (Fig. 3.2*A* and 3.2*B*).

The second injury pattern is the "two-column" injury seen in approximately 20% of the patients. This pattern of injury results in an anterior instability with a deforming kyphosis developing at the fracture site and spinal canal compromise secondary to bony compression. In these cases, a single anterior approach and instrumentation allows for correction of the kyphosis and canal decompression.

The third injury pattern is posterior ligament disruption occurring with an anterior disc herniation, posterior vertebral osteophyte, or fracture. Treatment of this type of injury pattern with a posterior procedure to treat the posterior instability would not have addressed the neural compression caused by the disc herniation or the vertebral osteophyte. In these cases, the authors recommend anterior decompression and plate stabilization as the only

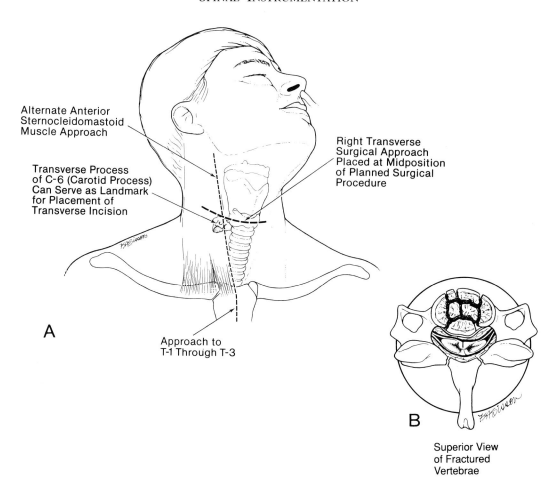

Alternate Anterior
Sternocleidomastoid
Muscle Approach

Transverse Process
of C-6 (Carotid Process)
Can Serve as Landmark
for Placement of
Transverse Incision

Right Transverse
Surgical Approach
Placed at Midposition
of Planned Surgical
Procedure

A

Approach to
T-1 Through T-3

B

Superior View
of Fractured
Vertebrae

Figure 3.3. *A,* Anterior approaches to the cervical spine. *B,* Unstable three-column injury. Superior view of comminuted vertebral body fracture, retrolisthesed fragment compromising the canal and posterior bilaminar fractures. *C,* Lateral view of cervical spine demonstrating unstable three-column injury with comminuted vertebral body fracture, retropulsed fragment compromising the canal and spinal cord, and posterior bone and ligamentous injury. Note the resulting kyphotic deformity. *D,* Transverse incision for anterior approach to the cervical spine. Important anatomical structures to identify are: the sternocleidomastoid and carotid sheath laterally, and the recurrent laryngeal nerve, thyroid cartilage, trachea, esophagus, and strap muscles medially. *E,* Transverse section of the neck viewed from above. "Finger" dissection of deep structures showing relationship of plane of dissection between the lateral carotid sheath and the medially retracted trachea and esophagus. The finger dissects down to the longus coli muscles on the anterior vertebral bodies. *F,* Diagram illustrates subtotal corpectomy of the body of C5 vertebra. The adjacent endplates of the vertebral bodies above and below are undercut to receive the tricortical graft. *G,* Superior view of subtotal corpectomy (removal of the central aspect of the affected vertebral body). This allows for complete decompression of the spinal canal and its contents without sacrificing the entire vertebral body. *H,* The tricortical bone graft is obtained from the anterior iliac crest. This is the usual source from the standpoint of both patient position for the anterior cervical fusion and the size and shape of the crest at this level (3–4 fingerbreadths posterior to the ASIS) to avoid the lateral femoral cutaneous nerve. *I,* Lateral view demonstrating vertebral body corpectomy, disc removal from adjacent endplates, and the use of a power burr to undercut the endplate of the adjacent vertebra to accommodate the tricortical graft. *J,* Inferior view demonstrating relationship of the endplate cut to the vertebral body. This cut helps to prevent posterior migration of the graft and allows for good bone contact/support. *K,* While traction is maintained, the superior end of the graft is inserted into the trough in the inferior endplate of the superior vertebra. The lower end of the graft is then inserted in the trough in the superior endplate of the vertebra inferior to the corpectomy. When in place, the traction is released. *L,* Anterior view of bone graft in place and traction removed. *M,* Superior view of iliac crest bone graft in place and its relationship to corporectomised vertebral body. Note graft depth is approximately 2/3 of the distance of the A-P diameter of the vertebral body. It is imperative that one maintain the anterior contour of the vertebral body and maintain the same relationship with the anterior body of the vertebral bodies above and below if a good plate/bone relationship is expected. *N,* Lateral view of graft in place and traction removed. Note the relationship of the graft to the corporectomised vertebra and the adjacent superior and inferior vertebral bodies. *O,* Anterior view of AO plate and screws added for graft and spine stability. *P,* Lateral

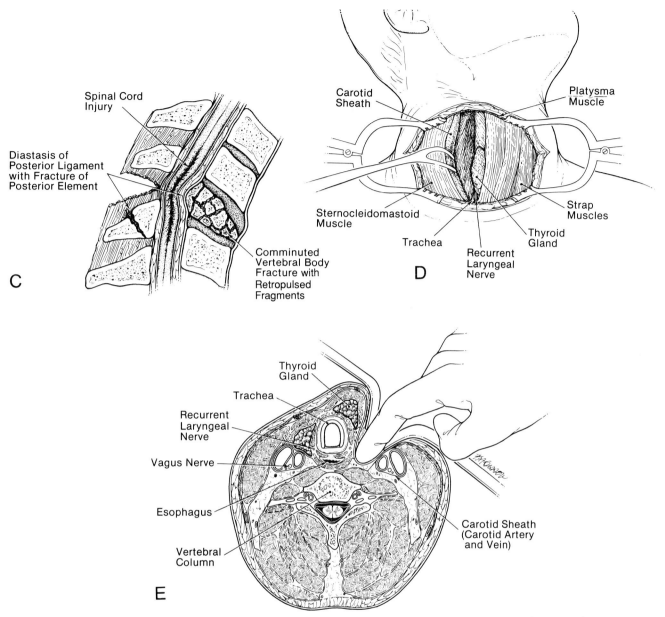

Figure 3.3. *C–E.*

view showing vertebral body corpectomy, iliac crest tricortical bone graft, and plate-screw fixation. Note that the superior and inferior screws that are in the adjacent vertebra to the corporectomised vertebra have bicortical purchase and engage the dorsal cortex of the vertebra. Those in the iliac crest tricortical graft extend only to the posterior aspect of the graft. Note that the plate fits uniformly along the anterior cortex of the superior vertebra, bone graft, and anterior cortex of the inferior vertebra.

Many times one must remove anterior osteophytes to get a good plate/bone relationship. This should be done judiciously with a rongeur or large (6–7 mm) burr, being careful not to compromise the strong anterior cortical bone. *Q*, Superior view demonstrating relationship of plate and screws with bicortical purchase. Note contour of plate to fit anterior vertebral body and iliac crest graft. The angle of the screws is 10–15° towards the midline, and proper length should give good engagement of the dorsal cortex.

single surgical procedure to address and treat the involved pathology. This injury pattern was seen in approximately 15% of the trauma patients at our center.

The fourth injury pattern is the extension-type injury seen most often in the elderly patients, causing disruption of the anterior ligamentous structures. This particular pattern was identified in approximately 5% of the trauma patients at our center.

The fifth injury pattern is the patient who sustains a cervical spine trauma without any evidence of instability

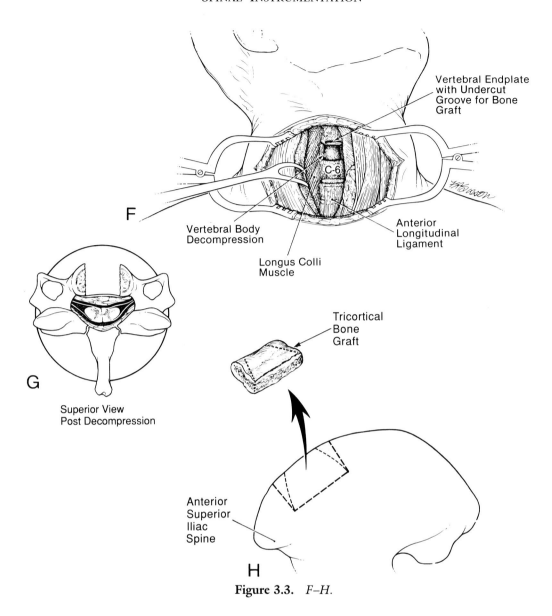

Figure 3.3. *F–H*.

or fracture, and after careful investigation, is found to have a neurologic injury secondary to a traumatically herniated disc. This injury pattern was identified in less than 5% of the trauma patients at our center. This pattern was treated by anterior disc excision and stabilization.

SURGICAL TECHNIQUE

All patients with suspected cervical spine instability are placed in skeletal traction applied via tongs upon admission. The patient is operated upon while in traction on a Stryker frame (Fig. 3.3). A standard anterior approach to the cervical spine is utilized (Fig. 3.1*A–D*, 3.2*E*). The right-sided approach is preferred by the authors. Depending on the level or extent of the exposure needed, a transverse incision or a longer anterior oblique incision anterior to the sternocleidomastoid is used. After the initial skin incision, the platysma muscle is split with blunt

dissection. Blunt dissection is carried down to the anterior cervical vertebrae, retracting the carotid sheath laterally.

Once the anterior exposure of the vertebral bodies is completed, the retractors are placed, and the superficial temporal artery pulse is verified by the anesthesiologist. The appropriate level is confirmed by x-ray. The cervical disc excision is then performed by sharply incising the anterior longitudinal ligament and curetting the disc and vertebral endplates. When cervical corpectomy is necessary, removal of the vertebral body is aided by the use of a high-speed burr. The adjacent vertebral endplates are then curetted free of cartilage and the diamond-tipped burr utilized to further debride the surfaces. Care is taken to leave the lateral vertebral walls to protect adjacent vascular structures. Also, care is taken to provide adequate nerve root decompression at the involved levels to promote neurologic return as much as possible.

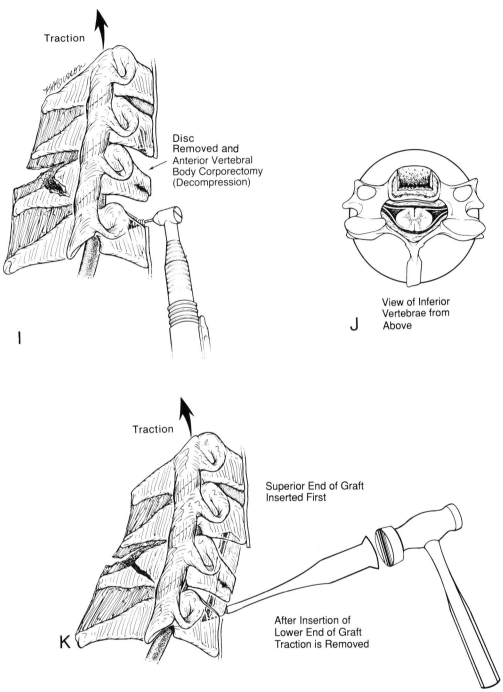

Traction

Disc
Removed and
Anterior Vertebral
Body Corporectomy
(Decompression)

I

View of Inferior
Vertebrae from
Above

J

Traction

Superior End of Graft
Inserted First

After Insertion of
Lower End of Graft
Traction is Removed

K

Figure 3.3. *I–K*.

Tricortical anterior iliac crest grafts are obtained utilizing an oscillating bone saw and contoured with the pneumatic burr. The graft is placed with cortical surfaces facing anteriorly and laterally and is measured prior to insertion so as not to exceed the anterior posterior dimensions of the adjacent intact vertebra. Prior to insertion of the graft, the anesthesiologist applies additional traction to the tongs by hand. This increases the distrac-

tion across the corpectomy site and allows easier placement of the tricortical graft. With the graft in place, all traction is released from the cervical spine, allowing for maximal compression of the graft itself. At this point, the appropriately sized cervical plate is selected so as to extend from the midportion of the superior uninvolved vertebra to the midportion of the adjacent inferior uninvolved vertebra. Care is taken to contour the plate to achieve

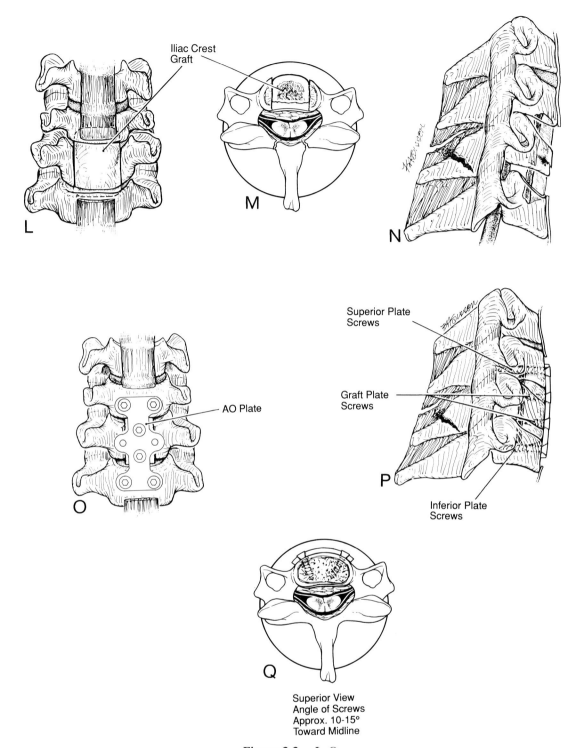

Figure 3.3. *L–Q.*

the normal cervical lordosis in the sagittal plane to allow maximal bony contact with the plate. Many times a ridge of anterior osteophyte is present on the vertebral bodies. These are carefully removed with the burr or rongeurs to allow maximum contact of the plate with the graft and vertebral bodies. The plate is then secured to the graft utilizing a centrally placed, unicortical, cortical or cancellous screw. This stabilizes the plate for placement of the peripheral screws and inhibits possible posterior migration of the graft.

With the plate centered and stabilized on the graft and vertebral midline, a 2-mm K-wire or 2-mm drill bit is utilized on an air-driven drill with an adjustable drill guide set to the previously measured anterior-posterior depth of the adjacent intact vertebra. This most often is between 18 and 20 mm. With the plate stabilized by the graft screw in the appropriate position, the K-wire/drill is drilled through the drill guide and plate into the intact cervical vertebra—to parallel both endplates of the vertebral body—and directed slightly toward the midline. With careful technique, the K-wire or drill can often be felt to encounter resistance as it abuts the posterior wall of the vertebra. Care must be exercised as the drill then penetrates through the posterior vertebral wall. Next, a depth gauge is introduced into the drill hole and carefully hooked over the posterior vertebral wall, staying very close to the anticipated length of between 18 and 20 mm. If bony resistance is encountered, the posterior vertebral wall has not been penetrated and the drill guide is adjusted to increase the length of the drill by 2 mm, and a repeat pass with the drill is made until the posterior wall is perforated. The hole is then tapped with the 3.5-mm cortical tap through both the anterior and posterior vertebral walls.

Careful calibration of the tap and tissue protector allows for accurate determinations of the depth that the tap has been inserted. Also, as in any bone, slight resistance is felt upon engaging the distal most cortex. At this point, the 3.5-mm cortical screw is inserted and lightly tightened.

This process is then repeated at the opposite side and end of the plate. The remaining screws are inserted in a similar fashion to provide paired cortical screws, with a total of four cortices of purchase (bicortical purchase) in each involved vertebra.

Anteroposterior and lateral x-rays are now obtained intraoperatively to confirm vertebral alignment, position of the graft, anterior plate, and appropriate screw length. All screws are firmly tightened and should be secure. Any indication of less than firm bite by any screw is reason to remove that screw and redirect it to obtain better purchase. If redirection does not obtain better purchase, i.e., poor quality osteoporotic bone, the use of methylmethacrylate for adjunctive screw fixation is indicated.

Upon completion of the procedure, the tongs are removed and the patient is placed in the appropriate orthosis. Most patients are able to begin to move to the erect position on the evening following the surgical procedure.

From July 1986 through December 1989, 151 patients

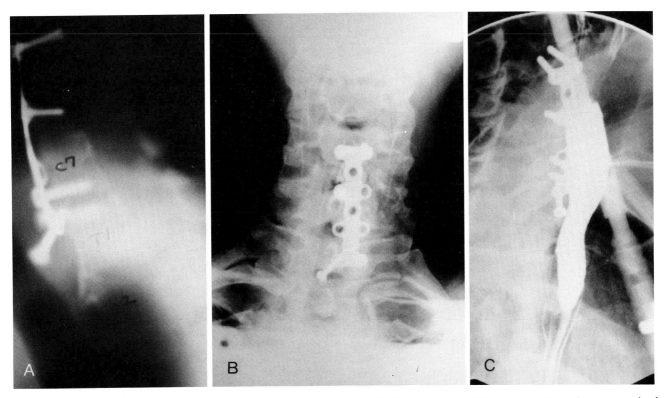

Figure 3.4. *A*, Postoperative lateral tomogram showing misplaced screw in disc space between C7 and T1, and screwback out. *B*, Postoperative AP x-ray, showing almost completely backed out screw. *C*, Barium swallow study.

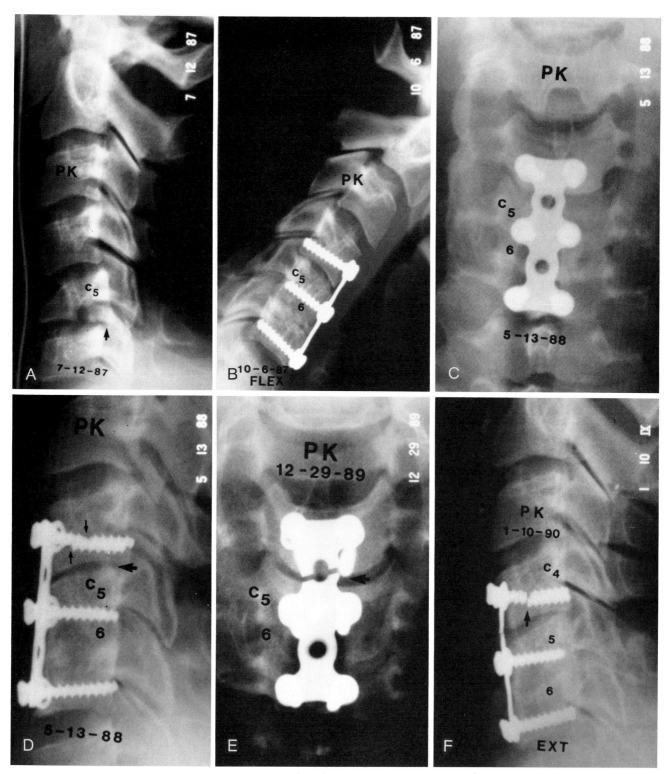

Figure 3.5. *A,* Preoperative lateral x-ray demonstrating a two-column injury with an anterior vertebral body fracture. Note the significant amount of kyphosis and the retrolisthesed bony fragment (*arrow*), causing spinal canal compromise. *B,* 3 months postoperative lateral x-ray. Patient demonstrating active flexion. Note the inadequate graft at the C4-C5 disc space interval. *C,* 10 months postoperative AP x-ray. Note plate is intact. *D,* 10 months postoperative lateral x-ray. Note the paucity of fusion at the C4-C5 disc space (*large arrowhead*) and the "fatigue" fracture of the upper level screws (*small arrows*). *E,* 26 months postoperative AP x-ray. The lack of a solid fusion (*large arrowhead*) failure of the screws and plate failure are readily apparent. *F,* 27 months postoperative lateral x-ray. The patient demonstrating active extension. Note the failed plate and screws (*arrows*), their position, and the increase in the anterior gap width of the failed fusion at the C4-C5 interval versus Figure 3.2B.

58

were treated via an anterior procedure which involved the application of anterior cervical vertebral plates and screws. These cases included traumatic injuries, stabilization of the cervical spine following tumor resection, spinal infections including tuberculosis, degenerative spine conditions, and the salvage of posttraumatic deformity treated unsuccessfully with a procedure/technique prior to the use of an anterior procedure (21).

Ninety-two patients had adequate clinical and radiographic follow-up for analysis. Criteria for inclusion consisted of minimum 1 year follow-up or to the point of solid arthrodesis as determined by a lack of motion on flexion-extension films with associated x-ray evidence of bridging bone across the entire length beneath the plate. In this series, all patients achieved arthrodesis in an average of 3.2 months (range 2.0–7.0 months). Average follow-up was 7.3 months (range 2.5–33 months).

Twelve patients (13%) had evidence of less than ideal hardware position. This consisted of: poor screw position (i.e., into adjacent disc), excessive length of screw, plate malposition involving an adjacent uninvolved disc, and improper graft technique (Figs. 3.4 and 3.5).

Evidence of loss of spinal alignment (i.e., greater than 2.5 mm) was identified in one patient; however, this did not preclude subsequent fusion. No patient had progressive kyphosis.

Four patients had x-ray findings suggestive of screw loosening (i.e., backout greater than two thread widths). Only one of these four patients had evidence of marked screw loosening with approximately 6 mm of backout. This patient developed symptoms of dysphagia approximately 8 weeks postoperatively and required subsequent repeat anterior exposure for the purpose of screw removal. This patient went on to achieve solid fusion without loss of correction following screw removal. In a review of original x-rays, the screw in question was found to be suboptimal in position, as it was partially placed into an unfused adjacent intervertebral disc (Figs. 3.4 and 3.5).

No patient had neurologic deterioration related to the use of anterior internal fixation. There were no deep wound infections. Two patients had evidence of transient recurrent laryngeal nerve palsies.

Four of the 104 patients were unable to be included in this series due to death from complications unrelated to the cervical procedure or fixation technique itself.

Other indications for anterior plate and screw fixation may include herniated discs, cervical spondylitic myelopathy, and tumors. In cases where anterior vertebral collapse exists without neurologic compromise, arguments could be made for posterior grafting and fixation as the sole procedure. However, it is the experience of the senior author that progressive loss of correction with resultant kyphosis to the injured levels can occur yielding unsatisfactory end results.

At present, the senior author's only absolute indication for posterior management of lower cervical spine trauma is a facet dislocation and/or fracture dislocations that cannot be reduced in a closed fashion prior to surgery. Even this indication may be disputed (17). Additional advantages of anterior plate-screw fixation is less rigid postoperative external immobilization (23,30). Our patients were placed in a cervico-thoracic orthosis or halo-vest postoperatively.

The safety of utilizing anterior plate and screw fixation to the surgeon inexperienced in this technique is of long-standing concern. Concerns regarding screw loosening that result in complications have largely been dispelled in more recent review articles regarding anterior fixation (2,4,6,7,10,12,15,20,28). Our experience confirms the extremely low incidence (2%) of significant complications related directly to the use of anterior plate and screw fixation. In those instances when significant screw loosening was recognized, it was found to be secondary to incorrect screw placement or improper plate position at the time of surgery. Thus, it could be implied that with strict adherence to the demanding technique of insertion, these complications may be avoided. The screw fixation should never cross an intact healthy intervertebral disc, as micro motions will also lead to screw loosening. When necessary, disc excision should be performed to allow for graft insertion when additional levels are felt to be added.

Certain authors have avoided fixation through the dorsal cortex in an attempt to reduce the likelihood of neurologic injury. In our institution, the majority of cases are performed with bicortical fixation without any evidence of iatrogenic neurologic compromise.

It is our belief that the ability to affix screws through both the anterior and posterior vertebral walls improves the stability of the construct and decreases the likelihood of complications secondary to loosening.

In summary, the single anterior procedure involving appropriate anterior decompression, tricortical inlay bone grafting, and the use of anteriorly applied cervical plates and screws for the treatment of acute lower cervical spine trauma in our study gave an excellent fusion rate of 98.9%, occurring on an average of 3.2 months postoperatively. If done properly, complications related to the use of anterior hardware are infrequent.

REFERENCES

1. Bailey RW, Badgley CE: Stabilization of the cervical spine by anterior fusion. J Bone Joint Surg 1960;42A:565–594.
2. Böhler J, Ganderhak T: Anterior plate stabilization for fracture-dislocations of lower cervical spine. J Trauma 1980;20:3.

3. Bohlman HH, Ducker TB, Lucas JT: Spine and spinal cord injuries. In: Rothman RH, Simeone FA, eds. The spine. 2nd ed. Philadelphia: WB Saunders, 1982;729–756.

4. Bremer AM, Nguyen TQ: Internal metal plate fixation combined with anterior interbody fusion in cases of cervical spine injury. Neurosurgery 1983;12:649–653.

5. Bynum D Jr, Ledbetter WB, Boyd CL, et al: Holding characteristics of fasteners in bone. Exp Mech 1971;353–369.

6. Cabanela ME, Ebersold MJ: Anterior plate stabilization for bursting teardrop fractures of the cervical spine. Spine 1988;13:888–891.

7. Caspar W: Die ventrale interkorporale Stabilisierung mit der HWS-Trapez-Osteosyntheseplatte. Indikation. Technik. Ergebnisse. Z Orthop 1984;122:121–124.

8. Cloward RB: Treatment of acute fractures and fracture-dislocations of the cervical spine by vertebral-body fusion: A report of eleven cases. J Neurosurg 1961;18:201–209.

9. Denis F: The three column spine and its significance in the classification of acute thoracolumbar spine injuries. Spine 1983;8:817–831.

10. de Oliveira J: Anterior plate fixation of traumatic lesions of the lower cervical spine. Spine 1987;12:324–329.

11. Ebraheim NA, Coombs R, Rusin JJ, et al: Reduction of postoperative CT artifacts of pelvic fractures by the use of titanium implants. Orthopaedics 13:1357–1358.

12. Gassman J, Seligson D: The anterior cervical plate. Spine 1983;8:700–707.

13. Holdsworth FW: Review Article: Fracture dislocations of the spine. J Bone and Joint Surgery. 1970;52A:1534–1551.

14. Koranyi E, Bowman EC, Knecht CD, et al: Holding power of orthopedic screws in bone. Clin Orthop 1970;72:283–286.

15. Lesoin F, Cama A, Lozes G, et al: The anterior approach and plates in lower cervical posttraumatic lesions. Surg Neurol 1984;21:581–587.

16. Morscher E, Sutter F, Jenny H, et al: Die vorder Verplattung der Halswirbelsaule mit dem Holschrauben-Plattensystem aus Titanium. Chirurgia 1986;57:702–707.

17. Oliveira JC: Anterior reduction of interlocking facets in the lower cervical spine. Spine 1979;4:195–202.

18. Orozco R, Llovet J: Osteosintesis en las fracturas del raquis cervical. Rev Ortop Traumatol 1970;14:285–288.

19. Meyer PR: Surgery of spine trauma. New York: Churchill Livingstone 1988.

20. Pasztor E, Lazar L, Benedek T, et al: Total body replacement with iliac bone graft and metal plate stabilization in the lower cervical spine. Acta Neurochir 1987;85:159–167.

21. Ripa D, Kowall MG, Meyer PR, et al: Series of 92 traumatic cervical spine injuries stabilized by anterior ASIF plate fusion technique. Presented 1990 AAOS Annual Meeting, New Orleans. Accepted for Publication, Spine, Sept. 1990.

22. Salvolaine ER, Ebraheim NA, Andreshak TG, et al: Anterior and posterior cervical spine fixation using titanium implants to facilitate magnetic resonance imaging evaluation. J Orthop Trauma 1989;3:295–299.

23. Sandor L: Die primare Stabilitat der AO-Platten-osteosynthese an der unteren Halswirbeisaule: Teil II. Vordere Spondyodsen mit H-Plattenosteosynthesen. Z Exp Chir Transplant Kunstliche Organe 1985;18:93–101.

24. Senegas J, Gauzere JM: Plaidoyer pour la chirurgie anterieure dans le traitement des traumatismes graves des cinq dernieres vertebres cervicales. Rev Chir Orthop 1976;62(Supple II):123–128.

25. Smith GW, Robinson RA: Treatment of certain cervical spine disorders by anterior removal of the intervertebral disc and interbody fusion. J Bone Joint Surg 1958;40A:607–623.

26. Stauffer ES, Kelly EG: Fracture-dislocations of the cervical spine: Instability and recurrent deformity following treatment by anterior interbody fusion. J Bone Joint Surg 1977;59A:45–48.

27. Tew JM, Mayfield FH: Complications of the anterior cervical spine. Clin Neurosurg 1979;23:424–439.

28. Tippets RH, Apfelbaum RI: Anterior cervical fusion with the caspar instrumentation system. Neurosurgery 1988;22:1008–1013.

29. Van Peteghem PK, Schweigel JF: The fractured cervical spine rendered unstable by anterior cervical fusion. J Trauma 1979;19:110–114.

30. Whitehill R, Richman JA, Glaser JA: Failure of immobilization of the cervical spine by the halo vest: A report of five cases. J Bone Joint Surg 1986;68A:326–332.

PART TWO

Anterior Instrumentation of the Cervical Spine

Paul R. Meyer, Jr., Joseph J. Rusin, and Michael H. Haak

INTRODUCTION

The primary function of the atlantoaxial articulation is rotation; approximately 50% of total lateral rotation has been attributed to C1-C2. The relationship between the vertebrae is a complex one with both significant bony and ligamentous contributions. Instability, with concurrent threat to vital neurologic structures, may occur secondary to failure of either or both components. The goal of treating conditions of the atlantoaxial articulation is restoration of stability and function. Newer surgical techniques of anterior fixation may now, in some applications, allow stabilization with maintenance of rotational function.

ANTERIOR C1-C2 SCREW STABILIZATION

The earliest surgical approaches to the upper cervical spine involved a transoral approach (16,21). The transoral approach of Fang and Ong (16), as well as the mandibular/tongue splitting approach of Kocher described by Hall (21) had significant infectious complications (up to 50%). This approach remains an option, and has been used by the senior author in limited application without infection.

The lateral retropharyngeal approach as developed by Whitesides permitted exposure of the C1-C3 region without increasing the risk of infection (31). This exposure was utilized by Barbour, Simmons, and Du Toit and Whitesides and Kelly for anterior fusion applications (6,15,28,30).

Barbour first described the application of bilateral transarticular screw fixation for atlantoaxial fusion for C1-C2 instability and fractures (6). This was further investigated by Simmons and Du Toit (5,28), who developed a drill guide to aid in correct screw placement. In cases of instability, some with previous failed posterior fusion by wire and bone graft methods, it created a rigid construct without the morbidity of attempting a repeat fusion in the previously operated area. In patients with absence of the posterior ring of C1 or with previous failed fusion, more extensive fusion to the occiput could be avoided. As in other conventional posterior fusions of C1 and C2, functional rotation will be lost.

Utilizing a "hockey stick" incision beginning at the tip of the mastoid process and following the anterior border of the sternocleidomastoid muscle, the dissection leads to the tips of the transverse processes.

The retropharyngeal approach is utilized as described by Whitesides (30). Dissection along the transverse process of the atlas leads to the lateral mass and atlantoaxial joint. The joint is cleared for placement of the lag screw.

The drill guide fabricated by Simmons and Du Toit guided the screw in the posteroinferior direction (25° inferiorly; 10° posteriorly). The atlantoaxial joint is then reduced and drilled to a depth of 25 mm; temporary stabilization by a Kirschner wire may be required in cases of severe instability. The drill hole is then tapped and a 26-mm AO lag screw inserted (Fig. 3.6). The joint is curetted and grafted prior to tightening. The procedure is then carried out on the other side in a similar fashion; the initially inserted screw may require loosening to allow

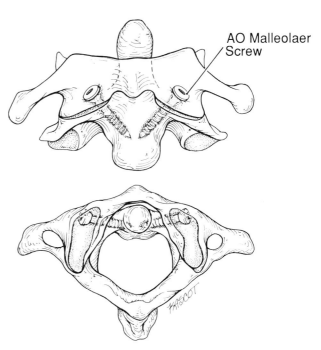

AO Malleolaer Screw

Figure 3.6. Lateral atlantoaxial arthrodesis shown in AP and axial views to demonstrate the screw orientation.

joint reduction. After routine closure, the patients were immobilized for 3 months.

As stated by the authors, this technique was applied in patients where no other alternative for limiting the fusion to C1-C2 existed (28). Although saving motion by not fusing other levels (e.g., occiput to C3), this approach has no functional advantage over conventional posterior procedures. The application of this technique may not be possible in all cases; patients with platybasia or very short necks will cause the drill to abut the mastoid process and prevent correct drill angulation. We have no experience with this particular technique. Bilateral procedures are required to prevent rotation around a single screw; this may lead the surgeon to prefer one of the many posterior fusion techniques utilizing wiring, clamps, or transarticular screws (13,17,18,20,24,29).

ANTERIOR SCREW STABILIZATION OF THE ODONTOID

The incidence of odontoid fractures in a review by Althoff has been reported to be 10–14% of cervical spine fractures (3). They were found in 8% of cervical spine fractures admitted to the Acute Spine Injury Service, Northwestern University. Of 130 odontoid fractures classified by the system of Anderson and D'Alonzo (4), 10 (7.69%) were type I; 89 (68.46%) were type II; 31 (23.85%) were type III (25) (Fig. 3.7). This classification system has been utilized to predict the success of treatment (fracture union), but many studies failed to evaluate displacement, which may be the major hindrance to acute fracture healing.

The traditional approach to treatment of odontoid fractures has been conservative, but operative fixation of selected fractures with preservation of atlantoaxial rotation has been described. Case studies describing anterior screw fixation of odontoid fractures were presented independently by Nakanishi (26) and Magerl (24). The largest early series was published by Böhler for both acute fractures and nonunions (9–11).

Multiple series have subsequently been published; these describe the experiences of numerous European centers (1,2,7,12,22,27). The approach and technique have found limited application in the United States.

The rationale for the direct anterior fixation is the restoration of anatomy with preservation of rotation, rigid fixation without the requirement for restrictive bracing, and avoidance of additional bone grafting complications. The anterior approach has been advocated as causing less morbidity and intraoperative blood loss.

The procedure described by Böhler is as follows: the operative approach is through the right anteromedial supracricoid interval; a 6–8-cm incision is utilized. The

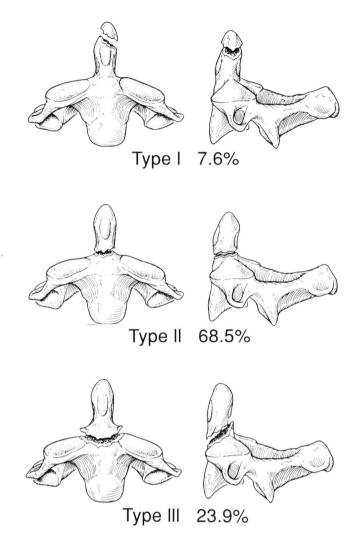

Type I   7.6%

Type II   68.5%

Type III   23.9%

Figure 3.7. Fracture type distribution at Northwestern University, Acute Spine Injury Center, 1972 to 1986. Classification after Anderson and D'Alonzo, 1974.

platysma muscle is split along the sternocleidomastoid border after undermining the skin slightly for mobility. The neurovascular bundle is identified, and the retropharyngeal space is accessed medial to the bundle. The dissection is carried out bluntly along the anterior longitudinal ligament to the level of the anterior tubercle of the atlas. The anterior longitudinal ligament is split over the body of the axis, exposing the odontoid and fracture site. Image intensification in both planes must be available, and reduction should be assessed radiographically and directly. Displaced fractures should be reduced by skeletal traction; unreduced displaced fractures may require mobilization with osteotomes prior to fixation. The anterior inferior border of the C2 body is selected for the starting point for drilling with 1.8-mm drill. The drill hole is tapped, and a 4.0-mm cancellous screw and washer inserted, extending just through the cortex at the tip of the dens. A second screw is inserted in identical fashion to complete fixation and prevent rotation about the axis of the single screw (Fig. 3.8A). The procedure for treatment of odontoid nonunion was similar; an anterior graft bridging C2 to C1 was utilized without formal resection of the granulation tissue. The nonunion patients in the early portion of this series had a posterior fusion as well.

Böhler's patients were treated in a plastic collar; in several cases where fixation was judged to be inadequate, a Minerva jacket was applied (10). Acute fracture patients demonstrated healing in 6–8 weeks, while delayed union patients required 10–16 weeks.

Böhler originally suggested the anterior screw technique for nonunion, either alone or in conjunction with a posterior fusion. He showed successful healing in conjunction with anterior bone grafting.

This application has been modified by the senior author (PRM) (25) (Fig. 3.8A and 3.8B). The drill holes are made under image intensification with 2.0-mm Kirschner wires; wires are withdrawn, screw holes tapped, and screws placed unilaterally with the remaining wire for stabilization. Once screws have been placed, a bone trough from the body of the axis to the odontoid is fashioned with a power burr, and bone grafted; alternatively, bone dowels may be placed into the trough up into the odontoid process. A halo-vest orthosis is utilized

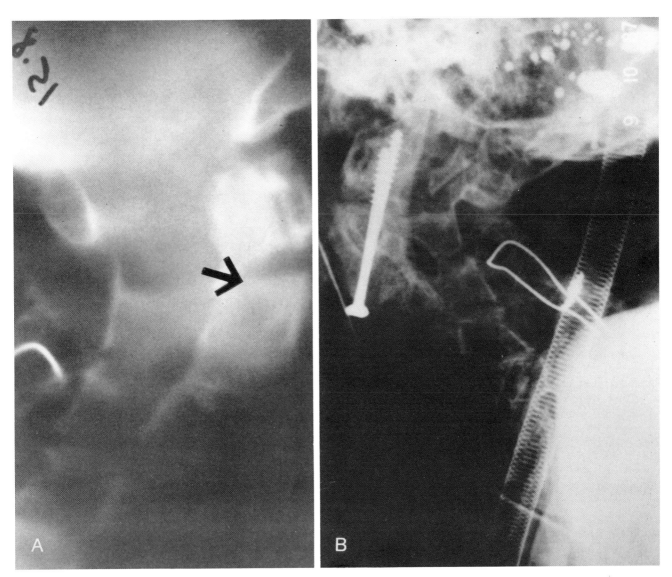

Figure 3.8. *A*, Tomogram of extension injury to the odontoid in previously operated patient with rheumatoid arthritis. *B*, Postoperative lateral radiograph showing fracture fixation with 4-mm malleolar screws across the C2 fracture.

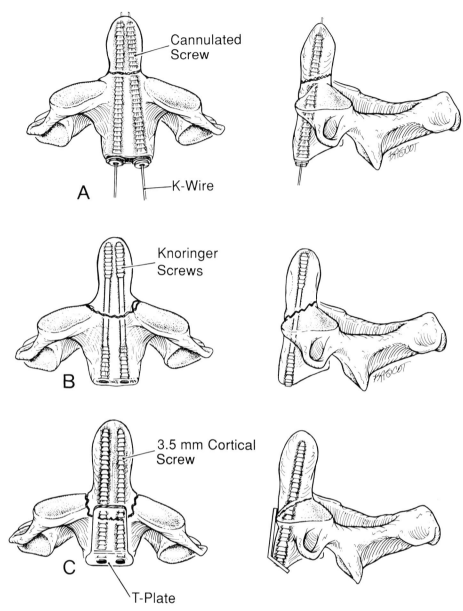

Figure 3.9. Variations on fixation technique. *A*, Utilization of cannulated screws; K-wire provides provisional stabilization and allows guided tapping and screw placement. *B*, Knöringer screws with variable pitch screw threads allows compression and prevents thread binding at the fracture site. *C*, Utilization of an inverted T-plate to limit forward displacement of oblique fracture with compression.

for postoperative immobilization. Böhler now advocates the anterior screw fixation for acute fractures only, surgical treatment taking place within 10 days of injury to prevent granulation tissue from filling the fracture and maintaining distractive forces (11).

The recommended screw insertion technique has also been refined; 2.0-mm K-wires are utilized for drilling. One K-wire is left in place to prevent rotation while tapping takes place. Cortical screws measuring 3.5 mm placed with lag technique are recommended over the 4-mm screws used previously, as the average odontoid diameter is approximately 8 mm, and screw "crowding" occurred (11). Screw length is usually about 40 mm; the tip should extend through the cortex of the odontoid tip. The drill starting point should be carefully selected on the anterior aspect of the inferior end plate of the axis; a starting point on the anterior surface is more likely to lead to posterior angulation and fracture malalignment.

This can sometimes be facilitated by removal of a small recess of C2-C3 disc, as well as by resecting a small corner of C2 or C3 with a burr. Washers or a two-hole plate should always be applied to distribute forces and prevent screw cut out; this is of particular concern in elderly and osteoporotic patients. Screw modifications have been proposed by several authors; Aebi et al. (1), have used a cannulated screw that can be introduced over the K-wires, (Fig. 3.9A), while Knöringer has developed a special screw with variable thread pitch at the ends to produce compression (Fig. 3.9B) (22,23).

This operative approach has been recommended by its proponents for type II and "high" type III injuries; these categories have the least success with nonoperative treatment. With asssociated C1 ring fractures or deficits limiting posterior fusion options, as well as displaced fractures, anterior screw fixation permits anatomic reduction and fixation with preservation of rotation. Anteriorly inclined oblique fractures had been a contraindication, but can be treated utilizing an inverted T plate to prevent the screws from displacing the fracture fragment anteriorly (Fig. 3.9C). Enough anterior body must be present for anchorage of the screws. Flexion-type fractures must be reduced preoperatively or with open reduction to purchase the odontoid fragment.

In the largest series to date, Böhler has treated a total of 75 patients with this technique. Utilizing two screws, patients have been treated postoperatively in plastic collars; other authors have applied a SOMI brace. On the average, the acute fractures are healed in 8–12 weeks. Böhler no longer recommends the anterior screw fixation technique for the treatment of nonunions (11).

The indications for this technically demanding technique would seem to be displaced odontoid fractures that cannot be reduced utilizing skeletal traction or a halo, as well as fractures associated with concomitant C1 ring fractures.

In rare cases, patients with congenital spina bifida at C1 may have the ring defect located unilaterally, allowing a modified posterior fusion by conventional techniques.

While it is no longer recommended by Böhler for nonunion, this has been successfully combined with an anterior bone graft in seven patients by the senior author (25). Fracture alignment must be achieved by traction or open reduction before drilling and screw placement. The technique is not applicable in patients with a large chest or fixed flexion deformity (ankylosing spondylitis) that may block appropriate drill orientation.

REFERENCES

1. Aebi M, Etter C, Coscia M: Fractures of the odontoid process: treatment with anterior screw fixation. Spine 1989;14:1065–1070.

2. Aebi M, Mohler J, Zaech GA, et al: Indication, surgical technique, and results of 100 surgically treated fractures and fracture-dislocations of the cervical spine. Clin Orthop 1986;203:244–257.

3. Althoff B: Fracture of the odontoid process. An experimental and clinical study. Acta Orthop Scand (Suppl) 1979;177:1–95.

4. Anderson LD, D'Alonzo RT: Fractures of the odontoid process of the axis. J Bone and Joint Surg 1974;56A:1663–1674.

5. Anderson LD, Clark CR: Fractures of the odontoid process of the axis. In: The cervical spine. Sherk HH and the Cervical Spine Research Society, eds. Philadelphia: JB Lippincott Company, 1989;325–341.

6. Barbour JR: Screw fixation and fractures of the odontoid process. S. Australian Clin 1971;5:20–24.

7. Barth H, Lang G: Die doppelte Kompressionsschraubenosteosynthese zur Behandlung Frischer Frakturen und Pseudarthrosen des Dens axis. Zentralblatt Chir 1989;114(4):263–270.

8. Böhler J: Fractures of the odontoid process. J Trauma 1965;5:386–389.

9. Böhler J: Schrauben Osteosynthese von Frakturen des Dens axis. Unfallheikunde 1981;84:221–223.

10. Böhler J: Anterior stabilization for acute fractures and nonunions of the dens. J Bone Joint Surg 1982;64A:18–27.

11. Böhler J: Lecture: 52nd AO Course (Spine), Davos, Switzerland, 1990.

12. Borne GM, Bedou GL, Pinaudeau M, et al: Odontoid process fracture osteosynthesis with a direct screw fixation technique in nine consecutive cases. J Neurosurg 1988;68:223–226.

13. Brooks AL, Jenkins EB: Atlanto-axial arthrodesis by the wedge compression method. J Bone Joint Surg 1978;60A:279–283.

14. Clark CR, White AA: Fracture of the dens: A multicenter study. J Bone Joint Surg 1985;67A:1340–1348.

15. Du Toit G: Lateral atlanto-axial arthrodesis. A screw fixation technique. S African J Surg 1976;14:9–12.

16. Fang HS, Ong GB: Direct anterior approach to the upper cervical spine. J Bone Joint Surg 1962;44A:1588–1604.

17. Fielding JW, Hawkins RJ, Ratzan SA: Spine fusion for atlanto-axial instability. J Bone Joint Surg 1976;58A:400–407.

18. Gallie WE: Fractures and dislocations of the cervical spine. Am J Surg 1939;46:495–499.

19. Griswold DM, Albright JA, Schiffman E, et al: Atlanto-axial fusion for instability. J Bone Joint Surg 1978;60A:285–292.

20. Grob D, Magerl F: Operative stabilisierung bei frakturen von C1 C2. Orthopade 1987;16:46–54.

21. Hall JE, Denis F, Murray J: Exposure of the upper cervical spine for spinal decompression by a mandible and tongue splitting approach. J Bone Joint Surg 1977;59A:121–123.

22. Knöringer P: Zur Behandlung frischer frakturen des dens axis durch kompressionsschraubenosteosynthese. Neurochirurgia 1984;27:68–72.

23. Knöringer P: Double threaded compression screws in osteosynthesis of acute fractures of the odontoid process. In: Voth D, Glees O, eds. Diseases of the cranio-cervical junction. Berlin-New York: De Gruyter, 1987;217.

24. Magerl F, Seeman PS: Stable posterior fusion of the atlas and axis by transarticular screw fixation. In: Kehr P, Weidner A, eds. Vienna: Springer-Verlag, 1987;322–327.

25. Meyer PR, Heim S: Surgical stabilization of the cervical spine. In: Meyer PR, ed. Surgery of spine trauma. New York: Churchill Livingstone, 1989;469–475.

26. Nakanishi T, Sasaki T, Tokita N, et al: Internal fixation the odontoid fracture. Orthopaedic Transactions 1982;6:176.

27. Pentelenyi T, Szarvas I, Bodrogi L: Screw fixation of odontoid fractures: Preliminary report. Injury 1988;19:139–142.

28. Simmons EH, Du Toit G: Lateral atlanto-axial arthrodesis. Orthop Clin North Am 1978;9:1101–1114.

29. Southwick WO: Current concepts review. Management of fractures of the dens (odontoid process). J Bone Joint Surg 1980;62A:482–486.

30. Whitesides TE, Kelly RP: Lateral approach to the upper cervical spine for anterior fusion. South Med J 1966;59:879.

31. Whitesides TE, McDonald AP: Lateral retropharyngeal approach to the upper cervical spine. Orthop Clin North Am 1978;9:1115–1127.

FOUR

Harrington Instrumentation and Modifications

Todd J. Albert, Howard S. An, Jerome M. Cotler, and Richard A. Balderston

INTRODUCTION

At the turn of the century, Dr. Hadra of Galveston used wires to stabilize a fracture dislocation of the cervical spine (26), and Albee and Hibbs reported a successful fusion in 1911 (7,34). However, it was not until the 1950s and 1960s that the Harrington rod for spinal instrumentation became available (28). Harrington's system originated in the early 1950s in Houston when Dr. Harrington assumed the care of children with progressive neuromuscular scoliosis secondary to polio. Poliomyelitis was epidemic at the time, and there were unacceptably high complication rates with Stagnara casting and the major operative procedures of the day. It was in this light that Dr. Harrington embarked on the development of the spinal instrumentation system employing hooks and rods to effect spinal fusion as well as correction of the deformed spine.

The initial operation that Dr. Harrington employed took 20 minutes and utilized facet screws through the vertebral bodies in the corrected position (30). Although the initial correction and results were satisfying, the results deteriorated postoperatively, leading to the abandonment of the facet screw fixation concept. The next step in the development of the present-day Harrington rod was to use a threaded rod and hook system to effect correction. This system could be used in either compression or distraction mode and was hand-made on the night prior to surgery by the investigator and an assistant. No bone grafting techniques or present-day fusion techniques were employed with these instrumentation systems, and hence two important concepts became apparent from the failures of Dr. Harrington's early work. First was the concept that dynamic correction without a good fusion could not work because of the high rate of hook disengagement as well as rod failure. These two complications led to a recurrence of deformity and failure of the procedure. The second concept was that greater durability was necessary in the design of the instrumentation, as

there was an extremely high rate of instrumentation failure through breakage. The investigators felt that the instrumentation would need to withstand at least 7 million cycles of loading before fatigue failure. Dr. Harrington arrived at this figure by doubling the estimated cycles for a 1-year period, assuming 10,000 cycles per day. In the early stages of development, these changes were accomplished by doubling the hardness and changing the fillet design of the ratchets in the rods.

It was not until Dr. Harrington presented his modified construct of the current Harrington rod system at the American Orthopaedic Association Meeting in 1960 that widespread use of the current Harrington system began. The modern Harrington rod represents over 47 changes since the original facet screw fixation system that Dr. Harrington developed in the early 1950s (28,30,31,35). Over the last 30 years, the Harrington rod system has been a gold standard for comparison of instrumentation systems used to effect spinal fusion in the treatment of scoliosis and the fractured spine, particularly at the thoracolumbar junction.

As the clinical indications for Harrington rod instrumentation expanded, modifications on the basic Harrington system were made to improve stability, capability, and adaptability. Dr. John Moe of Minneapolis attempted to achieve greater rotational control by squaring the distal hook and distal end of the rod of the Harrington system (16,53). The theory behind Moe's attempts to prevent loss of lordosis as well as better rotational control was that a square peg in a square hole would allow better control of contouring as well as rotation than Harrington's round tube in a round hole. Dr. Moe has also employed this system for subcutaneous distraction, particularly helpful in young scoliosis patients with significant residual growth potential (52,54).

Modifications in hook design were invoked in attempts to prevent hook dislodgement. Other modifications included a tongue to lock the sublaminar hook (38–40) as well as using two upper hooks in the proximal lamina

(6). The theory behind using a double hook model was to decrease individual hook site stress by 50% in distributing the stress between two hooks. Bifid facet hooks are available to gain purchase around the pedicle. Dr. Edwards of Baltimore has modified the Harrington system by altering the hook to match the anatomy of the lamina. He has further modified the system by improving modularity and employing universal rods, pedicle screws, and rod sleeves to effect forces in several directions in addition to distraction (18). This system is discussed in a later chapter of this book. These hook and rod modifications attempt to improve fixation from the original Harrington devices. In an effort to overcome the lack of axial stability of the Luque system and the lack of rotational control of the Harrington system, Winter has employed a hybrid consisting of Moe-modified Harrington distraction rods with Moe square-ended hooks combined with segmental

wiring, (Figure 4.1) ("Harriluque" technique) (76). All of the aforementioned modifications employed Dr. Harrington's original design and are a tribute to instrumentational change based on clinical experience.

INDICATIONS

The original major indication for the use of Harrington instrumentation was in the treatment of idiopathic scoliosis (28). Harrington instrumentation has been quite safe, with less than a 0.5% neurologic complication rate (62). Disadvantages reported for the Harrington construct include limited sagittal plane control, minimal derotating ability (1), and a relatively high pseudarthrosis rate for thoracolumbar and lumbar curves, approaching 4%. Also, hook dislocation rate has been relatively high, especially in the lumbar spine up to 3%. The need for

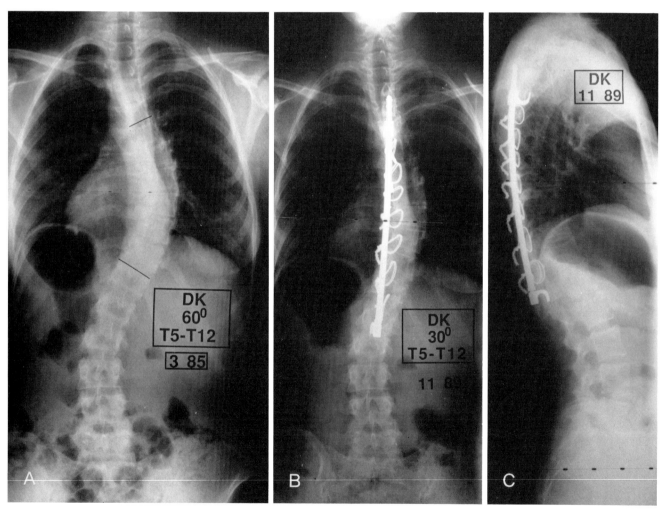

Figure 4.1. *A–C*, Excellent correction of a single thoracic curvature can be obtained with Moe-modified Harrington instrumentation and sublaminar wires or "Harriluque" technique.

external support has made the Harrington system less attractive, as newer systems have been developed that may obviate the need for external bracing or casting (62). "Harriluque" instrumentation with Moe modified square-ended hooks may also eliminate the need for postoperative bracing (13,14).

While Harrington instrumentation is indicated in any scoliotic pattern where distractive forces are a potential benefit, the spinal surgeon must not forget the major disadvantage of applying distraction across lordotic segments of the spine, particularly the low lumbar spine. Significant problems with loss of lordosis in the flatback syndrome have been reported with fusion employing Harrington distraction devices to the low lumbar spine (65). Decreasing lumbar lordosis causes an abnormal gait

as well as significant back pain and disability, and may require complex reconstructive procedures (32,45). Harrington instrumentation has also been used in the past for patients with neuromuscular scoliosis and adult scoliosis, but the results have been less than satisfactory, and greater complications have been noted compared with other newer spinal instrumentation. With availability of new devices, as described in other chapters, the spectrum of utility of Harrington instrumentation in the treatment of deformity is becoming limited to single thoracic and thoracolumbar curves that do not require fusion down to the lumbar spine.

Indications for the use of Harrington compression instrumentation in the treatment of deformity include placing compression rods on the convexity of the scoliotic

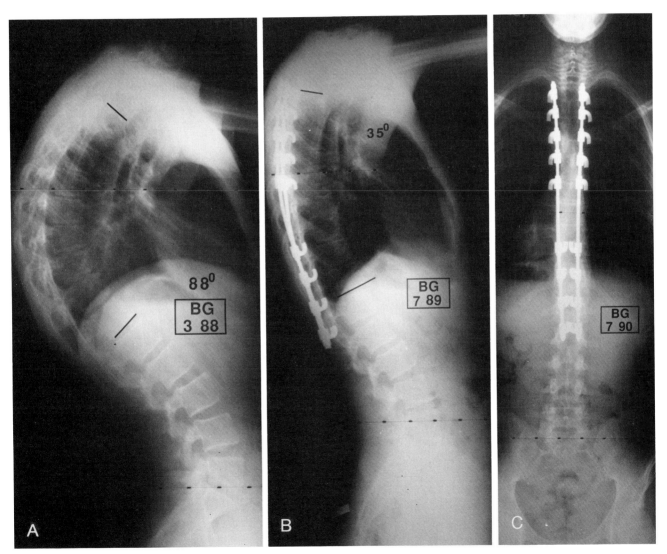

Figure 4.2. Harrington compression instrumentation for treatment of pure kyphosis as in this patient with Scheuermann's disease.

curve to help stabilize distraction instrumentation and decrease the rib hump deformity, particularly in thoracic curves. Compression rods may also be used in cases of thoracic kyphosis (Fig. 4.2). In the lumbar spine, compression rods help to preserve lordosis (Fig. 4.3). Compression rods are not indicated in thoracic lordosis because thoracic lordosis would worsen with compression instrumentation. In thoracic curves greater than 90°, compression rods limit the total correction possible by the distraction instrumentation (21,67).

Harrington constructs have been used extensively in the treatment of traumatic disorders (10,20). Dual Harrington distraction fixation offers excellent stability when an intact anterior longitudinal ligament exists. This is particularly true for axial loading injuries such as compression flexion and vertical compression injuries (19). Compression instrumentation can be very beneficial in the treatment of distractive flexion injuries, as in the Chance fracture of the lumbar spine. Assessment of middle column injury allows a good prediction of utility of

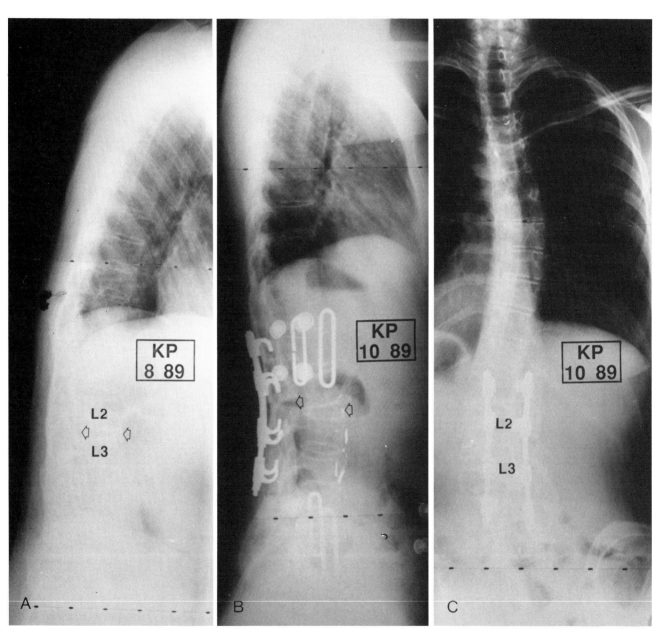

Figure 4.3. Compression instrumentation for stabilizing a spinal osteotomy after placement of an anterior graft. This patient had severe flatback deformity. Compression instrumentation helps to create and maintain lordosis.

the Harrington construct (51). With compression failure of the middle column, Harrington distraction instrumentation should be of benefit, and with distractive injury to the middle column, compression instrumentation has shown utility. With translational injury to the middle column or with an injury to the anterior longitudinal ligament, the risk of further neurologic injury with distraction prohibits the use of distraction instrumentation. Segmental spinal instrumentation is indicated in these three-column injuries.

Certain modifications to Harrington's original system have assisted in the treatment of spinal injuries. The development of a locking hook system and augmentation from the original Harrington rod system by Jacobs et al. has been reported to produce superior results in the treatment of posttraumatic injuries with regard to reduction, stability, and risk of hook pullout (36,37). The down side of the Jacobs system is a reported decrease in distraction force by two-thirds. However, the method does allow rod contouring, which is especially useful in contouring lordosis in the lumbar area. This feature allows better distraction, and anterior translation forces help preclude kyphosis and recurrence of vertebral body collapse. As mentioned earlier, the addition of sublaminar wiring improves torsional stability when used in combination with Moe modified square-ended hooks (76). These hooks are helpful in the treatment of traumatic disorders as well as in the treatment of scoliosis.

The addition of Edwards' polyethylene sleeves to the Harrington construct can also provide an anterior force that helps preserve lordotic moments and prevent late kyphotic collapse (18). All of these to achieve a lordosis presuppose an intact posterior bony column. Absence of the protection of a posterior bony column can predispose to iatrogenically imposed neural compromise when axial loading is initiated.

Again, Harrington compression rods as a treatment in traumatic conditions are indicated for posterior ligamentous disruptions, facet dislocations, and in the treatment of the flexion instability of a Chance fracture. However, compression instrumentation is contraindicated in any injury with axial instability. In the presence of axial instability, the application of the compression rods could lead to retropulsion of bone into the spinal canal, induction of iatrogenically created scoliosis, or the creation of further vertebral collapse with the induction of compression. If the surgeon has previously done an anterior decompressive procedure with middle column reconstruction with application of a bone graft into the middle column, compression instrumentation may be ideal. Care should be taken, as overcompression in this instance could lead to disc space narrowing, herniation, or collapse of the anterior graft if a stable construct was

not attained. Sublaminar wiring should be avoided with compression instrumentation, as the hooks may migrate anteriorly with wire tightening.

Many new instrumentation systems have been developed over the last 30 years, and some may have great utility and modularity in the treatment of spinal instability as well as deformity. The Harrington distraction and compression system, however, remains a gold standard for comparison of all new instrumentation systems. This is a tribute to the foresight and genius of its inventor, Dr. Paul Harrington. The lessons learned from the historical development of the Harrington instrumentation system and in its ongoing studies will enhance any new approaches to spinal instrumentation.

SURGICAL TECHNIQUES

Levels of Fusion

Although there is still controversy about levels of fusion in scoliosis, it is generally accepted at this time that most

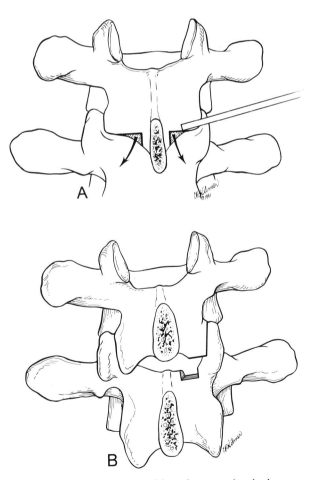

Figure 4.4. *A*, Preparation of facet for upper hook placement. *B*, Preparation of inferior laminar hook.

curves can be corrected by fusing the levels of the structural curve (42). The principles outlined by King et al. generally provide excellent curve correction and restoration of trunk balance. The decision to combine distraction on the concavity of scoliosis with compression on the convexity vs. the dual compression technique is based on the sagittal plane deformity. The compression rod assembly should be used with the distraction rod in scoliosis and in the maintenance of lordosis of the lumbar spine. The dual compression rods may be used in cases of pure kyphosis (55) (Fig. 4.2) or in stabilizing osteotomies with anterior grafts in place (Fig. 4.3).

When considering Harrington distraction and compression instrumentation, the surgeon must decide how many levels to instrument. In 1981, using 13 cadaveric specimens with Harrington distraction rods after creating ligamentous defects at T12-L1, Purcell demonstrated a significant increase in strength to failure (36%) by changing upper hook placement from two lamina above to three intact lamina above the injured vertebra (60). This study provided the basis of the "three lamina above/two lamina below" rule for hook placement of Harrington distraction instrumentation. However, the levels of fusion may vary, depending on the mechanism of injury, extent of injury and deformity, and type of instrumentation. Keep in mind that instrumentation is implanted to correct deformity until a bony fusion matures and that the primary goal is to create a bony fusion. This cannot be done without meticulous and effective fusion technique.

Hook Placement

Hook placement in the Harrington system involves preparation of the lamina, facet, or transverse process. For the distraction system in the thoracic spine, hooks may be placed into the facet or lamina. A ¼-inch osteotome is used to first prepare the inferior edge of the thoracic facet (Fig. 4.4A). The cut toward the lamina is made obliquely so that the medial margin of the cut is more cranially directed than the lateral margin. For placement of the lower hook in the distraction system, preparation of the lamina is carried out by removing a portion of the inferior facet, rongeuring or curetting the ligamentum flavum from its attachment to the lamina, and squaring the superior facet and laminar edge with a Kerrison punch (Fig. 4.4B). A Blount spreader or lamina spreader has also been utilized to assist with hook insertion by spreading the lamina away from the vertebral body above. After placement of both superior and inferior hooks, taking care to avoid false passage between the cortices of the lamina or facets, force should be applied with the hook holder both caudally and cranially for the laminar and thoracic hooks to ensure that these hooks will accept a significant distractive force. There are numerous modified

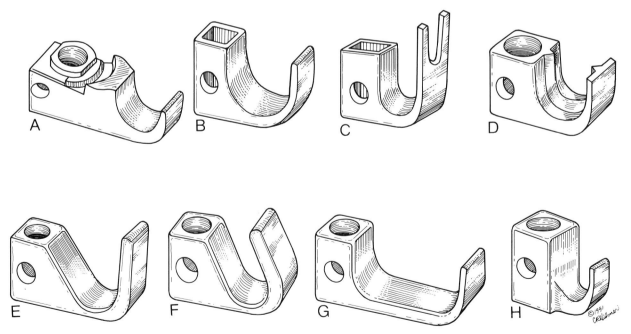

Figure 4.5. Modified hooks for Harrington distraction instrumentation. *A*, Bobechko's sliding barrell hook. *B*, Moe's square-ended hook. *C*, Zielke bifid hook. *D*, Ribbed hook. *E*, Leatherman hook. *F*, Andre hook. *G*, Moe alar hook. *H*, Pediatric hook.

hooks that are designed to reduce the risk of hook dislodgement or fracture of the facet or lamina (Fig. 4.5). Recently, Edwards also designed an anatomic hook that conforms to the lamina better to prevent hook dislodgement. The authors prefer this hook together with the Moe modified Harrington system, particularly in traumatic cases (Fig. 4.6).

Distraction Outrigger and Rod

While many surgeons prefer not to use the Harrington outrigger device, it can prove beneficial in cases of deformity with more severe curvature (>75°) and by allowing better exposure of the spine while undergoing correction with distractive forces. With the Harrington distraction outrigger in place, rod measurement for ultimate rod length can be facilitated. This is an important decision, as excessive ratchets should not be exposed above and below the upper hook.

After decortication and facet preparation on the concave side, the distraction rod is placed between the already mounted hooks. Distraction is carried out by using a Harrington spreader device between the upper hook and a ratchet on the rod. Experience dictates the point of safe maximum distraction. It is important to distract gradually to allow creep and to prevent overdistraction. The C ring is then placed and crimped around the uppermost ratchet just below the hook to prevent loss of distraction by rod slippage.

Harrington Compression Assembly

The compression assembly uses multiple hooks configured onto a fully threaded rod. There are two sizes of rod—⅛″ and ³⁄₁₆.″ While the smaller rod is more flexible and therefore easier to insert, it can undergo fatigue failure more readily than a larger rod. Two hooks are available for the compression system, which adapt to the two

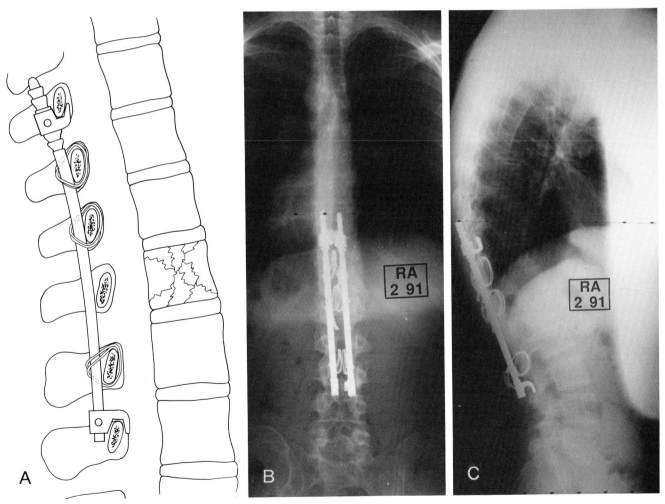

Figure 4.6. *A,* Diagram of Edwards' anatomic hooks with Moe rod and sublaminar wires for fracture stabilization. *B* and *C,* A flexion-compression injury of L1 treated with Moe distraction rods and sublaminar wires.

sizes of the fully threaded rods. Above T11, the hook may be placed over the transverse process or the lamina. From T11 caudally, it is preferable to place the hook underneath the lamina as close to the facet joint as possible. Before the entire assembly is inserted, the hooks are first placed temporarily over the selected transverse process as well as underneath the prepared lamina below T11 (Fig. 4.7). The sharp edge of the hook is used to cut the costotransverse ligament in the upper thoracic spine above T11. The transverse processes below T11 are

inadequate to accept the compression hooks. After transverse processes and lamina have been prepared to accept the assembly, the appropriate-size threaded rods with the hooks are attached. Generally, three caudad facing hooks above the apex and three cephalad facing hooks below the apex of the curve are placed with insertion of the assembly beginning at the upper level toward distally. Since the compression assembly is being inserted as a unit, it is imperative that all hook sites be well prepared so that the hook can be mounted to either the transverse process or the lamina in a 90° fashion. Tilting of the whole assembly to work the hook over the bone is impractical. The compression is initiated by using the Harrington rod holder of the appropriate size and using the Harrington spreader placed between the rod holder and the hook holder to effect compression. Nuts are then tightened down onto the hook using a hexagonal wrench.

Segmental Fixation and Rod Linkage with Harrington Instrumentation

Harrington instrumentation can be used with sublaminar or interspinous wires to further stabilize the construct. Recently, several rod linkage systems have also been available to connect the dual rods to make a rectangular construct. The addition of these systems allows the surgeon to continue using Harrington type instrumentations with good results (Fig. 4.8).

RESULTS

Deformity

The results of Harrington instrumentation and fusion in the treatment of spinal deformity are generally good (29,48,68). In the treatment of adolescent idiopathic scoliosis, the pseudarthrosis rate is 1–2%, and reported curve correction varies from 40–55%. Trunk balance in general is very well restored. The correction of the permanent rib hump is variable in the literature. Two-thirds of the patients who are seemingly much improved at the time of cast removal lose some of their rib hump correction by 4 years postoperatively (71). The benefit of the "Harriluque" system with Moe modified Harrington instrumentation is in the treatment of thoracic lordosis or hypokyphosis in association with scoliosis. The reported curve correction using this system is 39–50%, with minimal rotational correction (76). Daruwalla has demonstrated the benefit of the "Harriluque" system in correcting kyphotic deformity. In a retrospective review comparing the Harrington system alone (30 patients) with the Harriluque system (29 patients), he found no neurologic complications, but did note increased blood loss and increased operative time with the Harriluque

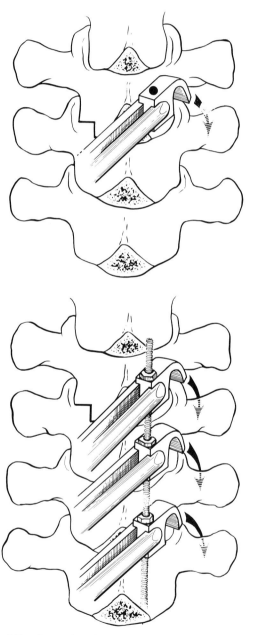

Figure 4.7. Preparing for insertion of the compression assembly on the transverse processes.

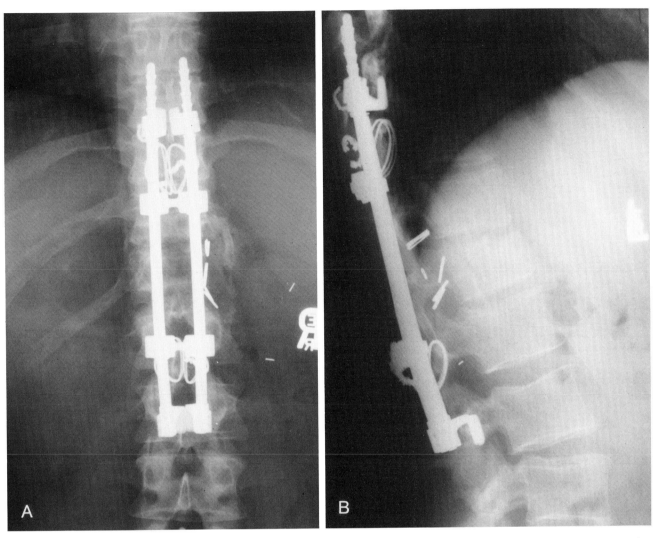

Figure 4.8. A flexion-compression injury of T12 treated with Moe distraction instrumentation, sublaminar wires, and rod-linking devices.

system. There was no difference in the correction of sco-liosis between the two systems. However, patients treated with the Harriluque system did have a better correction of kyphotic deformity as well as a quicker return to school (14). There were no pseudarthroses in this series. The other benefit noted with the Harriluque system is the lack of a need for bracing postoperatively. In another series by the same author, he noted no change in respiratory function as measured by the FVC or FEV1 in patients undergoing Harrington instrumentation alone vs. those who underwent a "Harriluque" technique (13).

Winter has also recorded a technique useful in main-taining lumbar lordosis when instrumenting with a Har-rington distraction rod into the L4 region (75). This technique involves spinous process wiring of the two lowest instrumented spinous processes as well as multiple

sublaminar wires throughout the construct. In over 30 years of use, Harrington instrumentation has less than a 0.5% neurologic complication rate. Its learning curve is certainly shorter than many of the newer instrumentation systems. While the hook cutout rate and pseudarthrosis rate is very low for single thoracic curvatures, these com-plications are more frequent in the thoracolumbar and lumbar spine (62).

Recently, Dickson et al. reviewed Dr. Harrington's patients with a follow-up average of 21 years, a response rate of 83% of 206 patients, and review of 111 x-rays (17). Comparing these patients to 100 controls, the au-thors found that fusions with Harrington instrumenta-tion at long-term follow-up had some increase in interscapular and thoracolumbar pain when compared to controls without fusion, but found no difference in the amount of low back or lumbosacral pain. Furthermore, pain and fatigue were not related to the type of curve, the size of the curve, the length of fusion, or to the presence or absence of broken rods.

As reported above, the overall results in the treatment of adolescent idiopathic scoliosis, especially for single and double thoracic curves, are very good with the use of Harrington instrumentation. However, the results with Harrington instrumentation in the treatment of adult scoliosis have not been as gratifying. Nuber and Schafer reviewed 62 adult scoliosis patients who underwent either Harrington instrumentation or Luque segmental instrumentation. They found a higher rate of complication and less correction and greater loss of correction with Harrington instrumentation vs. segmental spinal instrumentation (56). Complications in this group with Harrington rods included three pseudarthroses, three urinary tract infections, three instrumentation failures, one dural tear, one superior mesenteric artery syndrome, and one decubitus out of 19 patients treated with posterior Harrington instrumentation. Other studies show complication rates of 50–86% when using Harrington instrumentation in the treatment of adult scoliosis. Other common complications include psychotic problems, neurologic deficits, loss of lumbar lordosis, thromboembolic disease, and wound infection (44,59). In Dr. Harrington's series of adult scoliotics, over 70 complications were reported in 132 patients (59). The majority of these complications involve pseudarthroses. In an average follow-up of 3.5 years in 91 patients treated for adult scoliosis from the Twin Cities Scoliosis Center, the authors reported 38% correction at the time of surgery, which decreased to 32% at follow-up. They noticed a 33% complication rate with a pseudarthrosis rate of a 15% and hook dislodgement rate of 5% (69).

Another group of deformity patients where Harrington rod instrumentation has not led to excellent results are the neuromuscular scoliotics (11,33,58). After reviewing 40 patients, Herring and Wenger concluded that segmental instrumentation provided significant improvement in stability over conventional Harrington instrumentation in the treatment of neuromuscular scoliosis (33). Daher et al. reported two pseudarthroses and one patient with superior mesenteric artery syndrome after the treatment of 12 patients with Charcot-Marie Tooth disease, four of whom were treated surgically with Harrington instrumentation and one of these with segmental sublaminar wires (12). The same group from the Twin Cities Scoliosis Center have reported that there is a need for an anterior and posterior fusion in the treatment of myelomeningocele (58). The pseudarthrosis rate in this series was 46% when only posterior fusion and instrumentation were used. Swank et al., reporting on the treat-

ment of Duchenne's muscular dystrophy with Harrington instrumentation, found no pseudarthrosis but complications in eight of 13 patients (64). In treating scoliosis with associated spinal muscular atrophy, Daher reported that the Luque sublaminar wiring of Harrington or Luque rods without external support was the procedure of choice after reviewing 11 patients treated surgically, five with Harrington instrumentation, four with "Harri-luque" instrumentation, and two with Luque instrumentation alone (11). Although Harrington's original impetus in the development of his instrumentation system was the treatment of patients with scoliosis from poliomyelitis, segmental fixation such as Luque instrumentation is preferred in the treatment of patients with neuromuscular scoliosis.

Trauma

In 1958, Harrington first used posterior instrumentation and fusion for the stabilization of a fracture dislocation of the spine. Early work in studying the effect of instrumentation on spinal fracture emphasized the comparison of operative vs. nonoperative treatment for unstable thoracolumbar fractures. The conclusions drawn from the majority of these reports were that patients treated with internal fixation were easier to nurse, described less pain, and demonstrated less residual deformity than those treated nonoperatively (10,15,20,22,41,63,66). The best results with Harrington instrumentation in the treatment of traumatic disorders occur when a pure axial force is exerted to the middle column (Fig. 4.7). In translational injuries with associated disruption of the soft tissue envelope, the stabilization with Harrington distraction instrumentation is difficult and certainly more dangerous (10,51). The major complications associated with Harrington instrumentation in the treatment of fractures have been pseudarthroses and late rod disengagement (49). Gertzbein et al. have noted significant late loss of reduction, especially in the treatment of burst fractures (22). This loss of reduction was irrespective of original satisfactory reduction at the time of initial correction, delay before surgery, the length of the fusion, initial deformity, or neurologic deficit. He did note that technical errors, slippage of hooks, improper placement of hooks, and laminar fractures were the most frequent cause of failure with Harrington rod fixation (22,63).

Timing of instrumentation and decompression (early vs. late intervention) has not been studied prospectively as to its effect on neurologic recovery in incomplete patients, complications, or the ease of spinal realignment. Willen et al., in reviewing CT examination of the spine before and after Harrington instrumentation, noted that

Harrington rods restored the general spinal alignment. However, he also noted that even after surgery, the midsagittal diameter as well as the cross-sectional area of the spinal canal were still diminished by 26% (74). In that same study, the reduction of the spinal canal was improved significantly by early surgical intervention. This finding led the authors to recommend early surgery (within 3 days of injury).

The reduction force of Harrington distraction instrumentation when used in spinal fractures, as discussed earlier, is dependent on an intact anterior longitudinal ligament with a three-point bending moment exerted on the fracture site (a posterior distractive force acting in concert with the anterior tether). Disruption of the anterior longitudinal ligament, as possible in a rotational or translational injury, disrupts the anterior tether and causes unknown distraction on the neural elements. Therefore, it is exceedingly important to assess the soft tissue damage as part of preoperative planning. MRI can be helpful in this regard. The mechanistic classification of Ferguson and Allen is useful in predicting the integrity of the anterior longitudinal ligament. In compression-flexion and vertical compression injuries, the anterior structures are predominantly intact and offer an ideal environment for stability with distraction fixation. Conversely, torsional flexion and lateral flexion injuries lend themselves to complex soft tissue disruption and require special consideration and study before employing distraction instrumentation. Similar analyses of the soft tissue should be employed after distractive extension, distractive flexion and translational injuries to the thoracolumbar spine.

In terms of correction of both kyphotic deformity and lateral flexion, Cotler et al. found an improvement averaging 12.5° in kyphotic deformity after Harrington instrumentation for trauma, which fell to 10.1° at late follow-up (32). Lateral flexion improvement averaged 5.2°, with a loss of correction of 1.5° at late follow-up (10). In another series of 40 patients treated with Harrington instrumentation, 10 patients had anatomic reduction after Harrington instrumentation. In 34 of the 40 patients, there was a minimum loss of correction, most of which developed during immobilization and was less than 10°. In three of these 34 patients, kyphosis of 11°, 12°, and 16° developed during immobilization but progressed no further. Two additional patients had a late kyphosis of 9° and 15° after removal of external support and in whom pseudarthroses were discovered and repaired successfully with corrections to 7° and 4°, respectively (20). Recurrent deformity reiterates the importance of and the need for external support when using the Harrington system. We view external support

as an imperative adjunct to surgical treatment of spinal trauma patients with Harrington instrumentation.

Akbarnia explored the use of "Harriluque" instrumentation in the treatment of thoracolumbar fractures (4,5). He compared "Harriluque" technique with Harrington instrumentation alone and found equally satisfactory alignment in both groups, with a high rate of complications in both groups. He felt that the addition of sublaminar wires was useful only in eliminating the need for rigid external immobilization in those patients who could not tolerate a body cast. However, he also felt that the technique was a disadvantage when a short-length fusion was desired and added increased risk of neurologic complication in the passage of sublaminar wires.

In summary, Harrington instrumentation for the treatment of thoracolumbar traumatic injuries, when given the right indications, has enjoyed significant success in decreasing hospital stay, decreasing residual deformity, and improving rehabilitation potential in these patients. The majority of retrospective literature analyzing the success of Harrington instrumentation in the treatment of trauma has taught us that exacting indications, precise technical detail, and postoperative external support lead to improved results with regard to fusion rate and prevention of late deformity. Recent modifications of Harrington's original instrumentation provide more modularity, improvements in force application and hook design, while maintaining the original principles upon which Harrington based his instrumentation and which have led to great strides in the treatment of potentially devastating thoracolumbar injuries.

COMPLICATIONS OF HARRINGTON INSTRUMENTATION

McAfee and Bohlman stated that poor results of Harrington rod instrumentation for fractures are the results of poor Harrington instrumentation techique (49). They reported on 40 patients who underwent 45 Harrington rod instrumentation procedures, 30 of whom had greater than 2-year follow-up (49). Twenty-six of these patients required additional procedures; five had neurologic deterioration (one death); nine had inadequate translational reduction; 16 had dislodgement and loss of fixation; six had deep wound infection; three had wound dehiscence and metal showing; and 16 had unrecognized neural compression. The authors believed that the use of Harrington instrumentation in translation (flexion rotation) injuries, failure to obtain a contrast or CT study, failure to identify persistent neural compression, wound dehiscence, the use of distraction rods for thoracic kyphosis, and instrumenting across the lumbosacral joint all led to poor results with complications. As with many complications after a surgical procedure, the complication is not primarily the fault of the instrumentation, but of lack of preoperative planning and technical errors in the use of the instrumentation.

Loss of lumbar lordosis with the use of Harrington distraction instrumentation to the low lumbar spine or lumbosacral junction has been well described. Hasday noted no difference in the loss of lumbar lordosis between a "rod long-fuse short" group and the traditional "rod long-fuse long group" (32). The favored mechanism of compensation he noted was hip flexion and forward lean. Wasylenko noted that the loss of lumbar lordosis led to an increased lumbosacral angle when the joint was open with increased knee flexion and increased frontal and sagittal sway during gait (70). Aaro noted increased pain and rigidity after fusion below L3 with Harrington instrumentation (2). Recently, An et al. reported patients with fractures of low lumbar spine treated with various spinal instrumentations including Harrington rods, and observed poorer results with Harrington rods due to loss of lumbar lordosis and fusion of longer spinal segments (8). These reports and others have led to a heightened awareness and fear of fusion with Harrington distraction instrumentation to the low lumbar spine and lumbosacral junction. If fusion to this area is necessary, alternative fixation devices should be considered. Devices with pedicular fixation and rod or plate attachments allow sparing of motion segments in addition to rigid fixation and better lordotic contouring in the low lumbar spine.

The effect of placing metal hooks into the spinal canal has also been shown to cause sciatica and possible nerve root dysfunction of the lumbar and sacral nerve roots (24,27,43). Hales reported on hook migration into the canal in 18 patients with Harrington rod instrumentation. This subsequently resulted in sciatica and low back pain 2–32 months after implantation. The authors proposed that the migration was caused by a combination of the lumbosacral lordosis and mobility of the 5th lumbar vertebrae on the segment below, resulting in weakening of the lamina of the 5th lumbar vertebrae. All patients in Hale's series improved after removal of the hardware.

Certain theoretical complications exist with any instrumentation system. Coe and McAfee showed a significant increase in Wallerian degeneration of the dorsal columns, corticospinal tracts, and nerve roots, focal cystic degeneration, and intraspinal central cavitation in beagles after Harrington instrumentation when compared with noninstrumented but dorsally fused animals (9). The incidence of this neural histologic deterioration was 64% in instrumented animals, vs. 7% in noninstrumented animals. The authors proposed that subclinical neurologic injuries such as intraspinal and nerve root infarction in

posterior neural tissues may occur with the use of sublaminar hooks or wires. McAfee also has raised the issue of device-related osteoporosis, a theoretical complication of any instrumentation system (50). Using an adult beagle model, the authors investigated the effect of Harrington distraction, Luque rectangular, and Cotrel-Dubousset transpedicular fixation on the histology and biochemical qualities of the fusion mass. The authors showed that fusions performed in conjunction with spinal instrumentation were more rigid, but the volumetric density of bone was significantly lower (device-related osteoporosis) for fused vs. unfused spines. Harrington- and Cotrel-Dubousset-instrumented dogs were more osteoporotic than other groups (apparently related to the greater rigidity of these instrumentation systems). It should be noted that as the rigidity of the spinal instrumentation increased, there was an increased probability of successful spinal fusion. The authors concluded that the improved mechanical properties of spinal instrumentation on spinal arthrodesis more than compensate for the occurrence of device-related osteoporosis in the spine.

Other complications have been reported with the use of Harrington instrumentation. Disseminated intravascular coagulation (DIC) may be related to decortication during fusion surgery (61). The defibrination seen in two patients with this complication ceased at the end of surgery. Six other cases of DIC have been reported after orthopaedic surgery, and four of these six were during spinal arthrodesis. Treatment for this type of DIC is blood component replacement. Heparin should be avoided, as the complication ends with the completion of surgery. Superior mesenteric artery syndrome has been reported in patients as a postoperative complication of Harrington instrumentation for both the treatment of traumatic thoracolumbar fractures as well as in scoliosis surgery (57). It has been postulated that some degree of hyperlordosis of the spine may be responsible for this phenomenon. Air embolism and fat embolism leading to adult respiratory distress syndrome (ARDS), as well as iliofemoral thrombosis have all been reported after Harrington rod instrumentation (23,25,46). The incidence of these complications is very small. Vigilant and compulsive postoperative care and a high index of suspicion will lead to aggressive diagnosis and treatment of these uncommon complications, which can occur after any major surgical procedure such as Harrington rod instrumentation.

SUMMARY

The preceding information has reviewed the experience of Harrington instrumentation and Harrington modifications in the treatment of spinal deformity and trauma. Principles employed in the treatment of deformity and trauma can also be utilized in spinal stabilization after tumor surgery or treatments that destabilize the axial skeleton.

Harrington instrumentation (or Moe modifications) have proven most beneficial in the treatment of adolescent idiopathic scoliosis with single or double thoracic curves. Complications increased and results degenerated when using this instrumentation in adults with scoliosis or in the treatment of thoracolumbar or lumbar curves in adolescence. Distraction instrumentation is most useful in the concavity of the scoliotic curve. Compression instrumentation is useful to stabilize the distraction instrumentation as well as in preserving sagittal plane lordosis, particularly in the lumbar spine. Compression instrumentation in deformity surgery is useful in treating pure kyphosis.

In the treatment of traumatic spinal pathology, Harrington or modified systems help with quicker mobilization, the prevention of complications of recumbent treatment, and in the prevention of late deformity. Distraction instrumentation is indicated when the anterior longitudinal ligament is preserved, as in flexion-compression or vertical compression injuries. Distraction instrumentation is contraindicated with translational injury to the middle column. Harrington compression instrumentation is indicated for flexion–distraction type injuries and when a stable anterior graft has been placed (reconstituting the anterior column after anterior decompression).

Complications discussed in this chapter are in general the result of poor indications, improper surgical technique, or the failure to augment the instrumentation with external immobilization.

Harrington instrumentation revolutionized the surgical care of patients with spinal deformity and traumatic injuries to the spine. Most instrumentation systems available today are built upon concepts that have evolved from the development of Harrington instrumentation. All new instrumentation should be measured against Harrington instrumentation with regard to the biomechanical principles and the clinical results of that particular system. Finally, we must always remember that no instrumentation system can last without a solid fusion. Meticulous spinal fusion technique is necessary first, as instrumentation serves only as an adjunct means toward the goal of attaining a solid arthrodesis.

REFERENCES

1. Aaro S, Dahlborn M: The effect of Harrington instrumentation on the longitudinal axis of rotation of the apical vertebra and on the spinal and rib-cage deformity in idiopathic scoliosis studied by computerized tomography. Spine 1982;7:456–462.
2. Aaro S, Ohlen G: The effect of Harrington instrumentation on sagittal configuration and mobility of the spine in scoliosis. Spine 1983;8:570–575.
3. Aebi M, Mohler J, Zach G, et al: Analysis of 75 operated thoracolumbar fractures in fracture dislocations with and without neurological deficit. Arch Orthop Trauma Surg 1986;105:100–112.
4. Akbarnia BA, Fogarty JP, Smith KR, Jr.: New trends in surgical stabilization of thoracolumbar spinal fractures with emphasis for sublaminar wiring. Paraplegia 1985;23:27–33.
5. Akbarnia BA, Fogarty JP, Tayob AA: Contoured Harrington instrumentation in the treatment of unstable spinal fractures. The effect of supplementary sublaminar wires. Clin Orthop 1984;189:186–194.
6. Akeson J, Bobechko WP: Treatment of scoliosis by instrumentation with double upper hooks and posterior fusion [Abstract]. Orthop Trans 1986;10:35.
7. Albee FH: Transplantation of a portion of the tibia for Potts disease. JAMA 1911;57:885–886.
8. An HS, Vaccaro A, Cotler SM, Lin S: Low lumbar burst fractures: Comparison among body cast, Harrington Rod, Luque Rod, and Steffee Plate. Spine 1991;16:5440–5444.
9. Coe JD, Becker PS, McAfee PC, et al: Neuropathology with spinal instrumentation. J Orthop Res 1989;7:359–370.
10. Cotler JM, Vernace JV, Michalski JA: The use of Harrington rods in thoracolumbar fractures. Orthop Clin North Amer 1986;17:87–103.
11. Daher YH, Lonstein JE, Winter RB, et al: Spinal surgery in spinal musculo-atrophy. J Pediatr Orthop 1985;4:391–395.
12. Daher YH, Lonstein JE, Winter RB, et al: Spinal deformities in patients with Charcot-Marie Tooth Disease. A review of 12 patients. Clin Orthop 1986;202:219–222.
13. Daruwalla JS, Clark DW, Balasubramaniam P: Respiratory function in idiopathic scoliosis and adolescence treated by Harrington instrumentation with or without sublaminar segmental wiring. Revue De Chirurgie Orthopedigue Et Reparatrice De L Appareil Moteur 1989;75:490–492.
14. Daruwalla JS, Clark DW, Balasubramaniam P: Surgical treatment of scoliosis using Harrington instrumentation and arthrodesis. A comparison of two series with and without sublaminar segmental wiring. Rev De Chir Orthop Et Reparatrice De L Appareil Moteur 1989;75:537–341.
15. Denis F: Spinal instability as defined by the three column spine concept in acute spinal trauma. Clin Orthop 1984;189:65–76.
16. Denis F, Ruiz H, Searls K: Comparison between square ended distraction rods and standard round ended distraction rods in the treatment of thoracolumbar spinal injuries. A statistical analysis. Clin Orthop 1984;189:162–167.
17. Dickson JH, Erwin WD, Rossi D: Harrington instrumentation and arthrodesis for idiopathic scoliosis. A 21 year follow-up. J Bone Joint Surg 1990;72A:678–683.
18. Edwards CL, Levine AM: Early rod-sleeve stabilization of the injured thoracic and lumbar spine. Orthop Clin North Amer 1986;17:121–145.
19. Ferguson RL, Allen BL: A mechanistic classification of thoracolumbar spine fractures. Clin Orthop 1984;189:77.
20. Flesch JR, Leider LL, Erickson DL, et al: Harrington instrumentation and spine fusion for unstable fractures and fracture dislocations of the thoracic and lumbar spine. J Bone Joint Surg 1977;59 2:143–153.
21. Gaines RW, Leatherman KD: Benefits of the Harrington compression system in lumbar and thoracolumbar idiopathic scoliosis in adolescents and adults. Spine 1981;6:483–488.
22. Gertzbein SD, Michael D, Tile M: Harrington instrumentation as

a method of fixation in fractures of the spine. J Bone Joint Surg 1982;64B:526–529.

23. Gittman JE, Buchanan TA, Fisher BJ, et al: Fatal fat embolism after spinal fusion for scoliosis. JAMA 1983;249:779–781.

24. Gunzburg R, Fraser RD: Progressive sacral nerve root dysfunction, a possible complication of sublaminar hooks. A case report. Spine 1990;15:142–144.

25. Gurman W, Seimon LP: Iliofemoral thrombosis following Harrington spinal instrumentation. Report of a case. J Bone Joint Surg 1985;67A:1273–1274.

26. Hadra BE: Wearing of the spinous processes in Potts disease. Transamer Orthop Assoc 1891;4:206.

27. Hales DD, Dawson EG, Delamarter R: Late neurological complications of Harrington rod instrumentation. J Bone Joint Surg 1989;71A:1053–1057.

28. Harrington PR: Surgical instrumentation for management of scoliosis. J Bone Joint Surg 1960;42A:1448.

29. Harrington PR: Treatment of scoliosis: Correction and internal fixation by spine instrumentation. J Bone Joint Surg 1962; 44A:591–610.

30. Harrington PR: The history and development of Harrington instrumentation. Clin Orthop 1988;227:3.

31. Harrington PR, Dixon JH: An eleven year clinical investigation of Harrington instrumentation. A preliminary report on 578 cases. Clin Orthop 1973;93:113–130.

32. Hasday CA, Passoff TL, Perry J: Gait abnormalities arising from iatrogenic loss of lumbar lordosis secondary to Harrington instrumentation and lumbar fractures. Spine 1983;8:501–511.

33. Herring JA, Wenger DR: Segmental spinal instrumentation: A preliminary report of 40 consecutive cases. Spine 1982;7:285–298.

34. Hibbs RA: An operation for progressive spinal deformities. NY State J Med 1911;93:1013–1016.

35. Irwin WD, Dixon JH, Harrington PR: Clinical review of patients with broken Harrington rods. J Bone Joint Surg 1980;62A:1302–1307.

36. Jacobs RR, Asher MA, Snider RK: Thoracolumbar spinal injuries. A comparative study of recumbent and operative treatment in 100 patients. Spine 1980;5:463.

37. Jacobs RR, Dahners LE, Gertzbein SD, et al: A locking hook spinal rod—current status of development. Paraplegia 1983; 21:197–200.

38. Jacobs RR, Montesano PX: Development of the locking hook spinal rod system. Orthopaedics 1988;11:1415.

39. Jacobs RR, Nordwall A, Nachemson A: Reduction, stability and strength provided by internal fixation systems for thoracolumbar spinal injuries. Clin Orthop 1982;171:300–308.

40. Jacobs RR, Schlaepfer F, Mathys R Jr, et al: A locking hook spinal rod system for stabilization of fracture dislocations and correction of deformities of the dorsal lumbar spine. A biomechanical evaluation. Clin Orthop 1984;189:168–177.

41. Jodoin A, Dupuis P, Fraser M, et al: Unstable fractures of the thoracolumbar spine: A ten year experience at Sacre-Coeur Hospital. J Trauma 1985;25:197–202.

42. King HA, Moe JH, Bradford DS, et al: The selection of fusion levels in thoracic idiopathic scoliosis. J Bone Joint Surg 1983; 65A:1302–1313.

43. Kornberg M, Herndon WA, Rechtine GR: Lumbar nerve root compression at the site of hook insertion. Late complication of Harrington rod instrumentation for scoliosis. Spine 1985;10:853–855.

44. Kostuik JP, Israel J, Hall JE: Scoliosis surgery in adults. Clin Orthop 1973;93:225.

45. Lagrone MO, Bradford DS, Moe JH, et al: Treatment of symptomatic flatback after spinal fusion. J Bone Joint Surg 1988; 70:569.

46. Lang SA, Duncan PG, Dupuis PR: Fatal air embolism in an adolescent with Duchenne muscular dystrophy during Harrington instrumentation. Anest Analges 1989;69:132.

47. Lifeso RM, Arabie KM, Kadhi SK: Fractures of the thoracolumbar spine. Paraplegia 1985;23:207–224.

48. Lovallo JL, Banta JV, Renshaw TS: Adolescent idiopathic scoliosis treated by Harrington rod distraction and fusion. J Bone Joint Surg 1986;68A:1326–1330.

49. McAfee PC, Bohlman HH: Complications following Harrington instrumentation for fractures of the thoracolumbar spine. J Bone Joint Surg 1985;67A:672–686.

50. McAfee PC, Farey ID, Sutterlin CE, et al: 1989 Volvo award in basic science. Device-related osteoporosis with spinal instrumentation. Spine 1989;14:919–926.

51. McAfee PC, Yuan HA, Fredrickson BE, et al: The value of computed tomography in thoracolumbar fractures. An analysis of 100 consecutive cases and a new classification. J Bone Joint Surg 1983;65 4:461–473.

52. Moe JH, Cummine JL, Winter RB, et al: Harrington instrumentation without fusion combined with the Milwaukee brace for difficult scoliosis problems in young children [Abstract]. Orthop Trans 1979;3:59.

53. Moe JH, Denis F: The iatrogenic loss of lumbar lordosis [Abstract]. Orthop Trans. 1977;1:131.

54. Moe JH, Kharrat K, Winter RB, et al: Harrington instrumentation without fusion plus external orthotic support for the treatment of difficult curvature problems in young children. Clin Orthop 1984;185:35–45.

55. Moe JH, Winter RB, Bradford DS, et al. Scoliosis and other spinal deformities, ed. 1. Philadelphia: WB Saunders, 1978;143–150.

56. Nuber GW, Schafer NF: Surgical management of adult scoliosis. Clin Orthop 1986;208:228–337.

57. Ohery A, Zelig G, Shemesh Y: Acute intermittent arteriomesenteric occlusion of the duodenum after use of Harrington spinal instrumentation: Case report. Paraplegia 1988;26:350–354.

58. Osebold WR, Mayfield JK, Winter RB, et al: Surgical treatment of paralytic scoliosis associated with myelomeningocele. J Bone Joint Surg 1982;64A:831–856.

59. Ponder RC, Dickson JH, Harrington PR, et al: Results of Harrington instrumentation and fusion in the adult idiopathic scoliosis patient. J Bone Joint Surg 1975;57A:797.

60. Purcell GA, Markolf KL, Dawson EG: Twelfth thoracic-first lumbar vertebral mechanical stability of fractures after Harrington rod instrumentation. J Bone Joint Surg 1981;63A:71–78.

61. Raphael BG, Lackner H, Engler GL: Disseminated intravascular coagulation during surgery for scoliosis. Clin Orthop 1982; 162:41–46.

62. Renshaw TS: The role of Harrington instrumentation and posterior spine fusion in the management of adolescent idiopathic scoliosis. Orthop Clin N Amer 1988;19:257–267.

63. Rubenstein JD, Gertzbein S: Radiographic assessment of Harrington rod instrumentation for spinal fractures. J Canad Assoc Radiolog 1984;35:159–163.

64. Swank SM, Brown JC, Perry RE: Spinal fusion in Duchenne's muscular dystrophy. Spine 1982;7:484–491.

65. Swank SM, Mauri TM, Brown JC: The lumbar lordosis below Harrington instrumentation for scoliosis. Spine 1990;15:181–186.

66. Svensson O, Aaro S, Ohlen G: Harrington instrumentation for

thoracic and lumbar vertebral fractures. Acta Orthop Scand 1984;55:38–47.

67. Tolo V: Surgical treatment of adolescent scoliosis. In: Barr J, ed. Park Ridge, IL, AAOS, 1989;38.

68. Tolo V, Gillespie R: The use of shortened periods of rigid post-operative immobilization in the surgical treatment of idiopathic scoliosis. J Bone Joint Surg 1981;63A:1137–1145.

69. Van Dam BE, Bradford DS, Lonstein JE, et al: Adult idiopathic scoliosis treated by posterior spinal fusion and Harrington instrumentation. Spine 1987;12:32–36.

70. Wasylenko M, Skinner SR, Perry J, et al: An analysis of posture and gait following spinal fusion with Harrington instrumentation. Spine 1983;8:840–845.

71. Weatherley CR, Draycott V, O'Brien JF, et al: The rib deformity in adolescent idiopathic scoliosis: A prospective study to evaluate changes after Harrington distraction in posterior fusion. J Bone Joint Surg 1987;69B:179–182.

72. Willen J, Dahllof AG, Nordwall A: Paraplegia in unstable thora-columbar injuries. A study of conservative and operative treatment regarding neurological improvement and rehabilitation. Scand J of Rehab Med (Suppl) 1983;9:195–205.

73. Willen J, Lindahl S, Irstam L, et al: Unstable thoracolumbar fractures. A study by CT and conventional roentgenology of the reduction effect of Harrington instrumentation. Spine 1984;9:214–219.

74. Willen J, Lindahl S, Nordwall A: Unstable thoracolumbar fractures: A comparative clinical study of conservative treatment in Harrington instrumentation. Spine 1985;10:111–122.

75. Winter RB: Harrington instrumentation into the lumbar spine. Technique for preservation of normal lumbar lordosis. Spine 1986;11:633–635.

76. Winter RB, Lonstein JE, Vandenbrink K, et al: Harrington rod with sublaminar wires in the treatment of adolescent idiopathic thoracic scoliosis: A study of sagittal plane correction [Abstract]. Orthop Trans 1987;11:89.

Jacobs Locking Hook Spinal Rod Instrumentation

Franco P. Cerabona and Pasquale X. Montesano

INTRODUCTION

The use of posterior instrumentation has led to significant advances in the care and treatment of spinal fractures and deformity. The Harrington system, though a revolutionary step in spinal surgery, does have many deficiencies (16). Rod breakage due to the notches, hook pullout, lack of rotational control with loss of sagittal plane alignment and over distraction of the injured spine comprise some of the major problems with this type of instrumentation. These shortcomings supplied the major impetus for the development of newer spinal implant systems. Rotational control was partly addressed by the square-ended Moe system. However, using this system, precise determination of the hook placement and rod contouring was needed to ensure sagittal plane correction. Supplemental sublaminar wiring to control hook pullout resulted in higher risks of neurologic injury during insertion and removal of these wires. The use of pedicular fixation, which allows shorter fusion levels and preservation of more motion segments, is technically demanding and can cause neurologic injuries.

In 1979, Rae R. Jacobs, with the assistance of F. Schlaepfer, R. Mathys, and Alf Nachemson, designed a system to address these problems. A rod with hooks controlled by nuts and washers was used to allow positioning of the hook axially along the rod. This eliminated the need for deep notches in the rod with their weakening effect. Extra head 316-L stainless steel 5 mm × 7 mm rod was used to achieve maximum strength and increased fatigue life. The upper and lower hooks were in the anatomical configuration to conform to the lamina to which they are applied. A sliding cover is placed over the cranial aspect of the upper lamina to lock the upper hook in place (Fig. 5.1). This avoids the use of high distraction loads on the spine necessary for upper hook attachment. Both hooks are rotationally locked into the rod by meshing radial grooves of 6° increments into the hook and a washer that is keyed to the rod (Fig. 5.2). The hooks are locked into position by superior and inferior nuts which are crimped to the flat end of the rod. The system was developed to allow maintenance of sagittal plane correction, lessen upper hook pullout, increase strength, and allow for easier implant removal. The system was also

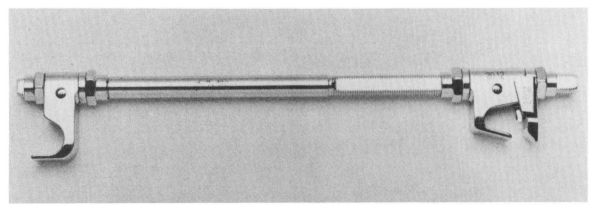

Figure 5.1. Preassembled Jacobs locking hook spinal rod (manufactured by the Synthes Corporation).

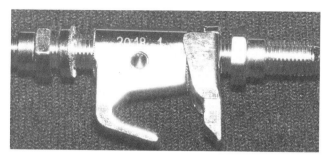

Figure 5.2. Upper hook with washers, nuts, and sliding cover.

designed to allow for the possibility of fusion of only the injured motion segment. Implant removal would then allow restoration of motion of the unfused segments after successful fusion and healing of the fractures (8). In canine models, there is evidence that unfused motion segments undergo degeneration. In the author's clinical practice, however, implant removal did not cause clinically significant back pain in the unfused segments (15).

The implant was tested in comparison with conventional Harrington instrumentation (10,12,14,18). The yield strength was 50% greater than that of the Harrington distraction rod (Fig. 5.3). Furthermore, when compared with Harrington instrumentation, the upper hook pullout strength was significantly increased (Table 5.1). The implant was also compared with long and short Harrington instrumentation in a three column injured spine. Long and short Harrington rods failed at 44 and 22 Nm respectively, but the Jacobs rod failed at 125 Nm, and provided better deformity correction in hyperextension (Table 5.2).

INDICATIONS

A primary indication for the Jacobs locking hook device is fractures of the thoracolumbar region. Currently, we believe that fractures about T9 or below L2 would better be handled by other available devices. Mid- to

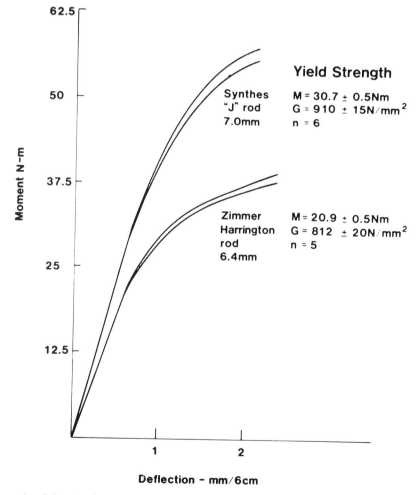

Figure 5.3. Yield strength of the Synthes 7-mm rod is 50% greater than 6.4-mm Harrington. (Reprinted with permission, Jacobs, et al., Clin Orthop 1984;189:173.)

Table 5.1.
Upper Hook Pullout[a]

	Harrington	Experimental
Applied distraction	40 kp	12.5 kp
Hook pullout force	81.1 ± 11.4 kp	130 ± 8 kp

[a]Reprinted with permission from Jacobs, et al: A locking spinal rod system for stabilization of fracture-dislocations and correction of deformities of the dorsolumbar spine: a biomechanical evaluation. Clin Orthop 1984;189:173.

upper thoracic fractures require instrumentation that would be beyond the apex of the thoracic kyphosis. Because of this bulky nature of the upper hooks in the system, this may result in prominence of the hardware and potential for skin breakdown or discomfort. Lower profile hooks are being considered to solve this problem and broaden the scope of the device. At present, the device is not indicated for fractures below L2 that would require placing the caudal hooks into L5 or S1. In general, hooks placed at the lower lumbosacral areas, especially S1, have a high failure rate and potential for neurologic injury.

Researchers are developing a rod with the ability to utilize pedicular screws and/or Galveston type iliac crest fixation. This would increase our ability to utilize this device for lower lumbar fractures, lumbosacral deformity, and degenerative problems. Specific fracture patterns may require supplementation with anterior surgery. The device has been utilized by the authors for tumors involving the vertebral body in conjunction with anterior decompression and fusion. It also has been used for scoliotic deformity by its developer, but presently neither author uses this device for this indication.

Table 5.2.
Combined Injury[a]

Implant	Load (Nm)[b]	Deformity (°)	Energy (J)
Harrington			
Dist. 2 + 2	22.2 + 2.4	23.8 + 3.4	2.30 + 0.4
Harrington			
Dist. 3 + 3	44.1 + 2.1	9.3 ± 1.9	5.7 ± 1.3
Jacobs 3 + 3	125.0 ± 17.0	2.5 ± 2.9	13.9 ± 3.7

[a]Reprinted with permission from Jacobs, et al: A locking spinal rod system for stabilization of fracture-dislocations and correction of deformities of the dorsocolumbar spine: a biomechanical evaluation. Clin Orthop 1984;189:173.
[b]Load at failure was nearly three times greater with the Jacobs locking hook spinal rod when compared with the Harrington device, with less deformity but more energy absorption because of reduction in hyperextension.

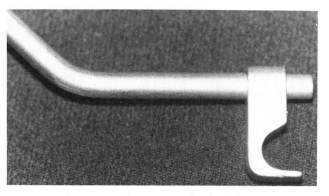

Figure 5.4. Lower hook trial.

SURGICAL TECHNIQUE

The primary consideration when utilizing the Jacobs hook device is to understand that this is not a Harrington rod. Some fundamental differences must be understood, especially for those surgeons who are very familiar with the Harrington rod system. The reduction of fractures is accomplished by four-point bending and not purely by distraction. Also, the tactile feedback from the seating and racheting the upper Harrington hook is very different. Distraction is used only to seat the upper hook in place and lock the hook to the rod. Most important, however, is the fact that the cranial Jacobs hook is inserted in the canal, not in the facet joints.

Surgical procedure is done with routine prone positioning. Initial reduction and lateral x-rays should be done at the time of positioning the patient, and any necessary correction using either hyperextension of the hips or adjustment of the frame should be done at this time. Surgical exposure is through a standard posterior midline approach. For a fracture of L1, for example, the spinous processes and the lamina from T9 to L3 are exposed. The lower hook site is prepared between the second and third vertebrae below the level of injury. The ligamentum flavum is removed in the standard fashion, and the supraspinous and infraspinous ligaments are left intact. This is important, especially if the rod long, fuse short method is being used. A small amount of bone at the upper edge

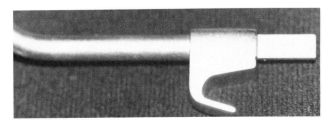

Figure 5.5. Upper hook trial.

Figure 5.6. Area of typical caudal lamina resection (darkened area).

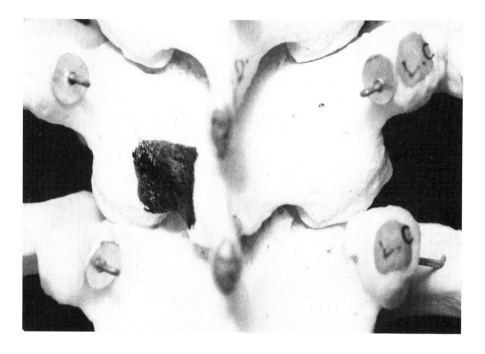

of the third lamina and medial border of the facet is removed. The trial lower hook inserter is placed utilizing rotation in the sagittal plane (Fig. 5.4). The hook placement should be done with rotation laterally, then medially, to set the trial hook. Posterior pressure is then applied to test placement. It may be necessary to remove some bone from the posterior lamina of the vertebrae immediately above especially if the angle of placement is anteriorly directed.

The upper hook site is prepared next. This is the essential part of the procedure. The lower border of the third lamina above the injury is removed. This allows for insertion of the trial hook into the spinal canal. The trial hook has a guide that will help determine how much bone must be removed inferiorly in order to allow for the locking cap to capture the superior lamina (Fig. 5.5). To allow this to happen, bone is taken from the weaker caudal portion of the lamina and not from the strong

cranial part (Fig. 5.6). The trial hook is inserted by directing it anterior and cranial but not by rotating in the sagittal plane, as with the lower hook. The lateral portion of the hook should be medial to the pedicle within the sublaminar area. No attempt should be made to seat the hook forcibly into the pedicle. The sliding cover should then fit over the top of the lamina. At times a very small amount of the cranial edge of the lamina may need to be resected for better placement of the locking cap. This

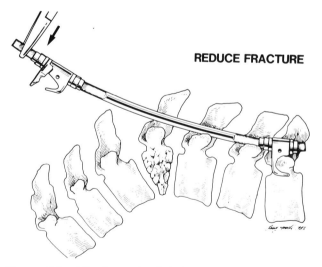

REDUCE FRACTURE

Figure 5.8. The lower hook is inserted first, and fracture reduction is completed by downward force on the upper end of the rod. (Reprinted with permission from Jacobs, et al: A locking hook spinal rod: Current status of development. Paraplegia 1983;21:197.)

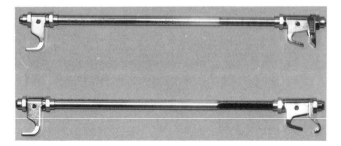

Figure 5.7. Conventional (*top*) and anatomical (*bottom*) locking hook spinal rod.

should be kept to a minimum. After the hook site is prepared, an appropriate length rod is selected. It is important that no rod should be below the lower hook at the level of the lamina and that the solid portion of the rod should be over the fracture site. These guides will help select the proper rod size. The rods and hooks come preassembled. Each rod should have two hooks, upper and lower, two locking washers, four nuts, and a straight locking cap, (an anatomically shaped cap has also been used and is being considered for greater capture of the lamina) (Fig 5.7). The rod is next prebent to conform to the normal spinal curve as compared with the post-reduction x-ray. Heavy-duty plate benders are suggested for this part of the procedure.

After bending the rod, the lower hook is placed through the interlaminar opening. The angular deformity is corrected by the use of the rod holder and application of a downwardly directed pressure on the rod (Fig. 5.8). Maintenance of the downward pressure with the rod holder is continued. The upper hook on its hook holder is then slid up the rod into place under the upper lamina. The hook holder is first directed perpendicular to the rod, then progressively angled downward to help slide the hook under the lamina (Fig. 5.9). The upper hook is then secured by tightening the nut just below the hook (Fig. 5.10). Care must be taken not to overdistract the spine by excessive tightening. This can occur if the locking cap is not secured. This rod is capable of generating strong distractive forces with nut tightening without the usual tactile feedback felt with Harrington racheting. As upper hook tightening proceeds, the locking cap is then alternately tightened as well. This will usually prevent overdistraction. After tightening the nuts, the rods are checked manually for tightness, and intraoperative x-rays are taken. If satisfactory, the nuts are then crimped to the flat surface of the rod with strong parallel pliers (Fig. 5.11). The fusion portion of the procedure should be

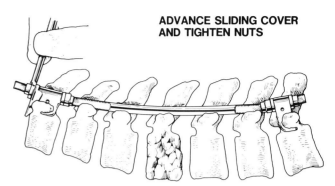

ADVANCE SLIDING COVER AND TIGHTEN NUTS

Figure 5.10. After evaluation of the reduction by x-rays, the sliding cover is advanced over the lamina, locking it to the hook. All nuts are tightened, thus locking the hooks to the rod in the selected position of rotation and amount of distraction. The sliding cover is also locked into position. (Reprinted with permission from Jacobs, et al: A locking hook spinal rod: Current status of development. Paraplegia 1983;21:197.)

done with meticulous care, as in all posterior spinal fusions. If a rod long, fuse short is performed, the facets and their capsules outside the fusion levels should be left undisturbed. Supplemental fixation with spinous process wiring or translaminar facet screws have also been utilized for extra rigidity but are not necessary in the majority of cases. Case examples are shown in Figures 5.12–5.14.

RESULTS

The largest published series of Jacobs locking hook spinal rod patients is by Gertzbein, Jacobs, et al. (8). In this series of 110 patients, 95 were treated in a prospective fashion. Seventy-two percent of the injuries were burst fractures, 19% fracture dislocations, and 9% were combinations of fracture dislocations and burst fractures. The level of injury was predominantly T12–L1, but a few

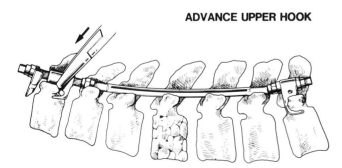

ADVANCE UPPER HOOK

Figure 5.9. The upper hook is advanced under the upper lamina with the upper hook holder. (Reprinted with permission from Jacobs, et al: A locking hook spinal rod: Current status of development. Paraplegia 1983;21:197.)

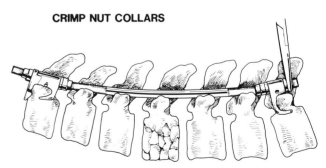

CRIMP NUT COLLARS

Figure 5.11. Nut collars are crimped into the flat sides of the rods. Care should be taken to avoid crimping the nuts themselves into an oval shape, since this may cause loosening. (Reprinted with permission from Jacobs, et al: A locking hook spinal rod: Current status of development. Paraplegia 1983; 21:197.)

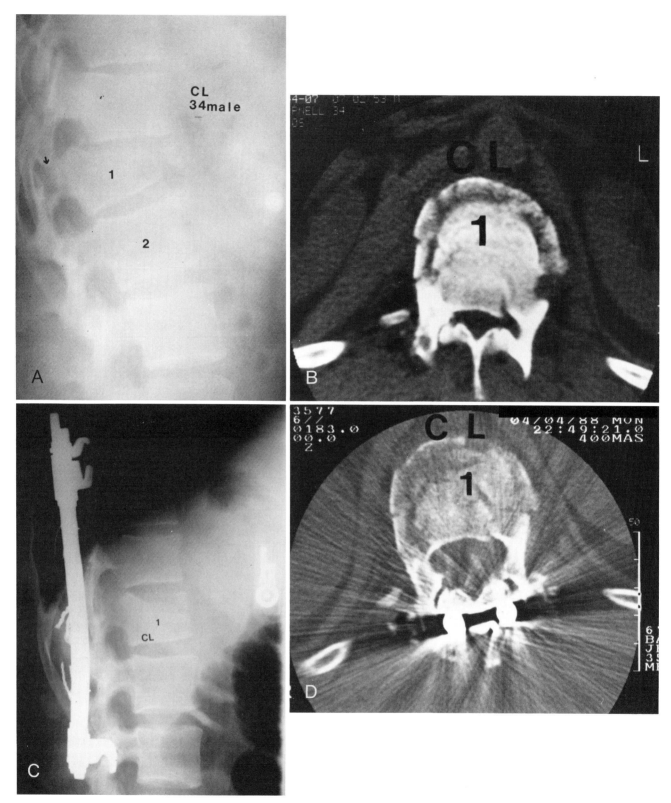

Figure 5.12. *A*, Lateral x-ray of an unstable Denis B burst fracture of L1. *B*, Preoperative CT seen showing 80% canal compromise. *C*, Postoperative lateral x-ray showing restoration of sagittal plane alignment and reconstruction of vertebral height. Note anatomical locking cap used. *D*, Postoperative CT with nearly complete restoration of spinal canal.

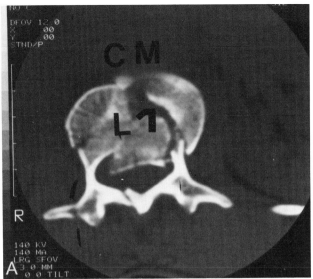

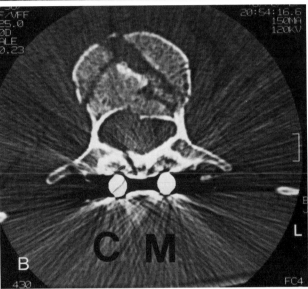

Figure 5.13. *A*, CT of a Denis type A fracture of L1 with 60% canal compromise. *B*, Postoperative CT with excellent canal restoration.

patients were as cranial as T4 and as caudal as L4. Initial kyphotic deformity was 21°, reduced postoperatively to 9°. At the time of rod removal, the deformity was 13°, and at 6 months postrod removal, the average kyphosis was 17°. Loss of vertebral height initially was 35%, reduced to 22% at final follow-up. The deformity tended to be less at follow-up if a brace was used for 3 months postoperatively. Complications were noted to be present in 13 patients. Two patients had wound infections that were treated. Thirteen patients had dislodgement of the rods, 11 at the upper and 2 at the lower end. Two of the patients had a fracture of the lamina which caused hook

dislodgement. In four of the patients, it was noted that there was a failure to crimp the nuts at the time of reoperation. If these cases are excluded, the overall loosening rate was 8.4%. There was no rod breakage, and there was no worsening of neurologic deficit. After rod removal, there was no significant incidence of back pain. Ninety-three percent of the patients had either little or no pain at follow-up. These results compare favorably to published data on correction and complaints of other posterior rod systems (2,3,7,9,17).

One author (Montesano) has recently compared the results of the Jacobs rod to his experience with the AO fixateur interne (1). The age, sex, follow-up time, mechanism of injury, type and level of injury, neurologic grade, and complications were compared. Radiographic analysis to show sagittal plane correction pre- and postoperatively and also after implant removal was done. There were 19 patients in the Jacobs locking spinal hook group and 29 in the AO group. Both groups were matched according to age, level, canal compromise, and initial kyphotic deformity. The most common fracture pattern in both groups was a Denis type B burst fracture (4). In the Jacobs rod group, the loss of initial height was 41% reduced to 23% postoperatively. Postrod removal, the loss of height increased from 27%, for a net 14% correction. The kyphotic deformity was 14° (1−28° to +28°). Postoperatively, kyphosis was reduced to an average of 1° (−0° to +15°). Of the patients who were studied and who had rod removal, the kyphosis increased an average of 5°. Therefore, net correction averaged was 9°. For comparison, the average AO group kyphotic deformity was 16° (−8° to −35°). Postoperatively, the sagittal kyphosis was corrected to minus 4° range (−26° to +14°). Of the 14 patients who had the hardware removed, the average sagittal angulation was 7° (−9° to +34°). Therefore, the net correction in this group was also 9°.

The complications in the Jacobs rod group included superior hook dislodgement in four patients. Of these four patients, two patients were not treated with an orthotic device. One patient had a bone graft site infection, and one patient developed a pressure sore over the rods, which resolved after rod removal. In the AO group, complications included screw breakage in four patients, deep wound infection in two patients, and screw loosening in two patients. There were no neurologic complications in either group.

This study demonstrates that there are comparable results with these systems in terms of correction of deformity. In this study there were no neurologic complications, but from a practical point of view, pedicle screw systems have a higher potential for neurologic in-

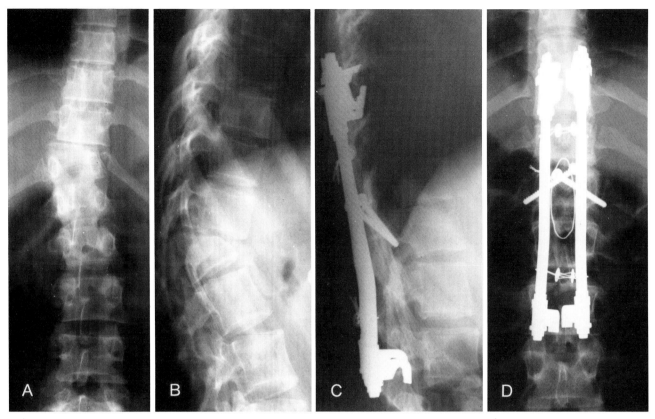

Figure 5.14. *A*, Unstable fracture dislocation, T12 AP view. *B*, Fracture dislocation, T12 lateral view. *C*, Postoperative AP. Note use of translaminar facet screws and Wisconsin wires for added stability. *D*, Lateral view with excellent restoration of sagittal plane alignment.

jury and rod hook systems have a significantly shorter learning curve.

In another study done by the author (Montesano), the cross-sectional area of decompression was compared (6). The posterior system showed greater percent decompression and no difference in the amount of intrusive material removed with the reduction as compared with a pedicular screw group. Review of both of the authors' present series reveals that the complications of hook pullout were markedly reduced with the use of a postoperative TLSO brace. Hook dislodgement also diminished as familiarity with

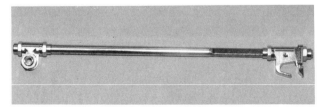

Figure 5.15. Jacobs locking hook spinal rod with AO fixateur interne Schanz screw coupling device.

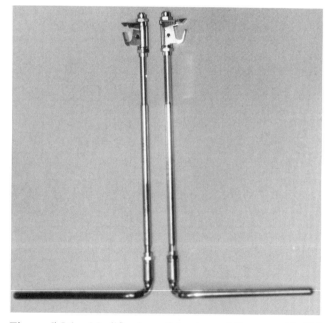

Figure 5.16. Modification of Jacobs rod for use with Galveston type fixation to the ilium.

implant placement was achieved. Lower hook pullout was observed in one case where instrumentation to L5 was done. In this instance, the L4 lamina was oriented in a rather vertical plane and the caudal portion of the rod failed to be bent enough to conform with this lamina. This was remedied by placement of the lower hook into the L4 lamina. The authors now feel that it is not optimal to place a hook in L5 or S1. The problems of hook prominence were not apparent when hook placement was kept below the T6 level. No neurologic deterioration had been noted in either of the authors' experience. No rod breakage or nut migration has been identified. Loss of correction does occur, but there has been no significant failure due to loss of correction that required reoperation.

SUMMARY

The Jacobs locking hook spinal rod is a system that is helpful in the stabilization and reduction of the thoracolumbar spine. It gives adequate correction and maintenance of correction with little risk of complications. It must be stressed that careful attention to detail, especially upper hook placement, is mandatory. Presently, the authors feel that the primary indication for the system is in the treatment of fractures from T9 to L2. Modifications of the system of the instrumentation may make insertion easier and also broaden the indications. There are prototypes in work to couple the system with pedicular screws (Fig. 5.15) and iliac fixation (Fig. 5.16). This would increase the current indications significantly and make the system a more versatile implant.

Acknowledgments. The authors wish to thank Lisa Feldman for her photography, Shannon Ackerman and Helene Caplan for the typing of this chapter, and Mildred Karpinski for proofreading.

REFERENCES

1. Boutin FJ, Burkus KJ, Sutherland T, et al: Jacobs locking hook spinal rod and the AO fixator intern for fractures of the thoracic and lumbar spine. Submitted for publication. Unpublished data.
2. Bradford DS, Akbarina BA, Winter RB, et al: Surgical stabilization of fractures and fracture dislocations of the thoracic spine. Spine 1977;2:185–196.
3. Crutcher JP, Anderson PA, King HA, et al: Indirect spinal canal decompression in patients with thoracolumbar burst fractures treated by posterior distraction rods. Read at 57th Annual American Academy of Orthopaedic Surgeons Meeting. New Orleans, Feb. 1990.
4. Denis F: The three column spine and its significance in the classification of acute thoracolumbar spinal injuries. Spine 1983; 8:817–831.
5. Dickson JH, Harrington PR, Erwin WD: Results of reduction and stabilization of the severely fractured thoracic and lumbar spine. J Bone Joint Surg 1978;60A:799–805.
6. Doerr TE, Montesano PX, Burkus JK, et al: Spinal canal decompression in traumatic thoracolumbar burst fractures; posterior distraction rods versus transpedicular screw fixation. Accepted, J Orthop Trauma.
7. Gertzbein SD, McMichael D, Tile M: Harrington instrumentation as a method of fixation in fractures of the spine: a critical analysis of deficiencies. J Bone Joint Surg 1982;64B:526–529.
8. Gertzbein SD, Jacobs RR, Stoll J, et al: Results of a locking hook spinal rod for fractures of the thoracic and lumbar spine. Spine 1990;15:4:275–280.
9. Jacobs RR, Asher MA, Snider RK: Thoracolumbar spinal injuries: A comparative study of recumbent and operative treatment in 100 patients. Spine 1980;5:463–477.
10. Jacobs RR, Nordwall A, Nachemson A: Reduction, stability and strength provided by internal fixation systems for thoracolumbar spinal injuries. Clin Orthop 1982;171:300–308.
11. Jacobs RR, Dahners LE, Gertzbein SD, et al: A locking hook-spinal rod: Current status of development. Paraplegia 1983; 21:197–200.
12. Jacobs RR, Schlaepfer F, Mathnys R Jr, et al: A locking spinal rod system for stabilization of fracture dislocations and correction of deformities of dorsolumbar spine: A biomechanical evaluation. Clin Orthop 1984;189:168–177.
13. Jacobs RR, Montesano PX: Development of the locking hook spinal rod system. Orthopaedics 1988;11:1415–1421.
14. Jacobs RR, Montesano PX, Jackson RP: The effect of lumbar spine fusions by the use of translaminar facet joint screws. Spine 1989;14:12–15.
15. Kahanovitz N, Bullough P, Jacobs RR: The effect of internal fixation without arthrodesis on human facet joint cartilage. Clin Orthop 1984;189:204–208.
16. McAfee PC, Bolman AA: Complications following Harrington instrumentation for fractures of thoracolumbar spine. J Bone Joint Surg 1985;67A:672–685.
17. McEvoy RD, Bradford DS: Management of burst fractures of the thoracolumbar spine and experience in 53 patients. Spine 1985;10:631–637.
18. Schlaepfer F, Magerl F, Jacobs RR, et al: In vivo measurements of loads on an external fixation device for human lumbar spine fractures. In: Engineering aspects of the spine. London: The Institution of Mechanical Engineers, 1980;59–64.

Six

Luque Instrumentation with Sublaminar Wiring

John G. Thometz and Howard S. An

INTRODUCTION

The use of sublaminar wiring to achieve multiple points of fixation to achieve spinal stabilization was developed by Luque over 20 years ago. Luque created his sublaminar wiring technique following observation of the use of sublaminar wiring for fusion of a fracture and dislocation of C3 on C4 (23). The advantages of sublaminar wiring were immediately apparent; it allowed firm fixation at multiple points along the instrumented area of the spine, distributing the corrective forces being applied to the spine and thereby diminishing the risk of osseous failure. A large percentage of his scoliotic patients had poliomyelitis with associated osteoporotic bone. In this patient population, he found that use of conventional Harrington instrumentation was associated with a high failure rate due to cutting out of the hooks. In addition, the socioeconomic situation of many of his patients made postoperative bracing difficult or impossible.

For the next several years, with increased clinical and laboratory experience, the technique underwent several modifications. At the end of this period, Dr. Luque reached several conclusions (23,24). He found that the use of double L rods with segmental sublaminar wiring along with good surgical technique led to a very high rate of arthrodesis. This construct provided excellent correction in both the frontal and sagittal planes. The multiple points of firm fixation allowed significant correction of the curves to occur; Luque cautioned that care must be taken in order to avoid very aggressive attempts at correction that could lead to neurologic compromise.

The concept of segmental fixation of the spine dates back to 1902 (21). Fritz Lange developed a technique for tuberculous spondylitis that was designed to prevent progressive kyphosis. His technique underwent many modifications, but eventually involved placing buried steel rods in the back which were fixed to the spinous processes with wires. His reception at the American Orthopaedic Association was rather skeptical; he was thanked for "bringing before the members a method of securing fixation of the spinal column without restraint of the respiratory organs of the body, but . . . it is questionable whether this method would be of much use . . . ." In 1963, Resina described a technique for the use of metal rods fixed to the spinous processes (33). He felt that it was most effective biomechanically for the corrective forces to work at right angles to the long axis of the rod. More recently, other methods of segmental fixation have been developed, which will not be covered here.

BIOMECHANICS

Multiple laboratory studies have proven increased stability of the sublaminar wiring technique over the previous Harrington instrumentation. Wenger, et al. studied 51 instrumented calf spines in vitro; with the single Harrington distraction rod, failure occurred at the metal-bone interface, while with the Luque technique, failure occurred outside the instrumented area (43). Wenger felt that the Luque technique provided a clear mechanical advantage over the traditional Harrington instrumentation, in that the sublaminar wiring provided stability in the frontal, sagittal, and transverse planes (42). Wenger's study also found that the 3/16"-diameter Luque rods would bend at 595 N of compressive loading. This flexibility indicates that these rods would probably not perform satisfactorily for either kyphosis or larger, more rigid curves. These larger curves could cause bending of the rods, either acutely or in follow-up. Clinically, the use of the smaller rod in extensive fusions with larger curves has been associated with significant incidence of rod breakage. Using a biomechanical injury model at the thoracolumbar junction, Panjabi et al. (31) also found that the Luque rods were more stable throughout flexion, extension, and lateral bending than the Harrington distraction system or the Harrington distraction-compression combination.

TECHNIQUE

Exposure

Once the spinous processes, lamina, and transverse processes have been completely cleared of soft tissue, excision of the ligamentum flavum is performed. A double-action rongeur is used to remove the bone overlying the ligamentum flavum in the thoracic spine; the superficial ligamentum flavum is gently removed until the epidural space is visualized. At this point a Penfield dissector may be inserted underneath the ligamentum flavum to protect the underlying dura and epidural vessels. A knife can then safely divide the ligamentum flavum. In order to provide for sufficient exposure for wire passage, the ligamentum flavum is excised with the use of small Kerrison rongeur. As with all techniques of spinal instrumentation, it is important to remember that the chief goal is to obtain a solid arthrodesis through decortication, facet excision, and the use of sufficient bone graft.

Wire Contour and Depth of Wire Penetration

The sublaminar wires are contoured in preparation for passage. Proper wire contour is critical to avoid injury to the underlying spinal cord or nerve roots. The optimal contour for the sublaminar wire obviously minimizes the depth of intraspinal wire penetration. Some authors have advocated a semicircular construct or even a rectangular configuration. Zindrick (49) developed a mathematical model which indicated that a semicircular model resulted in less canal penetration than the rectangular model. He also found that the larger the radius of the circle, the less the penetration into the canal.

Goll et al. (17) videotaped the passage of sublaminar wires to document the depth of wire penetration and came to the following conclusions: (*a*) passage of the sublaminar wire must remain strictly in the midline; (*b*) the tip at the bend of the sublaminar wire should not be at angle greater than 45°; otherwise, this will result in excessive penetration into the canal; (*c*) the radius of the curvature of the semicircular wire must be at least the width of the lamina. They also found that it was not advantageous to remove the osseus portions of the lamina in order to improve ease of passage of the wire. Exposure was, however, facilitated by removal of the spinous processes.

Concern about the presence of the sublaminar wire within the canal and the possibility of late wire breakage and cutting out of the wire through soft bone has led to the occasional use of a merceline tape in order to stabilize the Luque rods. The successful use in five cases was reported by Gaines (14).

Wire Passage and Stabilization

Once the sublaminar wire has been passed, the wire must be stabilized to prevent inadvertent trauma to the cord. A number of methods have been devised to handle the wires after passage, including clamping the ends of wires with hemostats and then threading a Luque rod through the finger loops (7). The method the authors have found most satisfactory is that of Yngve (48). The wire is passed in a caudal to cranial direction (Fig. 6.1). It is most important that the tip of the wire maintain contact with the undersurface of the lamina as the wire is advanced and rotated. An upward force on the wire must be continued throughout passage. If there is any resistance to passage of the sublaminar wire, it is best to gently remove the wire and to readvance it again in the midline position.

Passing a sublaminar wire is a two-handed technique. Once the tip of the wire is visible at the proximal end of the lamina, a large needle holder is used to grab the tip of the wire and gently advance the wire as the distal end of the wire is gently fed and controlled with the opposite hand (Fig. 6.2*A*). Once again, maintaining upward pressure on the wire as it passes through the canal is important to ensure that the wire does not spring back into the canal if the needle holder slips off the tip of the wire.

Once 6–8 cm of the tip of the wire is exposed, the tip of the wire is brought over the lamina, and one strand of the wire is placed on each side of the spinous process. It is contoured closely to the lamina. Once this has been accomplished, then the tails of the wire are brought proximally over the lamina in a cephalad direction and contoured firmly against the lamina. At the proximal end of the lamina, the tails are bent laterally out of the wound

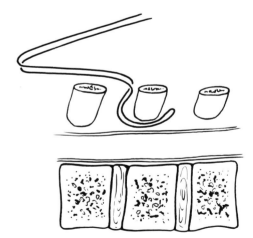

Figure 6.1. The tip of the sublaminar wire must remain in contact with the undersurface of the lamina to avoid injury to the underlying neural elements.

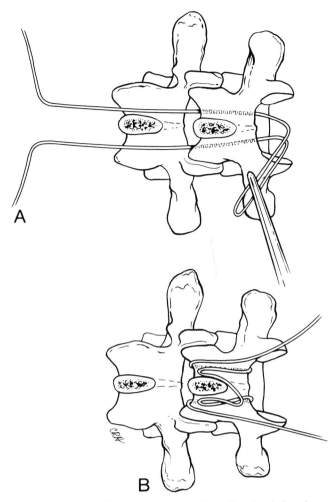

the superior portion is crimped lateral to the inferior wire. This helps stabilize the rod and prevent migration.

Rod Benders

Proper contouring of the rod so that it fits snugly against the lamina in the corrected position is critical. To achieve this, proper instrumentation is critical, particularly when using the Galveston technique wherein there are closely-adjacent bends and the angulation must be quite precise. One must have more than standard three-point plate benders, particularly when dealing with the ¼" rods (3, 35). It is quite helpful to have a bending unit with optional circle pins to change the radius and, therefore, the sharpness of the bend.

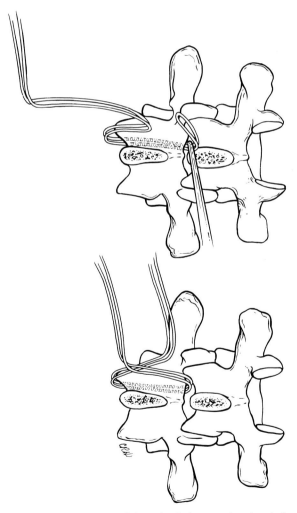

Figure 6.2. *A,* Kocher clamp may be utilized to help advance sublaminar wire. *B,* The tails of the sublaminar wire are brought proximally over the lamina; the tip of the sublaminar wire is brought distally and one strand is placed on each side of the spinous process.

(Fig. 6.2*B*). The doubled wires are also inserted in the same manner, and each end of the wire is bent and twisted about the lamina to prevent the wire from migrating down the canal (Fig. 6.3). For patients who have long, complex curves, particularly when the Galveston technique is utilized, this allows for easy placement of the rod. Once the rod is in place and appropriately contoured, the tips of the wires are cut off, and each end is twisted with its corresponding tail. This is done sequentially until appropriate correction has been achieved. At both the proximal and distal end of the instrumented area, two double wires should be used (Fig. 6.4). Allen and Ferguson (1) have noted that, to provide more secure fixation for the overlapping Luque rods at the end lamina,

Figure 6.3. Each end of the wire is bent and twisted about the lamina to prevent the wire from migrating down the canal.

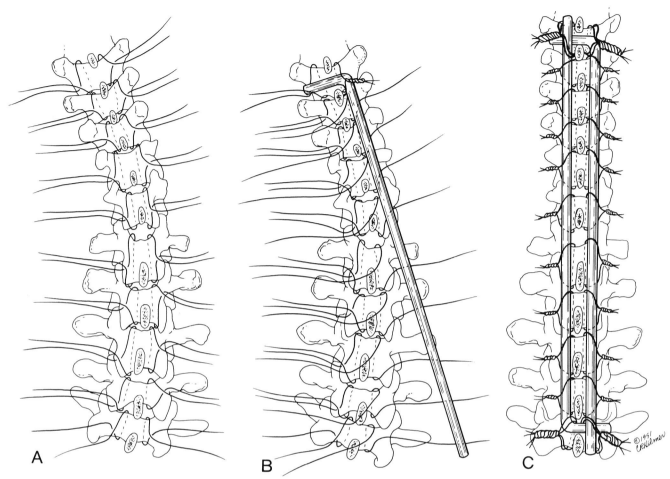

Figure 6.4. *A–C*, Following placement of sublaminar wires, correction can be obtained utilizing the convex technique with the Luque instrumentation.

Curve Correction

Correction of scoliosis with Luque instrumentation can be performed by several methods, including the convex technique and concave technique. The convex technique involves insertion of the Luque rod on the convex side of the curvature, and the correction of the scoliosis by sequential tightening of the wires (Fig. 6.4). After the rod has been placed in the convexity with the short arm of the L rod above the spinous process, the rod is fixed to the most proximal lamina involved in the fusion. Proceeding in a caudal direction, the next four or five lamina are fixed to the rod. The second rod can then be inserted on the concave side of the curve with the short arm of the L rod distal to the spinous process to be fused. Proceeding in a proximal direction, the concave rod is fixed to the next four or five lamina. The rods can then be levered in a parallel fashion to achieve correction of the curve, and the remaining sublaminar wires tightened against the rods. The convex technique is most useful in standard-type thoracic scoliosis when there is not significant thoracic lordosis present. This technique is also simpler to contour the appropriate lumbar lordosis.

On the other hand, in patients who have a significant lumbar curve, the concave technique is generally more appropriate. The concave technique is also more useful in thoracic scoliosis associated with significant thoracic lordosis. Severe deformities are also best corrected with the concave technique. With either technique, as one tightens down the wires, one must securely fix the end of the Luque rod, as significant rotatory forces may be applied to the implant. Rotation of the rod may lead to a loss of correction or even rotation of the rod tip toward the epidural space. After the rods have been fixed securely in place, the wires can be trimmed; they should be trimmed the length of at least 1 cm and then bent towards the midline.

Before cutting and bending the wires towards the midline, each wire should be checked carefully to ensure that it is not loose. Quite often tightening the wires two or three times is required to ensure a snug fit. One must observe the wire quite closely when tightening to avoid breakage. With both the convex and concave techniques, the amount of desired correction is what can be obtained from manually.

Crosslinkage

The L-shaped rod was designed to help prevent migration or rotation of the rod. Nonetheless, this can occur in spite of the L shape; rod migration can lead to painful prominence beneath the skin or even erosion through the skin. There can be loss of fixation with corresponding loss of correction. To inhibit this, the use of locking collar was described by McCarthy (27). The authors have found the crosslink system of the Texas Scottish Rite system to be very satisfactory in preventing rod migration and rotation.

Fusion to the Pelvis

The most popular method for achieving pelvic fixation is the method developed in Galveston by Allen and Fer-

guson (1). This is described as the triangular base, transverse bar configuration. Stabilization of the pelvis is achieved by driving a segment of the rod into each ilium (Fig. 6.5A–C). To accomplish this, both posterior iliac crests are exposed from the midline incision, roughly at the level of the posterior-superior iliac spine. The posterior iliac crests are exposed and followed by identification of the sciatic notch. Just proximal to the sciatic notch is the area that will provide the most satisfactory fixation (Fig. 6.6 A–C). A large, smooth Steinmann pin, corresponding to the size of the chosen rod, is then used to create a tunnel for the rod. Ideally, the amount of purchase in the ilium should be at least 6 cm (if the patient's size allows this). The pin can then be removed, and a malleable template can be used to aid in the contouring of the Luque rod. In patients with spina bifida or severe cerebral palsy, where the pelvis may be small and the ilium quite thin, another technique for achieving stabilization to the sacrum has been described by Dunn and McCarthy (26). In this technique, the patients' radiographs are used to make several sharply angulated curves

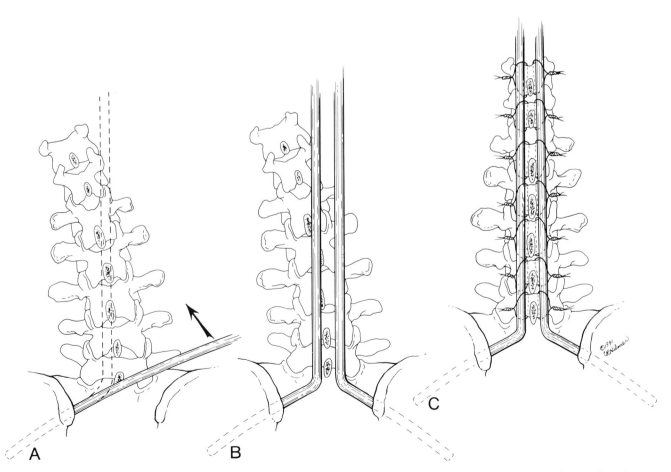

Figure 6.5. *A–C,* Galveston technique of triangular base transverse bar configuration to stabilize the pelvis to the spine.

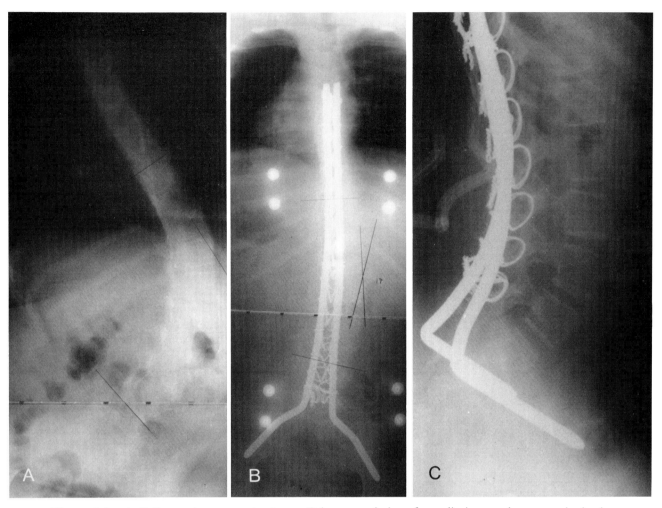

Figure 6.6. *A–C,* Pre- and postoperative Luque Galveston technique for scoliosis secondary to cerebral palsy.

preoperatively within the rod to contour over the top of the sacral ala. By this method, one can avoid placing the Luque rod through the iliac wing, and also avoid placing the rod across the sacroiliac joint. In patients who have instrumentation to the pelvis, rod breakage may occur distally even in the presence of a satisfactory lumbosacral fusion, as there is still motion at the sacroiliac joint.

Unit Rod

To avoid the difficulties in contouring in the appropriate thoracic kyphosis, lumbar lordosis, and appropriate pelvic shape from the Galveston technique, one can utilize a unit rod, wherein all the appropriate contours are already present (25). If necessary, minor modifications can be made in the frontal or sagittal contour. The unit rod is an excellent technique for correcting pelvic obliquity while maintaining lumbar lordosis (thereby avoiding

pressure concentrations over the ischiae, leading to ulcer) (10). With the use of the precontoured unit rod, it can be inserted into the pelvis securely between the inner and outer walls of the ilium. Once this is firmly seated, the proximal end of the rod can be used as a "rudder" to bring the distal end of the rod to the spine (Fig. 6.7). The most distal sublaminar wire is tightened. Tightening of the wires is then performed from a distal to a proximal direction. In this method, great correction can be achieved (Fig. 6.8*A–C*). Rinsky et al. found that the use of these unit rods helped to achieve greater correction as compared with a standard, double-rod technique (36).

Postoperative Immobilization

Luque initially felt that the use of the Luque instrumentation itself was sufficiently stable to avoid the need for postoperative immobilization. The authors feel that a

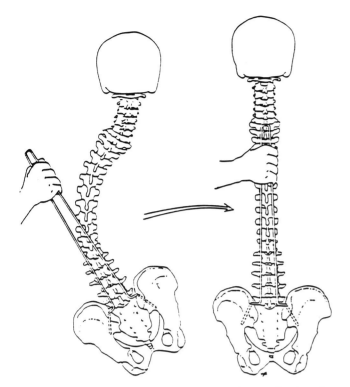

Figure 6.7.   Correction achieved through use of unit rod.

patient with severe curves, osteoporosis, spasticity, etc. should have postoperative immobilization for 4–6 months to prevent cutout with loss of correction, broken rods, and pseudarthrosis.

Instrumentation without Fusion

Segmental spinal instrumentation with the use of sublaminar wiring without fusion has been used in young neuromuscular patients in order to control the scoliosis and allow for further spinal growth. With this technique, neither the facet joints nor the transverse processes is exposed, and only the central portion of the ligamentum flavum is removed. In theory, this would correct and stabilize the scoliosis, and allow further spinal growth. In practice, however, the results with this technique have been discouraging (34). There has been a very high loss of intraoperative correction, less than impressive spinal growth, and a very high rate of instrumentation failure. It can be quite difficult to convert these cases to achieve satisfactory fusion due to technical problems; with the instrumentation in place, exposure of sufficient bone for arthrodesis is compromised.

Removal of Sublaminar Wires

Occasionally, these sublaminar wires must be removed for various reasons including sepsis, implant failure, spinal cord compromise, or pain. Once the sublaminar wire has been cut, great care must be taken upon its removal to prevent its sharp point from causing a dural laceration or trauma to the cord itself. Gaines reported a technique that he used to remove 100 sublaminar wires that had been in place for 22 months (30). With his technique, the wires are cut at the level of the fusion mass, and the opposite end of the wire is grasped by a heavy needle holder. The wire is then carefully rolled about the tip of the needle holder. Gastreau (29a), however, studied several techniques for extraction of sublaminar wires and evaluated these techniques with cineradiography. In his study, the roll-up technique caused the most erratic course of the wire within the spinal canal and occasionally went completely across the diameter of the spinal canal. Less dural compression occurred when the wire was extracted with an attempt made to keep it parallel with the lamina. When double wires are present, they should be removed independently. If they are removed simultaneously, they can assume independent pathways in an unpredictable fashion.

COMPLICATIONS

Neurologic Deficit

Neurologic loss can occur from direct trauma to the cord or nerve roots or from overcorrection. Wilber et al. (44) reviewed 49 patients who had Harrington rod instrumentation with sublaminar wiring and 20 patients who had the Luque rod instrumentation with sublaminar wiring. They noted neurologic changes in 17% of this patient group: 4% had a major spinal cord injury, and 13% had a transient sensory dysaesthesis. Forty-one percent of these patients had abnormal intraoperative somatosensory evoked potentials. Most cases of neurologic deficit tend to occur early in the "learning curve." The rate of neurologic deficit in this series is significantly higher than many others. More recently, however, multiple studies have reported the use of Luque instrumentation with no cases of neurologic loss (4,8,9,12,16,18,19,28,36, 39,45).

Neurologic deficit sometimes occurs acutely in the operating room, but it can also develop in a delayed fashion. Johnston (20) reported two cases of delayed paraplegia developing in patients who had an anterior release followed by second-stage posterior fusion with sublaminar wiring. If there is a significant kyphosis, this may narrow the spinal canal, and any edema occurring within the spinal cord can cause progressive neural loss. In patients with severe deformity and/or significant kyphosis, it may be best to attempt to preserve as many segmental vessels as possible to prevent the development of ischemic changes. If the segmental vessels are to be sacrificed, one may wish

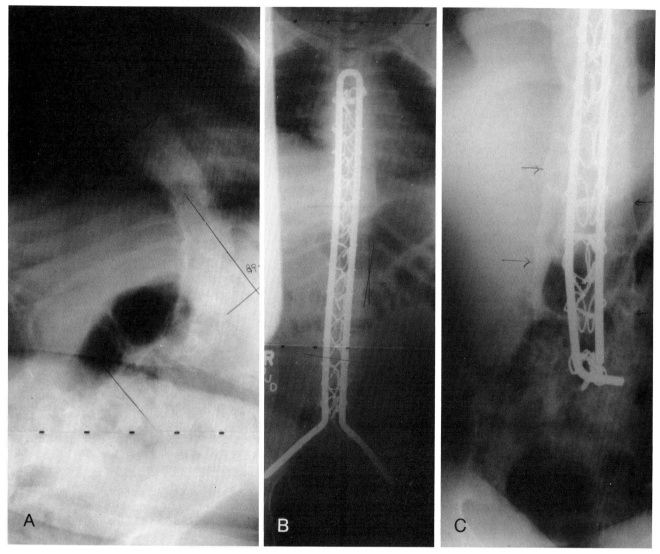

Figure 6.8. *A* and *B*, Pre- and postoperative anterior release, posterior spinal fusion with unit rod technique for rigid po- liomyelitic curve. *C*, Fusion to transverse process using auto- graft supplemented with allograft femoral head.

to first clamp them before transecting the vessels and observe the changes on the evoked potential monitor before proceeding.

Neurologic deficit may occur months to years later in cases of wire breakage (2). Corrosion also can occur at the junction between the sublaminar wire and the Luque rod, and repeated cyclical loading may ultimately lead to failure (32). One should avoid any kinking in the wire, as this will decrease its breaking strength significantly. Breakage is most likely occur at either end of the Luque rod construct.

The authors feel that the use of intraoperative soma- tosensory evoked potentials is helpful even in cases of neuromuscular deficit, only to ensure preservation of ad- equate bowel or bladder function. It is well known that the evoked potentials are not foolproof, and cases of par- aplegia have been reported in the face of normal intra- operative somatosensory evoked potentials (40). In addition, the evoked potential wave form may be affected by various factors, including blood pressure, temperature, etc. The patient who has a satisfactory intelligence and good motor control of the lower extremities should also have a wake-up test.

SURGICAL RESULTS

The successful use of Luque rod instrumentation in neu- romuscular scolisis has been reported by multiple groups.

Ferguson (12) reported on staged anterior release and fusion followed by second stage posterior Luque rod instrumentation and fusion. He found very satisfactory correction of the scoliosis and pelvic obliquity. Reviewing his cases and comparing them with other cases treated by an anterior Zielke, followed by posterior instrumentation and fusion, he concluded that the Zielke cases did not obtain more correction than those treated with simple anterior release and posterior instrumentation. Ferguson also noted that the anterior release improved the correctability of scoliosis significantly and that the anterior

instrumentation should not be used to force correction of the curve. Broom and Banta (6) reported on a group of 74 patients with neuromuscular scoliosis whose preoperative mean curve magnitude was 73° and corrected postoperatively to a mean of 38°. He found that in 25% of their patients where the fusion ended at the level of the 4th thoracic vertebra or distal to this, a progressive kyphosis developed proximal to the instrumented area. In one case, this led to a spastic parasesis over time. Broom and others noted that intraoperatively, there is a tendency to underestimate the amount of contouring that

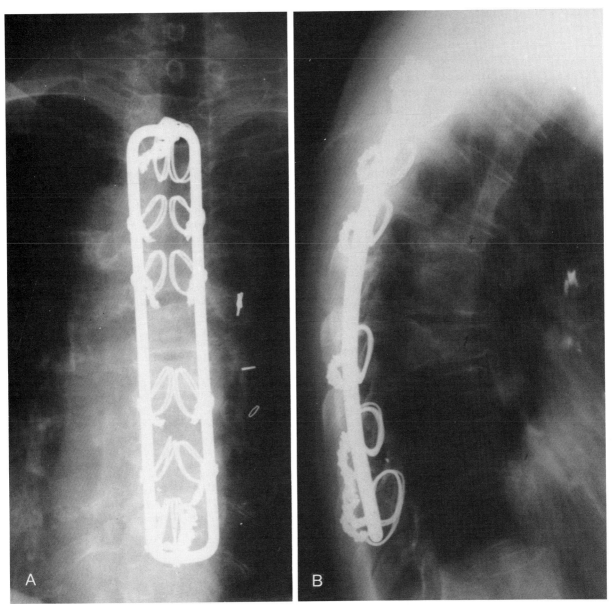

Figure 6.9. *A,* Postoperative anteroposterior and *B,* lateral roentgenograms of thoracic spine of a patient who underwent T3-T9 stabilization with boxed Luque rod and sublaminar wires after posterolateral decompression of metastatic tumor.

must be placed in the rod in order to preserve satisfactory lumbar lordosis. When the smaller $\frac{3}{16}''$-rods are utilized, they may lose correction due to their flexibility during the tightening process. In addition, when the patient is placed on the frame with the hips and the knees flexed, this may also diminish the amount of lumbar lordosis. The use of the smaller rod may allow for some bending to occur within the rod before fusion occurs.

Multiple authors, including Herndon (18), Ferguson (12), Swank (39), and Rinsky (36) noted a general trend toward increased use of anterior release and fusion without instrumentation prior to posterior fusion and instrumentation with the Luque rod.

The addition of sublaminar wiring to Harrington rod instrumentation successfully corrects thoracic lordosis or kyphosis (37,45,46,47). In a series comparing two comparable groups undergoing surgical treatment for idiopathic scoliosis (41), the results of the signal Harrington distraction rod with sublaminar wiring were compared with the single Harrington distraction rod with spinous process wiring. Both groups were found to have similar immediate postoperative correction and follow-up correction. The sublaminar wiring group was found to be more successful in correcting thoracic lordosis. Winter reported two cases of neurofibromatosis with significant thoracic lordosis treated successfully with Harrington rod instrumentation and sublaminar wiring (46). The use of sublaminar wiring in idiopathic scoliosis has decreased significantly, particularly with the success of Cotrel-Dubousset instrumentation in achieving normal thoracic contour (13). Luque instrumentation is used today primarily for neuromuscular scoliosis.

Since the principal use for Luque instrumentation is currently in patients with neuromuscular scoliosis, preoperative evaluation must be thorough to minimize the incidence of intraoperative and postoperative complications. First, one must be sure of the diagnosis in order to assess the risks vs. the benefits of a procedure of this magnitude. (It certainly becomes more questionable in a patient with a very rapidly progressive neurodegenerative process.) The pulmonary function is diminished in a great variety of neuromuscular diseases (29). Patients with very diminished ventilatory capacities may have great difficulty being weaned from the ventilator. Special attention must be paid to those patients with potential cardiomyopathy. Many patients with severe neurologic disorders are cachectic and in poor nutritional status. Drvaric and Roberts (11) found that most of the complications in a large series of cerebral palsy patients who underwent spinal fusion occurred in patients who had uncorrected gastroesophageal or nutritional abnormalities. A Nissen fundoplication and feeding via a gastrostomy tube may be required before the definitive spinal procedure. Predonation of

autologous blood and the use of the Cell-saver should be routine in most cases to minimize transfusion (5, 24). Use of bone bank bone via frozen femoral heads helps provide sufficient bone to ensure a satisfactory fusion.

Luque instrumentation with sublaminar wiring has also been applied to other problems such as fracture dislocations and tumors (Fig. 6.9A and B). Luque rods do not provide adequate resistance against axial loading and should be avoided in axial loading type or burst fractures. Luque rods provide good fixation for translational or shear-type injuries. Stabilization after decompression of the thoracolumbar spine in patients with neoplasms may also be done with Luque instrumentation (12a). When applying Luque rods for these problems, the surgeon should stabilize at least "three above and three below" the site of instability. The "boxed" configuration provides a better stability and is preferred over double L rods in these cases. Recently, the Cotrel-Dubousset system has lessened the use of Luque instrumentation with sublaminar wires; however, the Luque system still remains a good alternative if used in a proper setting.

REFERENCES

1. Allen B Jr, Ferguson R: L-rod instrumentation for scoliosis in cerebral palsy. J Ped Orthop 1982;2:87–96.
2. Bernard T Jr, Johnston C, Roberts J, et al: Late complications due to wire breakage in segmental spinal instrumentation. J Bone Joint Surg 1983;65A:1339–1344.
3. Black F, Rajan K, Armstrong G, et al: Rod bender for Luque instrumentation. Spine 1984;9:837–838.
4. Boachie-Adjel O, Lonstein J, Winter R, et al: Management of neuromuscular spinal deformities with Luque segmentation instrumentation. J Bone Joint Surg 1989;71A:548–562.
5. Borghi B, Binazzi R: Autotransfusion with intraoperative and postoperative blood recovery in posterior spine fusion. Paper #53 presented at Scoliosis Research Society Meeting.
6. Broom M, Banta J, Renshaw T: Spinal fusion augmented by Luque-rod instrumentation for neuromuscular scoliosis. J Bone Joint Surg 1989;71A:32–44.
7. Crawford A, Kiefhaber T, Crawford A Jr: Inoperative restraint for Luque wires. Spine 1984;9:96–97.
8. Daher Y, Lonstein J, Winter R, et al: Spinal deformities in patients with Charcot-Marie-Tooth disease. Clin Orthop Rel Res 1986; 202:219–222.
9. Daher Y, Lonstein J, Winter R, et al: Spinal surgery in spinal muscular atrophy. J Ped Orthop 1985;5:391–395.
10. Drummond D, Breed A, Narechania R: Relationship of spine deformity and pelvic obliquity on sitting pressure distributions and decubitus ulceration. J Ped Orthop 1985;5:396–402.
11. Drvaric D, Roberts J, Burke S, King A, Falterman K: Gastroesophageal evaluation in totally involved cerebral palsy patients. J Ped Orthop 1987;7:187–190.
12. Ferguson, R., Allen, B. Jr.: Staged correction of neuromuscular scoliosis. J Ped Orthop 1983;3:555–562.
12a. Flately TJ, Anderson MM, Anast GT: Spinal instability due to malignant disease. J Bone Joint Surg 1984;65A:47–52.
13. Fritch R, Turi M, Bowman B, et al: Comparison of Cotrel-Du-

bousett and Harrington rod instrumentation in idiopathic scoliosis. J Ped Orthop 1990;10:44–47.

14. Gaines R Jr, Abernathie D: Merseline tapes as a substitute for wire in segmental spinal instrumentation for children. Spine 1986;11:907–913.

15. Geremia G, Kim K, Cerullo L, et al: Complications of sublaminar wiring. Surg Neurol 1985;23:629–634.

16. Gershoff W, Renshaw T: The treatment of scoliosis in cerebral palsy by posterior spinal fusion with Luque-rod segmental instrumentation. J Bone Joint Surg 1988;70-A:41–44.

17. Goll S, Balderston R, Stambough J, et al: Depth of intraspinal wire penetration during passage of sublaminar wires. Spine 1988;13:503–509.

18. Herndon W, Sullivan A, Yngve D, et al: Segmental spinal instrumentation with sublaminar wires. J Bone Joint Surg 1987;69-A:851–859.

19. Harrington J, Wenger D: Segmental spinal instrumentation: a preliminary report of 40 consecutive cases. Spine 1982;7:285–298.

20. Johnston C, Happel L Jr, Norris R, et al: Delayed paraplegia complicating sublaminar segmental spinal fusion. J Bone Joint Surg 1986;68A:556–563.

21. Lange F: Support for the spondylitic spine by means of buried steel bars attached to the vertebrae. Am J Ortho Surg 1910;8:344–361.

22. Luque E: Segmental spinal instrumentation for correction of scoliosis. Clin Orthop Rel Res 1982;163:192–198.

23. Luque E: The anatomic basis and development of segmental spinal instrumentation. Spine 1982;7:256–259.

24. MacEwen D, Bennett E, Guille J: Autologous blood transfusions in children and young adults with low body weight undergoing spinal surgery. J Ped Orthop 1990;10:750–753.

25. Maloney W, Rinsky L, Gamble J: Simultaneous correction of pelvic obliquity, frontal plane, and sagittal plane deformities in neuromuscular scoliosis using a unit rod with segmental sublaminar wires: a preliminary report. J Ped Orthop 1990;10:742–749.

26. McCarthy R, Dunn H, McCullough F: Luque fixation to the sacral all using the Dunn-McCarthy modification. Spine 1989;14:281–283.

27. McCarthy R, McCullough F, Peek R, et al: A locking collar for Luque rods. Orthopaedics 1988;11:921–926.

28. Mielke C, Lonstein J, Denis F, et al: Surgical treatment of adolescent idiopathic scoliosis. J Bone Joint Surg 1989;71A:1170–1177.

29. Miller F, Moseley C, Koreska J, et al: Pulmonary function and scoliosis in Duchenne dystrophy. J Ped Orthop 1988;8:133–137.

29a. Nicastro JF, Hartjen CA, Traina J, et al: Intraspinal pathways taken by sublaminar wires during removal. J Bone Joint Surg 1986;68A:1206.

30. Ogilvie JW, Miller EA: Comparison of segmental spinal instrumentation devices in the correction of scoliosis. Spine 1983;8:416–419.

31. Panjabi M, Abumi K, Duranceau J, Crisco J: Biomechanical evaluation of spinal fixation devices: II. Stability provided by eight internal fixation devices. Spine 1988;13:1135–1140.

32. Prikryl M, Srivastava S, Viviani G, et al: Role of corrosion in Harrington and Luque rods failure. Biomaterials 1989;10:109–117.

33. Resina J, Alves A: A technique for correction and internal fixation for scoliosis. J Bone Joint Surg 1977;59 2:159–165.

34. Rinsky L, Gamble J, Bleck E: Segmental instrumentation without fusion in children with progressive scoliosis. J Ped Orthop 1985;5:687–690.

35. Rinsky L, Gamble J: A new bending device for Luque rods. Spine 1986;11:52–54.

36. Rinsky L: Surgery of spinal deformity in cerebral palsy. Clin Orthop Rel Res 1990;253:100–109.

37. Silverman B, Greenbarg P: Idiopathic scoliosis posterior spine fusion with Harrington rod and sublaminar wiring. Orthop Clin NA 1988;19:269–279.

38. Stephen J, Bodel J: Luque rod fixation in meningomyelocele kyphosis: A preliminary report. Aust NZ J Surg 1983;53:473–477.

39. Swank S, Lonstein JE, Moe JM, et al: Surgical treatment of adult scoliosis. J Bone Joint Surg 1981;63A:268–287.

40. Szalaly E, Carollo J, Roach J: Sensitivity of spinal cord monitoring to intraoperative events. J Ped Orthop 1986;6:437–441.

41. Thometz J, Emans J: A comparison between spinous process and sublaminar wiring combined with Harrington distraction instrumentation in the management of adolescent idiopathic scoliosis. J Ped Orthop 1988;8:129–132.

42. Wenger D, Carollo J, Wilkerson J Jr: Biomechanics of scoliosis correction by segmental spinal instrumentation. Spine 1982;7:260–264.

43. Wenger D, Carollo J, Wilkerson J Jr, et al: Laboratory testing of segmental spinal instrumentation versus traditional Harrington instrumentation for scoliosis treatment. Spine 1982;7:265–269.

44. Wilber R, Thompson G, Shaffer J, et al: Postoperative neurological deficits in segmental spinal instrumentation. J Bone Joint Surg 1984;66A:1178–1187.

45. Winter R, Lonstein J: Adult idiopathic scoliosis treated with Luque or Harrington rods and sublaminar wiring. J Bone Joint Surg 1989;71A:1308–1313.

46. Winter R: Thoracic lordosis in neurofibromatosis: Treatment by a Harrington rod with sublaminar wiring. J Bone Joint Surg 1984;66A:1102–1106.

47. Winter R: Thoracic lordoscoliosis in Marfan's syndrome. Spine 1990;15:233–235.

48. Yngve D, Burke S, Price C, Riddick M: Sublaminar wiring. J Ped Orthop 1986;6:605–608.

49. Zindrick MR, Knight GW, Bunch WH, et al: Factors influencing the penetration of wires into the neural canal during segmental wiring. J Bone Joint Surg 1989;71A:742–750.

SEVEN

Segmental Spinal Instrumentation with Spinous Process Wires

Denis S. Drummond

INTRODUCTION

Segmental spinal instrumentation with spinous process wires was developed for patients with idiopathic scoliosis as a safer alternative to instrumentation with sublaminar wires (1, 10). Our system evolved with three basic concepts. The first was to provide the stability afforded by segmental spinal instrumentation by applying an implant at every level of the instrumented spine. Second, this should be accomplished with maximum safety. To this end, we particularly wished to avoid the placement of sublaminar wires (7–9,16). Our final goal was to produce a technique that was easy to execute, while versatile enough to manage a wide variety of surgical problems. We proposed to accomplish this by a new technique, but with implants that were, for the most part, already available.

THEORETICAL CONSIDERATIONS

When we first developed our system, the two principal methods of correction available employed different applications of force. With Harrington instrumentation, forces are applied in a vertical direction, correcting by either distraction or compression. In contrast, the Luque system corrects with cantilever forces, which are horizontally directed. Theoretically, vertical forces are most efficient for the correction of large curves (greater than 40°), whereas horizontal forces are best for smaller curves (15).

THE IMPLANTS

We proposed to develop a system that combined the best of both existing systems. Accordingly, we decided to use a construct combining Harrington distraction and Luque segmental spinal instrumentation with the 316 L rod.

We began by selecting the base of the spinous process as the site for segmental purchase to the spine because it is readily available, easy to instrument, and there is usually adequate bond stock. Also, the spinous process had previously been used successfully for spinal fixation (12,13). We proposed to develop an implant that would provide more secure fixation with better load sharing than wiring alone. To this end, we developed a simple button-wire implant made of 316 L stainless steel (Fig. 7.1). The button plate is 8 mm in diameter and .8 mm thick. The wire is 18-gauge, attached to the plate and suaged at one end to form a smooth bead. This accomplishes a smooth passage for the wire through the bone at the base of the spinous process. Additionally, it prevents penetration of the surgical gloves. Because the implants are inserted in pairs, there is a hole in the button that allows the bead of one implant to pass through the other. In this way, two stable attachments are gained at each spinous process.

The implant is inserted at the base of the spinous process through a passage created ventral enough to pass through good bone stock but dorsal enough to avoid penetrating the spinal canal (Fig. 7.2). The preparation of the passage is shown in Figure 7.3. The rest of the instruments are readily available and include standard rod benders used to provide appropriate contours to the rod and wire twisters that secure the wires. Because the technique provides segmental fixation from the base of the spinous process, we call it interspinous segmental spinal instrumentation (ISSI).

SURGICAL TECHNIQUE

Autogenous bone graft for the spinal arthrodesis is harvested from the iliac crest and that wound closed. A standard subperiosteal approach is then made to the spine through a midline exposure. On the side of the concavity

Figure 7.1. The implant: A hole in the button plate accepts the beaded wire of the opposite paired implant.

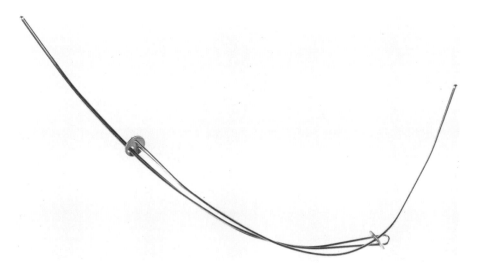

of the curve, the hook sites are prepared at the uppermost and lowest segmental levels selected for instrumentation. The upper level is prepared for a Harrington bifid (pedicular) hook by an osteotomy of the inferior articular facet. There are two bifid hooks, a sharp starter hook which cuts the path along the superior facet surface to

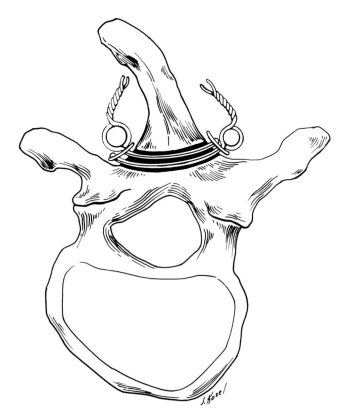

Figure 7.2. Depth of passage of implants through base of spinous process.

the pedicle. The blunt bifid hood can then be implanted into a stable position with the two limbs of the shoe of the hook surrounding the pedicle (Fig. 7.4).

The lower hook site is prepared by laminotomy and an André (anatomical) hook is inserted. The shoe of the Andre hook is designed to conform to the shape of the lumbar lamina so that its purchase becomes more stable as distraction forces are applied. At this time, it is convenient to complete the facet fusion, particularly in a small spine where prior placement of the button-wire implants could interfere with access to the facets.

With the completion of the facet arthrodesis, the implants are inserted at the base of the spinous process of each vertebra to be instrumented. The passage at the base of the process is prepared as outlined above (Figs. 7.2 and 7.3). Two implants are then passed at each level in opposite directions so that they share the loads imparted to the base of the spinous process. The only exception to this is at both ends of the instrumentation, where only one implant is inserted. This is directed from the concave to the convex side of the curve.

After all the button-wire implants are in place, a Moe modified Harrington distraction rod contoured to provide physiologic sagittal contours and loaded with two Texas Scottish Rite Hospital (TSRH) l-bolts is inserted by passing the rod through the open loops of wire and into the previously placed hooks. Gentle corrective distraction is then applied.

Following distraction, a malleable template is pressed against the convexity. This is a helpful guide to the contouring of the ³/₁₆ Luque rod. The L rod is also shaped to ensure an appropriate sagittal contour. Both ends of the rod are then bent at a right angle to its long axis to form a "C" shape so that the ends of the Luque rod will span the distraction hooks. The Luque rod, preloaded

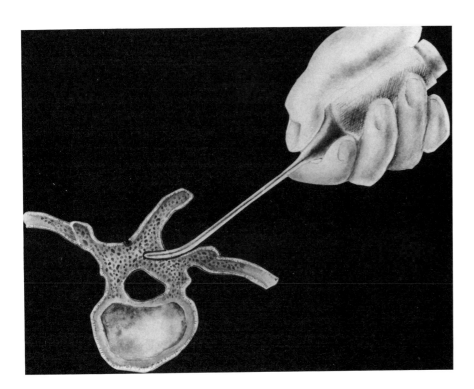

Figure 7.3. Preparation of the passage with curved awls.

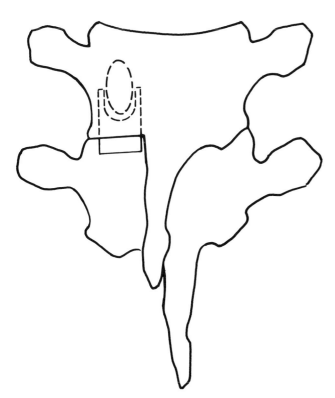

Figure 7.4. Preparation of the site for the bifid (pedicular) hook.

with two TSRH l-bolts, is then ready for insertion. This is accomplished by passing it through the open loops of the wires lying on the convexity and placing the short proximal limb of the rod under the ratchet part of the Harrington rod lying immediately superior and adjacent to the bifid (proximal) hook. The distal short limb should lie caudal and adjacent to the Andre hook (Figs. 7.5 and 7.6). The rod should then be pressed firmly against the spine with rod pushers and at each level fixed by twisting the wire. As with the distraction rod, correction should be achieved by pushing the rod firmly against the spine with the rod pusher and not by only twisting the wires, which can lead to wire breakage. To complete the instrumentation, any loose wires around the distraction rod are then twisted in order to segmentally secure this rod. It is important to apply the twist symmetrically to provide the strongest fixation with the least risk for fatigue failure of the wires (5).

The operation is completed by linking the rods together. We formerly wired them together. We now prefer to use the TSRH cross-link system (Fig. 7.7). The TSRH l-bolts, which were previously attached to both rods, are now fixed to the cross-plates with nuts using a torque wrench. We have found that the addition of the cross-link has added an increased stability to our procedure. Prior to closure, a C-clamp is applied to the ratchet section of the distraction rod adjacent to the upper hook and the rest of the bone graft is added.

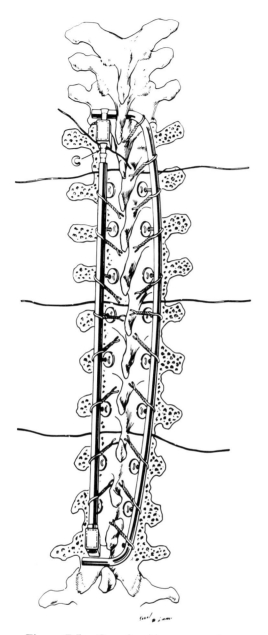

Figure 7.5. Completed instrumentation.

The postoperative regimen for most patients with idiopathic scoliosis is based on our biomechanical studies, which appear to demonstrate that the system provides enough stability that external support is not needed. Accordingly, most patients are encouraged to be walking brace-free by the third postoperative day and are discharged, on average, by the sixth day (6). They are allowed to return to school 3 weeks after their operation. Limited activities and long walks are allowed up until the first postoperative visit at 6 weeks. At this time, if the patient is free of pain and there has not been a significant loss of the correction achieved at surgery, activities such as jogging, bicycling, and lap swimming (without diving) can be permitted. Recreational sports such as tennis can be added at 6 months after surgery, and competitive or varsity sports at 1 year.

Exceptions to this brace-free regimen are made for problematic patients such as those with osteopenic spines. Also, because forces are high near the lumbosacral junction and because a greater risk for dislodgement exists for purchase sites placed at or below L4 (3), I advise the use of an orthosis when patients are instrumented to L4 or lower.

TECHNIQUE MODIFICATIONS

1. Thoracic Lordosis. When a thoracic lordosis or a significant hypokyphosis exists and appears to be the most problematic deformity, I advise that, prior to applying distraction to the curve, the wire loops around the Harrington rod at the apex of the curve be twisted. By tightening these first, the principal correction forces are applied to overcome the sagittal deformity rather than the scoliosis. Although this may compromise the frontal correction to some degree, it is usually not significant. Overall, this modification appears to give the best cosmetic and functional result for these patients.

2. Double Curves. The technique for double major curves is similar to that described above. The construct differs in that the distraction rod spans the concavity of both curves in a dollar-sign configuration. Also, the two Luque rods placed on the convex surfaces should overlap each other by at least two segmental levels to avoid stress loading the transition zone between the curves (Fig. 7.8).

3. Rigid Curves. For large and rigid curves, we have modified the technique by inserting two distraction rods into the concavity of the major curve. A small distraction rod is placed at the apex, and another spans the entire concavity. During distraction, each is alternatively tightened until both are snug. This maneuver provides load sharing between the four hooks and two rods and thus allow a more aggressive correction.

4. Spina Bifida. The implant has also proved to be very useful for the instrumentation of the dysplastic segment of spine deformities associated with myelomeningocele. My personal choice of technique for this problem is a standard sublaminar Luque instrumentation for the normally formed segments, modified by the button-wire implant, which is used to fix the bifid segments. After carefully dissecting the dural sac from the inner surface of the dysplastic pedicles, the implant is inserted from

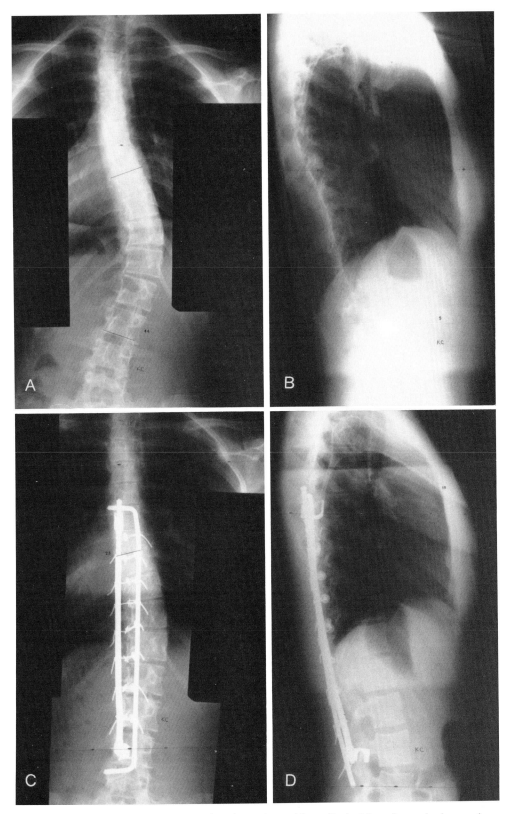

Figure 7.6. Pre- and postoperative radiographs of a patient with scoliosis. Note the sagittal curve improvement.

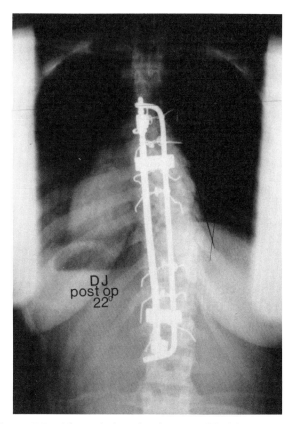

Figure 7.7. The technique has been modified by the use of TSRH cross-links.

within so that the button lies against the inner surface of the bifid defect. The beaded wire loops can then be opened to accept the rods which have been contoured to conform to the outer surface of the defect (Fig. 7.9).

5. Cervical Arthrodesis. Recent experience with the button-wire implant to help stabilize the spine when performing cervical arthrodesis has been rewarding. The implant, when inserted as a pair at the base of the spinous process, has an excellent purchase. I have used this method with intersegmental arthrodesis of the cervical spine and for occipitocervical fusions. Typically, with this latter technique, two implants are inserted at the base of the C2 spinous process and fastened over a corticocancellous autograft to two wires fixed to the occiput through burr holes. We have reviewed 10 consecutive cases so treated and have obtained successful fusion in all.

RESULTS

Laboratory Testing. The results of biochemical testing of the implant and the technique are reported in

detail elsewhere (2). Essentially, we have shown that the spinous process is thick enough to act as an adequate purchase for spinal instrumentation. Further, the implant increases the strength of fixation to the spinous process over wire alone by 48%. Although making the button even thicker stronger achieves fixation, experience has shown that this is unnecessary. Also, the bulkier implant would be difficult to work

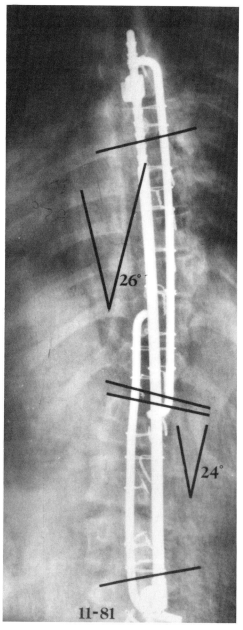

Figure 7.8. The construct used for double major curves. Note the two Luque rods overlap each other by at least two segmental levels.

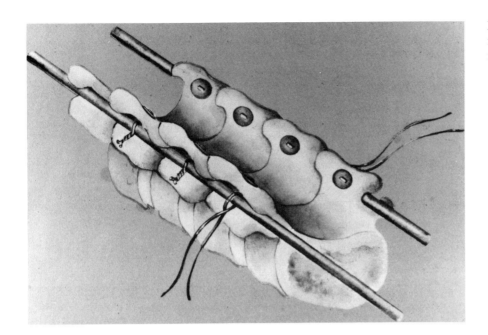

Figure 7.9. This construct is used for rigid curves. It provides load sharing during distraction.

with because it would conform poorly to the base of the spinous process.

ISSI has been tested on a scoliosis simulator and compared with Harrington distraction, Harrington distraction and compression with transverse approximation, and Luque instrumentation with sublaminar wires. The ISSI instrumented spines withstood compressive forces as well or better than the other systems tested to failure.

Clinical Results. We reviewed the first 110 patients with idiopathic scoliosis consecutively treated with ISSI and followed them for a minimum of 2 years (11). The average postoperative correction was 58% for both children and adults. The average loss of correction was 2%. Complications included one deep and one superficial infection, five broken wires in four patients, and one patient with dysesthesia, which resolved without permanent sequelae within 1 week. There were no other neurologic complications, rod failures, or pseudoarthroses observed.

Sagittal Deformity. Because flattening of already abnormal sagittal contours has been reported following distraction instrumentation in patients with idiopathic scoliosis, we have carefully shaped the rods to allow for physiological thoracic kyphosis and lumbar lordosis prior to inserting them. This is done to avoid thoracic hypokyphosis and lumbar flat back. The former deformity is associated with diminished pulmonary function (17) and the latter with disabling back pain (4). Further, because we were concerned that we

may have caused these sequelae in our patients, we reviewed the 110 patients described earlier and found that we had successfully prevented a deterioration of the sagittal contours. Preoperatively, the average kyphosis was 34° and reduced to 32° postoperatively. Also, these data included two patients with kyphosing scoliosis where we contoured the rods to reduce the kyphosis. The average lumbar lordosis was changed following surgery from 45° to 42.5°. When only the 77 children in the series were considered, the kyphosis was increased an average of 4°. In a smaller subgroup of patients, where a special effort was made to correct hypokyphosis by tightening the wires to the distraction rod near the apex of the curve prior to applying distraction, there was an improvement in the sagittal curve by an average of 10°. We concluded from this study that with careful contouring of the rod, the sagittal contours can be preserved. Further, with supple hypokyphotic spines, some improvement of this deformity can be achieved.

Neuromuscular Scoliosis. We have also found our technique helpful for managing scoliosis associated with cerebral palsy (14). We reviewed 34 institutionalized patients with spastic quadriplegia and severe scoliosis, managed by ISSI with Galveston type fixation to the pelvis (1). The average curve prior to ISSI was 82° and the average correction achieved was 51%. Also, despite the lack of external fixation for most patients, the average loss of correction was only 5°.

SUMMARY AND CONCLUSIONS

ISSI, in our hands, has proved to be an effective method of treating idiopathic scoliosis. It is safe, relatively easy to master, and provides a predictable result. This includes close to 60% correction, little loss of correction with time, protection of the sagittal contours, and few complications. In addition, the technique has proved to be versatile and applicable to a variety of surgical problems.

REFERENCES

1. Allen BL, Ferguson RL: The Galveston technique for L-rod instrumentation. Spine 1982;7:276–84.
2. Drummond DS, Guadagni J, Keene JS, et al: Interspinous process segmental spinal instrumentation. J Pediatr Orthop 1984;4:397–404.
3. Edwards LL, York JJ, Levin AM, et al: Determinants of spinal hook dislodgement. Read at the Twentieth Annual Meeting of the Scoliosis Research Society, Coronado, CA, 1985.
4. Ginsburg HH, Goldstein LA, Robinson S, et al: Back pain in postoperative idiopathic scoliosis. Orthop Trans 1979;3:50.
5. Guadagni JR, Drummond DS: Strength of surgical wire fixation: A laboratory study. Clin Orthop 1986;209:176–181.
6. Guadagni J, Drummond D, Breed A: Improved postoperative course following modified segmental instrumentation and posterior fusion for scoliosis. J Pediatr Orthop 1984;4:405–408.
7. Herring JA, Fitch RD, Wenger DR, et al: Segmental instrumentation: A review of early results and complications. Presented at the Annual Meeting of the Scoliosis Research Society, 1983.
8. Jones SJ, Edga NA, Ransford A, et al: A system for the electrophysiological monitoring of the spinal cord during operations. J Bone Joint Surg 1982;65B:134–139.
9. Lowe T: The morbidity and mortality report. Read at the Twenty-first Annual Meeting of the Scoliosis Research Society, Bermuda, 1986.
10. Luque ER: The anatomic basis and development of segmental spinal instrumentation. Spine 1982;7:256–259.
11. Neuwirth MG, Drummond DS: The results of interspinous segmental instrumentation in the sagittal plane. Read at the Twenty-Second Annual Meeting of the Scoliosis Research Society, Vancouver, B.C., Canada, 1987.
12. Perry J, Nickel VL, Bonnet C: Halo-button traction wire technique of spine fusion in the non-ambulatory respiratory patient with spine instability. J Bone Joint Surg 1968;5A:1059–1060.
13. Resina J, Ferreiira-Alvez A: A technique of correction and internal fixation for scoliosis. J Bone Joint Surg 1977;5B159–169.
14. Sponsellor PD, Whiffen JR, Drummond DS: Interspinous process spinal instrumentation for scoliosis in cerebral palsy. J Pediatr Orthop 1986;6:559–567.
15. Wenger DT, Carollo JJ, Wikerson JA, Wanthers K, Herring JA: The laboratory testing of segmental spinal instrumentation versus traditional Harrington instrumentation for scoliosis treatment. Spine 1982;7:265–269.
16. Wilber SR, Thompson SH, Shaffer JW, et al: Postoperative neurological deficits in segmental instrumentation. J Bone Joint Surg 1984;66A:1178–1187.
17. Winter RB, Lovell WW, Moe JH: Excessive thoracic lordosis and loss of pulmonary function in patients with idiopathic scoliosis. J Bone and Joint Surg 1975;57A:972.

EIGHT

Cotrel-Dubousset Instrumentation

Richard A. Balderston

INTRODUCTION

Since its introduction to the Scoliosis Research Society in 1984, Cotrel-Dubousset (C-D) instrumentation for the correction and stabilization of spinal deformity has generated tremendous excitement and applications. Both the Harrington and Luque systems were popular at that time, and their own versatility was gradually increasing. The biomechanics of their utilization, however, were confined to the application of unidirectional forces that achieved adequate correction, but often inadequate fixation. The addition of sublaminar wires, while safe in most experienced surgeons' hands, offers the potential for catastrophic complication. Indeed, many teachers of spinal surgery had great difficulty conveying the fundamentals of sublaminar wire technique without exposing patients to increased risk. The Cotrel-Dubousset device, with its ingenious rod design, has allowed for the unique utilization of multiple forces that attack spinal deformity on a more fundamental basis (2,4,5,9,12).

Most of the concepts elucidated in this chapter were not discussed or even considered a decade ago. Undoubtedly, this fixation device will continue to change our ideas concerning the treatment of patients with spinal deformity.

INSTRUMENTATION—ROD, HOOKS, AND DEVICE FOR TRANSVERSE TRACTION (DTT)

The standard Cotrel-Dubousset rod is composed of stainless steel and is 7 mm in diameter; a 5-mm pediatric rod is also available (Fig. 8.1). It is more supple and less brittle than either the Harrington or Luque rod. The entire surface is covered with diamond-shaped irregularities that allow for strong fixation of either hooks or pedicle screws through the use of bolting screws. The rods allow any degree of rotation of the hooks along the

rod. In addition, the hooks can be used in either direction to effect distraction or compression along the same rod. The rod has no weak points, and significant contouring can be accomplished throughout its entire length.

There are two types of hook or screw attachments to the rod. The first type is by means of a so-called closed hook; the rod is passed through the hook after the hook has been surgically positioned at the appropriate point on the spine. Closed hooks are most commonly used at the end of the surgical construct to provide maximum stability at the hook-rod interface. The second type of fixation is through the use of so-called open hooks. A clever sleeve mechanism, firmly attached to the rod, is slid into position within the open hook with a force applied in either distraction or compression (Fig. 8.2). The sleeve is then bolted down, fixing the rod to the sleeve and thus to the hook. The square portion of the

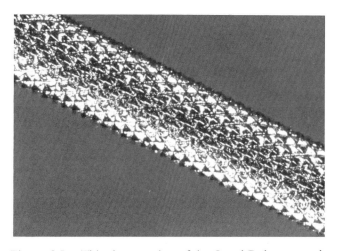

Figure 8.1. This close-up view of the Cotrel-Dubousset rod demonstrates the knurls and grooves that allow for fixation of hooks and screws by means of set screws that are tightened and then broken, forming a weld between the broken screw and the rod.

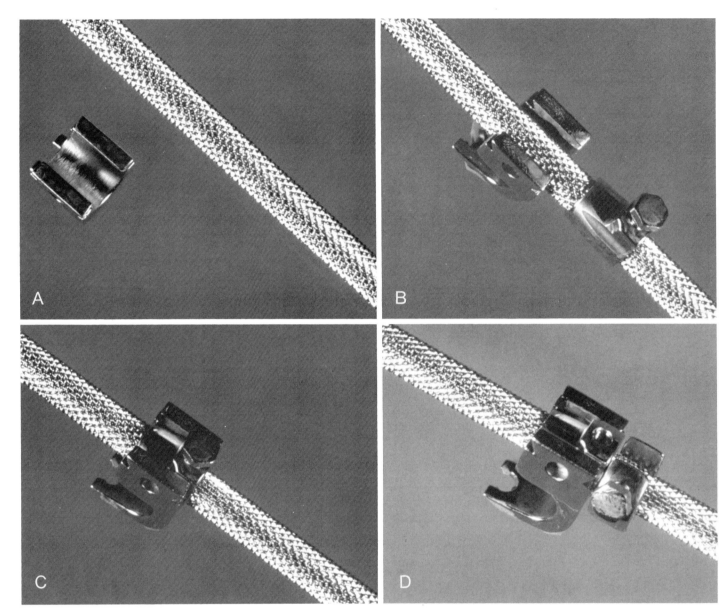

Figure 8.2. Insertion of the Cotrel-Dubousset rod into an open hook. *A,* This view demonstrates the relationship between the 7-mm Cotrel-Dubousset rod and the opening of the open pedicle hook. *B,* Shows the relationship of the rod as it is lowered into the open hook with the sleeve in position ready

to be driven into the open hook mount. *C,* Demonstrates the final position of the sleeve within the open hook. *D,* Demonstrates the position of the C-ring that is utilized for selected hooks before rod rotation.

sleeve is termed a blocker and blocks rotation of the hook on the sleeve.

Two types of hooks interface with bone (Figs. 8.3 and 8.4). The first is a pedicle hook designed with two prongs and a central notch to be guided into position along the inferior part of the pedicle. Once in position, the hook prongs prevent movement of the hook in the transverse plane. The second type of hook is the laminar hook, which has a round, blunted edge designed for insertion within the spinal canal with the shoe in contact with a vertebral

lamina. Also, this hook is used for transverse process fixation.

The device for transverse traction is used to couple rods in situ mechanically. Notches on the DTT hooks have been constructed to be the same size in reverse shape as the diamond notches in the rod. This arrangement gives a jawlike fixation to couple the rods together. The effect is to add rotatory stability of each individual rod by increasing the lever arm of stability to any rotatory force on either rod (10).

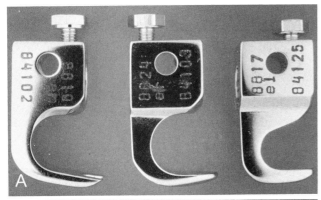

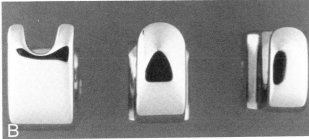

Figure 8.3. The early basic hook design for the Cotrel-Dubousset device. *A*, The lateral view of the closed pedicle hook on the left center closed laminar hook and on the right closed thoracic laminar hook. The thoracic laminar hook has a reduced shoe depth from the body of the hook. *B*, A view of the shoe of each hook. The pronged hook is the closed pedicle hook, and the solid shoe on the right is the thoracic laminar hook.

For each type of hook, either closed or open, there is an appropriate inserter. For pedicular fixation, a pedicular elevator is utilized to define the exact position and plane of pedicular hook insertion. For sliding sleeves along the rods in situ, a number 1 and number 2 pusher have been devised to first seat the sleeve in appropriate rotation, and then to drive the sleeve into its final position within the open hook. Strong rod grippers have claws similar to the hooks on the DTT that combine for excellent stability of the gripper-rod interface and the ability to control the rod precisely with respect to rotation and translation. Closed hooks and open hook-sleeve combinations can be advanced where appropriate with either a distractor or compressor.

BIOMECHANICS

Several laboratories have documented the rigidity and fixation strength of the C-D device. In a vertebrectomy model, Farcy et al. tested the Harrington, Luque, and C-D constructs (6). Two C-D configurations were utilized, one with a single vertebra claw pattern above and below the vertebrectomy, and another with a two-level claw necessitating fixation two levels above and below

the vertebrectomy defect. With respect to axial stability, the two-level C-D device had four to five times greater axial stability than the Harrington instrumentation. With torsional testing, the Harrington device was only 13% as rigid, while the Luque device was 65% as rigid as a two-level C-D construct.

Gurr et al. have tested the Cotrel pedicle screw system in an L3 vertebrectomy model (9). Compared with the Steffee and Luque devices, the C-D had better rotational and axial rigidity and fixation.

Johnston et al. studied the torsional stiffness of the

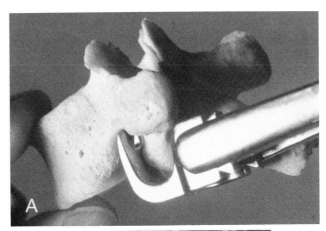

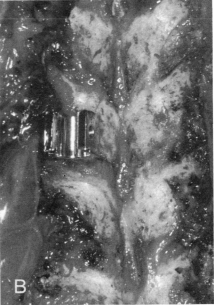

Figure 8.4. Positioning of the pedicle hook. *A*, Demonstrates on a model the position of the pedicle hook as it is inserted on a normal thoracic vertebrae. The length of the shoe corresponds to the distance between the inferior edge of the inferior facet and the inferior border of the pedicle. The spokes of the prong should sit on either side of the pedicle for optimum fixation. *B*, Demonstrates the position of an open pedicle hook in situ.

C-D rods, with and without the DTT, in a bovine spine (11). They found that the torsional stiffness of the construct was improved by 50% when the DTT was utilized to span the two Cotrel rods in a box configuration.

THEORETICAL CONSIDERATIONS FOR APPLICATION

The biomechanics of the Harrington rod are based on the racheting system that allows for distraction between two points. With the addition of either interspinous or sublaminar wires to the Harrington rod, an additional component of force, translation, could be added. With the precontoured Luque rod, the surgeon applies force through the use of wires in an effort to draw the vertebral body to the rod. The wire's final position on the rod is based on the construct's most stable position in the operating room. However, neither the final position of the wire on the rod, nor its direction can be controlled once the wound is closed and the patient is ambulating. Indeed, through relaxation of the tissues, the actual force holding the rod to the vertebral lamina may be significantly diminished after several days. Thus, for the Harrington and Luque devices, the forces of correction are quite powerful, while the long-term bone-instrumentation interface is much more unstable.

The CD device forces the surgeon to consider a much greater armamentarium in the quest for correction of spinal deformity. At the end of each rod, the closed hooks function in a traditional manner affecting two-point distraction or compression between the vertebrae at the end of the rod. At this point, the surgeon may add intermediate hooks with a wide choice of possible positions. The primary utility of the intermediate hooks with this device is for more potent application of force at the level of greatest deformity. In the right thoracic curve pattern, bending films will demonstrate discs that do not change significantly in their deformity. Generally, there will be one–three discs where the majority of the scoliotic deformity is concentrated (Fig. 8.5). The remaining vertebrae within the curvature are relatively more flexible. Through the use of intermediate hooks spanning two–four vertebral segments, so-called apical distraction may be carried out to apply maximum force to the area of maximum deformity (Fig. 8.5). Similarly, for thoracolumbar and lumbar curves, apical compression may be applied at the convexity of the curvature again to effect maximum force where the deformity is the worst. For double major curves where apical distraction is required for the right thoracic curve, and apical compression is required on the left thoracolumbar or lumbar curve, the application of a single rod may be utilized to correct both deformities.

With previous fixation devices, the sagittal plane was often ignored because the surgeon had little choice with respect to the possibilities for maintaining sagittal alignment. Many of the instrumentation constructs designed for scoliosis of the lumbar spine produced worsening of the spinal deformity in the sagittal plane. The C-D device forces active consideration of the lateral roentgenograph. Often, the apex of the deformity in the coronal plane does not correspond to the apex of deformity in the sagittal plane. The C-D device allows the surgeon to consider both roentgenographic views to produce a more normal sagittal contour and, simultaneously, a maximally corrected coronal plane.

Through the use of rod rotation the surgeon may also create a more physiologic kyphosis or lordosis. Thus lordosis may be created with compression and rod rotation, while kyphosis may be created with posterior element distraction and rod rotation. In addition, the relationship between the contours of the two rods effects derotation of the spine and may help to diminish the rib hump deformity.

The aforementioned considerations pertain to the surgical correction of deformity, but perhaps the even greater contribution of this instrumentation occurs when the surgical options for *fixation* are considered. At the end of any instrumentation procedure, the surgeon must consider the chances of loss of fixation. The usual positions for loss of fixation include the ends of the surgical construct with respect to hook dislocation or pullout, and the loss of correction that may occur with failure of intermediate level fixation. The C-D device offers the surgeon increased surface area of bone-metal interface at multiple vertebrae. For instance, one common construct is the pedicular-transverse process claw, where two hooks are utilized in a compression manner, one a pedicle hook, and the other a laminar hook about the transverse process to create a grip on one particular vertebrae. Laminar hooks present a traditional interface to the lamina, but the surgeon has the option of creating a claw configuration where two laminar hooks may be used facing each other and capturing one or two lamina in their grasp. Roach et al. have shown that the two-vertebrae claw configuration is stronger than the single laminar claw configuration (13). More recently, the use of a pedicle screw with an oblique hook allows for two separate fixation modes on the same vertebrae. All of these options allow the surgeon to maximize the fixation component of the instrumentation to supplement the corrective forces that had been utilized earlier.

HOOK PLACEMENT FOR SPECIFIC CURVES

Given the much broader range of forces available to the surgeon with this new instrumentation, it is not surpris-

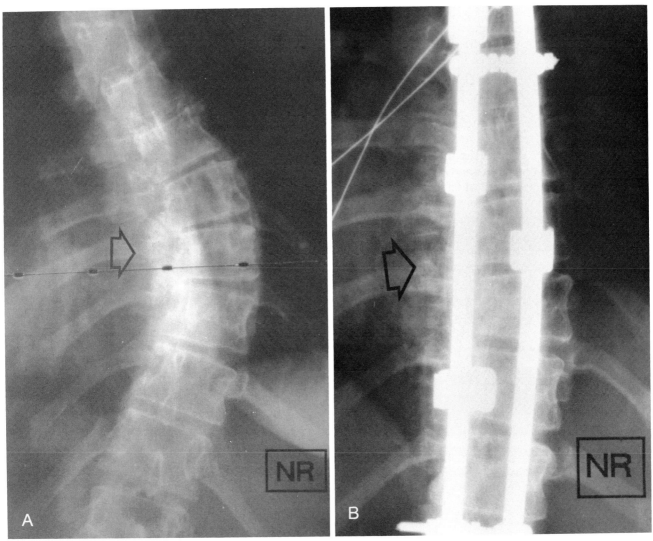

Figure 8.5. Apical distraction for right thoracic curves. *A,* Demonstrates the apex of a right thoracic curve in a 22-year-old female. Note the asymmetry of the disc heights at the apical three discs. *B,* Demonstrates a close-up of the apical distraction that has been achieved over the same three apical discs. Note the power of the correction of these three discs by the open pedicle hook above and the open laminar hook below on the left-sided rod.

ing that there has been a slow evolution in the hook patterns that have been utilized for each specific curvature. As each surgeon of spinal deformity knows, there are no two curves that are exactly alike, so that a cookbook approach will not be successful in every case. What follows is a rationale for the placement of hooks and the techniques of rod insertion for several broad common categories of idiopathic scoliosis. Obviously, for patients with congenital deformity, these recommendations will need to be modified.

Right Thoracic Curve with Hypokyphosis

This type of thoracic scoliosis, a King type III curve, forms a good starting point for the student of C-D in-

strumentation. The fundamentals of the surgical management of this curve type provide the groundwork for the consideration of other curve patterns.

The first considerations for hook placement are the end vertebrae for the left concave rod. The upper hook in the end vertebrae is a closed pedicle hook. It is classically placed in a position similar to the upper hook of the Harrington device. Bending films will determine the end vertebrae of the upper curve, and placement should be in part predicted on the creation of a balanced spine in the coronal plane. Consideration of the lateral x-rays is also important to determine the amount of kyphosis present over the upper segment. Should there be a focal kyphosis at the area where the hook would normally be placed, consideration should be given to a more cranial placement than would normally be considered on the AP view. Lower hook position is determined by left bending film to determine the opening of the disc spaces. The disc space below the fusion should be mobile to become horizontal on bending. There have been a few reports of progressive junctional kyphosis if this lower hook, a closed laminar hook, is placed at T12 so that the usual most cranial placement is L1. Occasionally, for the uncomplicated type III curve, fusion must be extended down to L2 (Fig. 8.6). Cephalad and caudal hook should not be at a curve apex on both AP and lateral radiographs. Additionally, the cephalad and caudal vertebrae should fall within Harrington's stable zone.

The position of the intermediate hooks is determined by the right side bending film. Those discs that do not correct appreciably and appear most rigid are spanned by an open pedicle hook and an open laminar hook, usually over three or four levels.

Hook placement of the right convex rod is as follows: at the upper end vertebra, either a transverse process-pedicle claw with a closed laminar and closed pedicle hook may be utilized, or a closed thoracic laminar hook above the right upper lamina in a downgoing position. An intermediate open pedicle hook is utilized at the apex of the curve, primarily to assist as a derotation pressure point with convex rod insertion, and to further stabilize the rod itself. A two-segment claw will complete the hook construct at the right lower vertebra with a cranially facing closed laminar hook on the end vertebra and an open laminar hook downgoing on the vertebra above.

The concave rod is inserted first and contoured for mild scoliosis. Sleeves are utilized for the open hooks, and with the rod in position, rotation is carried out, usually through 90°. In adult patients this rotation may not be possible due to tissue stiffness and facet arthritis. Hook seating is then carried out by distraction of the intermediate hooks, first to achieve maximal correction of the curve apex. Finally, the end vertebrae are distracted into position. The right rod is contoured into slightly less kyphosis than is present with the first rod construct

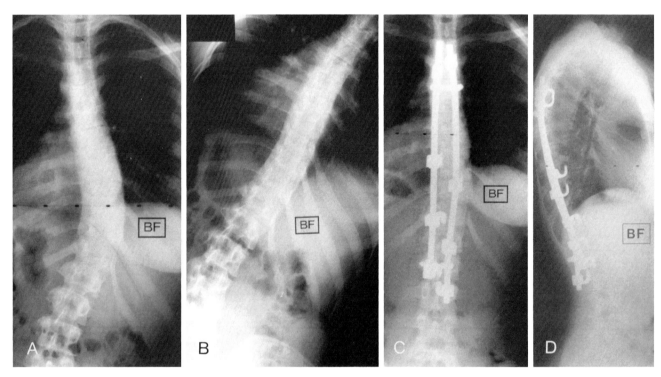

Figure 8.6. King type III right thoracic curve treated with the Cotrel-Dubousset device. *A*, Preoperative PA roentgenograph in a 16-year-old female with a 45° right thoracic curve. *B*, Demonstrates significant correction on side bending. *C*, Demonstrates fixation of the King type III right thoracic curve with the Cotrel-Dubousset device. The left-sided rod was placed first, and 90° of rod rotation was achieved. Apical distraction was then carried out between T9 and T12. Closed pedicle hook at T5 and closed laminar hook at L2 complete the configuration. For the right-sided rod, a downgoing closed thoracic laminar hook is used at T5, open pedicle hook at T10, open laminar hook downgoing at L1, and a closed laminar hook upgoing at L2. DTTs above and below complete the instrumentation. *D*, Demonstrates the lateral view with maintenance of normal contours both of the thoracic spine and at the thoracolumbar junction.

and is inserted as a derotation device by applying pressure at the open pedicle intermediate hook on the apex of the curve.

Right Thoracic Curve with Junctional Kyphosis

If significant kyphosis is present either at the thoracolumbar junction or at the upper thoracic spine on the lateral view, then the rods must be extended to add a compression force across the kyphosis. Thus, in the case of thoracolumbar kyphosis, the rods are extended to the L2 level, and hooks may be added to effect bilateral compression across one or two discs at the lower end of the construct. With significant kyphosis along the entire thoracic spine, there are several options available to the surgeon. The first is to utilize the construct for the type III curve with hypokyphosis and merely not obtain as much correction with rotation. The hooks are inserted, and distraction is carried out in a routine fashion with only 20° or 30° of rotation. However, the surgeon must be extremely careful to factor in the lengthening of the posterior column with the distraction maneuver; and indeed, simply using the left rod without any rotation will cause an increase in kyphosis. Evaluation of the hyperextension lateral x-ray is extremely critical at this time. Should correction of the kyphotic component of the deformity not be significant with hyperextension, then an anterior surgery will be necessary to section the anterior longitudinal ligament and provide an acceptable result with respect to sagittal contours. One other technique is to utilize a temporary right-sided rod inserted in compression in an effort to decrease the kyphosis before the left concave rod is placed. With kyphosis diminished as the result of a temporary convex rod, the left rod may be inserted, and then the right rod removed, and rotation carried out with seating of the hooks. The left rod will then be correcting the scoliosis and maintaining the kyphosis in a reduced position. The right rod may then be inserted with the addition of one or two pedicular-transverse claws or sequential thoracic laminar hooks superiorly.

Thoracolumbar and Lumbar Curves

The basic principle behind the treatment of thoracolumbar, lumbar, or the lumbar component of double major curves lies in compression of the apical vertebrae. It has been the fault of previous instrumentation systems that posterior column shortening, or creation of a lordotic moment, was not easy to achieve. The apex of a curve must be determined, and then hooks are placed above and below the apex. Depending upon the curvature, intermediate hooks may include a downgoing open laminar hook on the vertebrae above the apex, and an upgoing open laminar hook on the vertebrae below the apex. Additional hooks may be used sequentially, such that the apex may have a hook in the downgoing position on it as well as a segment below the lowest intermediate hook may be instrumented with another open laminar hook. The lower end vertebrae are determined by a side bending view. If the curve is a left convex one, then a forced right side bending will demonstrate which vertebra reaches a neutral position with correction of the compensatory lumbosacral curve to its fullest extent. This vertebra usually does not correspond to the stable vertebrae as defined by King; generally, there are more open disc segments that are allowed utilizing this technique.

For upper hook placement, consideration is given to instrumenting a variable distance of the concavity of the compensatory right thoracic curve. The same principles for the King type III curve should be utilized at this point, and the closed pedicle hook at the top of the instrumentation should be placed well within or above any area of kyphosis as seen on the lateral x-ray. For the concave rod, hooks are inserted to neutralize the lordosing effect of the convex rod. Thus, the lower end vertebra is instrumented with a downgoing closed laminar hook, and the upper end vertebra is instrumented with either a transverse process pedicle claw or a closed thoracic laminar hook in a downgoing position. The highest downgoing open laminar hook on the convex rod is neutralized by an upgoing open laminar hook on the opposite side. A second intermediate hook is usually placed at what would be the apex of the compensatory thoracic curve. Thus, the convex rod usually requires six–seven hooks, while the concave rod requires four–five hooks.

The convex rod is then contoured into the desired sagittal plane alignment and placed into the hooks with all sleeves attached. Occasionally, a rod introducer is necessary for this step. Rotation is then achieved with C-washers placed at the apical hooks to prevent migration of these hooks during rotation. Hooks are tightened sequentially about the apex to achieve apical compression first from those hooks nearest the apex to those hooks farthest from the apex. Finally, the upper hook is seated in distraction. The neutralization rod is then tightened into position, but this rod, in contrast to the thoracic curve patterns, does not have a derotation effect on the lumbar vertebrae.

Double Major Curve Patterns—Right Thoracic Left Lumbar or Right Thoracic Left Thoracolumbar

This hook configuration forms the basis for the classic King type I curvature. Hook selection is based upon a combination of the right thoracic type III pattern and the thoracolumbar and lumbar curve patterns. For these curves, the fortuitous ingenious design of the C-D instrumentation is most effective. The end vertebrae for the left-sided rod are determined by the same criteria as for the individual curve patterns. The intermediate vertebrae of the thoracic curve again are chosen as they are chosen for type III pattern. The lumbar or thoracolumbar pattern is chosen with the use of open laminar hooks centered about the apex of the curvature. The same hooks at the cranial side of the apex that function to compress the apex also serve as the anchor for distraction of the thoracic pattern. In general, six–eight hooks are utilized on the left-sided rod. The right-sided rod is inserted with the usual end vertebrae hooks. The intermediate hooks include an open pedicle hook at the apex of the thoracic curve and an open laminar hook opposing the uppermost downgoing hook of the left-sided rod. Additional open laminar hooks may be placed within the instrumented thoracolumbar or lumbar curve (Fig. 8.7).

The left rod is inserted first with the desired sagittal plane contour. Rotation is achieved and produces simultaneous posterior column lengthening of the thoracic curve and posterior column shortening of the left thoracolumbar or lumbar curve. Great care must be taken at this time to be sure that maximum compression is achieved at the apex of the lower curve. Once apical compression has been carried out, distraction is achieved through the intermediate hooks of the thoracic curve. The last hook tightened is the left upper end vertebra. The right rod is then inserted with the possibility present for derotation of the thoracic curve. Usually, no additional derotation is achieved in the lumbar spine.

Type II Curve Patterns

It was originally suggested that type II curves with significant flexibility of the lower lumbar or thoracolumbar component be instrumented in a similar manner to the recommendations of King et al. However, several authors have noted that there was increased decompensation of the entire spine produced with this rod and hook configuration (12,14,15). The solution to this problem includes a partial instrumentation and fusion of the flexible thoracolumbar or lumbar curve. For a left flexible thoracolumbar or lumbar curve, the forced right side bending film is examined. The uppermost vertebra that achieves total correction of the disc space with correction of rotation may serve as the lower end vertebra for the construct. In general, this vertebra is L2 or L3; in the standing PA view, however, this vertebra may not fall into the stable zone. Hook configuration on the left concave rod is the same as for type III curves, except that

the rod is extended down to the level of the preselected end vertebra and compression is carried out with an added fifth hook upgoing on the lower end vertebra. Thus, the hook selection includes upper end vertebra closed pedicle, intermediate hooks at the apex (open pedicle and open laminar), and open laminar hook on the lower end vertebra of the right thoracic curve. The closed laminar fifth hook is upgoing to act as a compression lordosis at the thoracolumbar junction with partial correction of the flexible compensatory curve. Insertion of a neutral rod is then carried out with hook placement the same as for the double major curve pattern.

Double Thoracic Curves

In general, these curve patterns correspond to the King type V configuration where there is a significant upper left thoracic scoliosis; utilization of the usual type III configuration would produce increasing decompensation and shoulder asymmetry. Hook placement is similar to that of the double major curve; however, it must be remembered that compression of the posterior column at the level of the left upper curve will increase the lordosis of this segment. In general, a temporary right-sided rod must be placed into the upper curve to distract and increase the kyphosis of the upper thoracic curve, and at the same time, partially correct the scoliosis. The hook pattern for the concave rod for the lower right thoracic curve is as for the typical type III configuration. One or two hooks are added to correct the left thoracic curve, and thus a total of five or six hooks are required on each rod. With the temporary rod in position on the right side, the left-sided rod is then inserted. If there is a significant curvature of the upper thoracic curve that is placed into the rod before rotation, then 90° of rotation will dramatically increase the lordosis of that curve. This arrangement is not ideal and must be counteracted with significant correction by the right temporary rod. In general, an attempt is made to insert the upper left rod as straight as possible, thus diminishing the lordotic moment arm created with rotation and correction of the lower right thoracic curve. The right-sided neutralization rod is as for type III, except there is extension superiorly with a closed pedicle hook at the upper end vertebra.

Severe Rigid Right Thoracic Curves

For right thoracic curves that are greater than 90–100°, occasionally the hooks will be aligned so that the insertion of one rod will be impossible. In these cases, the surgeon may decide to utilize two rods to separate and maximize the correction achieved by the intermediate hooks, as well as the end vertebrae hooks. With these rigid curves, the

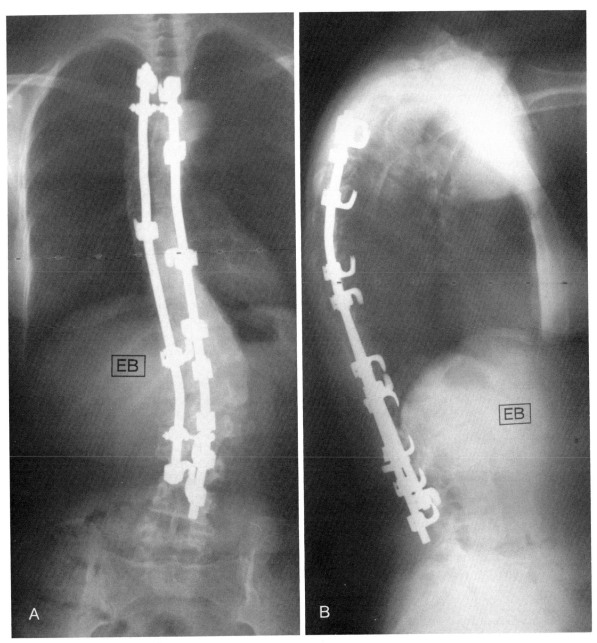

Figure 8.7. Fixation of King type I curve. *A*, AP roentgenograph. The rod on the right demonstrates multiple hook configuration to create curve correction and lordosis at the thoracolumbar junction. The three lowest hooks on the right are all upgoing laminar hooks. The next three hooks on the right-sided rod are all downgoing laminar hooks. Thus, compression is initially achieved from T10 to L3. The upper two hooks on the right-sided rod add distraction to the concavity of the thoracic curve. Thus, with initial placement of the right-sided rod, compression of the thoracolumbar curve and distraction of the thoracic curve are achieved simultaneously. *B*, Demonstrates the lateral view with maintenance of lordosis in the lumbar spine with normal sagittal alignment in the thoracic spine.

right side bending view usually demonstrates four, five, or possibly six segments that are rigid. The apex of a curve is identified, and two, three, or four hook sites are chosen, depending upon the curvature. The end vertebrae are chosen in routine fashion. For the short concave rod, closed pedicle hooks and closed laminar hooks are used at the end of the construct and open pedicle or laminar hooks, as indicated, are used in the middle of the rod. At the end vertebra, closed laminar hooks are used below and a closed pedicle hook above. The short rod is inserted first, and maximal correction is achieved. Distraction of the end vertebra is then carried out with a longer rod, and the two rods connected with two DTTs if possible. The right-sided neutralization convex rod is inserted like the type III configuration.

With a double major component, this combination may be extended utilizing the same principles as discussed before.

SPECIAL CONSIDERATIONS FOR ADULT SCOLIOSIS SURGERY

Surgery in the adult poses a greater challenge because of a hardening of the normally soft tissue structures of the disc and facet joints in the adult. Osteopenia, facet arthritis, and disc degeneration force the surgeon to be more careful in the adult patient.

For curvatures where a significant correction is achieved, there is significant pressure at the end vertebrae. These vertebrae are subject to fracture with loss of fixation at the bone-metal interface. A technical factor to consider in patients with osteopenia is the addition of extra hooks for fixation sites at the end vertebrae, including one- or two-level claw patterns (Fig. 8.8). In addition, pedicle screw fixation may be utilized to enhance end vertebrae fixation.

Another consideration is the amount of expected correction. The C-D allows the surgeon to create significant force for the realignment of scoliosis. In patients with significant facet and disc disease, this correction may not be possible, and the surgeon should not expect a correction similar to the adolescent patient. Adult patients should be warned of this outcome.

Evaluation of the sagittal plane is much more critical in the adult than the adolescent patient. These patients have an increased tendency for progressive kyphosis at the junction of their instrumentation with the remaining mobile segments, both above and below the fusion. Hyperextension lateral films are recommended in most adult patients who require fusion for scoliosis.

Another problem that the surgeon must confront in the adult patient is decompensation in the coronal plane. The discs that are left free in the adolescent often allow the surgeon more latitude by accommodating to the new configuration above them, and allow the patient to maintain balance. The lower discs in the adult may be degenerated, and coronal plane balance may not result if the configuration and arthritis of the lower discs are not taken into account.

The question of degeneration of the disc at the lowest level of the fusion has not been resolved. Currently, we do not recommend discograms to determine the lowest level of the fusion. Obviously, if a fusion is to be taken into the lower lumbar spine, oblique x-rays are mandatory to determine if a spondylolysis or spondylolisthesis is present. Currently, we try to avoid degenerative changes per se as criteria for selection of the lower end vertebrae of the fusion. However, newer developments in the refinement of the discogram or magnetic resonance imaging may alter these conclusions.

PEDICLE SCREW INSTRUMENTATION

The design for C-D pedicle screws has undergone extensive changes in the last several years. The early design demonstrated significant problems with bending and breakage of the screws (2). The current design has a large diameter, as well as a sturdy thread-head interface. The most popular screw designs include the closed, posterior opening, and side opening configurations.

The technique of insertion of the pedicle screws utilizes the standard techniques of locating the posterior aspect of the pedicle and its projection to the junction of the pars, transverse process, and lateral border of the superior facet. After removal of cortical bone at this junction, a probe in the form of an awl or joystick may be inserted. Before this step, a lateral x-ray is usually taken with a pin to determine position of the pedicle in the lateral view. The pedicle system does not require a tap, and the screws are then inserted directly. Compared with other designs, the thread of the C-D screw is much blunter, and the danger of cortical penetration of the pedicle is diminished. The rod placement within the pedicle screws can be utilized as either an extension of one rod connected to hooks in the thoracic spine, or a separate rod may be utilized and connected to a more superior rod with a double-barrelled connector (Fig. 8.9).

RESULTS OF SURGERY

Cotrel et al. first reported 2-year follow-up results on 250 patients operated upon between 1983 and 1985 (2). For a mixed population of adolescent and adult idiopathic scoliosis, the mean angular Cobb correction was 66°. Thoracic lordosis was improved at least minimally in all patients. When they compared the sagittal alignment with previous patients operated with the Luque or Harrington technique, the lumbar lordosis was maintained in a much better position. Utilizing CT scans and Perdriolle ruler, the authors demonstrated that in flexible curves, vertebral rotation could be corrected by 40%. Two patients developed neurologic complications, while six patients had dislodgement of upper hooks. At follow-up, there was minimal loss of correction in those patients who had no technical mistakes. If there was hook migration or other failure of the bone-metal interface, loss of correction was

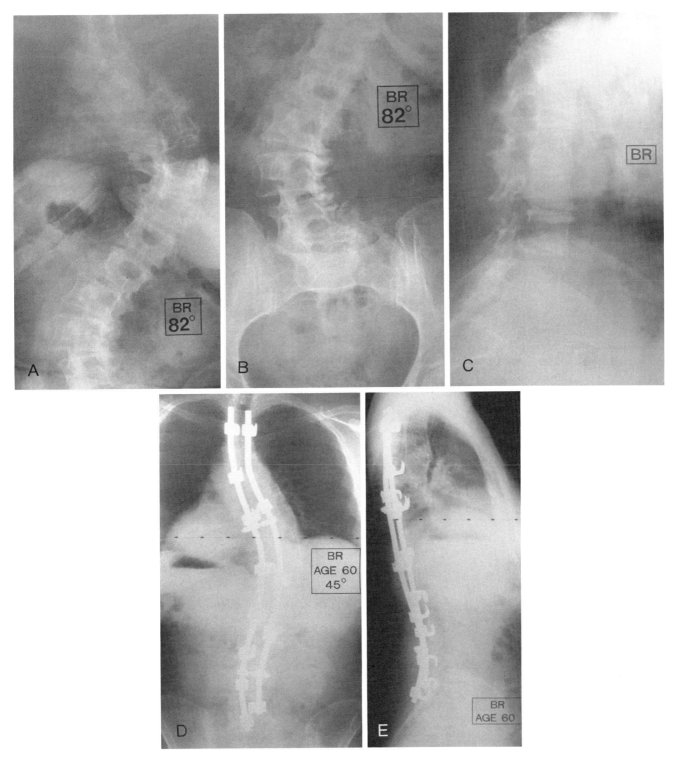

Figure 8.8. Use of the Cotrel-Dubousset device in a 60-year-old female. *A*, Demonstrates the PA standing films of a 60-year-old woman with progressive idiopathic scoliosis and increasing decompensation. *B*, Supine view of the lumbar spine demonstrating significant degenerative changes with rotatory subluxation. *C*, Shows a lateral view of the lumbar spine with significant loss of lumbar lordosis. *D*, The postoperative roentgenograph showing stabilization of the right thoracic curve with a return of compensation in the coronal plane. *E*, Shows the lateral view with increase of the lumbar lordosis and a well-compensated spine.

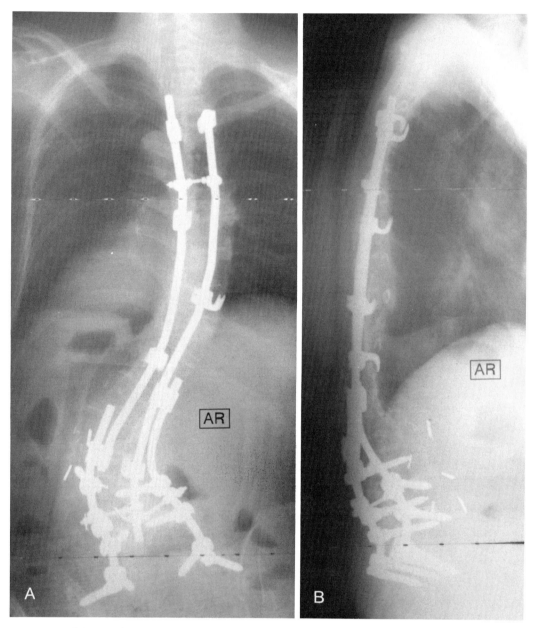

Figure 8.9. Extension of the Cotrel-Dubousset device to include pedicular fixation and sacral fixation. This patient had undergone two previous surgical procedures for fixation of a thoracolumbar curve. Increasing decompensation and loss of posterior elements necessitated the use of pedicle screw fixation in the lower lumbar spine and to the sacrum. Pedicle screws may be inserted in multiple directions into the sacrum for increased fixation. In addition, double-barrelled dominoes may be used to join rods to create a rigid construct. *A,* The PA view. *B,* The lateral view.

greater than 10° in three, and between 5–10° in two additional patients.

The issue of rotation was addressed by Ecker et al., who obtained CT scans in 30 patients who were treated for adolescent idiopathic scoliosis (5). With respect to the apical vertebrae, a sagittal line was constructed on the transverse image of a CT scan; vertebral rotation improved from 15° to 13°. For curves less than 25°, kyphosis

increased by a mean of 10°. Bridwell et al. evaluated 160 patients who had Cotrel-Dubousset instrumentation (1). They examined the thoracolumbar junction in patients who had spinal fusion down to the level of L2. The sagittal alignment was better maintained with a short compression on the left-sided concave rod at the level of the thoracolumbar junction. For fusions below the level of L2, lumbar lordosis was not worsened, although they did not see a significant amount of lumbar lordosis enhancement when this goal was attempted at surgery.

At the Rothman Institute between September, 1985 and December, 1989, 90 consecutive patients with adult spinal deformity were treated using C-D instrumentation. All patients were followed in a prospective manner. The age of the patients was from 20 to 61 years, and the average follow-up was 1.6 years. The diagnosis was idiopathic scoliosis in 82, congenital scoliosis in 3, neuromuscular scoliosis in 1, and Scheuermann's kyphosis in 4. Within the idiopathic scoliosis group, there were 12 thoracolumbar curves, King type I, 26; King type II, 15 patients; King type III, 21 patients; and King type V, 8 patients. Eighty-seven patients underwent primary surgery, and there were 5 revision operations, 2 on the first group of the original 87, and 3 revisions from previous Harrington procedures. The revision rate for this group of patients was 2.3%. The average curve correction at follow-up was 52%.

The complications within the series included one fracture of C-D rods associated with pseudarthrosis at greater than 2-year follow-up. Of 10 patients with type II curves treated with early suggested hook configuration, one was decompensated more than 2 cm. There were three cases of upper claw vertebral fracture, and two patients who had painful prominent hooks and rods at the top of their instrumentation. Four patients had subluxation or dislocation of their lower hooks, below type I curve patterns with instrumentation into the lower lumbar spine. Of the first 20 type I curves instrumented, this represented a 20% complication rate. Subsequently, more hooks have been added to the convex lower rod so that the average number of hooks utilized to control the lower curve has increased from four to six hooks (Fig. 8.7). Fracture of the convex cranial end claw through the transverse process has been eliminated by the use of an upper right convex closed thoracic laminar hook. Since this hook has been utilized, there have been no dislocations in over 50 patients. Of the two patients with prominent instrumentation superiorly, both had instrumentation to the T8 level or below. Currently, all patients who require instrumentation above the thoracolumbar junction are being fused to the level T6 or above.

COMPLICATIONS

In its morbidity report of 1987, the Scoliosis Research Society compared the different instrumentation techniques for idiopathic scoliosis with respect to their rate of neurologic injury. The Harrington technique had the lowest complication rate at the level of 0.1%, the Luque and the C-D techniques were comparable at 1.8% for the Luque, and 1.5% for the C-D. Those surgeons who utilized pedicle screw fixation had a neurologic injury rate of 3.2%.

In 1988, the Society again examined the complication rates of C-D, and found that major deficits occurred in 0.2% of patients. There were minor neurologic deficits produced in 1.7%. Implant failure was described to have occurred in 2.2%, and reoperations were required in 3.1% of patients. Of course, the follow-up on these patients was averaged less than 1 year.

Failure of the instrumentation system can be classified into three groups: (1) failure of the bone-metal interface; (2) failure at the hook-rod interface; (3) fracture of one of the metal components. Early surgical series have reported an extremely low rate of rod fracture. With admittedly short-term follow-up, the rate has been less than one in a thousand.

Failure at the bone-prosthesis interface has been the most common problem. This set of complications includes pedicle and lamina fracture due to excessive stress, or hook dislocation secondary to inadequate fixation. Because of its mobility, the lumbar spine is more prone to hook subluxation or frank dislocation, as evidenced by the series from Pennsylvania Hospital.

Failure of the rod-hook interface has taken several forms. The first failure of fixation that may occur is sliding of the hook in spite of a tightening of the set hex screw. For end closed hooks, this complication may be minimized by breaking off two screws in both set holes of the closed screw. Sleeve migration within the open hook has occurred infrequently and may lead to loss of fixation. Rarely, open hooks will back out of their fixation point and lose appropriate contact with their sleeve.

CONTRAINDICATIONS TO THE USE OF COTREL-DUBOUSSET (C-D) INSTRUMENTATION

The C-D device is a much more rigid form of spinal fixation than the spinal surgeon may be accustomed to. For patients with significant osteopenia where force modulation is important, flexion with a device utilizing sublaminar wires may assist the surgeon in titrating the force so that the end vertebra stress is significantly diminished. Other than this single relative contraindication, the C-D device is extremely versatile in all aspects of spinal deformity surgery.

Of course, the same contraindications that hold for other instrumentation systems may be applicable to the C-D device. For patients with congenital scoliosis, great caution must be taken in the reduction of spinal deformity. An extensive work-up including myelography and magnetic resonance imaging should be done to be sure that there are no intracanal anomalies, such as diastematomyelia. Caution must be taken with the patient with active infection, particularly of the lumbar spine, where the introduction of a foreign body might not be appropriate when compared with fusion in situ.

NEWER GENERATION COTREL-DUBOUSSET INSTRUMENTATION

The use of the C-D device has been expanding into all fields of spinal surgery. One of the greatest problems that has yet to be solved is the issue of distal fixation to the sacrum. The iliosacral screw has been utilized for several years, but there are no good, long-term follow-up studies to document its usage. Some have devised a sacral block to be imbedded in the sacrum to allow increased distribution of fixation forces for rods that will proceed cranially. The "tulip" pedicle screw may offer increased fixation at the level of the sacrum and lumbar spine. Other screw modifications are also being evaluated.

For fractures and degenerative stabilization, multiple offset and oblique hooks have been devised to complement pedicle screw fixation. In addition, the shoe of the laminar hook has been diversified into caudally and cranially directed devices.

SUMMARY

The C-D device has introduced a significant increase in the number of available surgical options for the patient with spinal deformity. The use of apical distraction or compression, the ability to distract and compress along the same rod, the advantages of rod coupling through the use of DTT, and the newer generation devices that offer exciting potentials for fixation to the sacrum and pelvis are major milestones in the operative treatment of spinal deformity. Currently, the use of the device is expanding into the field of degenerative spinal disorders and spinal trauma. With tens of thousands of cases now performed worldwide, the Cotrel-Dubousset device has proved to be a safe and effective method in the treatment of scoliosis.

REFERENCES

1. Bridwell KH, Betz R, Capelli AM, et al: Sagittal plane analysis in idiopathic scoliosis patients treated with Cotrel-Dubousset instrumentation. Trans Orthop 1990;14:559.
2. Cotrel Y, Dubousset J, Guillaumat M: New universal instrumentation in spinal surgery. Clin Orthop 1988;227:10–23.
3. Cundy PJ, Paterson DC, Hillier TM, et al: Cotrel-Dubousset instrumentation and vertebral rotation in adolescent idiopathic scoliosis. JBJS 1990;72:670–674.
4. Denis F: Cotrel-Dubousset instrumentation in the treatment of idiopathic scoliosis. Orthop Clin North Am 1988;19:291–311.
5. Ecker ML, Betz RR, Trent PS, et al: Computer tomography evaluation of Cotrel-Dubousset instrumentation in idiopathic scoliosis. Spine 1988;13:1141–1144.
6. Farcy JP, Weidenbaum M, Michelsen CB, et al: A comparative biomechanical study of spinal fixation using Cotrel-Dubousset instrumentation. Spine 1987;12:877–881.
7. Fitch RD, Turi M, Bowman BE, et al: Comparison of Cotrel-Dubousset and Harrington rod instrumentations in idiopathic scoliosis. J Pediatr Orthop 1990;10:44–47.
8. Gurr KR, McAfee PC: Cotrel-Dubousset instrumentation in adults. A preliminary report. Spine 1988;13:510–520.
9. Gurr KR, McAfee PC, Warden KE, et al: A roentgenographic and biomechanical analysis of spinal fusions; A canine model. Baltimore: Scoliosis Research Society, 1988;77–78.
10. Holt RT, Johnson JR: Cotrel-Dubousset instrumentation in neurofibromatosis spine curves. A preliminary report. Clin Orthop 1989;245:19–23.
11. Johnston CE, Ashman RB, Corin JD: Mechanical effects of crosslinking rods in Cotrel-Dubousset instrumentation. Hamilton, Bermuda: Scoliosis Research Society, 1986;77–78.
12. Richards BS, Birch JG, Herring JA, et al: Frontal plane and sagittal plane balance following Cotrel-Dubousset instrumentation for idiopathic scoliosis. Spine 1989;14:733–737.
13. Roach JW, Ashman RB, Allard RN: The strength of a CD claw at one verses two spinal levels. Amsterdam: Scoliosis Research Society, 1989;46.
14. Shufflebarger HL, Clark CE: Cotrel-Dubousset instrumentation. Orthopaedics 1988;11:1435–1440.
15. Shufflebarger HL, Crawford AH: Is Cotrel-Dubousset instrumentation the treatment of choice for idiopathic scoliosis in the adolescent who has an operative thoracic curve? Orthopedics 1988;11:1579–1588.
16. Wojcik AS, Webb JK, Burwell RG: Harrington-Luque and Cotrel-Dubousset instrumentation for idiopathic thoracic scoliosis. A postoperative comparison using segmental radiologic analysis. Spine 1990;15:424–431.

NINE

Texas Scottish Rite Hospital (TSRH) Universal Spinal Instrumentation System

Charles E. Johnston, II, J. Anthony Herring, Richard B. Ashman

INTRODUCTION

A truly universal spinal instrumentation system should be applicable to any area of the spine (cervical, thoracolumbar, sacropelvis), and to any spinal pathology for which stabilizing or corrective instrumentation is indicated. Such a system has been developed over the past 5 years at the Texas Scottish Rite Hospital (TSRH). Originally designed as an adjunctive implant for Luque sublaminar segmental instrumentation (SSI), the original Crosslink™ device has become part of a complete, versatile system for correction of adolescent spinal deformity, utilizing and expanding the principles of the Cotrel-Dubousset system, while simultaneously improving certain technical aspects of implantation and, perhaps more importantly, improving the ease of *removing* and *revising* instrumentation already implanted.

With the addition of vertebral screws, anterior *and* transpedicular fixation are possible, thus greatly expanding the uses of the instrumentation to pathologies other than adolescent deformity, including all types of adult degenerative, traumatic, or neoplastic instabilities. With the addition of smaller, pediatric-sized hooks, deformity in very young or skeletally dysplastic patients can be instrumented safely, as well as certain cervical spine instabilities. With its ability to extend existing instrumentation cephalad or caudad by the axial crosslinking plates, the TSRH system has evolved into a *truly* universal system for instrumenting the spine.

CROSSLINK DEVELOPMENT

Postoperative rod migration in segmental spinal instrumentation (SSI) was the original problem addressed in 1985. The Luque procedure (18) revolutionized the treatment of neuromuscular spinal deformity in the 1970s, but in spite of the increased stability provided by segmental fixation, loss of fixation with rod migration secondary to cyclic loading still occurred (Fig. 9.1) (1,5,7,20). The problem most commonly occurred in neuromuscular deformities, where osteopenia prevented secure wire-rod fixation to the posterior elements when there was no meaningful connection between one rod and the other.

Through studies of the load-carrying capacities of SSI constructs on a computer model, Weiler proposed the concept of cross-bracing of spinal rods (25). The rigid plate implant, now available as the TSRH Crosslink, was developed in 1985 to bring this concept of rigid cross-bracing to the surgeon's armamentarium. Using an eyebolt and locking nut, a three-point interference clamp mechanism was created (Fig. 9.2), so that when the threaded nut was progressively tightened, the crosslink plate was clamped securely to a rod. Using calf spines as an anatomic scaffolding, the mechanical performance of crosslinks was evaluated by testing the axial and torsional stiffness of spinal rod constructs with significant contouring built into the rods (15). The axial stiffness of an SSI construct was significantly improved by the simple addition of crosslinking. With the movement between rods essentially eliminated, the increased stiffness to axial load proved an important benefit of crosslinking, especially in severe deformities in which significant rod contouring was required because of residual deformity, and which had produced an alarming loss of construct stiffness (15). The first surgical case using Crosslinks was performed in 1985 with custom implants (Fig. 9.3).

The introduction of the rotational maneuver to correct scoliosis by Cotrel and Dubousset was a breakthrough in deformity surgery (10), and it was logical to assume that a system using rotational correction should be evaluated mechanically by testing its ability to resist torsional loading. The Cotrel-Dubousset (C-D) system already uti-

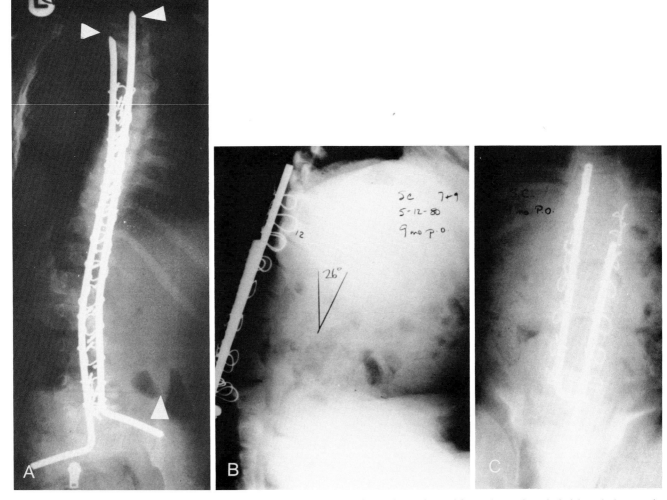

Figure 9.1. *A–C,* Immediate postoperative loss of fixation with Luque rod migration. Postoperative shift in SSI to the pelvis. The right rod has migrated cephalad in relation to the left, with recurrence of pelvic obliquity.

lized a dynamic transverse traction (DTT) device to crosslink the 7-mm knurled rods (Fig. 9.4*A*). When standard C-D constructs were subjected to torsional testing unlinked, crosslinked with the DTT device, and crosslinked with the TSRH plate, it was revealed that the DTT enhanced the torsional stiffness of a construct only minimally over unlinked rods, especially when the interrod distance exceeded 2.5 cm. In contrast, the torsional stiffness of a C-D construct crosslinked with the TSRH plate actually increased as the distance between the rods increased (Fig. 9.4*B*) (14).

The original crosslink design underwent modifications to increase the thickness of the plate and to decrease the size of the oval holes, allowing a thicker isthmus to be placed between them (Fig. 9.5). The isthmus allows contouring of the plate to accommodate rods that are not parallel or are in significantly different planes due to con-

tours required by the spinal deformity, while decreasing the susceptibility to plate fracture. Although the plate was made thicker, it carries a low profile compared with the earlier implant and with the DTT device (Fig. 9.5) by decreasing the height of the nut. Clinical use of this device is over 150 cases with a minimum follow-up of 1 year has demonstrated its utility in stabilizing all types of spinal rod systems, with a negligible incidence of loosening or failure (16). The spiral lock thread of the eyebolt and the necessity of tightening the nuts to 17 Nm of torque are primarily responsible for the low incidence of nut loosening.

CONSTRUCT RESEARCH

Rigid crosslinking increases the *axial* stiffness of rod-wire constructs in which the only rod-bone connection is by

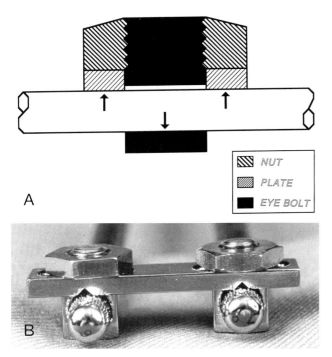

Figure 9.2. *A*, The eyebolt in cross-section. Three points of rod contact produce the clamping mechanism. *B*, The original crosslink design (end view).

a twisted wire, such as in traditional SSI (15). It is also known to increase the *torsional* stiffness of rod-wire constructs and rod-hook constructs where the rod-bone connection is via a hook with a set screw or ratchet-jamming mechanism (14,15). However, the clinical efficacy of increased spinal construct stiffness, while ostensibly appropriate, has never been studied in terms of the effect of the construct stiffness on the process of biological arthrodesis. Gurr and coworkers demonstrated an increased incidence of arthrodesis when spinal fusions were augmented with implants in dogs (12), but the *quality* of the fusion mass as a function of the stiffness of the construct has never been evaluated.

Results of an in-vivo spinal fusion study of goats reveal that stiffer constructs increase the axial and torsional stiffness of the ensuing fusion mass (13). Standardized 10-segment posterior fusions with segmental wiring using Drummond button-wire implants (11) were carried out, attempting to increase the overall construct stiffness by using rods of larger diameter and adding Crosslinks. Although rod-wire slippage during cyclic loading (20) in vivo prevented significant additional axial stiffness to be imparted by rods of larger diameter or by crosslinking. 6.4-mm rods did produce fusion masses significantly stiffer in axial testing than 3.2-mm rods. Unlike axial testing, in torsional testing rod-wire slippage was not critical,

because both larger rod diameter and rigid crosslinking increased the torsional stiffness of the ensuring fusion masses. This finding was predicted by earlier experimental mechanical testing (2,13,14). These results offered evidence linking the quality of the fusion mass to the stiffness of the internal fixation construct. Accordingly, from the purely biological standpoint of seeking a more robust fusion mass, stiffer spinal constructs are preferred. At the same time, the fusion mass obtained from 4.8-mm rods rigidly crosslinked (Fig. 9.6A) was just as stiff as the fusion mass produced by unlinked 6.4-mm rods, suggesting that smaller diameter, more easily implanted rods, when crosslinked, provide the same fusion mass stiffness as unlinked, heavier rods, which may be more difficult to contour and implant.

Additional studies have shown *no* significant changes in fusion stiffnesses resulting from varying the stiffness of constructs in short, three-segment fusions (Fig. 9.6B and 9.6C, unpublished data). This suggests that increased construct stiffness, producing stiffer fusion masses in the longer, 10-segment model (simulating a scoliosis operation) is not so critical in a short-segment fusion (simulating a degenerative lumbar fusion) when meticulous arthrodesis technique is followed.

HOOKS, SCREWS, AND RODS

The three-point clamping mechanism provided by the eyebolt was logically extended to the attachment of a hook or screw to a rod (Fig. 9.7). The hooks are designed so that a rod can be inserted from above for easy assembly of the construct intraoperatively; thus, all hooks are "open." A small recess on each side of the rod groove in the hook (Fig. 9.7A) allows the rod to be "trapped" within the hook while the eyebolt nut is still only partially tight. This tightness is sufficient to keep the rod seated in the hook, but is loose enough to allow compression, distraction, or rotation maneuvers to be performed without additional adjunctive implants or devices to keep the rods seated during these maneuvers. Hook holders are attached at the side of the hook opposite where the nut will be tightened so that they will neither impede rod entrance into the hook from above nor subsequent nut tightening by a wrench (Fig. 9.7B).

Mechanical studies comparing the axial and torsional force required to disengage an eyebolt from a smooth rod have documented the integrity of this clamping mechanism (Fig. 9.8). One perceived disadvantage of a smooth rod is that hook or screw attachments may slip. The axial and torsional loosening strength of the TSRH eyebolt is equal to or better than any of the various C-D devices using either one or two set screws. The importance of the spiral lock thread on the eyebolt and the requirement

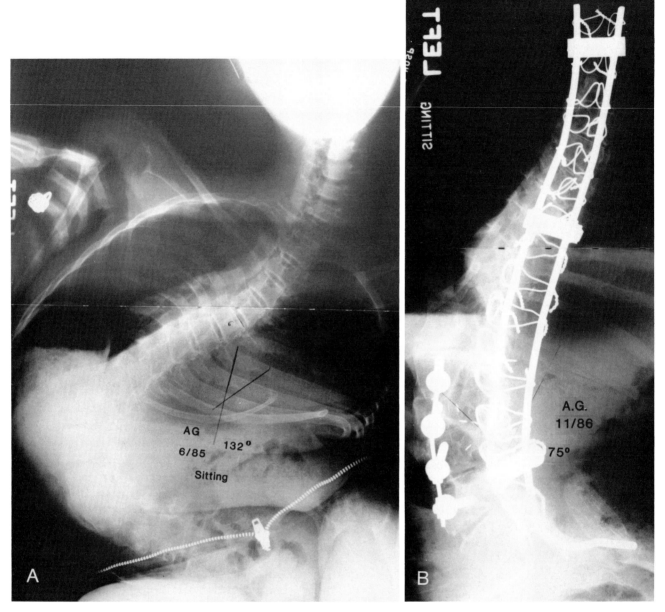

Figure 9.3. *A*, Preoperative radiograph with 14-year-old boy with Duchenne muscular dystrophy and a neglected spinal deformity. Bend films showed passive correction to 90°. FEV$_1$ was estimated at 28% of predicted value. *B*, Simultaneous anterior and posterior correction was performed because of the patient's anticipated inability to tolerate staged procedures. Correction to 75° was achieved. At 1-year follow-up, there is no shift of rods or loss of correction. Three Crosslinks stabilized this markedly contoured, relatively flexible construct. The patient survived for 4 years without loss of correction.

of tightening the nut to at least 17 Nm of torque cannot be overemphasized.

Why should a smooth rod be used? First, there is less friction or binding between a smooth rod and a hook body during a rotational maneuver than with a rough knurled rod. Excessive friction between a knurled rod and hook body might prevent satisfactory rod rotation, or more seriously, might cause hook displacement during the rotational maneuver if the binding were too great. Pedicle hook dislodgment into the spinal canal during the rotational maneuver has been suspected in some cases of neurologic injury associated with C-D instrumentation

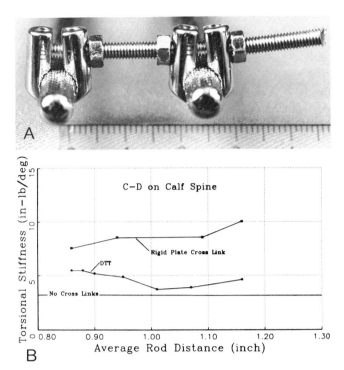

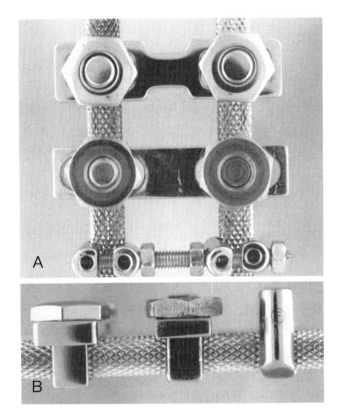

Three additional laminar hooks are used in the system. The buttressed laminar hook (Fig. 9.10) has the same design as the pedicle hook, with a buttressed axilla producing anatomic contact with the lamina and preventing intrusion of the hook shoe into the neural canal. This hook is usually placed through a laminotomy over the superior edge of a lamina and faces caudally. The larger, circular laminar hook (Fig. 9.11) can be utilized over the superior edge of the lamina when its thickness is too great for the buttressed lamina hook, and can also be utilized facing cephalad under a lamina or over a transverse process. The laminar hook with offset top (Fig. 9.12) is useful when the plane of the hook is more anterior than the plane of the rod, as it extends the height of the hook more dorsally.

Side-opening laminar hooks (Fig. 9.13) are available and quite useful when translating the rod toward the spine from the side, as in a cantilever correction of thoracolumbar deformity with posterior instrumentation. Since the eyebolt nut is tightened from directly above with this hook, it is ideal in areas of difficult exposure.

Figure 9.4. *A*, Dynamic transverse traction (DTT) implant. *B*, Graph of torsional stiffness vs. interrod distance for C-D construct unlinked, crosslinked with DTT, and crosslinked with TSRH implants. Torsional stiffness imparted by TSRH Crosslink increases as the interrod distance increases.

(23). A smooth rod is less likely to displace pedicle hooks during the rotational maneuver because of a lack of binding.

Another important factor for neurologic safety during the rotational maneuver is the stability to rotation of the pedicle hooks. Increased stability has been achieved by widening and deepening the radius between tines so that they may more firmly "grasp" the pedicle (Fig. 9.9*A*). In addition, the shape of the axilla of the hook has been modified so that the inferior lamina edge and articular process can be grasped by an anatomic, rather than circular design (Fig. 9.9*B*, 9.9*C*). In each of three testing protocols, where hook contact with the pedicle or lamina surface was varied from minimal to ideal, TSRH pedicle hook stability was significantly improved over other hook designs (Fig. 9.9*D*) (4). Additionally, the TSRH hook design allows less intrusion into the canal should the hook rotate off the pedicle and displace medially. Thus, the smooth rod decreases the chance of binding between the rod and hook during the rotational maneuver, and the pedicle hook design modifications improve stability to rotational force, theoretically decreasing the chance for neurologic injury intraoperatively.

Figure 9.5. *A*, Current TSRH Crosslink (*top*) in profile with the obsolete first-generation implant (*middle*) and the DTT device. *B*, Note the low profile of the present implant (*left*).

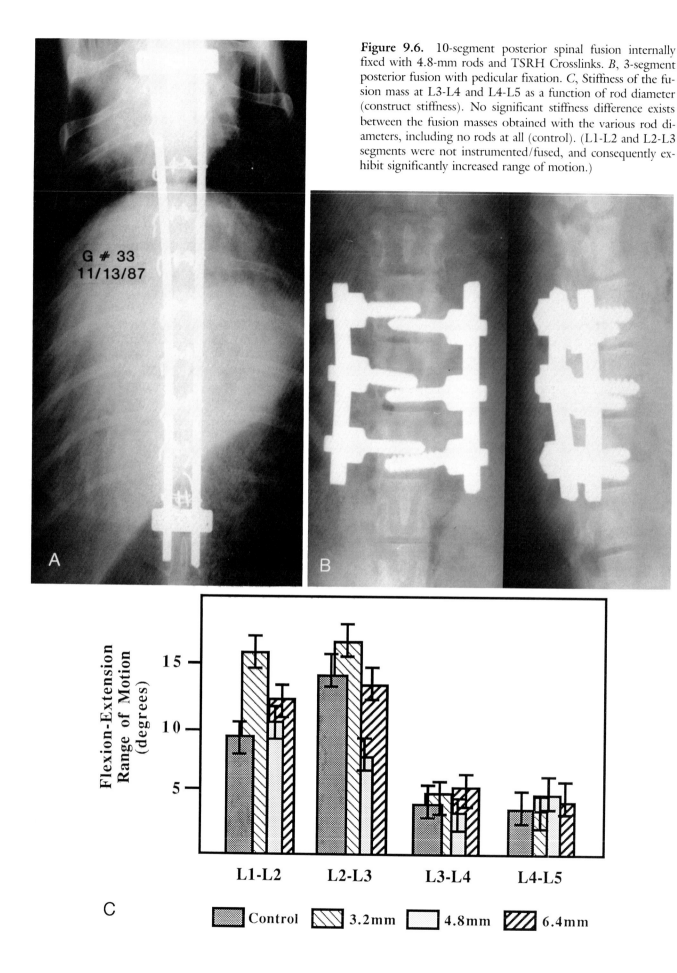

Figure 9.6. 10-segment posterior spinal fusion internally fixed with 4.8-mm rods and TSRH Crosslinks. *B,* 3-segment posterior fusion with pedicular fixation. *C,* Stiffness of the fusion mass at L3-L4 and L4-L5 as a function of rod diameter (construct stiffness). No significant stiffness difference exists between the fusion masses obtained with the various rod diameters, including no rods at all (control). (L1-L2 and L2-L3 segments were not instrumented/fused, and consequently exhibit significantly increased range of motion.)

A closed transverse process hook (the only closed hook in the system) is useful as the cephalad hook on the convexity of a scoliosis construct (Fig. 9.14). Once the rod has been threaded through the eyebolt and closed hook, it cannot dislodge from the hook even though no nut tightening is performed. This is a useful convenience when exposure and space are limited.

The circular laminar hooks have been downsized for use in constructs where two laminar hooks might be placed side by side in the spinal canal at the same level, facing either cephalad or caudad. The shoe of these hooks has been narrowed considerably (Fig. 9.15A) and the hooks have half-tops to reduce bulkiness and width. These "fracture" hooks are most useful when used as part of a laminar-laminar claw, or a pedicle screw-laminar claw, as in a posterior one-above, one-below fracture construct. The fracture hook with the multispan top accommodates a laterally placed pedicle screw to produce a claw when directed cephalad in the lumbar spine. Normally,

a laminar hook under the same lamina as the pedicle screw would be placed medially (Fig. 9.15B), requiring the multispan top to allow this one-level claw to be realized. Biomechanically, the screw-laminar claw construct increases by 50% the pullout strength of a construct with pedicle screws alone (Fig. 9.15C), an invaluable improvement in managing lumbar spine fractures by fusing as few segments as possible and hopefully avoiding pedicle screw failure complications (Fig. 9.16).

Pediatric hooks are also available (Fig. 9.17). These small hooks have a single central upright, that allows rod attachment from either side; they are of an appropriate size for the young patient (under age 8), and are also useful in the cervical spine. Along with a single pedicle hook, there are two designs of the laminar hook. The eyebolts are downsized and accommodate the 4.8-mm rod. Clinical examples using these hooks will be discussed at the end of this chapter.

Analysis of available pedicle screw systems demon-

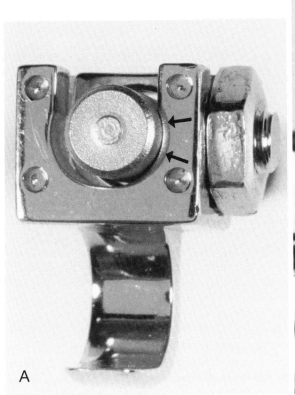
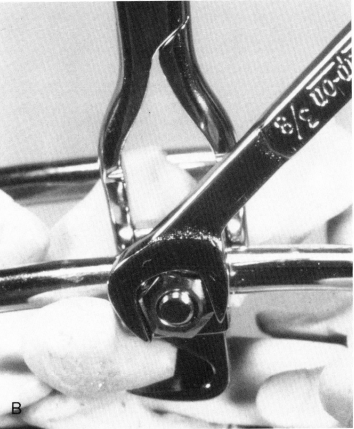

Figure 9.7. *A,* End view of hook attached to a rod by the eyebolt mechanism. Notice recesses on each side of the rod groove (*arrow*). *B,* Tightening of the locking nut. Access to the nut is not impeded by the hook holder.

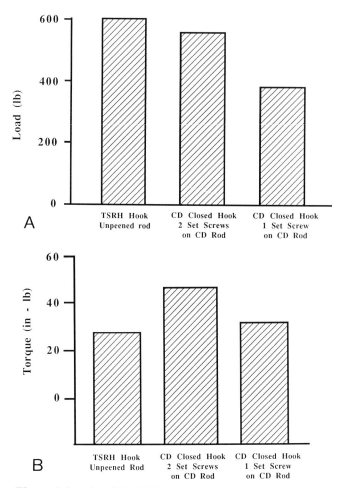

Figure 9.8. *A* and *B*, Axial and torsional loosening strengths of TSRH hook and eyebolt on a smooth unpeened rod, compared with a C-D closed hook with one or two set screws.

strained (e.g., Luque plates, AO notched plate) systems (Fig. 9.18*B*). If used as a transpedicular device, the TSRH screw design is satisfactory for withstanding cantilever bending (tensile) stresses in the short term at the screw-rod junction, with fatigue characteristics in bench testing similar to *non*constrained systems. Of course, the importance of obtaining a solid arthrodesis cannot be overemphasized, since all screws will eventually fatigue if cyclical motion is not eliminated in a finite time period by fusion (9). Comparison of constrained pedicle screw systems in cyclical fatigue tests has shown the TSRH screw and smooth rod system to exceed other constrained systems in resisting fatigue fractures (Fig. 9.18*C*). In difficult lumbosacral fixations, pivoting screw top attachments (vertical or horizontal rod attachment) add an important "nonconstrained" versatility to the armamentarium (Fig. 9.18*D*).

TSRH screws may be used for anterior fixation of the spine. Both screw diameters (6.5 and 5.5 mm) have cancellous threads, suitable for fixation in the vertebral body. An example of anterior implantation might be stabilization after vertebrectomy for anterior cord impingement due to trauma or pathologic fracture (Fig. 9.19). For anterior short-segment stabilization, the double-rod construct on the anterolateral spine, with Crosslink, is as mechanically stable as other devices (e.g., Kaneda device) specifically designed for such an anterior application (26). The TSRH anterior construct has additional advantages of utilizing rods that are easily contoured, as well as easily distracted, compressed, or rotated, providing the surgeon greater versatility.

In certain lumbar and thoracolumbar scoliosis patterns, anterior instrumentation and fusion allow the surgeon to fuse fewer levels, an important benefit when the deformity extends caudally into the lumbar spine. TSRH instrumentation is quite effective as an anterior scoliosis instrumentation, using vertebral screws and the solid 4.8- or 6.4-mm rod to produce rotational correction while maintaining lordosis (Fig. 9.20).

Although experimental studies suggest that stiffer spinal constructs produce stiffer fusion masses in scoliotic deformities (13), the use of an extremely stiff rod can be difficult or even dangerous. Rotational correction of scoliosis requires that the rod be stiff enough that the spine conforms to the contouring of the rod and that the kyphosis provided by the rod contour is maintained after the rotational maneuver. Many surgeons using C-D instrumentation have noted that C-D rod flexibility often does not maintain the original amount of kyphosis contoured into the rods. This is because the rods deform intraoperatively during the rotation maneuver in response to the stiffness of the deformity. Obviously, rod flexibility provides a safety factor during the rotation maneuver in

strated the need for important improvements in design of screws used in a constrained system to decrease the incidence of fatigue fracture. Ashman and colleagues have identified the root of the screw at its junction with the rod or plate as the point of maximal stress concentration and the predictable point of failure in constrained pedicle screw systems (3). TSRH vertebral screws have incorporated into the design a large-diameter, nonthreaded neck of the screw to minimize stress concentration at the site of greatest vulnerability, namely, the junction between the shank and the root of the screw where the rod/eyebolt mechanism attaches (Fig. 9.18*A*). Cyclic testing to produce fatigue fracture (±440 N axial load at 2 Hz) demonstrated that the 6.5-mm screws show no failure at greater than 1 million cycles, similar to the other constrained (e.g., AO fixateur interne) and noncon-

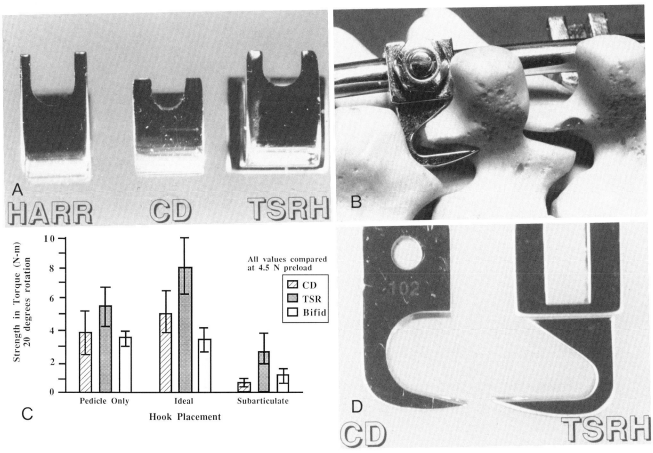

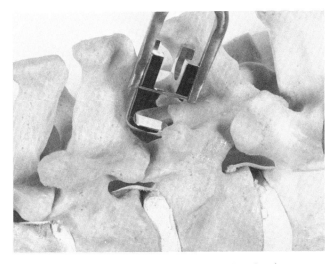

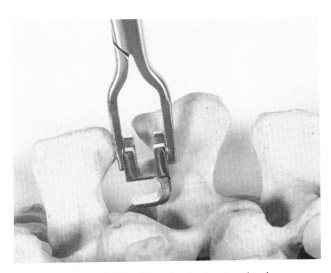

Figure 9.9. *A*, Tines of various pedicle hooks. TSRH design includes a wider and deeper radius to "grasp" the pedicle rather than simply contact it. Harrington (HARR) tines are easily deformed during insertion, and their length allows possible medial protrusion into the spinal canal. *B*, Anatomic design of the TSRH hook, designed to fit the laminar surface precisely.

C, Circular design of some pedicle hooks (*left*) do not provide the same anatomic, "press-fit" grasp of the laminar surface, increasing rotational instability. *D*, Experimental rotational stability in torque of three hook designs. "Pedicle only" and "subarticulate" placements provide suboptimal contact between lamina, pedicle, and hook.

Figure 9.10. The buttressed laminar hook.

Figure 9.11. The circular laminar hook.

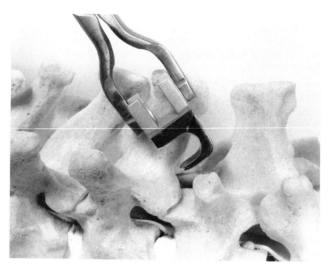

Figure 9.12. The offset circular laminar hook.

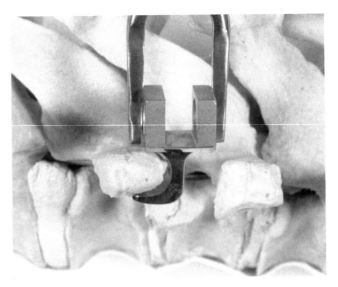

Figure 9.14. Closed transverse process hook.

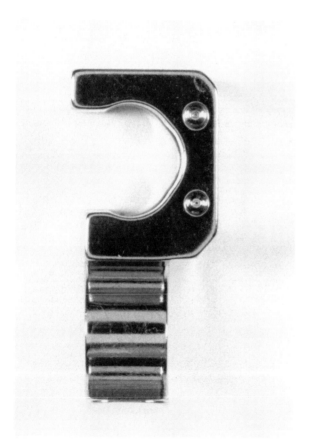

Figure 9.13. Side-opening laminar hook.

case the kyphosis contoured into the rod is excessive or the deformity too stiff to allow full rotational correction.

To resolve this predicament, the TSRH instrumentation provides three levels of rod stiffness (4.8 mm, flexible 6.4 mm, stiff 6.4 mm) (Fig. 9.21*A*). The stiff rod on the concavity allows the surgeon to seek maximal rotational correction without loss of the rod-imposed kyphosis, and is most applicable in a severe deformity that is moderately flexible. If significant stiffness of the deformity prevents such correction, the more flexible rod is appropriate, primarily for ease of implantation. The same considerations apply to the correction and fixation of posttraumatic or degenerative deformities. All TSRH rods have a shot-peening surface treatment that increases their fatigue life (Fig. 9.21*B*). All rods have a hexagonal-shaped end that allows rotational force to be used at one end of the rod with an appropriate wrench (Fig. 9.21*C*). Because the hooks, screws, and Crosslinks use the same locking mechanism for attachment to the rod, namely, the eyebolt, the versatility of the TSRH system is perhaps its greatest advantage over other systems. The eyebolt mechanism makes the system extremely easy to remove or revise—the locking nut is loosened, and the system can be immediately disassembled. Because all the hooks and screws are "open," a dislodged hook can be easily replaced, the rod reseated (with a corkscrew, for example), and the eyebolt retightened, without having to disassemble the entire construct and start over. Revision of previously operated cases is often simplified because surgical exposure can be limited to a local area of pseudar-

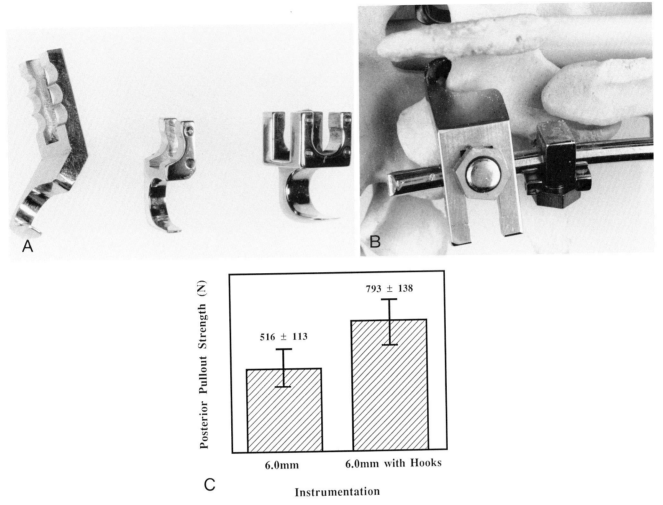

Figure 9.15. *A*, Fracture hooks with half-top (*center*), and multispan top (*left*). The narrow shoe of these hooks is compared with a standard laminar hook shoe (*right*). *B*, Close-up of pedicle screw-laminar claw using multispan fracture hook. *C*, Posterior pullout strength of pedicle screw constructs ("one-above, one-below") without and with laminar hooks to produce pedicle-screw/laminar clawing at cephalad and caudal segments.

throsis or implant failure. Reinstrumentation can be applied without having to remove intact instrumentation above or below the level of revision (Fig. 9.22). When extending an existing instrumentation cephalad or caudad, the extension is accomplished without disturbing the existing instrumentation (Fig. 9.16).

The ability to link rods axially is extremely advantageous when performing Galveston fixation (1) to the pelvis in patients with neuromuscular deformity. Correction of pelvic obliquity is performed as a separate step in the operative procedure (Fig. 9.23). This technique eliminates the extremely complex rod contours (Galves-

ton bends) required to place a rod in the iliac wing while simultaneously accommodating deformities in the thoracolumbar spine above (8). Once separate sets of thoracolumbar rods and pelvic rods have been linked together axially, pelvic obliquity may be corrected, for example, by distracting on the high side. Care must be taken to contour accurately any Crosslinks connecting rods that are nonparallel, and final tightening of the nuts on axial Crosslinks is performed only after assuring that the two rods linked together enter the grooves in the Crosslink plates perpendicularly to ensure proper three-point clamping fixation (Fig. 9.24).

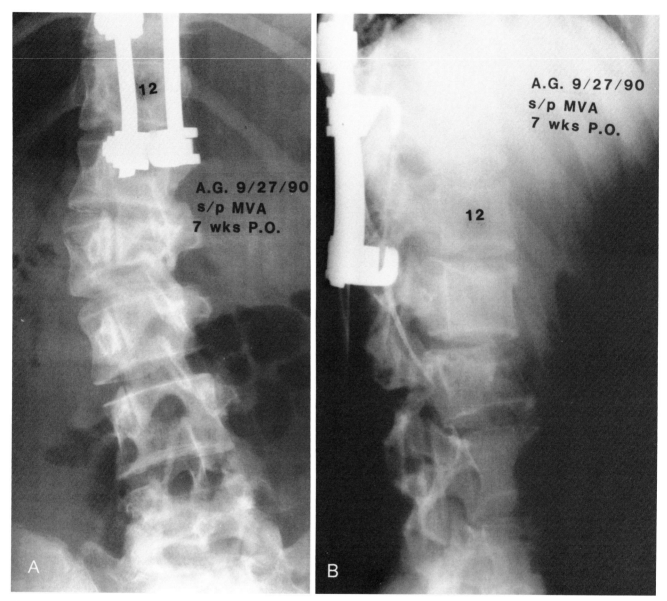

Figure 9.16. *A* and *B*, A 16-year-old female, 7 weeks following instrumentation and fusion to T12 for idiopathic scoliosis, suffered an L2 burst-distraction injury in a motor vehicle accident. *C*, Intraoperative view of distraction (Chance fracture) component in L2 posterior elements. Cephalad-facing hooks under T12 lamina (from previous scoliosis surgery) are at left. *D* and *E*, Instrumentation was extended to L3 using pedicle screws with multispan fracture hook claw at the same level. By crosslinking to the existing instrumentation ending at T12, and distracting the concavity (right side) of the fracture deformity while compressing and lordosing the convexity (left side), the fracture was reduced and stabilized, while only extending instrumentation one level distal to the injury. The pedicle-screw-laminar claw is essential for this short extension caudal to the injury.

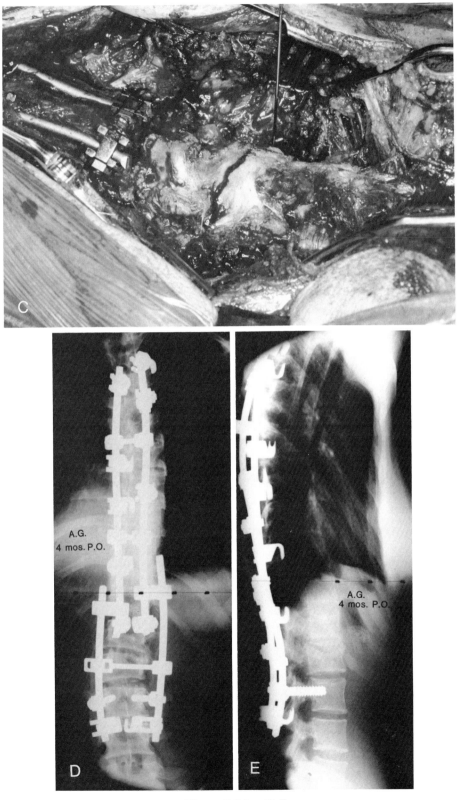

Figure 9.16. *C–E.*

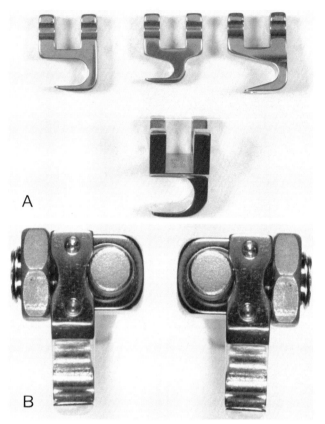

Figure 9.17. *A,* Pediatric hooks (standard adult hook for comparison). *B,* A 4.8-mm rod may be attached to either side of the central post.

INSERTION EQUIPMENT

The following devices are used to insert the components of the TSRH instrumentation system.

Hook Holders. Hook holders attach to the hooks parallel to the rod entrance into the hook, a feature that allows the holders to remain on the hook while the rod is inserted (Fig. 9.7*B*). Access to the tightening nut is not impeded by the hook holder either.

Hook Inserter. The hook inserter fits inside the hook (in the rod groove) to provide control during hook insertion.

Trial Hooks. The trial hooks are identical to the implants but are rigidly attached to a color-coded handle (Fig. 9.25). This is particularly important for seating

pedicle hooks. After the trial hook has been inserted satisfactorily, it is not necessary to then insert an implant hook to confirm a satisfactory insertion, since the trial hook and implant hook are identical.

Corkscrew. A corkscrew device is used to push the rod and eyebolt into a hook (Fig. 26). The device is a modified hook holder with a threaded pusher rod. The endplate of the pusher must be placed precisely on the rod and eyebolt to maintain control of the eyebolt during insertion (Fig. 9.26*B*).

Mini-corkscrew. The mini-corkscrew attaches to an ordinary hook holder (Fig. 9.27*A*). Thus, a standard hook holder need not be removed intraoperatively in order to use a corkscrew device. The curved extension on the pusher rod may be used either at the crotch of the hook holder close to the spine (Fig. 9.27*B*), or may be placed at the ratchet closure of the hook holder well away from the spine for better visualization (Fig. 9.27*A*).

Eyebolt Spreader. This instrument pushes the rod and eyebolt into the hook by spreading between the crotch of the hook holder and the eyebolt (Fig. 9.28). This is useful for moving the eyebolt and rod a short distance to obtain perfect seating in the hook.

Wrenches. Several wrenches are available to tighten the nuts (Fig. 9.7*B*). Whenever possible, the T-handled torque wrench (Fig. 9.29) is most convenient to tighten a nut rapidly, and is extremely important in ensuring that the minimum-required 17 Nm of torque is achieved when final tightening is performed. Additionally, there is a hexagonal-ended wrench for rod rotation (Fig. 9.21*C*).

SURGICAL TECHNIQUE
Deformity Correction

The sequence of surgical correction of spinal deformity includes: (a) exposure; (b) level identification (radiographically); (c) hook site preparation; (d) bilateral facetectomy; (e) rod contouring (usually concave); (f) decortication on the side of first rod placement (usually concave); (g) hook insertion and placement of the first rod; (h) rotation, distraction, or compression of first rod; (i) decortication of the second side; (j) hook placement on the second side; (k) rod contouring (second rod) and insertion (l) distraction or compression of second rod;

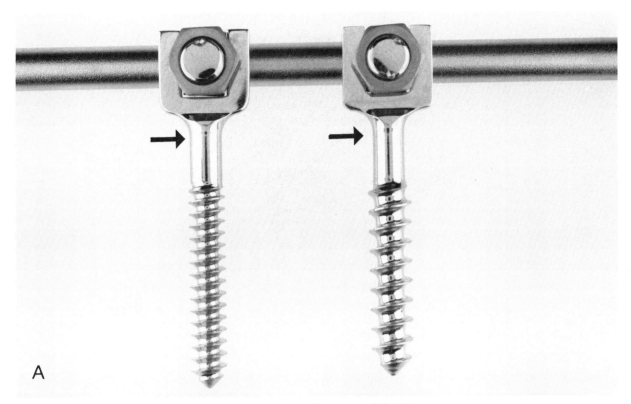

A

Cyclical Loading to Failure
+/- 440 N

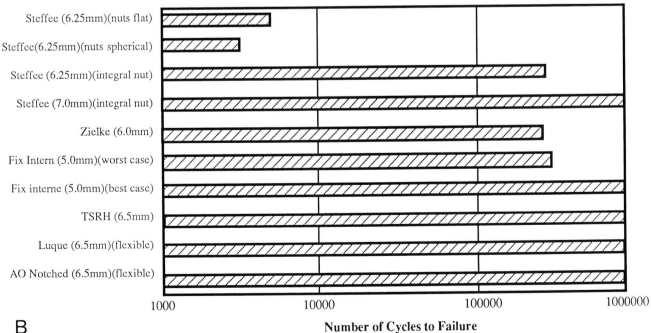

B

Number of Cycles to Failure

Figure 9.18. *A*, Large-diameter, nonthreaded root of the TSRH screw decreases vulnerability of the screw-rod junction to fatigue failure by decreasing stress concentration (*arrows*). *B*, Number of cycles to failure of various screw designs. *C*, Cyclical fatigue tests (load vs. number of cycles to failure) of constrained pedicle screw systems (implant failure or disengagement). *D*, Vertebral screws with pivoting tops, for nonconstrained rod attachment.

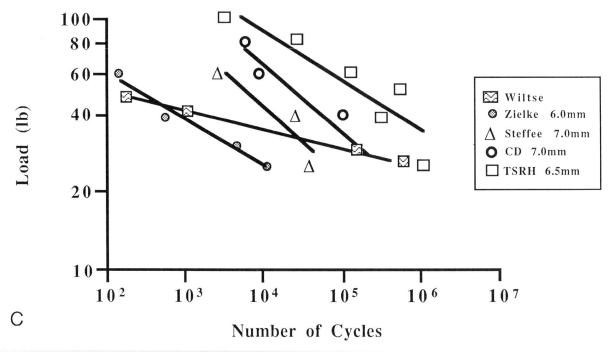

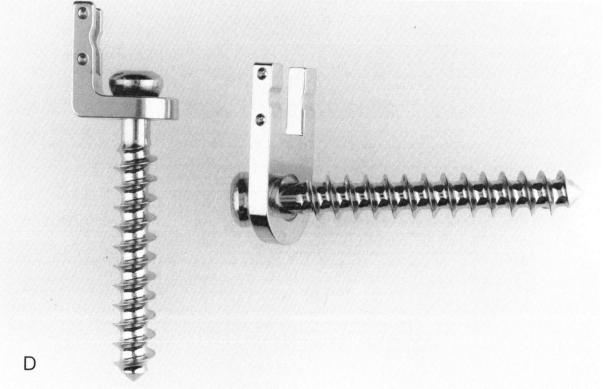

Figure 9.18.   *C–D.*

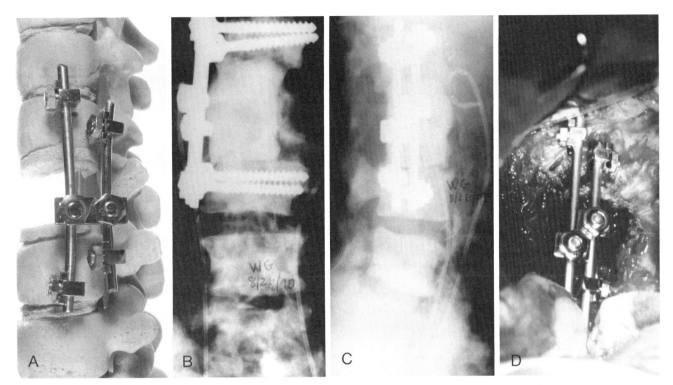

Figure 9.19. *A*, Anterior short-segment stabilization following vertebrectomy, using a double-rod construct with Crosslink. The more anterior rod can be distracted for reduction and lordosis, while the more posterior rod can be compressed to lock in bone graft. *B* and *C*, A 70-year-old male with progressive kyphosis and paraparesis from a pathologic fracture of L2 due to metastatic carcinoma of the prostate. Bone retropulsion was noted on the MRI. The patient was decompressed and stabilized using anterior TSRH double-rod construct with methylmethacrylate spacer. (Case courtesy of Gary L. Lowery, M.D.). *D*, Intraoperative view of double-rod construct with vertebrectomy (anterior-left).

(m) crosslinking of the rods; (n) placement of autogenous iliac graft; (o) closure.

Single Thoracic Scoliosis, King Type III

This deformity will be corrected by rotation of a concave rod with a four hook construct (Fig. 9.30) (10). The two end vertebrae to be instrumented should be identified from the radiograph. With a King III curve, the upper neutral vertebra, or one level cephalad to neutral, usually is chosen for the most proximal hook. Distally, the vertebra next most cephalad to the stable vertebra (17) is tentatively chosen as the end vertebra. The lateral radiograph should then be evaluated for the presence of a junctional kyphosis, a mildly kyphotic transition at the thoracolumbar junction. Normally, the thoracolumbar junction is neither kyphotic nor lordotic. The end vertebra chosen tentatively should not be used if it occurs at the apex of a junctional kyphosis. If a junctional kyphosis is present, instrumentation one to two levels below the apex of the kyphotic segment is recommended. A hook reversal pattern may be necessary in the upper lumbar spine to extend beyond a junctional kyphosis and initiate upper lumbar lordosis (6,24).

Next, the apex of the deformity is identified, and the concave intermediate hook sites are selected. Usually, one vertebra proximal and one vertebra distal to the apex of the curve are chosen for these intermediate hook sites. The bending radiographs help make this decision. The vertebrae at the end of the stiff apical segment—the first vertebrae at which the disc spaces proximal and distal to the apex open with bending—are appropriate for these intermediate hook sites.

Convex hook sites are chosen as follows: the upper end vertebra should be instrumented by a "claw" configuration, usually placing a transverse process hook facing caudally at this level, and creating a claw by placing a pedicle hook cranially—facing at the next distal level. The claw should be split in this fashion over two levels for the added strength of fixation, the ease of insertion, and the ability to perform a facet fusion between these two hooks (22). At the apical vertebra on the convexity, a cephalad-

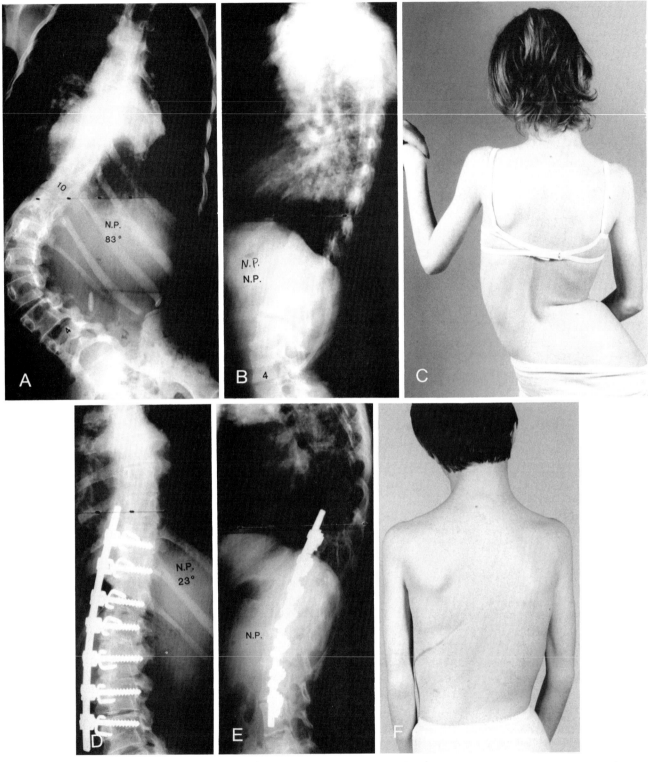

Figure 9.20. *A* and *B*, A 16-year-old autistic female with progressive lumbar scoliosis and pelvic obliquity, threatening her ambulatory status. *C*, Preoperative clinical appearance. *D* and *E*, Postoperative correction using anterior TSRH instru-mentation T10 to L4. Note preservation of lordosis. *F*, Clinical appearance postoperatively. The patient had *no* postoperative immobilization.

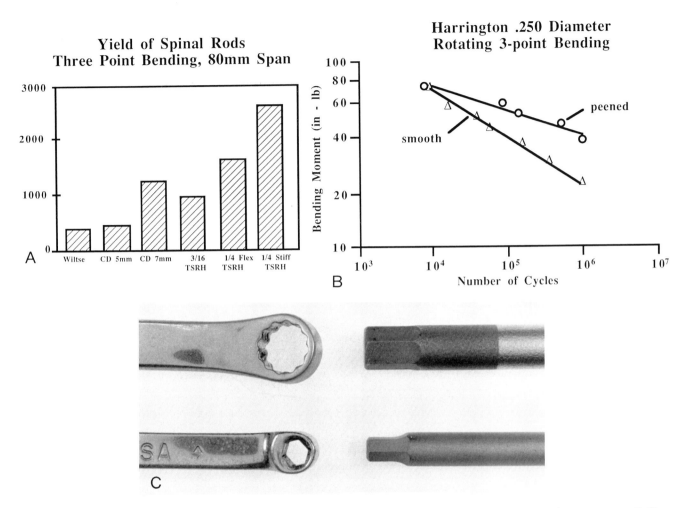

Figure 9.21. *A*, Relative stiffnesses of TSRH rods compared with other spinal rods. *B*, Effect of shot-peening surface treatment on fatigue failure of the rod-ratchet junction of a Harrington rod. The fatigue life of the junction (notorious for fatigue fracture) is increased by the surface treatment. *C*, Shot-peening surface treatment and hexagonal shaped end of TSRH rods.

directed hook for compression is selected, and the final hook is at the lower end vertebra, also cephalad-directed in compression (10).

Pedicle hook sites are created at the upper end and intermediate vertebrae on the concavity as well as part of the upper convex claw and at the convex apical vertebra. A conservative excision of the distal portion of the inferior articular process is performed to expose a small amount of articular cartilage from the superior facet of the next more caudal vertebra. A small elevator may be used to probe and open the joint, and then the pedicle hook trial is inserted to seat the buttressed axilla of the hook against the resected inferior portion of the superior process. If the proper amount of bone has been removed, the tines of the pedicle hook should also engage the pedicle, thus providing the greatest stability of this hook to rotational force (Fig. 9.9) (4).

The transverse process hook creating the pedicle-transverse claw on the convexity is placed by passing the trial hook over the intended transverse process in a subperiosteal plane. Care should be taken during this maneuver to avoid intraosseous penetration of the base of the transverse process, which would weaken the hook site (10).

Laminar hooks are placed at the lower intermediate and lower end vertebrae on the concavity, and will be placed facing caudally in the spinal canal. A significant amount of bone from the spinous process and inferior articular process of the vertebra immediately cephalad is excised to create a large laminotomy. The ligamentum flavum is opened and removed with a Kerrison ronguer.

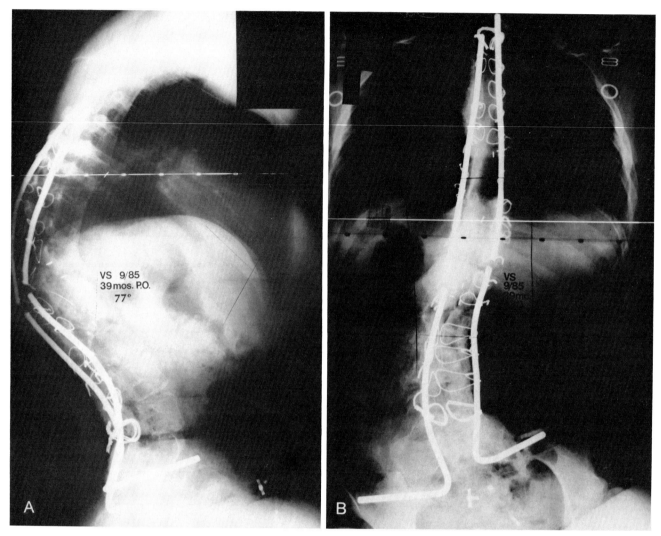

Figure 9.22. *A* and *B*, A 16-year-old paraplegic female 3 years after staged anterior-posterior fusion with SSI to correct a post-laminectomy, postradiation kyphosis caused by spinal cord astrocytoma. Recurrent deformity and pain occurred with rod fracture. *C*, Intraoperative view of rod repair with axial plates and eyebolts and additional compression instrumentation across the pseudarthrosis. *D* and *E*, One year later, the correction and fusion are maintained with only a short posterior revision and pseudarthrosis repair without having to revise the entire SSI construct.

Usually, the buttressed (thoracic) laminar hook is selected for placement over the superior edge of the instrumented lamina because of its anatomic fit (Fig. 9.10). The larger circular laminar hooks may be used in the presence of a very thick lamina. Regardless of which laminar hook is chosen, the surgeon must determine that the hook fits securely on the superior surface of the lamina, and that the hook is not freely intruding and moving in the spinal canal. Normally, laminar hooks in the canal are removed at this time, so that they are not resting near neural elements during facet removal and decortication procedures where a mallet may be used.

Cephalad-directed laminar hooks, such as would be placed in compression at the convex and vertebra distally, are seated by using the laminar elevator and laminar trial instruments under the inferior edge of the vertebra to be instrumented. The inferior edge of this vertebra should be exposed carefully without disturbing the interspinous ligaments and ligamentum flavum in the interspace just caudal to the hook site. This helps to prevent a junctional kyphosis from developing at the end of the instrumentation. The hook path at this level should be superficial to the ligamentum flavum. This hook is the most likely to disengage of the eight-hook construct normally uti-

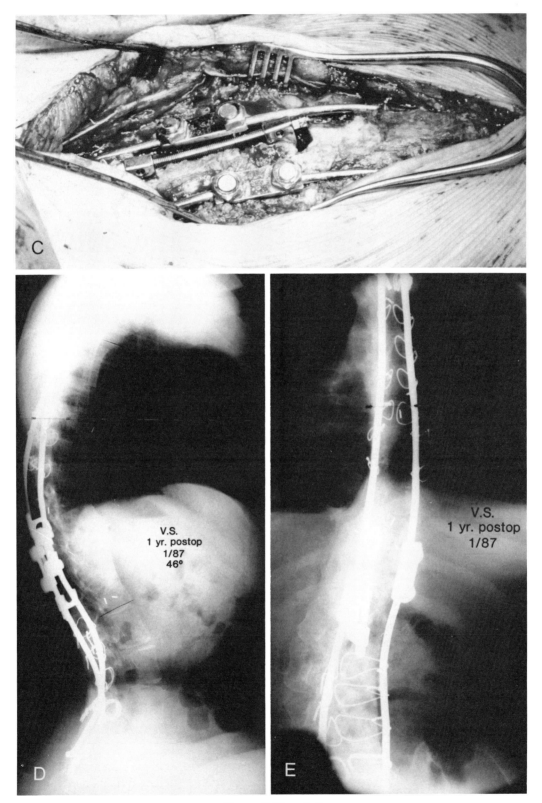

Figure 9.22. *C–E.*

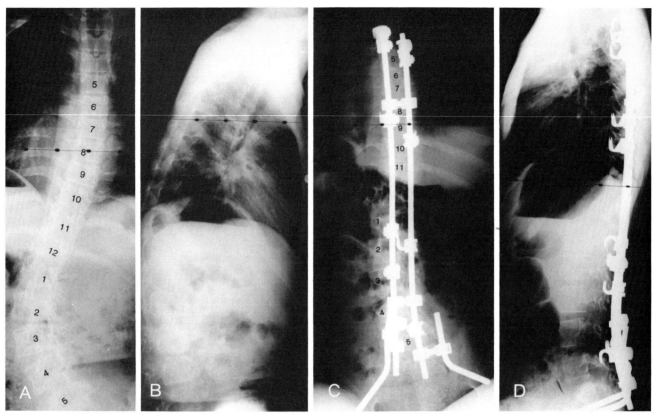

Figure 9.23. *A* and *B*, 14-year-old male with Duchenne muscular dystrophy and progressive scoliosis and pelvic obliquity. *C* and *D*, Postoperative correction using two sets of double-rods. Instrumentation from T4-L5 is accomplished first to obtain balance in the sagittal plane, and then is linked to separate "Galveston" iliac rods using TSRH Crosslinks. Pelvic obliquity is corrected as a separate step by distracting the high side of the pelvis against the construct already implanted above.

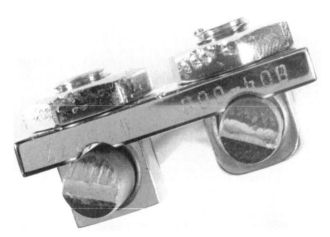

Figure 9.24. Secure fixation cannot be achieved unless the rods fit precisely in the grooves of the plate (*right*). Insecure fixation appears on the left—the rod is not centered in the plate groove.

lized for a King III deformity, and if there is any concern on the surgeon's part that this hook is not well seated, careful sublaminar exposure can be done, again avoiding disturbing the interspinous ligaments if possible. Alternatively, a caudally facing laminar hook may be placed in the sublaminar space at this level, or the next more cephalad level, to create a laminar-laminar claw at the inferior end of the concave rod, stabilizing this end compression hook.

After hooks have been seated and facetectomy/decortication performed, a rod is contoured (usually 6.4 mm flexible) and eyebolts placed on the rod for the appropriate hook positions, not forgetting to include two eyebolts for the Crosslink placement. The rod should then be seated in a sequential fashion, usually beginning at the cephalad end of the construct, seating each eyebolt into each hook in order, and tentatively tightening each nut to ensure the eyebolt does not escape from the hook in which it has just been seated while maneuvering the rod

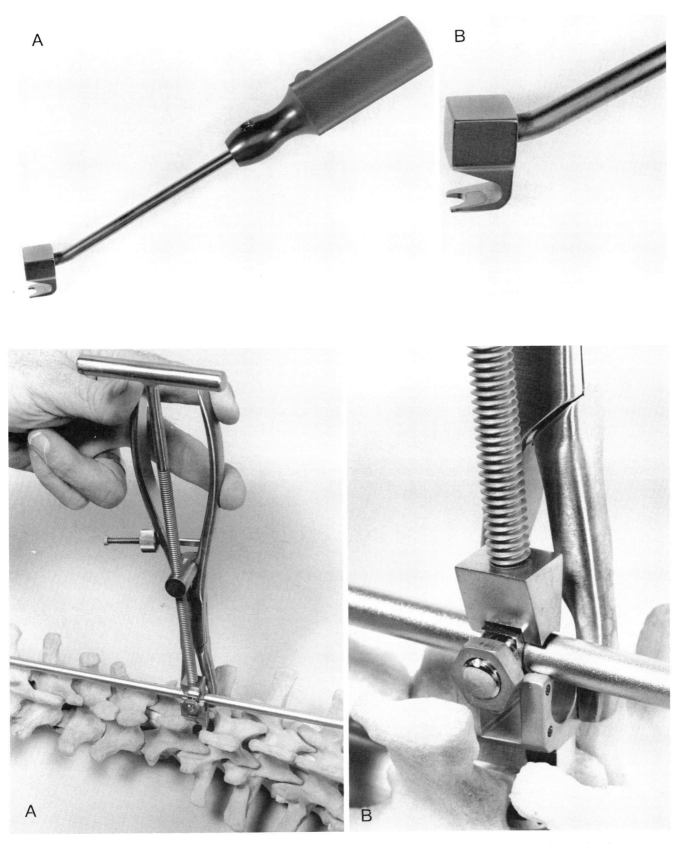

Figure 9.26. *A*, The corkscrew in use. *B*, Close-up of the pusher rod directing eyebolt and rod into a hook.

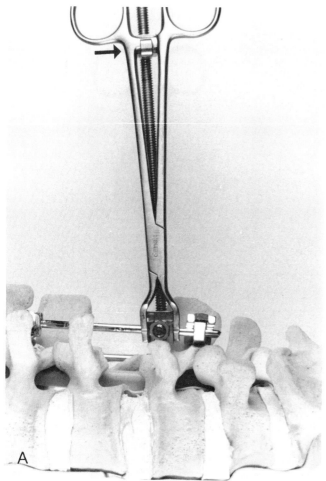

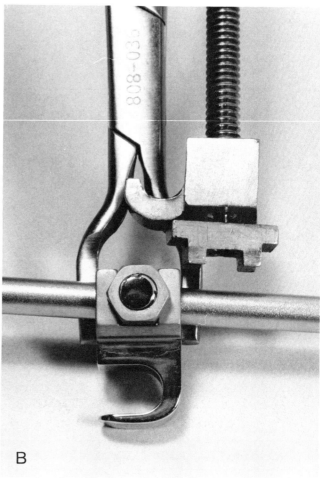

A

B

Figure 9.27. *A*, The mini-corkscrew, attached to a hook holder at the ratchet closure (*arrow*). *B*, Mini-corkscrew. The curved extension of the pusher rod will be attached at the crotch of the hook holder.

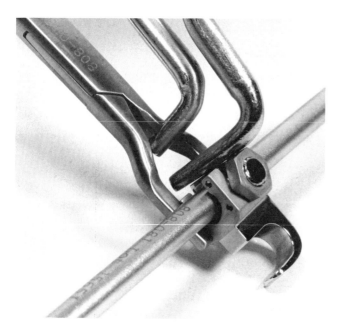

Figure 9.28. The eyebolt spreader.

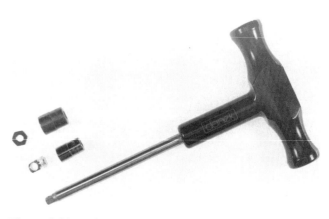

Figure 9.29. The T-handled torque wrench. Two sockets are available, one for the Crosslink nuts, and one for the smaller hook/screw eyebolt nuts.

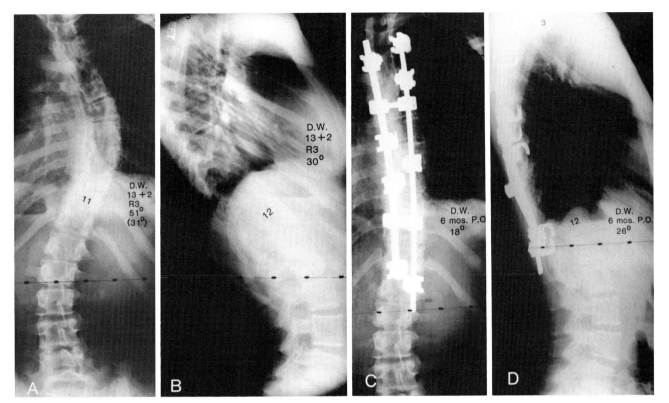

Figure 9.30. King III curve instrumentation. *A*, Preoperative radiograph of a 51° right thoracic scoliosis (bending flexibility to 31°). The stable vertebra is L1. *B*, Lateral radiograph showing no junctional kyphosis. *C*, Postoperative radiograph. The standard four-hook pattern on the concavity consists of cephalad-directed pedicle hooks at T4 and T7, and caudad-directed laminar hooks at T9 and T12 (the latter hook is one level proximal for seating in the next more caudal hook. Corkscrews and rod pushers are useful to direct the rod into each hook in sequence. After all hooks are seated, a small amount of distraction is applied to each hook with the nuts partially tightened to seat hooks well and maintain slight distraction. The rod is then rotated to convert the scoliosis into kyphosis in the thoracic spine (10), using the hex-ended wrench at the cephalad end of the rod, and an additional vise grips distally on the rod if the surgeon feels more control is required. After completion of rotation, each hook is again distracted, at this time for correction of deformity, and then sequentially locked to the rod using the wrenches.

The convex rod is then contoured and placed into its respective hooks in a similar fashion, again following a sequence from one end of the rod to the other. Since most of the corrective force has already been applied to the deformity with the first rod, the second (convex) rod is felt to provide only additional points of fixation to the to stable). The standard four-hook compression pattern for the convexity consists of a T4-T5 transverse process-pedicle claw (a two-level claw (22)), a cephalad-directed pedicle hook at T8, and a cephalad-directed laminar hook at T12. *D*, Postoperative lateral radiograph showing no instrumentation-produced junctional kyphosis.

spine and the first rod (via Crosslinks). A 4.8-mm rod—easily contoured and implanted—is often used (Fig. 9.30*C*). It is most convenient to seat the pedicle-transverse claw at the cephalad end first, and after locking these nuts tentatively, to seat the remaining two hooks further distally. After all hooks are seated, compression is achieved by moving the apical and distal end vertebra toward the proximal claw. Finally, appropriate-length Crosslinks are attached to the prepositioned eyebolts, and all nuts of both hooks and Crosslinks are maximally tightened using the torque wrench when possible.

Low Single Thoracic Curve

The thoracic curve with an apex at or below T9 will require instrumentation to cross the thoracolumbar junction (Fig. 9.31). The caudal end vertebra should either be the stable vertebra or the next more cephalad vertebra. Because the instrumentation must cross the thoraco-

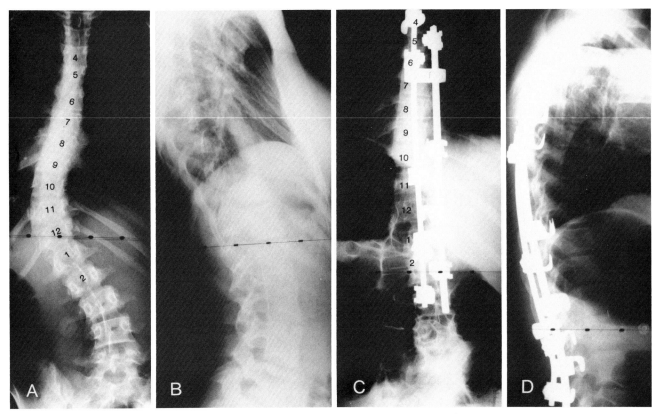

Figure 9.31. Instrumentation for a low thoracic scoliosis. *A,* Anteroposterior radiograph of a left thoracic scoliosis, apex T10. *B,* Lateral radiographs, showing thoracic hypokyphosis, and normal upper lumbar lordosis. *C,* Postoperative radiograph. The convex (*right*) rod has a standard four-hook construct in distraction, an unphysiologic technique to cross the thoracolumbar junction (caudal-directed hook at L2). The convex (*left*) rod has a laminar-laminar claw at L1-L2, allowing some compression in the upper lumbar region. Coronal balance is satisfactory. *D,* Postoperative lateral radiograph. Hook reversal (6,24) at the caudal end of the instrumentation might have provided better initiation of lordosis in the upper lumbar segments. The thoracic kyphosis, however, is improved.

lumbar junction, it is necessary to use compression to initiate a slightly lordotic contour at the T11-L2 area. Therefore, concave hooks are placed so that there is distraction between the upper thoracic hooks and T11 or T12, and compression between T11 or T12 and the lower end vertebra. The rod must be contoured for a thoracic kyphosis and upper lumbar lordosis, and consequently will not match a single scoliotic deformity in the coronal plane. Because the rod contour does not match the scoliosis, some lateral translation of the rod will be required to seat it in the hooks (see discussion of cantilever correction of thoracolumbar curves). Proper correction of this curve requires contouring the rod for the sagittal correction anticipated, and ignoring to some degree the coronal deformity. By a combination of rotation and lateral translation of the rod, the single scoliotic deformity will be satisfactorily corrected by the hook-reversing technique (6,24) across the thoracolumbar junction.

The convex rod is applied with compression over the thoracic curve and distraction across the thoracolumbar curve. This technique seats the hooks and stabilizes the internal fixation, but does not truly change the sagittal contour already set by the first rod.

Double Thoracic Curve, King Type V

The double thoracic curve pattern is corrected by a combination of rotatory correction of the lower thoracic curve (Fig. 9.32), and distraction-compression correction of the upper curve (17). Instrumentation at the cephalad end must be carried to T1 or T2 if there is significant tilting toward the concavity of this curve. The caudal end vertebra is usually the neutral vertebra, identical to the end vertebra for a single thoracic King type III deformity. Hook placement for the lower thoracic curve is also identical to a King III four-hook pattern on the concavity.

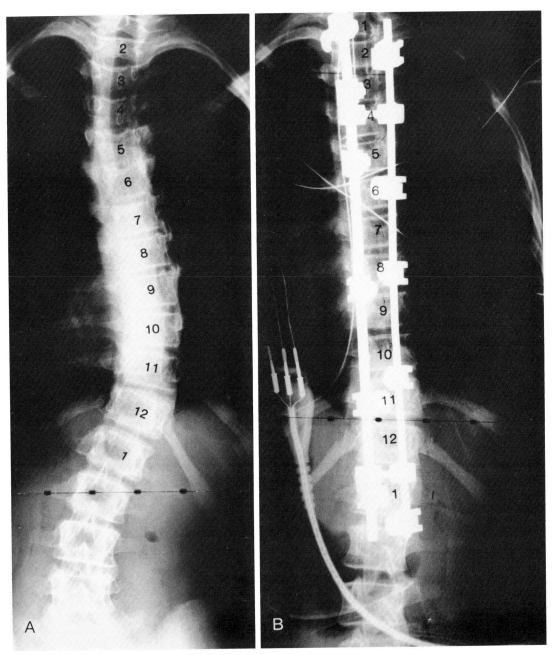

Figure 9.32. Instrumentation for a double thoracic scoliosis. *A,* Anteroposterior radiograph. Hypokyphosis of both thoracic deformities was noted on the lateral. *B,* Postoperative radiograph shows instrumentation T2 to L1. The left rod was placed first, having been contoured to a physiologic kyphosis. There is a transverse process hook at T2, pedicle hooks at T3, T5, and T8, and buttressed laminar hooks at T11 and L1. The left rod was inserted into the lower curve hooks first, rotated, and cantilevered into the upper hooks. The right rod has a pedicle hook at T2 and circular laminar hooks at T6, T8, T10, and L1.

Additional caudally-facing compression hooks (transverse process or sublaminar) are included on the convexity of the upper thoracic curve on the same side, with one hook at the apex and another hook facing caudally at the upper end vertebra. On the concavity of the upper thoracic curve, a distraction hook directed cephalad will be placed at the end vertebra with the remaining hooks in the standard fashion for the convexity of a single thoracic curve.

The rod contour is that of a normal kyphosis, and the rod is placed in the lower curve hooks first and rotated in the normal fashion. The upper curve hooks are then seated, either by lateral translation or by using corkscrews.

Since all the hooks are open, either from the top or the side, it is usually possible to translate the rod without difficulty to seat these upper hooks. Once all hooks are seated, the upper curve is compressed and the lower hooks distracted. The convex rod is seated, again allowing for single kyphotic contour and using lateral translation as necessary to seat all hooks prior to distraction or compression.

An alternative method to correct a double thoracic curve utilizes two separate rods on the first side, a rod for the lower thoracic curve that is rotated, and a second rod for the upper thoracic curve that is simply compressed. The two rods are then linked together using an axial crosslink.

Double Curves, King Type II

Significant balance problems have been reported with rotational correction and selective thoracic instrumentation of the King II curve (17,19,21). In mild deformities (thoracic curve less than 60°, lumbar curve less than 45°) and in those with a trunk shift to the right, selective fusion of the thoracic curve may be appropriate, provided there is no junctional kyphosis. Correction with a standard rotational maneuver and hook pattern may be chosen usually, but not always, with satisfactory results. In certain cases with more severe deformity, or with a preoperative left decompensation, rotation alone may produce worsening of the left decompensation. In this situation, the thoracic curve may be selectively instrumented using a distraction-compression technique, perhaps augmented with transverse loading, but in which no rotational maneuver is performed. In deformities resembling true double major patterns, or if there is a junctional kyphosis, instrumentation of both curves is indicated.

Selective Thoracic Fusion with Rotational Correction

This deformity is instrumented as in the single thoracic curve, with the lower end vertebra being one proximal to the stable vertebra (17,19,21). Junctional kyphosis must not be present for this pattern to be appropriate (Fig. 9.33).

Selective Thoracic Fusion without Rotation

This technique and hook pattern (Fig. 9.34) recalls the success reported by King et al. for selective thoracic fusion with Harrington instrumentation (17). A distraction construct with hooks only on the end vertebra of the concave side is created. The rod is contoured for a normal thoracic kyphosis. Fixation on the concavity may be augmented

with spinous process wires, as described by Drummond (11). The wires are tightened around the concave rod to load the curve transversely. The convex rod is placed in a standard four-hook construct. Crosslinks complete this simple technique to avoid instrumentational decompensation as theoretically, at least, distraction-compression forces are applied from the stable vertebra, and hence should maintain balance as described for Harrington instrumentation (17).

Instrumentation of Thoracic and Lumbar Curves in King II Pattern

In deformities where the lumbar component is either of large magnitude (greater than 45°) or relatively inflexible, experience with rotational correction has produced truncal decompensation (19, 21). Both curves should therefore be instrumented to maintain balance (Fig. 9.35). The technique for instrumentation of both curves begins with placement of the rod on the concave side of the thoracic curve, using the normal four-hook construct. The end vertebra of the thoracic curve serves as the proximal hook for the lumbar curve which is instrumented primarily in compression. Depending on the number of lumbar levels requiring fixation, the convexity of the lumbar curve will have four hooks, or perhaps three. The configuration generally includes a laminar-laminar claw at the distal end, in order to achieve lordosis at this mid-lumbar level (usually L2-L3), and also to assure stability of the lower end of the construct.

The rod is contoured for a normal kyphosis-lordosis for the levels to be instrumented. The rod is seated in the usual sequence and fashion, but prior to rotation of this rod, compression must be applied to the lumbar curve hooks to ensure that lordosis is produced in this segment. Additionally, prior to rotation and compressing of the left-sided rod, the distraction hook on the end vertebra of the concavity of the lumbar curve must be placed via laminotomy; otherwise, after compressing the convex lumbar segments, it may not be possible to insert this hook once the laminotomy site has been closed by the compressive maneuver.

The right-sided rod (thoracic convex, lumbar concave) is placed in the usual sequence and fashion, with the cephalad-facing distal end hook of the thoracic curve doubling as the distraction hook on the upper end vertebra of the lumbar curve. Usually, an intermediate vertebra hook is placed in distraction at the apex of the lumbar curve concavity and, as already mentioned, a distraction hook on the end vertebra of the lumbar concavity. The second rod provides stability and additional points of segmental fixation, by distracting the lumbar curve against the rod that has already been placed, rotated, and

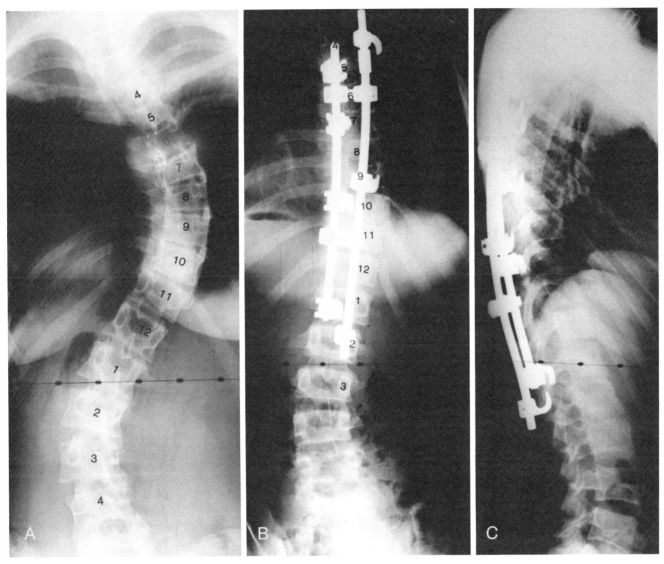

Figure 9.33. Instrumentation of a King II double curve, thoracic component only. *A*, Anteroposterior radiograph. The lumbar component was 100% corrected on bend film. There was no junctional kyphosis. *B*, Postoperative result, selective fusion to L1. A standard concave and convex pattern (as for King III deformity) to the stable vertebra maintained coronal balance. (Left rod, TSRH instruments; right rod, C-D instruments). *C*, Lateral postoperative radiograph. Normal thoracic kyphosis is seen.

compressed. A 4.8-mm rod is often used for ease of implantation. Crosslinks are added to complete the fixation.

Thoracolumbar Curve

Posterior Instrumentation. Thoracolumbar curves and King type IV (17) thoracic curves instrumented posteriorly require a completely different hook and rod sequence from single thoracic or double thoracic-lumbar deformities. It is impossible to produce a kyphosis-lordosis contour across the thoracolumbar junction *and*

a corrective single frontal plane contour by rotation from the concavity. Correction is therefore produced by a cantilever mechanism (Fig. 9.36). The concave rod is contoured for the *sagittal* correction desired. It is inserted into the caudal two or three hooks, which are distracted to seat them well, with the rod rotated so that the sagittal lordosis contour fits the lumbar scoliosis deformity. This requires that the cephalad portion of the rod is displaced well to the right of the upper spine (Fig. 9.36*A*). The rod is then rotated to turn the lumbar scoliosis into lordosis, and simultaneously and progressively translated to

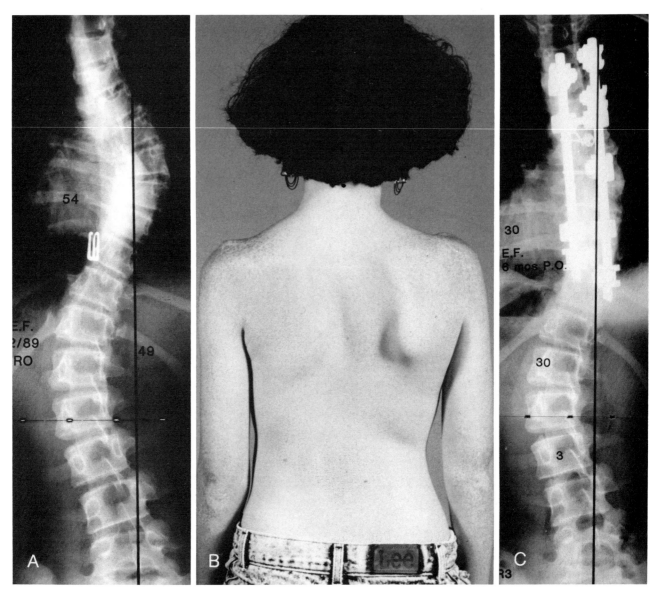

Figure 9.34. Instrumentation of a King II double curve, using distraction instrumentation and selective thoracic fusion. *A,* Anteroposterior radiograph shows the double curve pattern and left-sided decompensation of the patient. There was no junctional kyphosis on lateral. *B,* Clinical appearance of the patient showing preoperative left decompensation with a prominent right rib deformity. *C,* Postoperative radiograph 16 months later, showing selective instrumentation T4 to T10. There is no worsening of the patient's imbalance to the left. The left rod has a pedicle hook at T4, and a buttressed laminar hook at T10, with spinous process wires at the apical three segments. The right rod has a standard four-hook construct with a pedicle-transverse process claw at T4-T5, a pedicle hook at T7, and a laminar hook at T10.

the next more cephalad hook(s). Since all hooks are "open," the rod can be sequentially seated in each more cephalad hook. The shifted spine (and trunk) are gradually corrected by this cantilever maneuver using rod pushers and corkscrews to translate the rod to the hooks. The rod should be fully rotated into the sagittal plane contours by the time the most cephalad hook is seated (Fig. 9.36*B*).

The convex rod is placed after an appropriate sagittal contour is created. Because the lumbar hooks on the concave side have been distracted for seating and initial correction purposes, and because distraction across the thoracolumbar junction is not physiologic, these concave hooks should be released once the convex rod is seated in all of its hooks (Fig. 9.36*C*). The convex hooks should then be compressed across the thoracolumbar junction.

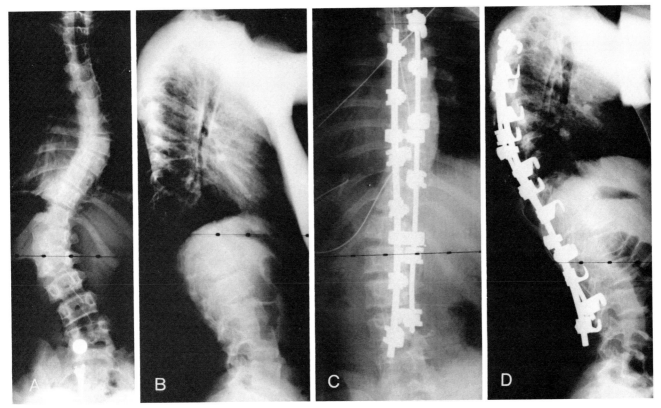

Figure 9.35. Instrumentation for a King II double curve. *A,* Anteroposterior radiograph showing double curves of equal magnitude. *B,* Lateral radiograph demonstrates a junctional kyphosis at the thoracolumbar junction. *C,* Postoperative anteroposterior radiograph showing instrumentation T4-L3. The left rod is inserted first. There are pedicle hooks at T4 and T6, laminar hooks at T10, T12, L2, and L3. The left rod was inserted first and rotated for correction. On the right, there is a transverse process hook at T4, pedicle hooks at T5 and T8, laminar hooks at T10 and L1, and a buttressed laminar hook at L3. *D,* Postoperative lateral radiograph. Note the contour of the kyphosis-lordosis across the thoracolumbar junction, and the offset laminar hook facing cephalad on L3 (for ease of rod insertion).

The concave hooks are then gently redistracted to seat them properly, but further distraction should be avoided. Crosslinks are added as the final stabilizing step.

An alternative technique may be used to avoid the necessity of releasing the distracted concave lumbar hooks prior to compressing the convex hooks (Fig. 9.36G). A concave hook pattern producing both compression and a "claw" may be produced by reversing the direction of the end vertebra hook and adding another distraction hook downwards at the next level cephalad. Lordosis of the lumbar segment may be secured during and after completing the cantilever correction, with the lower laminar-laminar claw adding stability of purchase during the cantilever correction maneuver (recommended in stiffer deformities).

Thoracolumbar Curve

Anterior Correction. In thoracolumbar and lumbar major curves, the TSRH system may be used anteriorly much like the Zielke-VDS system (Fig. 9.20). After exposure of the levels to be instrumented via a thoracoabdominal approach, meticulous removal of the intervertebral discs, endplates, and anterior longitudinal ligament should be accomplished, not only to provide segmental mobilization of the deformity, but also to obtain interbody arthrodesis. Vertebral screws of appropriate lengths are inserted through vertebral staples or circular collars. Whenever possible, staple fixation is recommended to supplement screw resistance to cantilever (compression) pullout (Fig. 9.37). A 4.8- or 6.4-mm rod (flexible) is usually selected and contoured for the lordotic posture in the lumbar portion of the curve. The thoracolumbar junction is usually left straight. After seating each eyebolt in each screw head, the rod is rotated to convert the scoliosis into lordosis. It is generally more convenient to place the rod posterior to the heads of the vertebral screws, so that the eyebolt nuts face anteriorly toward the abdominal contents for ease of tightening. If necessary, however, the rod may be placed anterior to the

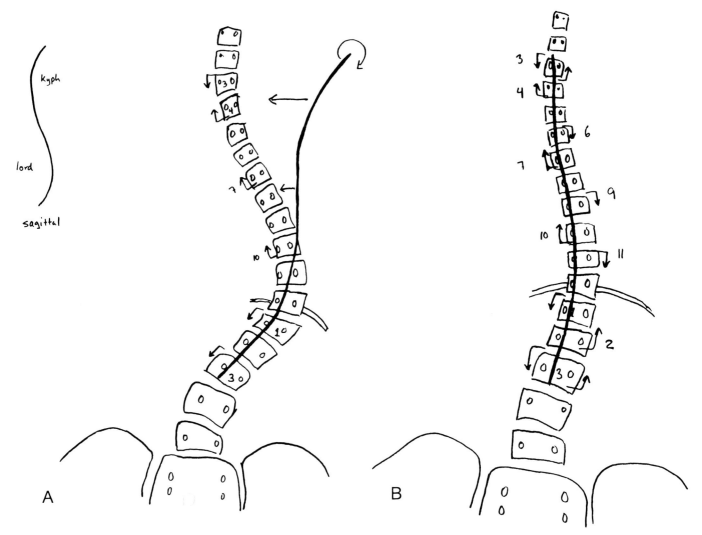

Figure 9.36. Thoracolumbar curve, posterior instrumentation. *A*, A standard single thoracic hook pattern, centered on the T11-T12 apex, includes cephalad-facing concave T10 and T7 hooks, and caudal-facing hooks at L1 and L3; pedicle transverse claw at T3-T4 completes this hook pattern for the upper thoracic compensatory curve. The rod is contoured for appropriate kyphosis-lordosis and inserted in the L1 and L3 hooks. The rod is displaced to the right of the spine above, and is translated leftward and rotated to seat the T10 and T7 hooks sequentially. The L3 hook must remain well seated and must not migrate to the right of the L3 spinous process during translation. *B*, The completed concave instrumentation/translation. Convex cephalad-facing hooks are placed at L3, L2 (or L1), and caudally-directed at T11 and T9. This produces compres-

sion at the thoracolumbar junction. Hooks at T6 and T3 complete the pattern for the upper curve. *C*, Prior to compressing on the convexity between T11 and L3, distraction is released from the concave lumbar hooks. *D*, Anteroposterior radiograph of right thoracolumbar major curve with compensatory upper thoracic curve. The lateral radiograph showed extension of lordosis into the lower thoracic area. *E* and *F*, Postoperative radiographs following cantilever correction. *G*, Alternative pattern to produce/maintain lordosis with the concave rod. A laminar-laminar claw at L2-L3 is created eliminating the necessity to release these hooks prior to compressing on the convexity, and adding stability at the L2-L3 hooks during the cantilever correction.

screws to translate a vertebral body more anteriorly during sequential seating. After completion of rotation, morselized bone graft from the rib resected during the exposure is placed in each disc space, and all discs are compressed toward the apical screw, and finally tightened. Because the rod is solid, this compression maneuver

does not produce a kyphosis, as the lordosis is maintained by the precontoured lordosis of the rod. Careful attention to the fit of the rod perpendicularly in the grooves of the screw head must be paid to ensure secure fixation at each level at final nut tightening (Fig. 9.38).

Preliminary results in the first 35 cases of scoliosis cor-

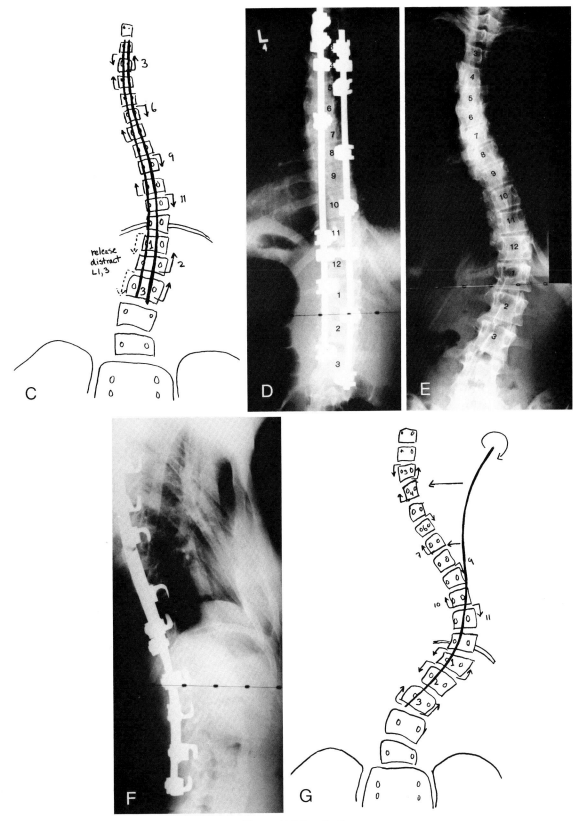

Figure 9.36. *C–G.*

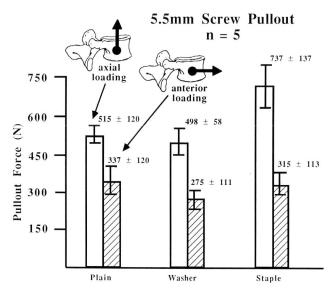

5.5mm Screw Pullout
n = 5

Figure 9.37. Increased resistance to cantilever (axial) screw pullout provided by staple fixation (compared with washer or no additional screw stabilizer).

rected anteriorly by the TSRH instrumentation system have proved this to be one of the most effective methods of deformity correction. The importance of obtaining correction of thoracolumbar or lumbar deformities anteriorly by a method that maintains lordosis is self-evident. In addition, experience has demonstrated that, with adequate bone-screw fixation at each level, postoperative immobilization is unnecessary. Clear radiographic documentation of interbody arthrodesis has been noted as early as 3 months postoperatively.

Pediatric System. The dimunitive size of the pediatric implants (Fig. 9.17) allows internal fixation and some corrective ability for deformities in small children or patients with skeletal dysplasia. Because of weak bone due to size, immaturity, or diagnosis, *correction* with the pediatric system may be limited, but the ability to fix deformities that have undergone correction by other means (e.g., traction) is often invaluable (Fig. 9.39). The eyebolts are also smaller to accommodate the smaller hook tops, and only the 4.8-mm rod is used, which can be attached to the hook tops on either side (Fig. 9.17*B*).

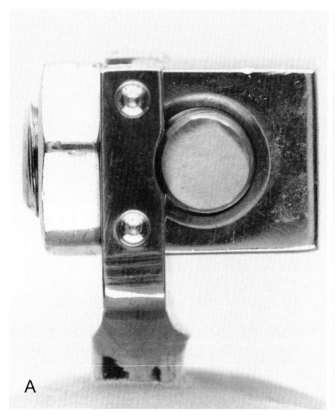

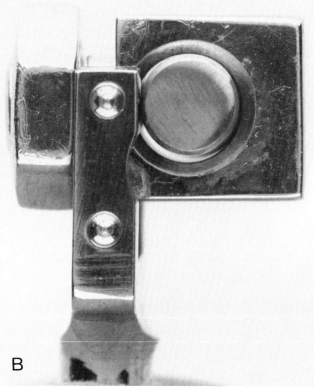

A

B

Figure 9.38. *A,* Screw-rod stability requires that the rod be perfectly aligned in the grooves of the screw head prior to tightening the eyebolt. *B,* If the rod does not engage the grooves precisely, disengagement will occur regardless of how tight the nut is tightened.

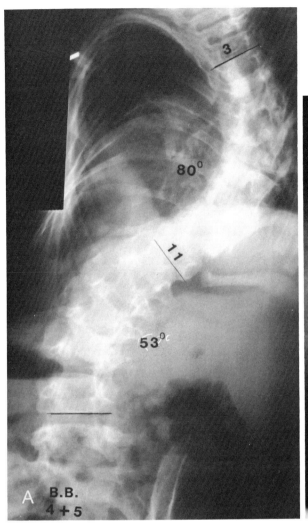

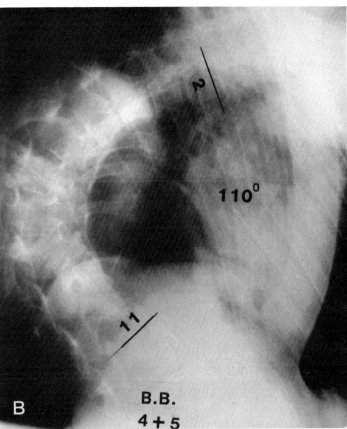

Figure 9.39. *A* and *B*, A 4-year-old child with severe collapsing kyphoscoliosis secondary to spinal muscular atrophy. *C* and *D*, Clinical appearance of the deformity. *E* and *F*, Correction obtained after 4 months of halo-wheelchair continuous traction, the only method which appeared to offer safe correction in this diminutive, osteopenic child with muscular weakness. *G* and *H*, Postoperative radiographs demonstrating maintenance of correction using pediatric hooks. No rod was inserted on the convexity of the deformity because of hardware prominence. (Courtesy John G. Birch, M.D.)

Because of their small size, the pediatric hooks are very useful for laminar positions in the cervical spine, where they fit conveniently over or under laminar surfaces without encroachment (Fig. 9.40). When using the 4.8-mm rod, pediatric and adult hooks can be *combined* on the same rod (by using the appropriate eyebolts for their respective hooks). This may be helpful when adult hooks might be too prominent in a kyphotic area where skin closure might be compromised by the larger hooks (Fig. 9.41).

CONCLUSION

The TSRH universal spine instrumentation system has evolved over 5 years from an adjunctive rod-stabilizing implant (the Crosslink) to the versatile, complete spinal instrumentation described and illustrated in this chapter. The *techniques* of implantation are nearly identical to techniques developed previously by others. The implants themselves, and their method of intraoperative assembly and locking, have been developed to simplify the increasing complexity of modern spinal procedures, while enhancing stability of fixation, neurologic safety, and resistance to fatigue failure. The versatility of the system is perhaps best illustrated by the ease of its removal or revision simply by loosening the locking nuts, allowing the surgeon to dismantle the entire construct, or to dismantle it at only one end and, by adding additional eyebolts, then proceed with extending the instrumentation. Metal-cutting power equipment is unnecessary, and the

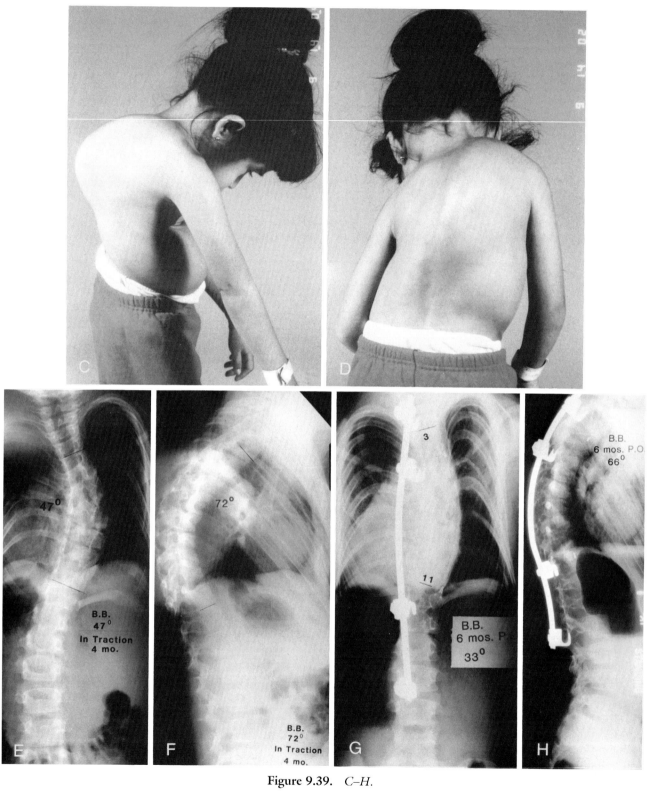

Figure 9.39.   *C–H.*

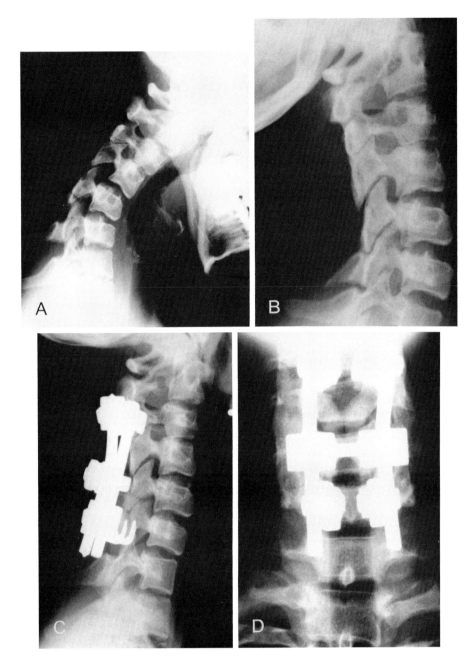

Figure 9.40. *A* and *B*, A 17-year-old female 3 years status postcervical laminectomy to remove a diastematomyelia. The patient's scoliosis secondary to her dysraphic lesion had been previously corrected. She developed the insidious onset of neck pain and shoulder girdle weakness. Postlaminectomy instability at C4-C5 and perhaps C5-C6 were felt to exist in flexion. *C* and *D*, Postoperative radiographs 6 weeks following C3-C6 instrumentation and fusion with TSRH pediatric hooks. Laminar hooks were placed over the superior laminar of C3, and in the facet joints at C6, where enough lamina remained for instrumentation. The robust fusion mass already present at 6 weeks postoperative is easily appreciated on the anteroposterior radiograph.

destructive (to the fusion mass) and time-consuming rod removal becomes simpler. Broken existing hardware can be repaired in situ or revised by extending it, thus eliminating the need for total removal of non-TSRH rod systems in order to reinstrument. No other spinal implant system provides this option, to repair or revise the implants of another manufacturer left in situ.

The ability to instrument *all* areas of the spine (cervical, thoracolumbar, sacropelvis), in *all* sizes of patients (including small and skeletally dysplastic ones), from either

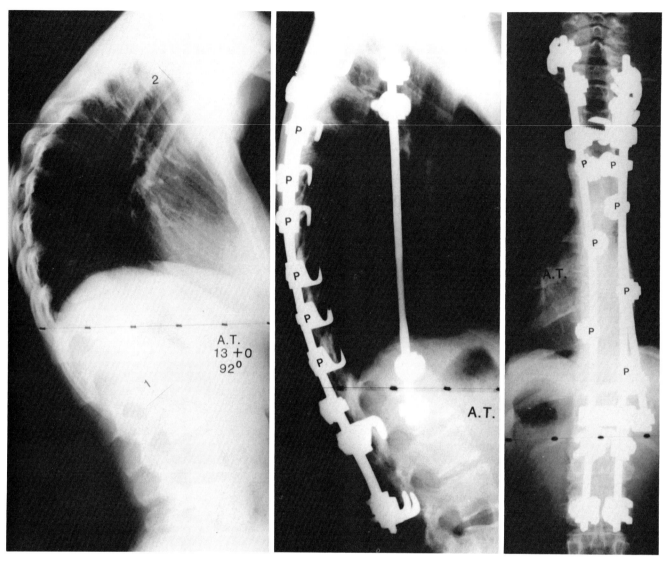

Figure 9.41. *Left,* Lateral radiograph of a 13-year-old female with progressive Scheuermann's kyphosis. *Middle,* Postoperative lateral radiograph following two-stage instrumentation and correction. Anterior correction with TSRH vertebral screws at T3, T4, T11, and T12 and a distraction rod (4.8 mm) was performed in conjunction with discectomy and fusion. Second-stage correction utilized posterior instrumentation from T1 to L1 with two 4.8-mm rods. Adult hooks were used in "claw" configuration at the most cephalad and caudad aspects of the instrumentation, with several intermediate pediatric hooks (*P*) used because of their low profile and ease of closure at the apex of this patient's severe kyphus. No postoperative immobilization was necessary. *Right,* AP radiograph of the postoperative result.

anterior or posterior approaches using screws or hooks, makes the TSRH system truly universal, especially in light of the fact that *all* implants use the same method of attachment to the rod(s), namely the eyebolt with threaded locking nut. This attachment, when tightened appropriately, is mechanically sound and as strong as other methods, and is always easily reversible (i.e., can be loosened without total removal), again, an option not available when using set screws, for example. The TSRH system therefore fulfills the criteria of stability, simplicity, safety, versatility, and ability to remove or revise easily, which defines it as the most ideal spinal instrumentation available.

REFERENCES

1. Allen BL, Ferguson RL: The Galveston technique for L-rod instrumentation of the scoliotic spine. Spine 1982;7:276–284.
2. Ashman RB, Birch JG, Bone LB, et al: Mechanical testing of spinal instrumentation. Clin Orthop 1988;227:113–125.
3. Ashman RB, Galpin RD, Corin JD, et al: Biomechanical analysis

of pedicle screw instrumentation systems in a corpectomy model. Spine 1989;14:1398–1405.

4. Birch JG, Camp JF, Corin J, et al: Rotational stability of various pedicle hook designs—an in vitro analysis. Presented at the Annual Meeting of the Scoliosis Research Society, Amsterdam, The Netherlands, September 17–22, 1989.

5. Boachie-Adjei O, Lonstein JE, Winter RB, et al: Management of neuromuscular spinal deformities with Luque segmental instrumentation. J Bone Joint Surg 1989;71A:548.

6. Bridwell KH, Betz R, Capelli AM, et al: Sagittal plane analysis in idiopathic scoliosis patients treated with Cotrel-Dubousset instrumentation. Spine 1990;15:644–649.

7. Broom MJ, Banta JV, Renshaw TS: Spinal fusion augmented by Luque-rod segmental instrumentation for neuromuscular scoliosis. J Bone Joint Surg 1989;71:32–44.

8. Camp JF, Roach JW: Immediate complications of Cotrel-Dubousset instrumentation to the sacropelvis: a clinical and biomechanical study. Spine 1990;15:932–941.

9. Collins JA: High-cycle fatigue. In: Failure of materials in mechanical design: analysis, prediction, prevention. New York: John Wiley & Sons, 1981.

10. Cotrel Y, Dubousset J, Guillaumat M: Nouvelle technique de correction des deviations du rachis. Technique C.D. de Yves Cotrel et Jean Dubousset. In: Cotrel Y, ed: Nouvelle instrumentation pour chirurgie du rachis. London: Freund Publishing House Ltd, 1986;61–66.

11. Drummond D, Guadagni J, Keene JS, et al: Interspinous process segmental spinal instrumentation. J Pediatr Orthop 1984;4:397–404.

12. Gurr KR, McAfee PC, Warden KE, et al: Roentgenographic and biomechanical analysis of lumbar fusions: a canine model. J Orthop Res 1989;7:838–848.

13. Johnston CE II, Ashman RB, Baird AM, et al: Effect of spinal construct stiffness on early fusion mass incorporation. Spine 1990;15:908–912.

14. Johnston CE II. Ashman RB, Corin JD: Mechanical effects of cross-linking rods in Cotrel-Dubousset instrumentation. Ortho Trans 1987;11:96.

15. Johnston CE II, Ashman RB, Sherman MC, et al: Mechanical consequences of rod contouring and residual scoliosis in sublaminar segmental instrumentation. J Orthop Res 1987;5:206–216.

16. Johnston CE II, Haideri N, Ashman RB: Early experience with rigid crosslinking. Presented at the Annual Meeting of the Scoliosis Research Society, Honolulu, Hawaii, September 23–27, 1990.

17. King HA, Moe JH, Bradford DS, et al: The selection of fusion levels in thoracic idiopathic scoliosis. J Bone Joint Surg 1983;65A:1302–1313.

18. Luque ER: The anatomic basis and development of segmental spinal instrumentation. Spine 1982;7:256–259.

19. McAllister JW, Bridwell KH, Betz R, et al: Coronal decompensation produced by Cotrel-Dubousset derotation maneuver for idiopathic right thoracic scoliosis. Orthop Trans 1989;13:79.

20. Nasca RJ, Hollis JM, Lemmons JE, et al: Cyclic axial loading of spinal implants. Spine 1985;10:792–798.

21. Richards BS, Birch JG, Herring JA, et al: Frontal plane and sagittal plane balance following Cotrel-Dubousset instrumentation for idiopathic scoliosis. Spine 1989;14:733–737.

22. Roach JW, Ashman RB, Allard RN: The strength of a posterior element claw at one versus two spinal levels. J Spinal Disord 1990;3:259–261.

23. Shufflebarger HL: Neurologic injury with Cotrel-Dubousset instrumentation. Report to Scoliosis Research Society, Membership Survey on Morbidity, 1989.

24. Shufflebarger HL, Clark CE: Fusion levels and hook patterns in thoracic scoliosis with Cotrel-Dubousset instrumentation. Spine 1990;15:916–920.

25. Weiler PJ: Buckling analysis of spinal implant devices used for the surgical treatment of scoliosis. Thesis, Department of Mechanical Engineering, University of Waterloo, Waterloo, Ontario, 1983.

26. Zdeblick TA, Wayden KE, Zou D, et al: Anterior spinal fixators: a biomechanical in vitro study. Presented at the Annual Meeting of the Scoliosis Research Society, Honolulu, Hawaii, September 23–27, 1990.

TEN

Roy-Camille Posterior Screw Plate Fixation for Cervical, Thoracic, Lumbar Spine and Sacrum

Raymond Roy-Camille, Christian Mazel, and Claude Laville

INTRODUCTION

The posterior approach of the spine is relatively simple. Thus, posterior fixation with plates and screws has been developed in the cervical, thoracic, and lumbar spine. Posterior cervical fixation with plates has been developed over 25 years by one of us (RRC), followed by a pedicular screw plating system in the thoracolumbar spine. The evolution of the instrumentation has now solved almost all difficulties and technical problems of stabilization of the spine, whatever the pathology.

The approach to the spine is the routine midline incision. This instrumentation has been developed based on the knowledge of the anatomy and logical biomechanical principles of rigid fixation. Most importantly, the technique has to be precise to prevent malimplantations, and the surgeon must be well trained to perform it safely.

INSTRUMENTATION

Cervical Spine. For the cervical spine, the plates are prebent to adapt to the cervical lordotic curvature and are 1 cm wide, 4 mm thick, with a hole every 13 or 15 mm. The plates are available with 2, 3, 4, or 5 holes. Fixation of the plates is achieved into the articular masses with screws that are 3.5 mm in diameter and range from 12–16 mm in length (Fig. 10.1).

Special tileplates are used to take the place of broken articular facets (Fig. 10.2).

Upper Cervical Spine. In the upper cervical spine, for occipitocervical fixation, we use special plates that are contoured to restore the normal occipitocervical junction sagittal alignment with a curvature of 105° (Fig. 10.3). The fixation is achieved with short screws (4 mm long) in the occipital bone and the usual screws (12–16 mm long) in the articular masses of the cervical spine.

Thoracic and Thoracolumbar Levels. For thoracic and thoracolumbar levels, the plates are 1 cm wide in order to fit into the posterior thoracolumbar vertebral grooves (Fig. 10.4). The interface between the holes is 13 mm. This distance has been selected because the mean distance between two vertebral pedicles is approximately 26 mm with only slight differences along the entire length of the spine. To prevent plate breakage, we have developed the plates with reinforced holes. This reinforcement around the holes diminishes stress concentration at the holes so that the relative strength of the plate is the same all along its length. When bending a long plate, the contour will be smooth and very regular along the entire plate without any abrupt bends at the screw holes. They are precontoured to adapt to the normal sagittal curvature of the posterior aspect of the spine. For the thoracic level, they have a sagittal contour to fit the normal kyphosis. For lumbar levels, they have the proper curvature to reproduce the average lumbar lordosis. The same plate can be adapted for use in the thoracic and lumbar level. The surgeon simply has to place the plate with the reinforced side facing the spine for the thoracic levels and the flat side facing the spine in the lumbar levels. For the thoracolumbar junction, the plates are usually longer and are precontoured with a slight kyphosis at the superior end of the plate and a lordosis at the inferior end. Therefore, the plate will fit the normal sagittal contours of this transitional zone of the thoracolumbar junction. This precontoured shape is very important because when one implants the plates and as the screws are tightened into the pedicles, the spine will be drawn back toward the plates, and its normal curvature will be restored.

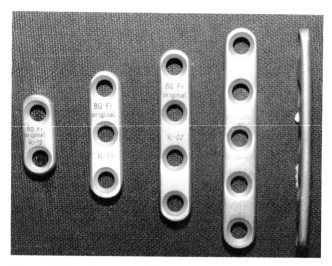

Figure 10.1. Four sizes of posterior plates. There is a small bending of the plate to adapt to cervical lordosis.

Lumbar Level. For the lumbar level, the same plates can also be used for long fixation. However, we often use what is known as the "three-vertebra plate" which fits the height of three lumbar vertebrae, and it has the holes in a slightly different position (Fig. 10.4). At both ends of the plate, there are three holes with a distance of 9 mm between them and one hole at the midpoint of the plate. The three holes at both ends are used to implant two screws into one pedicle through two adjacent holes. The lumbar vertebral pedicles are broad enough to allow placement of two screws into one pedicle.

Lumbosacral Junction. For the lumbosacral junction, the superior part of the plate has the standard 13 mm

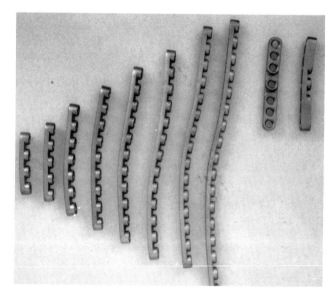

Figure 10.3. Occipitocervical plates. Two sizes are available. Occiput-C4, Occiput-C5. The 105° angle preserves the correct position of the head.

spacing with reinforced holes. The inferior part is flat with three holes facing obliquely in a lateral direction, so there are right- and left-hand plates. Screws can be implanted through the inferior holes into the bony lateral part of the sacrum for stronger fixation (Fig. 10.5).

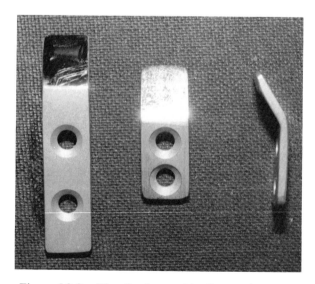

Figure 10.2. The tile plate enables facet replacement.

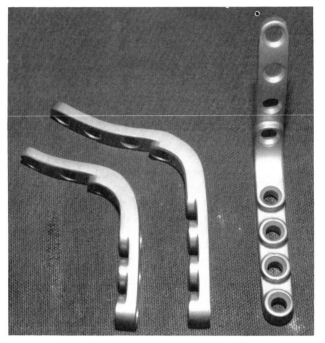

Figure 10.4. Thoracolumbar plates. Interspace hole is 13 mm. Each hole has a reinforcement ring to give additional stability to adapt to the normal thoracolumbar contour. In the upper right of the figure is the short three-vertebra plate.

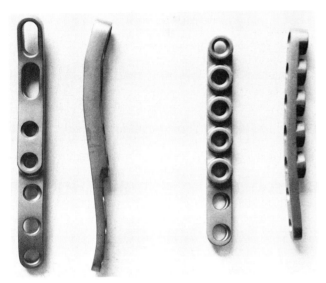

Figure 10.5. Lumbosacral plates. On the right is an L4-S2 plate. On the left is a spondylolisthesis reduction plate.

For the sacrum and specifically for the suicidal jumper's fracture, we used a special plate. It is turned on the longitudinal axis with a rotation of 45° between the two halves. This fracture separates two fragments—the superior one being the lumbar spine and the body of S1 and S2; the inferior one being the pelvis, the lower sacrum, and the alars. The fracture line is U-shaped between the two fragments. After reduction, the fixation is achieved on the superior fragment with screws implanted in the pedicles of L4, L5, and S1 and on the inferior fragment with oblique screws through the fracture line for one and two screws and directly below through the lateral part of sacrum, the S-I joint and the posterior part of iliac bone.

At the lumbosacral junction we also use special plates to reduce and stabilize spondylolisthesis with great displacement. Their special shape and curvature of the plate allow for pulling back on L4 and L5 vertebrae with special screws, inducing a cork-screw effect (Fig. 10.5).

The screw-plate interface at the reinforced hole is not rigidly constrained with slight clearance in order to allow a small amount of motion to prevent screw breakage. Two types of screws are available with the system. The first type are standard bone screws (Philips Vitallium or Maconor screws) available in the following diameters: 3.5 mm, 4.0 mm, 4.5 mm. The second type of screw (Mille Pattes) is specifically made for implantation into the pedicles (Fig. 10.6). These screws are composed of two sections. The first section to be implanted into the vertebral body has a large thread and comes with a diameter of 3.5, 4.0, 4.5, or 5.5 mm. They are available from 30–45 mm in length. The end of the screw that goes through the plate has a standard diameter of 5.00

mm and a fine thread to receive a lock nut. A correction of a displacement or of a deformity can be done with special instruments that can provide distraction or compression between two adjacent screws when seating the plate. In this screw type as well, a clearance is preserved between screws and plates, decreasing screw breakage, and this is a basic element of our philosophy of spinal plating.

TECHNIQUE OF POSTERIOR PLATING

Cervical Spine. In the cervical spine, the screws are implanted into the articular masses and not into the pedicles (Fig. 10.7).

The landmarks are extremely precise. The posterior approach must expose the levels to be instrumented out to the lateral border of the articular masses (Fig. 10.8). When completely exposed, the posterior aspect of the lower cervical spine can be described as having the spinous processes in the midline, with the lamina sloping laterally to the articular masses, which bulge posteriorly like hills. Between the hills and the laminae, there is a longitudinal depression that we compare to the bed of the river. In front of the river is the vertebral artery that one must avoid. Therefore, the screws are implanted laterally on the top of the hills, thus in the center of the

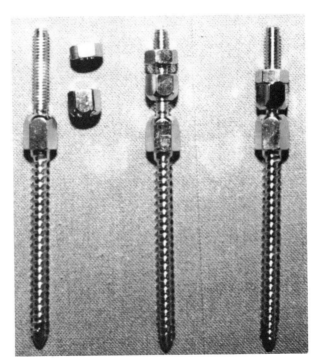

Figure 10.6. "Mille Pattes" screws. Reduction of local deformity can be achieved on these screws by acting on the upper part with special clamps.

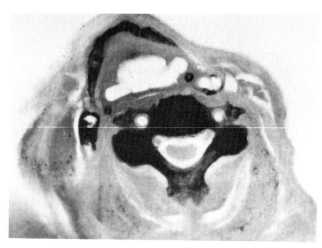

Figure 10.7. Transversal section of the spine. Articular masses are far apart from the cord. Vertebral artery is medial and anterior to it.

articular masses. The drill should be directed perpendicular to the vertebra in the inferior/superior direction and 10° laterally in the medial/lateral direction. With this orientation in the center of the articular masses, the screws will avoid the nerve roots running through the foramen in the gutter above the pedicle. The screws are going through the two cortices of the articular masses.

BIOMECHANICAL

This study was performed with the help of Rollin Johnson in New Haven at the Veterans Administration Hospital. In it, we investigated mechanical properties of cervical plates, in flexion and extension stress.

Two cervical vertebrae from a fresh cadaver were fixed posteriorly with a symmetrical pair of two-hole plates. The lower vertebra embedded, and stress was applied to the upper vertebra. Displacements were analyzed during stress with displacement gauges. The whole experiment was performed in a large glass box in order to keep a constant hygrometic level and to stay as close as possible to in vivo characteristics. Displacements were measured as well as radiographed.

The average breaking load in extension stress is 52.5 kg (515 N). This represents 60% of the load necessary to dislocate two normal cervical vertebrae. These results have been compared with the other methods of posterior cervical fixation. For an extension stress, a posterior wiring of the spinous processes or in the articular masses is inefficient in the stabilization of the spine. The posterior plates fixation gives an increase of 60% to the normal stability. A methylmethacrylate fixation on the spinous processes gives a 99% increase in stability.

For a flexion stress, the posterior wiring between the spinous processes gives a 33% increase in stability. The

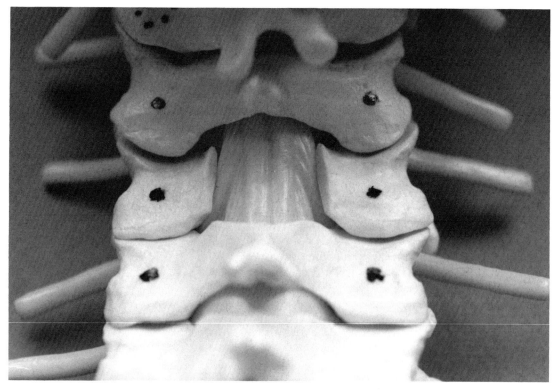

Figure 10.8. Screw implantation at cervical level is down in the middle of the articular mass (*black point*).

same wiring, but around a complementary bone graft gives a 55% increase in stability; the increase is 88% when the wiring is going through the articular masses. The plate fixation gives a 92% increase in stability.

The tileplate is used to replace a broken articular facet. Through the posterior approach, the space between the two articular masses is opened with a Penfield elevator in order to remove the broken fragment of the facet which may have caused a compression of the root. The tileplate is introduced into the facet joint, and the lower part of the plate is pushed forward toward the articular mass, thus with this maneuver reducing the rotatory displacement of the vertebra above. Instead of using a single tileplate, we routinely prefer to do the "porte-manteau" procedure (Fig. 10.9). In this procedure, after insertion of the tileplate, a regular two-hole plate is applied over it. The fixation is performed with a lower screw going through the lower holes of both plates, and the superior

screw is placed in the superior hole of the regular two-hole plate. On the opposite side, a regular two-hole plate is implanted symmetrically in the routine fashion.

In some cases, such as a fracture separation of the articular mass, the tileplate can be longer, and it bridges the articulation below the broken articular mass. The porte-manteau procedure then necessitates a three-hole plate over this long tileplate.

Another construct is possible in case of fracture-separation of the articular mass. A three-hole plate will bridge over the fractured mass. Pushing frontward will reduce the displacement. Then the screws will be implanted in the following manner (Fig. 10.10):

In the middle hole, the screw is directed obliquely downward to get across the facet joint below, and the screws in the superior hole and the lower hole are placed in the routine fashion perpendicular to the articular mass.

With this type of instrumentation, the fractured mass is directly fixed on the adjacent masses above and below. A symmetrical three-hole plate is placed on the opposite side.

Thoracic and Thoracolumbar Levels. For the thoracic and thoracolumbar levels, the secret of posterior spinal plating is the pedicle. The anatomic features of the pedicles must be extremely familiar: height, width, length, and orientation in order to determine the appropriate point of entry and to implant the screws accurately.

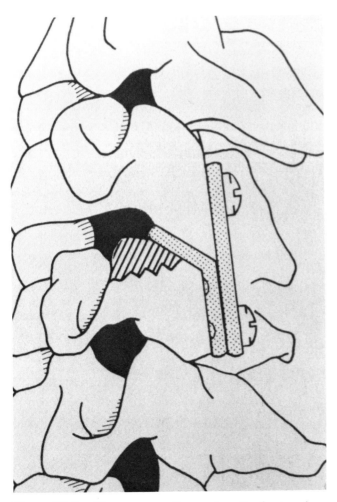

Figure 10.9. "Porte manteau" procedure for facet replacement. The tile prevents recurrence of the deformity. A second plate is placed on top of it.

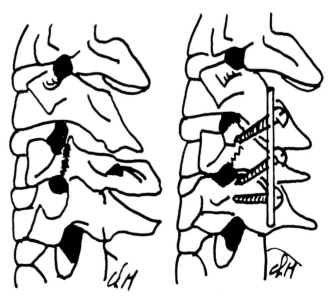

Figure 10.10. Articular mass separation fracture. *A*, The fracture lines are anterior in the pedicle and posterior on the lamina. The articular mass positioned itself horizontally. *B*, Fixation with a three-hole plate. The upper screw is oblique through the facet joint. The middle screw is also oblique downward. The lower screw is routinely implanted straightforward.

In our institution, the rules are simple and always constant. The screws are implanted perpendicular to the vertebra at which the surgeon is working and straightforward from the point of entry. The pedicle is at the junction of the transverse process and the lamina and connects to the superior articular facet just below its inferior edge. When one has exposed the facet joint line, the point of entry is just 1 mm below this facet joint. In case of a difficult insertion such as in the presence of osteophytes, it may be necessary to remove the capsule, expose the articular cartilage of the superior facet, which is the very precise landmark, and the point of entry is 1 mm below the inferior edge of this cartilage. The facet joint is in a frontal plane, and the point of entry must be exactly in the midline of the joint. This point is at the base of the transverse process, where there is usually a small crest of bone sloping down medially. This crest can be another landmark for the point of entry.

Another way to determine the correct location for screw placement is at the junction of two crosslines (Fig. 10.11). One is a vertical line in the midpart of the facet joint, and the other is a horizontal line going through the upper part of the base of the two transverse processes. In the thoracic spine, the diameter of pedicles is small, and the smallest is T5, which is between 3.5–4 mm wide, so that one must use screws measuring no more than 3.5 mm in diameter. Such small screws may be used without the risk of breakage since in this system the screw/plate interface is not extremely rigid, thus limiting the stresses imparted to the screws. In the thoracic spine, the length of the screws is between 30–35 mm.

Thoracolumbar Junction. At the thoracolumbar junction, the anatomic configuration of the pedicles is the same as the thoracic spine. The superior articular facet is supported by the superior border of the posterior part of the pedicle. However, at T12-L1 and in the lumbar spine (Fig. 10.12), the orientation of the facet joints is more sagittal than coronal. The point of entry is still 1 mm below the inferior edge of the facet joint and on the line of the facet joint. The point of entry of the pedicle can also be located, as in the thoracic spine, at the junction of the same two crosslines. Another very good landmark in the lumbar level is a crest going up from the lower facet, lateral to the isthmus. This crest ascends up to the level of the point of entry, and it is often necessary to flatten it with a rongeur before drilling into it with the drill bit. The screws for the thoracolumbar junction are 4 mm in diameter and 40 mm long.

Lumbosacral Spine. For the lumbosacral spine, the landmarks are the same in the lumbar level as in the spine above, and for the sacrum, S1 is considered to have a normal pedicle. The point of penetration is also 1 mm below the middle of the facet joint, which is oblique both inferiorly and laterally. Therefore, the vertical landmark line will be in the middle of the oblique joint line. S1 facets are rather big with a dimple hidden by fat just below it. This is the location of the point of entry. The screws are directed either perpendicular to the posterior aspect of S1 and straight anteriorly or slightly superiorly trying to gain purchase in the dense bone below the S1 superior endplate (Fig. 10.13). The lower screws in the

Figure 10.11. Thoracic pedicle markers. Pedicle entrance point is located at the middle of two crosslines: A vertical line in the midpart of the facet joint; a horizontal line through the upper part aspect of the transverse process.

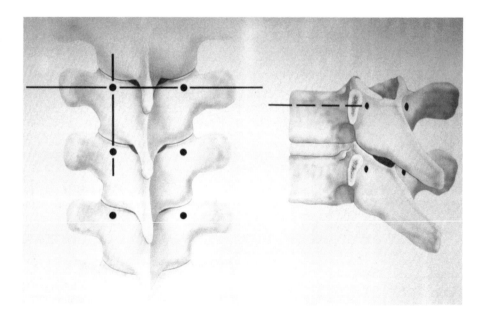

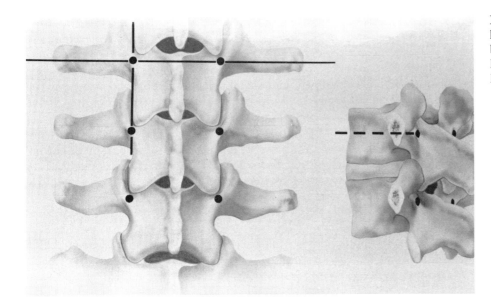

Figure 10.12. Lumbar pedicle markers. Pedicle entrance point is 1 mm below the tip of the joint at the crossline of the same horizontal and vertical lines as in thoracic spine.

sacrum are introduced oriented in a lateral direction through the oblique holes of the plate. If these lower screws are placed straightforward, they will enter either the sacral foramen or the sacral canal. The bone is thicker laterally in the sacral ala, and this is where the screws must be implanted. The lower sacral screws are 4 mm in diameter and 40 mm long, with a smaller 6-mm head in order to prevent prominence. Bulky hardware in this location may lead to skin breakdown, as there is often little subcutaneous tissue at this level. For the lumbar spine, the screws are 4.5 mm in diameter and 45 mm long. We may alternately use screws of 5.5 mm in diameter, mainly in case of revision surgery.

At any level of the spine, we never use extremely long screws because the holding power and pullout strength is predominantly from the pedicle itself. Therefore, it is necessary to penetrate into the midpart of the vertebral body and not any further forward. Perforation of the

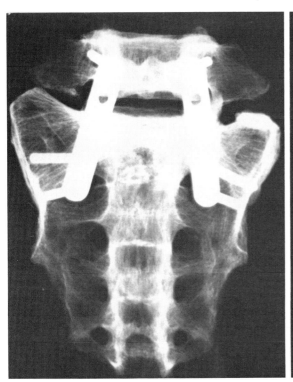
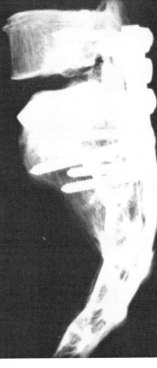

Figure 10.13. L5-S2 fusion. Screws are implanted into L5 and S1 pedicles. Two lower screws are implanted into the sacrum alar.

anterior cortex of the vertebral body carries the potential morbidity of injury to the great vessels with subsequent hemorrhage.

INDICATIONS FOR POSTERIOR SPINAL PLATING (PSP)

Trauma

In our own practice, posterior spinal plating is the most commonly used technique when surgery is indicated for spinal trauma.

The first indication is neurologic involvement with cord damage. The best decompression is achieved by the reduction of the displacement with or without a laminectomy. After the decompression, the fixation that we perform with spinal plates is very important to prevent secondary displacement and to reestablish the stability of the spine (Fig. 10.14).

The second indication for spinal plating is unstable lesions of the spine even without neurologic involvement. This is important because of the risk of a secondary acute, progressive or chronic displacement which can induce a

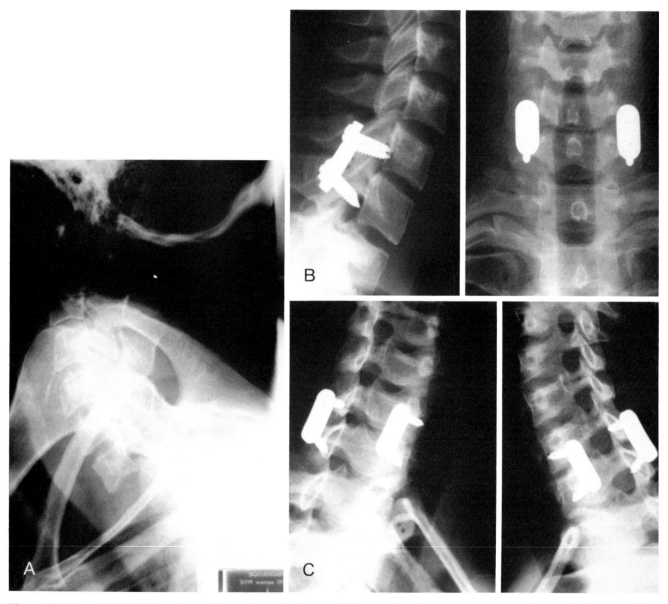

Figure 10.14. *A*, C6-C7 dislocation with tetraplegia. *B*, Posterior reduction and instrumentation AP and lateral view. *C*, Oblique view demonstrates the position and relations of the screws and the foramina.

late neurologic deterioration. We usually analyze the spine according to three vertical and two horizontal segments. The midvertical segments are the posterior wall, pedicles, and articular facets, and the mobile horizontal segments are the disc and ligaments. Their damage will induce instability, particularly if the disc and ligaments are disrupted due to poor healing.

The third indication is significant displacement with deformity of the spine even without a cord syndrome. Patients in whom the spinal injuries have this significant displacement have a tendency to increase the deformity progressively. In some cases, magnetic resonance imaging (MRI) has demonstrated evidence of a secondary post-traumatic syringomyelia of the cord at the level of a marked kyphosis. To prevent the development of such a chronic cord syndrome, it may be best to correct the initial deformity of the spine in cases with specific types of malalignment. Indications for treatment include the following presentations:

- Kyphosis of more than 20°;
- Displacement, which narrows the surface area of the spinal canal by more than 50%; or
- A posterior fragment protruding in the spinal canal with the same decrease in canal area.

It is obvious that if the deformity can be corrected by conservative treatment, as in Boehler's reduction of a traumatic thoracolumbar kyphosis, surgery is not indicated.

In addition, for each of the different levels of the spine, we have specific indications for spinal plating.

A specific indication is for a hangman's fracture with a fracture of the pedicles of C2 associated with an anterior dislocation of the posterior arch of C2 over the articular facets of C3. In such cases, after a posterior reduction of the displacement, the most elegant and precise instrumentation is achieved with bilateral 35-mm screws drilled directly into the pedicles through the fracture line. These screws are placed bilaterally through two-hole plates in order to bridge the C2-C3 facet joints posteriorly. The lower screws are implanted into the articular masses of C3.

Thoracolumbar Spine. In the thoracolumbar spine, posterior plating is well adapted to the treatment of spinal trauma. The vertebral body will usually be restored to its normal height and shape. To achieve adequate stability and lever arms for reduction, posterior plating usually requires inclusion of two vertebra above and two vertebra below the lesion (Fig. 10.15). With this long fixation, we usually do a short posterolateral fusion, bridging just one disc above the fractured vertebra, or two discs (one above and one below the fractured vertebra).

Lumbar Spine. In the lumbar spine, posterior plating must be kept as short as possible in order to prevent a significant decrease in the mobility of the lumbar spine. Posterior plating should include, as frequently as possible, only one vertebra above and one vertebra below the injury level, and the fusion should be of the same length.

In some cases in both the thoracolumbar and lumbar spine, the surgical restoration of the height of the anterior column of the vertebral body or, more importantly, of the adjacent disc is unsatisfactory. In such cases, a complementary anterior grafting and fixation is often necessary.

General Considerations for Spinal Plating in Trauma

The patients are placed in the prone position on a Judet orthopaedic table. This reduction is achieved with the help of the table by pulling on the lower limbs with counterpressure applied through axillary supports. The traction lengthens the spine and reduces the axial compression component of the vertebral injury. Then the lower limbs are lifted toward the ceiling, inducing a lumbar and thoracolumbar lordosis that reduces the kyphotic deformity. The full reduction is completed after the incision is opened by manipulation of the vertebra with elevators and clamps. If necessary, a decompression of the dural sac is performed through a laminectomy, which may be enlarged when needed to include the facets and the pedicle. This approach allows reduction or removal of a posterior fragment of the vertebral body protruding into the canal.

When reduction and decompression are achieved, the displacement of the posterior wall of the vertebral body is assessed with ultrasound. Then the plates are implanted. If regular screws are used, it is first necessary to drill all the pedicles at the point of entry where the screws will be implanted. Then a K-wire is put into each pedicle hole. The two plates are usually applied sequentially and not simultaneously. The K-wires are placed through the appropriate holes in the plate in such a position to allow for completion of the reduction and stable fixation. Each K-wire is then sequentially removed and the screw implanted in its place. The screws closest to the fracture level are inserted first, working progressively to the ends of the plate. A second symmetrical plate is then placed on the contralateral side. The progressive tightening of the screws achieves a few more degrees of reduction as the spine is pulled back toward the plates, which are prebent to the normal sagittal configuration.

When special screws (Mille Pattes) for spinal pedicles are used, the technique is somewhat different. It is not necessary to drill the holes to the depth of the entire

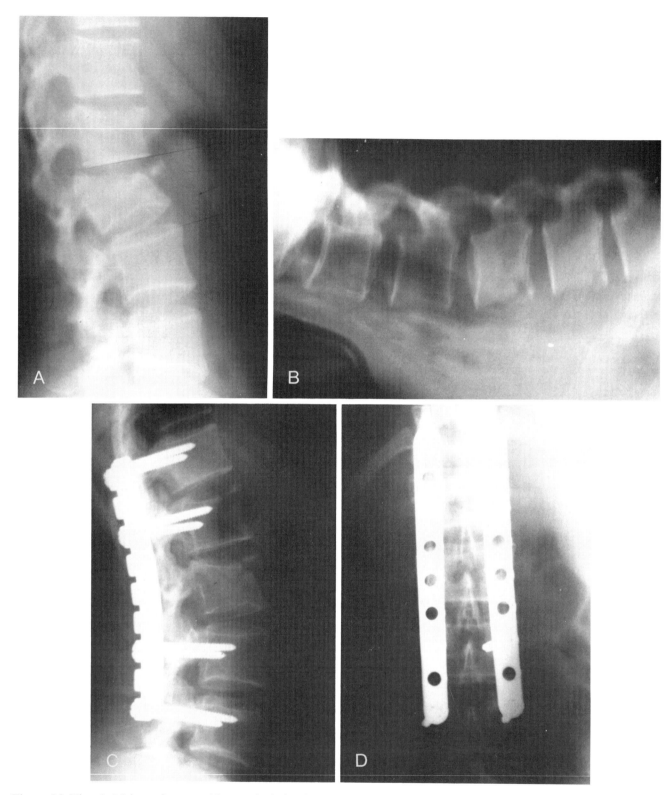

Figure 10.15. *A*, L2 burst fracture with neurologic involvement. *B*, Reduction on the operating table in prone position. *C–D*, Posterior instrumentation. Long fixation taking two vertebra above and below the injured level.

length of the screws. The surgeon determines the point of entry of the screw, and then with an awl begins the hole in the pedicle only to a depth of 3 or 4 mm. From this starting point, he/she inserts the spinal screw directly, as it is self-tapping. The screw will find its own way in the center of the pedicle through the cancellous bone between the cortices, and the risk of malimplantation out of the pedicle is lessened. When all the screws are inserted, the reduction of the fracture is completed with the special instruments for distraction or compression. The posterior part of each screw is placed through the corresponding hole in the plate, and the nuts are tightened and the fixations achieved.

In postoperative cases with medullary syndrome, the spinal stabilization is strong enough to allow early ambulation of the patients with an orthosis: cervical collar for severe sprains and simple dislocations of the C-spine, minerva for fracture dislocations, minerva corset for thoracic spine injuries above T6, and 3-point corset for lower injuries.

In 123 consecutive cases of thoracic and lumbar spine injuries, the mean loss of kyphosis was 4.4° when the plates were in place and 6.3° when the plates were removed at 1 year follow-up. Specifically, 39% maintained correction, 19% had 5°, 36% had 5–10°, and 6% had 10–20° of secondary kyphosis.

At the lower cervical spine in 221 patients, the results were excellent without nonsecondary kyphosis in 85.2%. Five degrees of secondary kyphosis were found in 8 (8% of the cases), 5–10° of secondary kyphosis in 3% of the cases, and 10–20° of secondary kyphosis in 3% of the cases.

TUMORS

Metastasis

Posterior spinal plating (PSP) is very efficient in the treatment of spinal metastasis with pain and neurologic involvement from C1 to sacrum. It is usually associated with a fairly extensive laminectomy and removal of metastatic epidural mass. The patients are painless and comfortable for the remaining period of life, which is the goal.

The stabilization of the occipitocervical junction with two plates and graft is particularly helpful for the upper cervical spine metastasis. At the lower cervical spine, the problems include instability and cord compression. So a posterior fixation is first achieved with or without laminectomy. Then an anterior corpectomy is usually performed to have a more complete cord compression.

At the thoracic spine, the epidural metastasis spreads easily along the cord over more than one vertebral level, so a large laminectomy is often necessary through a pos-

terior approach. The instability induced by the bony lytic lesion is corrected with two long pedicular plates.

At the lumbar level, the instability is the main problem of metastasis with radicular pain. A posterior approach allows root liberation when necessary and fixation with pedicular screw plates (Fig. 10.16).

In all the cases when the neurologic status allows it, the patients are walking immediately postoperatively with a minerva or a corset. The complementary treatment with radio- or chemotherapy is performed a few weeks after. In a series of 189 spinal metastases (27–79 years old) the general results obtained were survival over 1 year (up to 6 years) in 50% of the patients and pain improvement in 94%. Sixty-eight out of 72 patients with radicular deficits improved postoperatively.

Neurologically, 21 of 62 patients with cord compression improved, 33 remained stable, and 8 worsened postoperatively. There were 6 infections and 2 hardware failures.

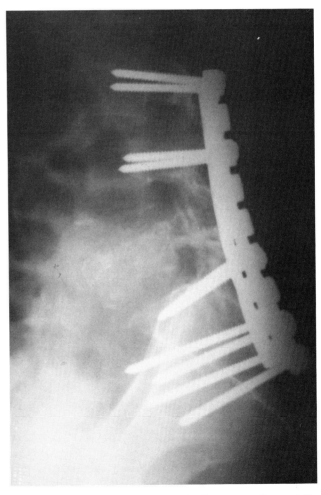

Figure 10.16. L5 breast metastasis. Decompression and fixation through a posterior approach.

PRIMARY TUMORS

En bloc vertebrectomy for primary tumors can be achieved at the thoracic spine through one posterior approach equivalent of a double costotransversectomy. At the lumbar spine, a posterior approach allows removal of the whole posterior arch including the pedicles down to the vertebral body. The vertebra is then excised en bloc through a lateral retroperitoneal exposure. Before any destabilization of the spine and to prevent any possible damage of the cord, it is mandatory to implant one pedicular screw plate on one side. Then, when the tumor resection is achieved, the spinal reconstruction is completed with a second symmetrical plate associated to a strong anterior interbody grafting plus posterolateral grafts if necessary. The patients walk 1 week after surgery with a minerva corset or a 3-point corset.

We have performed 34 such constructs after spinal tumoral resection. We had three cases of secondary early bending of the anterior graft with a crack, which led us to use stronger grafts. Tibial or femoral bone bank filled in the medulla with autologous cancellous bone is used. The posterior instrumentation remained the same.

RHEUMATOID DISEASES AND DEGENERATIVE DISORDERS

Cervical Spine

The occipitocervical plates and the long cervical plates are very helpful in rheumatoid diseases because of the quality of their purchase in the occipital bone and in multiple articular masses. We first attempt to obtain a correction of the displacement with a skull traction, followed by the fixation (occipito-C4 more often than C1-C2) with, if necessary, a resection of C1 posterior arch. If there is a persistent compression of the dens with neurologic involvement, we achieve a resection of the odontoid process more often through a lateral retropharyngeal approach than through a transoral approach.

Lumbosacral Fusion

It is important to understand the two different elements of the technique we use.

The Spinal Fixation. It may be performed with two symmetrical plates implanted, as indicated above. This is the good technique after a Gill's procedure or a large laminectomy.

It may also be performed with one plate on one side and screws implanted directly across the facet joints on the opposite side. It is simpler and as efficient. This technique gives more room for the grafting.

The Grafting. We prefer to avoid the classical posterolateral fusion because to prepare it, one must damage the muscles of the lumbar grooves and their vascularization coming specially from an arterial branch overlapping the transverse process at each level. Thus, we like to ensure the fusion with (Fig. 10.17): (*a*) a direct, bilateral, careful grafting of each articular joint; and (*b*) a posterior and lateral decortication of the articular facets, laminae, and sacral alars reaching just the base of implantation of the transverse processes in order to avoid the muscular vascularization. The spinous processes and laminae are also prepared as Hibb's. The cancellous bone will be located in a posterior and a lateral situation. Postoperatively, the obliteration of the facet joint lines on the oblique radiographs will be good proof of the fusion.

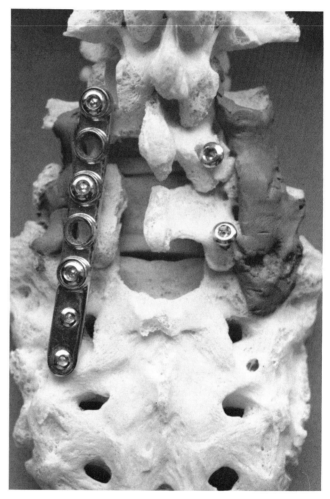

Figure 10.17. L4 sacrum fusion. Laminectomy and root exploration is on the side of the plate. Bone graft is posterolateral on this side. Interspinous ligament and spinous processes are preserved; two direct screws are implanted into the facet joint. Bone graft is laid on the posterior and the posterolateral groove.

In a recent series (by Roy-Camille) of 272 cases, the rate of fusion was 93.4%. Eleven cases were reoperated with success, and seven cases were followed without further surgery.

Spondylolisthesis with Significant Displacement

Using our special instrumentation, the posterior approach permits removal of L5 posterior arch (Gill's procedure), distraction between L4 inferior and S1 superior facets to expose L5 nerve roots, release of bilateral L5 nerve roots by resecting the L5 pedicle hooks, implant of the special plates in the sacrum, their superior part distance from L4 and L5 posterior aspect, pulling back of L4 and L5 vertebra with a cork-screw effect, and achieving a bilateral posterolateral fusion.

In a recent series of 29 cases, 19 cases were grade III, eight cases were grade IV, and two cases were spondyloptosis. The mean preoperative displacement was 69%, ranging from 54–100%, and the postoperative displacement was 44%, ranging from 0–56%. The mean preoperative slip angle was 31°, ranging from 20–66°, and it improved to 19° postoperatively, ranging from 13–24°. The fusion was successful in 28 out of 29 cases, and one required secondary fusion.

Four partial and transient L5 roots paralyses were observed in this series. One must observe the L5 roots under direct visualization, and one must prevent tension of the roots and accept less reduction in many cases to avoid neurologic deficits.

Adult Scoliosis

From 1986, we started to correct, fix, and fuse this difficult type of scoliosis using adapted plates and the special pedicular screws. We called it the "Mille Pattes" technique because it involves bilateral implantation of pedicular screws in each vertebra all along the instrumented spine. It is a multisegmental instrumentation, similar to Dwyer's or Luque's, and results in a good correction of the deformity.

The regular plates are flattened at their extremity to permit an overlapping of two plates that will be fastened by two adjacent pedicular screws (Fig. 10.18). The usual instrumentation extends from T6-T8 to sacrum. The technique is usually performed in two sittings 1 week apart in order to decrease the blood loss and morbidity.

The first sitting includes a large dissection of the posterior aspect of the vertebra up to the top of the transverse processes and the implantation of the pedicular screws with preparation of the facet joints fusion. Then, a pelvic-halo traction is maintained for 1 week.

During the second sitting, the plates are positioned. The correction of the deformity is achieved with distraction and compression applied at the base of the screws with the special instruments. The first instrumentation is placed bilaterally from L3-S2 in accordance with our usual and reliable technique of lumbosacral fusion. Then, overlapping plates are placed from L4-T8 or T6. One plate is placed after the other from the bottom to the top. The ancillary instrumentation is simple with a pusher for the plate and another one fork-shaped for the screws.

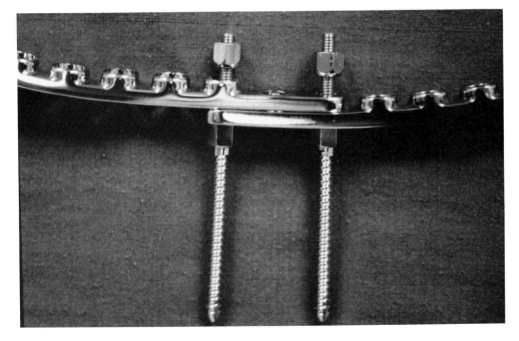

Figure 10.18. Scoliosis treatment (Mille Pattes instrumentation). Plates are flattened at both ends to enable enveloping.

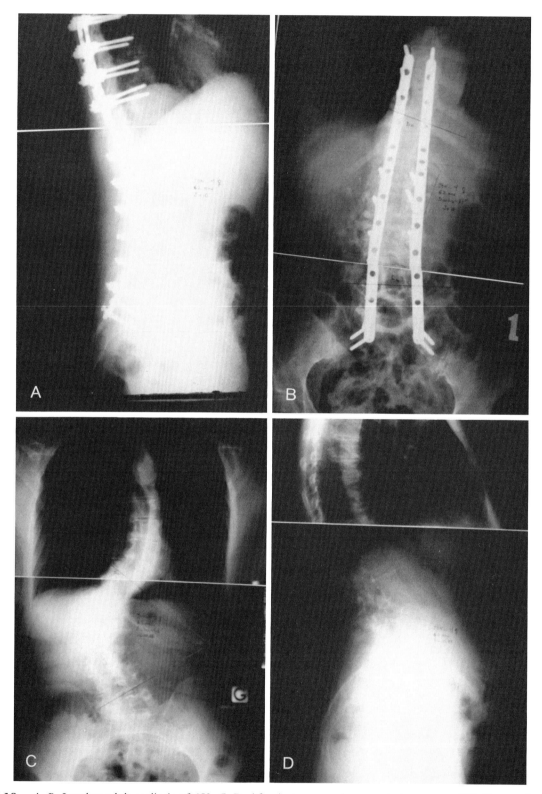

Figure 10.19. *A–B*, Lumbar adult scoliosis of 68°. *C–D*, After instrumentation: cervical curvature 17°. Restoration of lumbar sagittal lordosis and thoracolumbar curvature.

Working successively on each screw of each level, the stress is never too great, and the correction is progressively achieved. If necessary, a third pair of plates is used to reach the vertebra above up to C7. The usual screw dimensions are those indicated above for trauma cases. Between the two plates and lateral to them, there is a large area for a good graft (Fig. 10.19).

Postoperatively, the patients will wear an adapted 3-point corset, which is helpful for these osteoporotic vertebrae. Deambulation is progressively started during the two postoperative weeks.

In our series of 44 patients ranging from 24–74 years of age, the results revealed improvement from 38° (ranging from 20–60°) to 13.5° (ranging from 0–30°) in isolated lumbar curves. In double curves, preoperative angles were 51° (ranging from 14–65°) and 45° (ranging from 18–75°) for thoracic and lumbar curves, respectively. Postoperatively, thoracic curves improved to 25° (ranging from 10–40°), and lumbar curves improved to 14.5° (ranging from 0–30°). There was one infection, and there was one nonunion.

CONCLUSION

In our technique, the basic element is the point of implantation of the screws. Screws are implanted in the articular masses in the cervical spine, and in the pedicles in the thoracic and lumbar spines.

The fixation is strong but not rigid because of the clearance of the screws in the hole plates. This will prevent screw breakage. This technique may be used at the lumbar spine and at the thoracic spine. The diameter of screws must change as the size of pedicles changes from thoracic to lumbar region.

With such instrumentation, the surgeon is always able to solve any problem of instability of the spine and is always able to reconstruct in a stable manner.

SUGGESTED READINGS

1. Roy-Camille R, Roy-Camille M, Demeulenaere C: Ostéosynthèse du rachis dorsal, lombaire et lombosacré par plaques métalliques vissées dans les pédicules vertébraux et les apophyses articulaires. Presse Méd, 1970; 78:1447–1448.
2. Roy-Camille R, Saillant G, Mazel C: Plating of thoracic, thoracolumbar and lumbar injuries. Orthop Clin North Amer 1986; 17:147–161.
3. Roy-Camille R, Saillant G, Mazel C: Internal fixation of the lumbar spine. Clin Orthop 1986;203:7–17.
4. Roy-Camille R, Saillant G, Mazel C: Internal fixation of the unstable cervical spine by a posterior osteosynthesis with plates. In: Sherk MM, ed. The cervical spine. Philadelphia, JB Lippincott, 1989;390–421.
5. Roy-Camille R, Mazel C, Saillant G, et al: Rationale and techniques of internal fixation in trauma of the cervical spine. In: Treatment of surgical spine disease. New York, Springer-Verlag, 1990;163–191.
6. Roy-Camille R, Mazel C, Saillant G, et al: Treatment of malignant tumors of the spine with posterior instrumentation. In: Sundaresan N, Schmidek MM, Schiller AL, et al, eds. Tumors of the spine: diagnosis and clinical management. Philadelphia: WB Saunders, 1990;473–487.

ELEVEN

Spinal Internal Fixation with Louis Instrumentation

Réné Louis

INTRODUCTION

Following the works of Roy-Camille, published in 1969, on posterior vertebral osteosynthesis by pedicle screw plate, we adopted this method in order to stabilize certain vertebral lesions. After 2 years of experience with this procedure, we decided to implement our own method with different material while maintaining the use of pedicle screws. Transarticular screws did not seem to be useful and could even be dangerous for the contents of the foramen. In addition, the screw holes were too far apart to regularly allow for exact positioning of the pedicular screws. To avoid a systematic second operation with ablation of the material, the author chose short and solid osteosyntheses accompanied by fusion of the posterior joints covered by the osteosynthesis. We also modified the method for screw insertion in order to decrease the surgeon's exposure to x-rays. Finally, our conception of vertical stability with three vertical columns, one anterior and two posterior, led us to perform anterior osteosyntheses or even combined posterior and anterior osteosyntheses to repair and stabilize each of the columns with the same type of plate.

This chapter will include a section on the equipment and the installation procedures we used, and a discussion of the outcomes.

EQUIPMENT

We began to insert our own plates in 1972. The first plates were made of vitallium, chosen for its excellent tolerance. However, the screws proved to be brittle, and in 1985, we chose stainless steel. Our equipment includes the plates, screws, and ancillary material.

The plates we have designed vary according to the vertebral region in question. For L5-S1 osteosynthesis, we have conceived butterfly-shaped monoblock plates that resemble the posterior arch and are equipped with four holes (Fig. 11.1). The two superior holes are oval-shaped for the two L5 pedicular screws, and the two inferior holes are slanted obliquely at 45° outward and caudally to allow for fixation in the sacral ala. These plates come in three sizes (small, medium, large), depending on the interpedicular distance in patients. Regardless of the model, the sacral holes have been studied according to anatomical data so that the sacral screws can always be positioned away from the S1, S2 roots. For osteosynthesis extending from L4 or L3 to the sacrum, we have opted for a pair of symmetrical plates, each having a superior hole for sagittal screwing into L3 or L4 pedicles and two inferior screws for oblique screwing in the sacral ala. In their middle section, the plates are equipped with closely spaced holes, four in the L4-S1 plate and eight in the L3-S1 plate, allowing for precision screwing of the intermediate pedicles.

For pedicular screwing of the first thoracic vertebra until L5, we use a pair of symmetrical bone plates with sagittal screwing and closely spaced holes (Fig. 11.2). Plate width is 11.5 mm, thickness is 4.0 mm, and the length ranges from 3–35 holes. Each hole has a diameter of 6 mm, and the centers of two neighboring holes are separated by 9 mm. All of these stainless steel plates can be modeled with a pair of 3-point pliers to fit any kyphosis or lordosis. Finally, these plates can be sectioned with a large pair of pincers in order to adapt their length to that of the projected osteosynthesis. All of these plates can also be used for osteosynthesis of the posterior columns as well as the anterior column. For the thoracic anterior column presenting a physiologic kyphosis, we have conceived a plate that is slightly curved at the edges with a length corresponding to 14 holes.

Cervical plates are different for posterior osteosynthesis and anterior osteosynthesis (Fig. 11.3). For posterior osteosynthesis of the cervical vertebrae, we have designed a pair of symmetrical plates with closely spaced holes and a slightly reduced thickness of 3 mm and a length of 3–10 holes with a small curvature in lordosis. For the an-

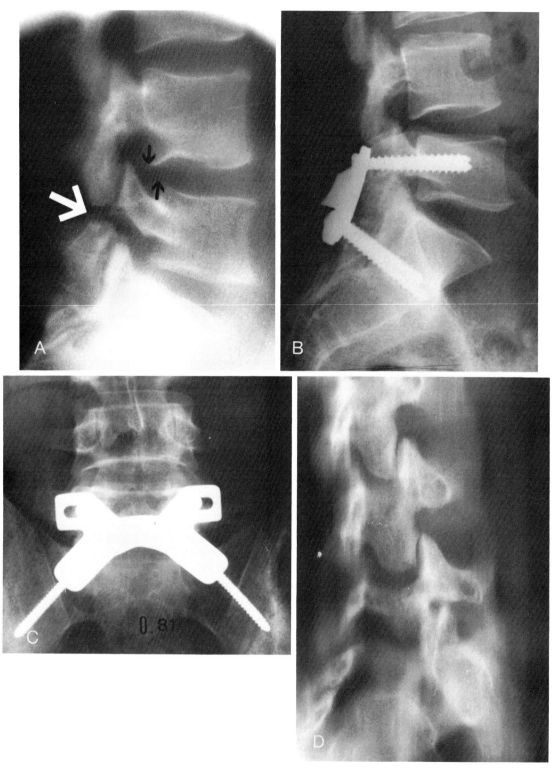

Figure 11.1. Our procedure of pars reconstruction for painful spondylolysis. *A*, Preoperative lateral x-rays, showing spondylotic defect (*large arrow*). *B* and *C*, Postoperative aspects with bone grafting of defects and temporary fixation with our "butterfly"-plate. *D*, Final tomogram after plate removal by the 6th month and sound repair of the pars.

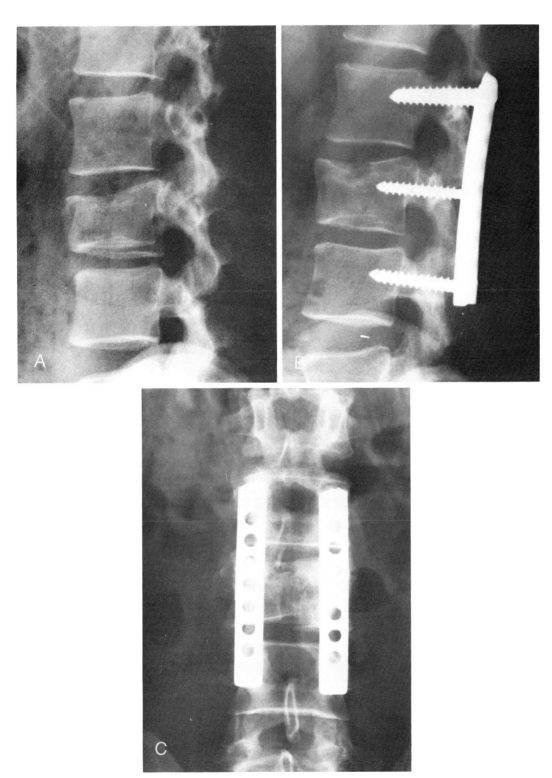

Figure 11.2. *A*, Lateral x-ray, showing a burst fracture of L3 with radiculopathy. *B* and *C*, Posterior decompression stabili- zation with two posterior plates with fusion of intermediate posterior joints.

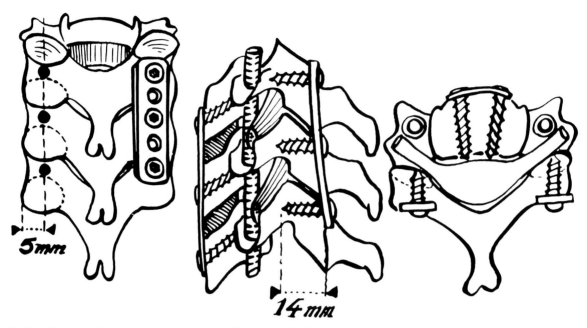

Figure 11.3. Drawings for demonstrating internal fixation of the lower cervical spine by either our anterior or posterior plates. For severe instability, a combined procedure can be indicated.

terior cervical spine, we have designed two types of plates that are rectangular and slightly curved transversely and longitudinally to adapt to the anterior convexity of the cervical spine. For osteosynthesis of two vertebral bodies with an intermediate disc, the plates are equipped with five holes: two superior holes, two inferior holes, and a central hole to attach the intersomatic graft. Plate holes are 5 mm in diameter for 4.5-mm screws. A second plate for osteosynthesis of three cervical vertebrae and fusion of two intervertebral discs has been designed with three pairs of horizontal holes and two intermediate median holes for grafts. The distance between the centers of the holes for the vertebral bodies is 18 mm.

For the craniocervical junction by transbuccal approach, we use two plates, one for osteosynthesis of the odontoid process in the form of an upside-down T with two inferior holes at the same level and a superior hole with two fork-shaped prongs to block the lateral aspects of the odontoid process (Fig. 11.3). In order to perform a C1-C2 arthrodesis, we have designed a rectangular plate, molded with two superior holes for the anterior arch of the atlas, two inferior holes for the axis body, and an intermediate hole for the base of the odontoid process.

For the material made of vitallium, we used Phillips-head screws with a diameter of 4.5 mm. However, given the frequency of vitallium screw deformation by torsion, we created three models in stainless steel (Fig. 11.4). The first model has a diameter of 5.5 mm and is used for posterior and anterior thoracolumbosacral plates. Their length varies from 15–60 mm, and the required drill bit is 3.2 mm. Given the specificity of vertebral bone structure, we have made an intermediate thread between the cancellous and cortical screws. The very solid hold that we currently obtain has given us complete satisfaction with this choice. The second model has a diameter of 4.5 mm and has the same morphologic characteristics as the first model. A 2.8-mm drill bit should be used for this screw. These first two models have hemispheric heads with a hexagonal perforation for insertion of the screwdriver. The 4.5-mm screws are especially intended for the superior thoracic pedicles and posterior cervical plates. The third screw model has a diameter of 4.5 mm but with a modified head in order to avoid any projection on the anterior cervical plates behind the soft organs. These heads are flattened with a cross-groove for the screwdriver and a threaded central hole for screwdriver grasping by an axial threaded rod.

Ancillary instruments are composed of screwdrivers, compression-distraction instruments, and instruments for spondylolisthesis reduction.

There are two types of screwdrivers. The first is hexagonal with an autoblocking cylinder to hold 4.5-mm or 5.5-mm screws. We have designed the second screwdriver with a cross for anterior cervical screws. To grasp these screws, this screwdriver is equipped with an axial tunnel in which one can insert a threaded rod that screws directly onto the head of the screw. After screwing, it is only necessary to unscrew the axial part of the screwdriver to free the screw.

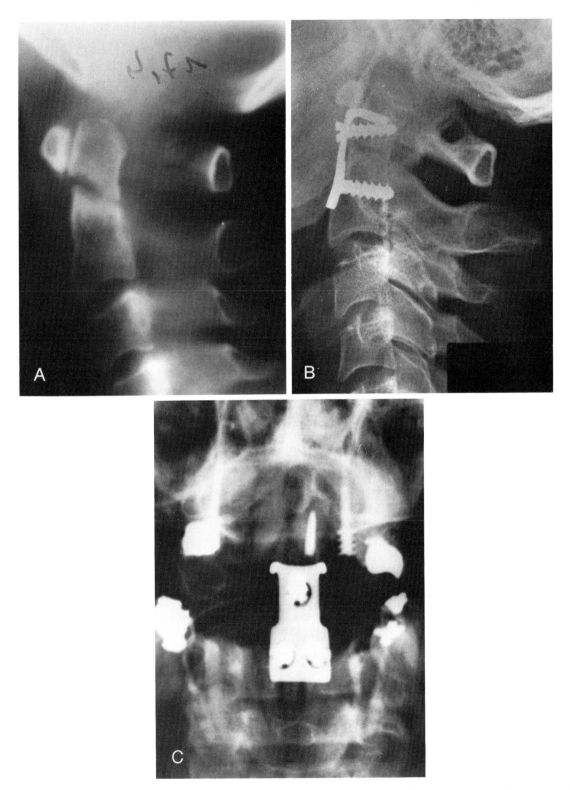

Figure 11.4. *A*, A fracture at the base of the odontoid. *B* and *C*, Transoral osteosynthesis of the dens with our special plate supplemented by median bone grafting. There is no fusion of C1-C2 joints, and no material removal is necessary.

We have designed two devices for perioperative reduction; one for compression and the other for distraction (Fig. 11.5A). Each of these devices is equipped with a threaded axis with a nut at the end for adaption of a universal wrench. There are two long hooks on this threaded axis, one of which can take hold in a plate hole and the other on the inferior edge of a lamina or a facet. An antirotation device adapts onto the hook and the plate. The distraction system is made in the same manner but with inversed screw threads on each half of the threaded rod. For reduction, each plate is screwed to one of its ends, and the device is applied from a plate hole toward a vertebral lamina situated beyond the other end of the plate. Compression-distraction makes it possible to slide the plate and at the end of reduction, position it

flush to one or several pedicles. The screws are then inserted directly through the plate holes and into the corresponding pedicles. It should be noted that for most reductions in kyphosis or lordosis, we use concomitant three-point vertebral traction. The patient's feet are attached to the operating table by orthopedic boots, his head is positioned in a leather helmet connected to a dynamometer and to a hoop that is attached to the cephalic part of the operating table (Fig. 11.5B). This axial traction is completed by a third force, perpendicular to the first two, represented by the angulation of the table under the operative area. With an average force of 5–15 kg, one obtains easy reduction of the areas in kyphosis, in either the supine or prone positions.

For instrumenting for spondylolisthesis reduction, we

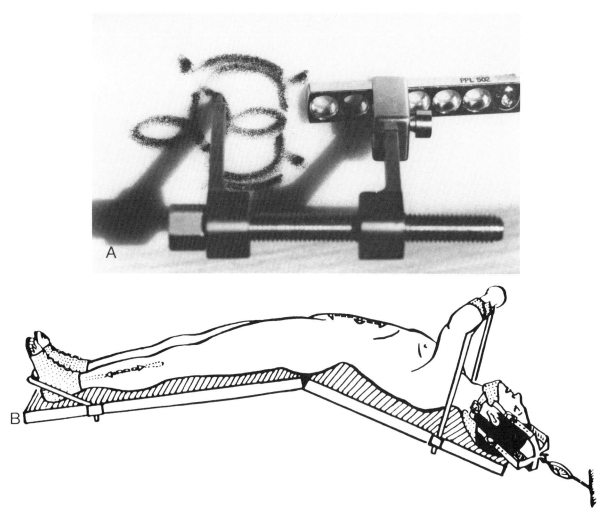

Figure 11.5.   Our two procedures for perioperative reduction of spinal deformity. A, Personally-designed device for compression or distraction. The posterior plates fixed by one top are displaced from or toward an anchorage point of the device upon a lamina through a hook. B, The patient is subjected to three gentle forces (5–15 Kg) perpendicular to the two others just behind the kyphosis due to table angulation.

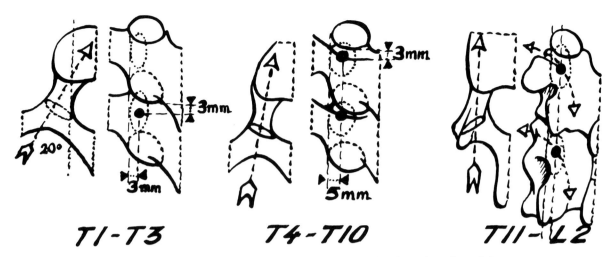

Figure 11.6. Landmarks for posterior screw insertion into thoracic pedicles.

have had elevators made in order to separate the olisthetic vertebra from the sacrum. These elevators are at angles that range from 90–180°. In addition, we have a reducer for retropulsion of the olisthetic vertebra that is composed of: a central part that fastens through the L5-S1 interspace onto the posterior edge of the sacral plateau and a peripheral part with a stopchuck that pushes the L5 body backward after screwing.

INSTALLATION PROCEDURES
Thoracolumbar Spine

Our methods of vertebral osteosynthesis by screw plates can be characterized by specific installation sites, tactics, and associated maneuvers. The precise pedicle landmark is the key to proper instrumentation (Fig. 11.6).

At the level of the first three thoracic vertebrae, pedicular screwing is performed 3 mm below the posterior joints and at 3 mm from their lateral edge. The screws are slanted medially from 15–20°. Screw length is from 25–30 mm.

From T4–T10, pedicle penetration is made at the intersection of a ridge that medially extends the superior edge of the transverse processes and a vertical line drawn at 5 mm from the lateral edge of the posterior joints. Screwing is strictly sagittal, and the screws should penetrate to a depth of 30–40 mm. At the level of the lumbar spine, screwing is again sagittal and is at the intersection of three lines: the first, a vertical line from the external edge of the articular interspace; the second, a horizontal line from 1 or 2 mm above the inferior edge of the articular facets; and the third, a curved line projected at 4 mm above and inside the notch at the outside limit of the pars interarticularis (Fig. 11.7). In any case, the ver-

tical line can be modified according to the more or less sagittal or coronal appearance of the articular facets, which must be verified by anteroposterior x-ray of the patient.

For difficult spinal surgery such as revision or for any surgeon beginning in vertebral osteosynthesis, it is better to identify, before screw insertion, the proper location of the pedicles by temporary insertion of small Kirschner pins of 3–4 cm in length. These pins are positioned on only one side of the spine undergoing osteosynthesis and are checked by the image intensifier. We always begin by positioning the superior pedicular screw. Then, the plate is aligned on the posterior joints so that it is parallel to the median sagittal plane. The hole for the inferior pedicular screw is drilled directly through the plate hole over the pedicular landmark. The positioning of the intermediary pedicular screws is determined by the opposite pedicular landmarks. The hole is therefore drilled directly through the plate hole, and the screw is inserted immediately after. The plate on the opposite side is assembled in the same sequence.

For the vertebral bodies, the screws must be inserted in their lateral aspect at 10 or 15 mm from the foramina (Figs. 11.8, 11.9, and 11.10). The screws are inserted at a slightly oblique backward direction toward the contralateral side without transgressing it. At the level of the thoracic spine or lumbar spine, screw plates are temporarily positioned by placing them on the lateral aspect of the vertebral bodies so that their medial edge is flush to the plane of their anterior aspect. The plates are temporarily held in place by two Steinmann pins in the holes at each extremity. Then, the holes are successively drilled and the screws are inserted in an almost coronal plane. It is not necessary to reach the opposite cortex in order

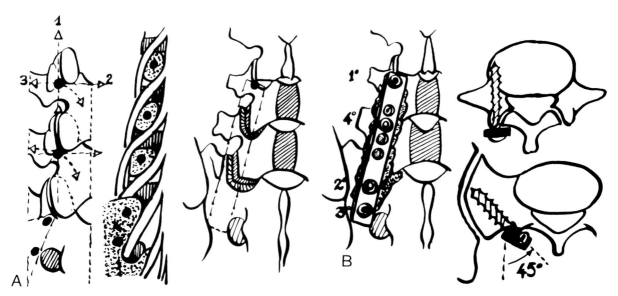

Figure 11.7. Landmarks for posterior fixation of our L4-S1 screw plates. *A,* The posterior facet joints to be fused are prepared with packing of bone grafts taken in situ from spinous processes. The upper pedicular screw is inserted and the plate aligned over the facet joints. *B,* The second screw to be inserted is the upper sacral screw directly through the plate hole. The third screw is the lower sacral one, and finally, the intermediate screw for L5 pedicle is inserted through the plate hole corresponding to opposite L5 pedicle landmarks.

to avoid vascular injury. It is not at all advisable to position a plate behind a large vessel—vena cava, aorta, iliac arteries and veins—due to the risk of further injury by screw displacement.

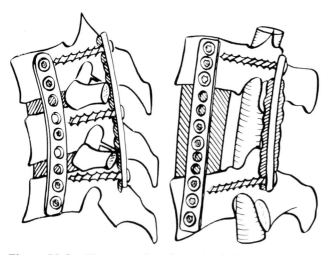

Figure 11.8. Two examples of anterior fusion of the thoracolumbar spine with lateral fixation. On the left, two interbody fusions with a curved laterally screwed plate. On the right, montage after total vertebrectomy for malignant tumor with reconstruction of the three pillars of the spine. The anterior pillar is reconstructed with 2 to 3 vertical pieces of fibular struts and a laterally screwed plate. The two posterior pillars are reconstructed with iliac bone grafts and bilateral plates.

Lumbosacral Spine

Sacral screws are anchored directly into the sacral ala in a manner that avoids all radicular contact. In older patients, one can encounter bony rarefaction areas. However, our new 5.5-mm diameter screw makes good penetration possible in all cases on the condition that the direction of the screw is changed to a more sagittal direction if one encounters an area of less resistance. The length of the first sacral screws is an average of 45 mm with the second screws at 35 mm.

In order to install our "butterfly" plate, we begin by drilling two L5 pedicular holes after having shortened the inferior facet (Fig. 11.11 *A–E*). Bayonet-shaped pins are inserted into the holes, and the interpedicular distance makes it possible to select the proper plate. The plate is then slipped over the pins and held in position by an assistant so that each pin remains in the middle of the plate hole. Each pin is successively replaced by a screw that is held by a grasping screwdriver. For the sacrum, the holes are drilled directly through the plate holes with the screw inserted in the same manner. For the L4-S1 or L3-S1 lumbosacral plates, one begins by positioning the two superior screws by aligning the plate along the posterior articular interspaces, i.e., in a manner that slightly diverges at the level of the sacrum. Then the first sacral screws are inserted after drilling their holes directly through the plate, followed by insertion of the second sacral screws. The intermediary pedicular holes are lo-

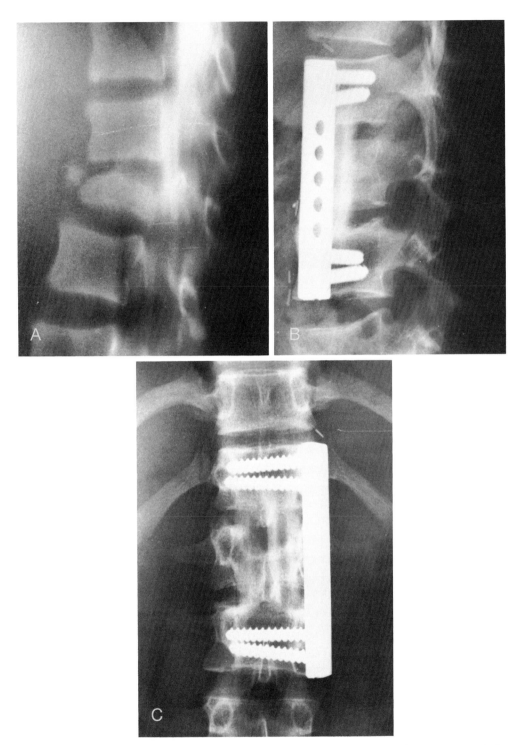

Figure 11.9. *A*, Example of anterior decompression for partial neurologic compromise due to severe L1 fracture. *B* and *C*, Stabilization with fibular struts and laterally screwed plate.

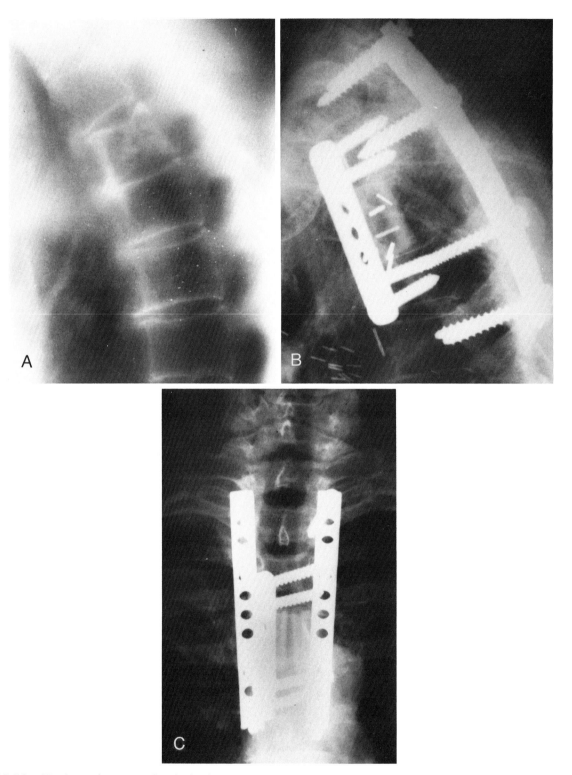

Figure 11.10. Total vertebrectomy for single thoracic metastasis from chest carcinoma. *A*, a lateral tomogram showing the thoracic involvement. *B*, Lateral, *C*, anteroposterior roentgenograms showing total vertebrectomy and reconstruction with anterior and posterior plates and screws.

cated by comparing the opposite side in order to select the plate hole that best corresponds.

Cervical Spine

Posterior screwing is not performed in the cervical pedicles but rather in the articular pillars. Penetration is also sagittal, perpendicular to the lamina at 5 mm from the lateral edge of the facets and at an equal distance above and below the facet joints, generally 3–4 mm below the overlying interspace. Screw penetration should go 10–14 mm into the bone for 14–18-mm screws. Our landmark permits the head of the screw to be positioned at the base of the pedicle, thus avoiding penetration in the foramen and in the intertransversal space where the vertebral artery is situated.

The anterior screw plates are sagittally screwed with a slightly ascending direction in the vertebral bodies for an average length of 16–20 mm, depending on the patient. One can either stop at the posterior cortex or go through it by 1 to 2 mm.

Cervical body plates are positioned by placing a superior screw. Then, the plate is properly aligned on the midline, followed by insertion of the second inferior screw. We verify correct screw penetration by an image intensifier and modify it if required. The other screws are then inserted, the central screw for the graft and the two remaining end screws.

Associated Maneuvers

Vertebral osteosynthesis can be associated with reduction and/or arthrodesis.

For reduction, we regularly use bipolar vertebral traction with a third perpendicular force represented by the angulation of the table under the operative area. These three forces enable us to reduce all deformations, especially deformations in kyphosis. If reduction is required during osteosynthesis, we use our compression or distraction device.

We almost always perform arthrodesis in association with vertebral osteosynthesis. We do not practice intertransversal fusion but prefer intraarticular arthrodesis. For this, the accessible part of the articular interspace is excised from its cartilage, and corticocancellous shavings removed from the spinous processes are packed into the joint. The spinous processes are an excellent material for grafts on the condition that they be cut in horizontal slices, cut in half, and, finally, stripped of all soft tissue. At the level of the anterior column of the spine, we use iliac grafts for the cervical region and sagittal segments of fibular shaft extemporaneously removed from the pa-

tient. A fibular peg is required for the thoracic spine, two or three pegs for the thoracolumbar spine, and three or four for the lower lumbar region. A good montage with fibular material requires that the ends of the graft be against two healthy endplates, above and below. The endplates should have their cortex intact but should be stripped of all cartilage or fibrous tissue.

DISCUSSION

We will now consider the complications encountered with our method, the quality of fusions, and the advantages of our method as compared with others.

Complications

When we used vitallium, we had up to 13% of the patients with screw alterations. These were either cases of screw displacement of a few millimeters or torsion or even rupture of the extraosseous part of the screw. Since we began using 5.5-mm stainless steel screws with a thread that is more adapted to the spine, we have had practically no other such complications.

Installation difficulties with such plates could come from changes in tactics. Indeed, with our plates, one must not first drill all of the pedicular holes and then try to match them with the plate holes. It is essential to follow the installation protocol as described above. In difficult cases, previous positioning of small Kirschner pins directly above the pedicular landmarks is an excellent solution.

Vitallium has a reputation for better tolerance than stainless steel, but in the 5 years that we have been using stainless steel, we have yet to find any chemical reaction for the techniques that require material ablation such as pars interarticularis reconstruction for spondylolysis.

As far as the strength and reliability of anchoring points are concerned, sagittal pedicular screwing appears to us to be much more solid than oblique pedicular screwing, which attempts to remain parallel to the axis of the pedicles. Indeed, screwing into the pedicle walls is much more solid than axial screwing. The reliability of our landmarks is excellent. We have had no major problems for screw positioning after 19 years of practice. During the first 2 years, while seeking these landmarks, we had some cases of malinsertion that occasionally injured a root, causing intolerable pain in the patient on recovery. We would then withdraw the offending screw, either under general anesthesia or under local anesthesia. This is now no longer a problem, as perioperative monitoring of screw position makes it possible to avoid such incidents.

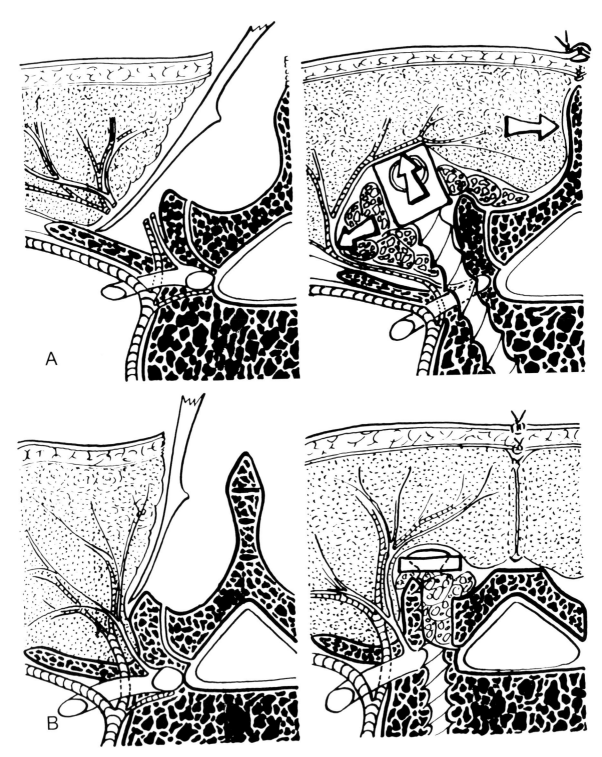

Figure 11.11. *A*, The procedures associating huge material laterally fixed into pedicles and intertransverse bone grafting threaten or destroy erector spinae muscle nerve and blood supply. *B*, Our procedure with flat screw plates, sagittal pedicular screws, and intraarticular bone grafting respects erector spinae muscle nerve and blood supply. *C–E*, Example of our technique for reduction and combined fusion for severe spondylolisthesis.

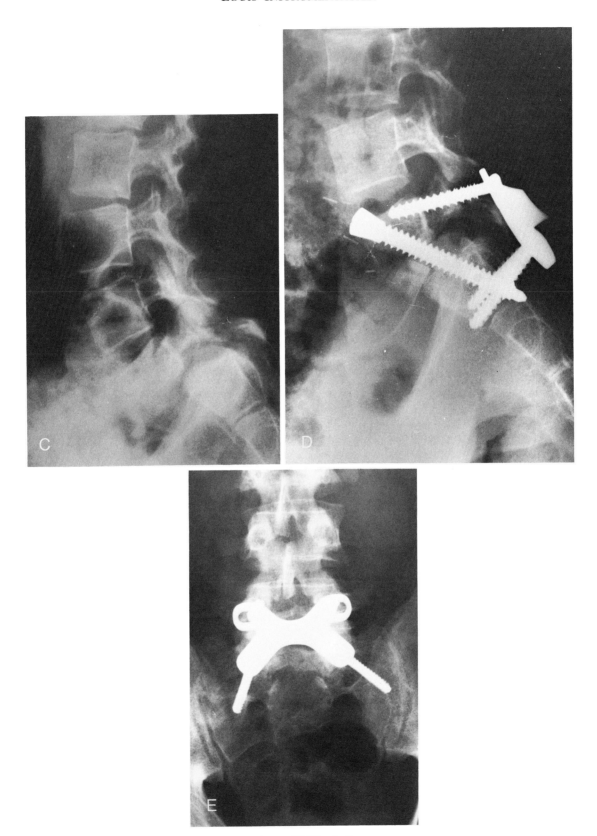

Figure 11.11. *C–E.*

Fusion

With our osteosynthesis and fusion of the posterior joints by spinous grafts, we have obtained fusions for the lumbosacral region at a rate of 94.5% in a series of more than 500 cases presented in 1982. For combined lumbosacral arthrodeses, we have obtained a fusion rate of almost 100%. Our montage therefore seems to be sufficiently rigid without being excessive, avoiding rupture of the material.

Advantages of Our Method

Our material is the least voluminous of the currently available material for osteosynthesis of the spine. The other materials, additionally equipped with a reduction device by screwing or sliding on a rod, are all very voluminous and require on closure of the muscular folds, a pressure that could damage the vascularization of the erector spinae muscles. Projection of the material can therefore be a problem in thin patients. With our method, which consists of not exceeding the external edges of the posterior joints in the exposure of the posterior arches, we never touch the neurovascular bundles of the erector spinae muscles that run beside the pars interarticularis areas. Oblique screwing into the bases of the transverse processes as well as using a median approach of intertransversal arthrodesis with large iliac corticocancellous bone fragments are bound to sacrifice several neurovascular bundles, which are incompatible to proper erect vertebral function in man. We are convinced that many complications following vertebral surgery are most often due to these neurovascular sacrifices than to so-called epineuritis. Finally, installation of this material is rapid with, for example, lumbosacral osteosynthesis in less than an hour. As our method leaves the posterior vessels intact, there is almost no blood loss and therefore no need for transfusion. The positioning of the plates on the posterior joints permits subsequent operations for decompression of the vertebral canal. Finally, this stainless steel material with very little ancillary instrumentation as well as the plates for both posterior and anterior osteosynthesis costs very little. A lumbosacral osteosynthesis with our material costs 10% of the price of the more expensive materials.

CONCLUSION

Our system of screw plates for anterior and posterior vertebral osteosynthesis permits short and solid stabilization of the three stabilizing columns of the spine. The association of a posterior intraarticular or anterior intersomatic arthrodesis is usually indispensible. The reliability of our montage and its excellent fusion rate with a moderate cost are the principal advantages of this method. This process, along with perioperative reduction maneuvers either by vertebral traction or by ancillary instrumentation, make it possible to treat all vertebral deformations in the sagittal plane.

SUGGESTED READINGS

1. Louis R., Maresca C: Les arthrodèses stables de la charnière lombosacrée. Rev Chir Orthop Suppl II 1976;62:70–79.
2. Louis R, Maresca C, Bel P: Les fractures instables, la réduction orthopédique. Rev Chir Orthop 1977;65:449–451.
3. Louis R: Lumbo-sacral fusion by internal fixation. Clin Orthop Rel Res 1985;203:18–33.
4. Louis R: Spinal stability as defined by our three column spine concept. Anatomia Clinica 1985;7:33–42.
5. Roy-Camille R: Ostéosynthèse du rachis dorsal, lombaire et lombosacré par plaques métalliques vissées dans les pédicules vertébraux et les apophyses articulaires. Pres Méd 1970;78:1447.

TWELVE

Transpedicular Fixation of the Spine Using the Variable Screw Placement System

Alexander R. Vaccaro, Howard S. An, and Jerome M. Cotler

INTRODUCTION

There is much debate in the literature over the optimum spinal internal fixation device that affords the surgeon the benefit of rigid stabilization for fusion maturation while preserving the normal contouring and biomechanics of the spine. For years, the gold standard was the Harrington rod and hook system. This system allowed the surgeon to manipulate the spinal deformity in the coronal plane but included excess motion segments in the fusion mass with the additional loss of optimum sagittal contouring. Today, there is great interest in utilizing the pedicle as a means of rigidly instrumenting all three columns of the spine, especially in the presence of posterior element deficiency. The addition of spinal plates attached to the pedicle screws allows the surgeon the ability to perform wide, aggressive decompressions of the spine while stabilizing a limited number of spinal segments with preservation of the normal contours of the spine.

In 1944, King (21) first developed the concept of using the pedicle as a means of spinal fixation, and it wasn't until 1959 that Boucher (4,38) reported on the actual success of obtaining a posterior fusion by passing screws through the lamina and pedicle into the vertebral body. Since the early 1960s, numerous surgeons have developed spinal fixation systems using the pedicle as a major component of fixation (13,18,22,24–26,30,31, 48–50,52).

In 1986, Arthur D. Steffee introduced the variable screw placement system (VSP) as a means of transpedicular fixation of the unstable spine (1,38). He described the efficacy of this system in patients suffering from spinal instability, severe back pain unresponsive to conservative treatment, and patients with back pain relieved by immobilization (38). In his earliest article on VSP plating, he described the concept of the "force nucleus," the junc-

tion of the pedicle, superior and inferior facets, the pars, transverse process and lamina, a channel where all forces posteriorly can be transmitted anteriorly through the pedicle to the anterior column of the spine (38). The functional importance of the pedicle's anatomic location is further enforced by the proximity of the lumbar multifidus and longissimus attachments (mammary and accessory process, respectively), both important in segmental movement of the spine (38). Steffee's early attempt at fixation of the "force nucleus" consisted of an AO neutralization plate and cancellous bone screws, but he soon discovered the lack of flexibility between the fixed circular plate hole and the hex head of the cancellous screw. This led to the development of the variable screw placement system.

The VSP system consists of two bilaterally placed stainless steel plates with nested slots, allowing precise placement of specifically designed screws at any angle necessary for rigid fixation (Fig. 12.1) (40). The screws consist of a long cancellous threaded portion that enters the pedicle and a machine-threaded section on its shank with an integrated hex nut between both portions assisting in level placement of the slotted plates (Fig. 12.2). The screw lengths (cancellous portion) vary from 16–55 mm, with screw diameters of 5.5, 6.25, and 7.0 mm. Three different plate spacer washers (3 mm, 5 mm, and tapered) are used between the hex head of the cancellous portion of the screws and the undersurface of the plate to achieve level metal-to-metal contact between the plate and screw shank. A VSP tapered nut is used to secure the plate to the pedicle screw, and a VSP lock nut is then used on all VSP screws to secure the entire fixation device (Fig. 12.3). The VSP instruments consist of a VSP T-handle screw wrench with a 3.18-mm hex socket for all VSP screws, a VSP T-handle nut wrench with a 9.5-mm hex socket for tapered nuts, and an 8-mm hex socket for

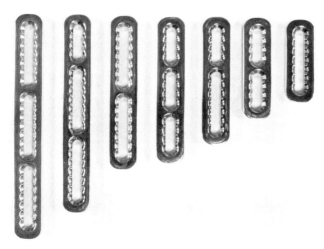

Figure 12.1. VSP bone plate selection. Plates are 16 mm in width and vary from 44–166 mm in length. There are 1–5 slots per plate, increasing in ½ slot increments. (From AcroMed Corp.)

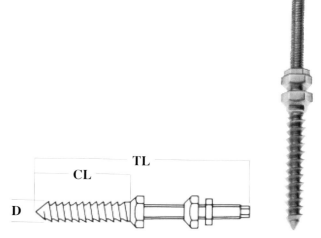

Figure 12.2. VSP pedicular screws. (From AcroMed Corp.)

locking nuts. The set also includes a VSP screw alignment bar and rod, a VSP pedicle probe (gearshift), a VSP aluminum template set, a VSP sounding probe, and a VSP bone tap (Fig. 12.4).

INDICATIONS FOR VSP INSTRUMENTATION

The VSP system is being used today for various pathologic disorders but, unfortunately, very little published literature is available in support of its application in specific spinal disorders. The clinical situations cited in the literature for VSP instrumentation include: (*a*) conditions of spinal instability secondary to extensive surgical posterior decompressions for spinal stenosis and degenerative or herniated disc disease; (*b*) multilevel laminectomies with decompression (3); (*c*) the failed back patient with a documented pseudarthrosis; (*d*) spinal decompression with deficient posterior elements (3); (*e*) lower thoracic or lumbar burst fractures and fracture dislocations; (*f*) the reduction or stabilization of symptomatic spondylolisthesis (48); (*g*) stabilization of spinal tumor resections (48); and (*h*) at times, for severe disabling back pain relieved by immobilization (38).

ADVANTAGES OF VSP INSTRUMENTATION

VSP instrumentation allows short, rigid immobilization of the spinal column with good sacral fixation (48) without the need for canal encroachment. The shorter fixation of spinal motion segments and preservation of sagittal contouring may possibly decrease the incidence of low

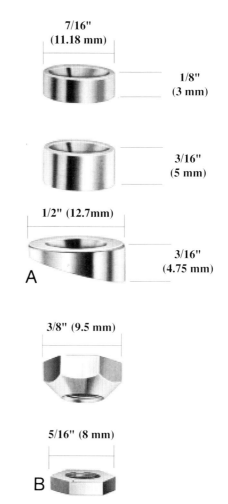

Figure 12.3. *A*, VSP plate spacer washers (sizes 3 mm, 5 mm, and tapered). *B*, VSP lock nut. (From AcroMed Corp.)

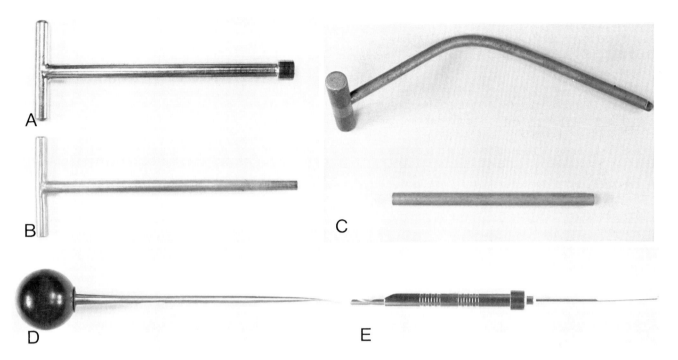

Figure 12.4. *A*, VSP T-handled screw wrench. *B*, VSP T-handled nut wrench. *C*, VSP screw alignment bar and rod. *D*, VSP pedicular probe (gearshift). *E*, VSP aluminum contouring template set.

back pain (48,53). The rigid nature of the VSP fixation constructs may indeed improve fusion rates (1,55) and remove the need of postoperative immobilization or prolonged bed rest except in certain specific clinical situations (38).

The VSP spinal instrumentation system is not without its documented disadvantages. The system is comparatively large and bulky, and at times, especially in slim patients, can result in overlying soft tissue irritation. It is a technically difficult system to master, usually resulting in increased operative time, increased blood loss, and a small, but documented increased postoperative infection rate (55).

ANATOMY

The pedicle is considered the strongest part of the vertebra (1). Roy-Camille (32), in 1986, dissected 35 cadavers to illustrate the various horizontal and vertical diameters of the lower cervical, thoracic, and lumbar spinal pedicles (Fig. 12.5). In 1985, Krag (24) described the sagittal anatomic alignment of the lower thoracic and lumbar vertebral pedicles and found the pedicles at T12 to be −0.6° from the sagittal midline (slightly anterolateral angulation) compared with +27.2° at L5. In terms of size, the average adult pedicle measures from 0.7 cm in horizontal diameter at T10 to 1.5 cm at L5, and from 0.7 cm at T12 to 1.6 cm at L5 in its vertical diameter

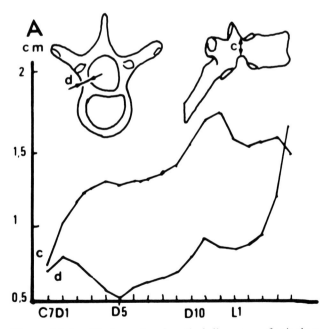

Figure 12.5. Horizontal and vertical diameters of spinal pedicles in 35 cadaveric dissections. (From Roy-Camille R, Saillant G, Mazel C: Internal fixation of the lumbar spine with pedicle screw plating. Clin Orthop 1986;203:7.)

(33). The interval between adjoining pedicles averages about 2.6 cm, with the dural sac measuring approximately 0.2–0.3 cm from the medial wall of the thoracolumbar pedicles (33).

VSP instrumentation has been useful in the complicated arena of sacral fixation. Until recently, the hazards of sacral screw placement were known but not anatomically well illustrated. Mirkovic (28) recently described sacral pedicle screw fixation in 30 human cadaveric specimens. He found that the internal iliac vein, artery, and the L4-L5 nerve roots were at great risk from screws protruding through the anterior sacral cortex, while the long mesentery of the sigmoid colon protected this organ from injury. Screws placed into the S1 pedicle and through the anterior cortex were least likely to cause neurovascular damage, while screws placed directly into the S2 pedicle were in direct alignment with the neurovascular bundles. In 1986, Zindrick (54) tested the biomechanical strengths of various pedicle screw constructs and found that S1 pedicle screws yielded the greatest fixation strength, while screws placed in the S2 pedicle yielded the weakest fixation. He also found that screws angled 45° laterally into the sacral alae yielded optimum

fixation ability. Mirkovic (28) further tested commonly quoted angles used in placing sacral screws and found that screws aimed inferior to the S1 facet, 25° inferiorly and 30° laterally, placed the internal iliac vein at risk 30% of the time, and screws placed 25° inferiorly and 45° laterally, placed the lumbosacral trunk at risk 55% of the time (28).

OPERATIVE TECHNIQUE

The operative approach to the posterior spine is performed in the standard fashion with subtle variations according to the individual surgeon. Preoperative planning should consider the use of somatosensory evoked potentials (SSEP) if any direct or indirect manipulation of the cord or conus is expected. Additionally, due to the potential for bloodborne transmission of infectious disease, the use of hypotensive surgery, and the presence of intraoperative cell saver may lessen the need for postoperative homologous blood transfusions (32). The collection of preoperative autologous blood should also be considered to lessen the further need for foreign blood transfusion.

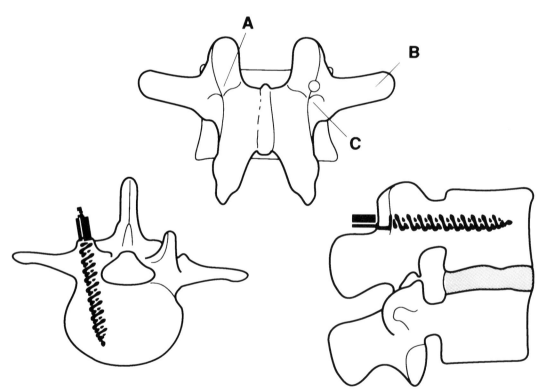

Figure 12.6. Landmarks to locate pedicles. *A*, Transverse process corresponds to level of the pedicle. *B*, Caudal tip of the inferior facet. *C*, Junction of the facet, transverse process, lamina. (From White AH, Rothman RH, Ray CD: Lumbar spine surgery techniques and complications. St. Louis: CV Mosby, 1987:322–338).

Surgical Exposure

The patient is placed prone in a kneeling position (1,38,48), allowing the abdomen to be free of any compression, indirectly decompressing the epidural venous plexus. Skin and dermis may be injected with 0.5% bupivacaine and 1/200,000 epinephrine in line with the intended skin incision (1). A midline incision is made down to the level of the spinous processes with all soft tissue dissected subperiosteally off the posterior elements out to the tips of the transverse process, leaving the intertransverse membrane intact. If no midline decompression is needed, the paraspinal muscle splitting approach may be performed, allowing easier placement of the pedicular instrumentation. The appropriate spinal level is identified either anatomically or with radiographic assistance, and an appropriate laminectomy and decompression is performed, depending on the clinical situation. Preparation for the posterior lateral bone graft bed is performed by exposing the appropriate facet joints and transverse processes with burring of all exposed cortical bone.

Attention is now directed toward the pedicle screw insertion. The pedicle in the lumbar spine is located at the junction of the transverse process, lamina, pars interarticularis, and caudal tip of the inferior facet (Fig. 12.6). A burr (¼″) is used to penetrate the posterior cortex of the pedicle, and the pedicle probe ("gearshift") is used to carefully follow the path of least resistance into the cancellous bone of the pedicle (Fig. 12.7). The pedicle sounding probe is then placed into the pedicle palpating in a complete 360° circle to make sure there are no cortical perforations (Fig. 12.8).

The surgeon should be aware of the potential complications from pedicle cortex disruption (1). If the pedicular cortex is violated superiorly, the intervertebral disc will be penetrated with resultant poor screw fixation. If the inferior cortex is perforated, the nerve root is at risk. If the medial cortex is disrupted, the canal will be violated, and if the screw goes out laterally, the segmental vessels are at risk as well as poor purchase for screw fixation. A laterally placed screw hole can lead to an erroneous long screw length measurement off the depth gauge due to the slippage of the depth gauge off the side of the ver-

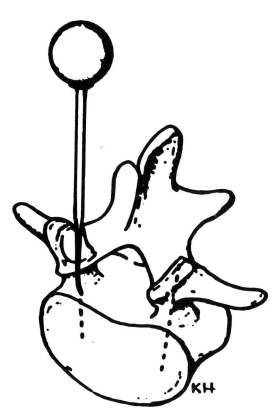

Figure 12.7. Pedicle probe is advancing through pedicle into vertebral body. (From White AH, Rothman RH, Ray CD: Lumbar spine surgery techniques and complications. St. Louis: CV Mosby, 1987:322–338.)

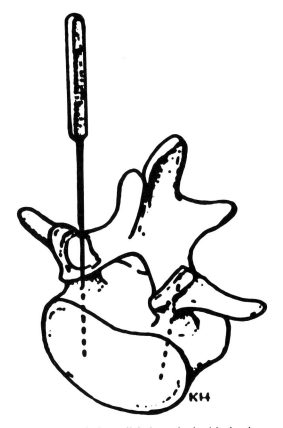

Figure 12.8. Hole in pedicle is probed with depth gauge to be sure that it is surrounded by bone 360°. (From White AH, Rothman RH, Ray CD: Lumbar spine surgery techniques and complications. St. Louis: CV Mosby, 1987:322–338.)

tebral body with possible retroperitoneal penetration (38). Weiland and McAfee (45) compared Cotrell-Dubousset (C-D) pedicular instrumentation (49 patients) with Steffee instrumentation (51 patients), placing a total of 473 pedicle screws with a 2-year follow-up. The authors cited no adverse sequelae of screw placement and no intracanal penetration. They emphasize to the surgeon performing pedicular screw fixation a thorough understanding of the vertebral landmarks, visualization of the intracanal pedicular wall, and the use of a pedicular probe for better localization of the pedicle canal rather than a drill.

Following the use of pedicular probes, different sized Steinmann pins are placed bilaterally in each pedicular hole with their positions confirmed by a plain roentgenogram (1). The pedicle screw path is then tapped, and an appropriate length pedicle screw is placed. We recommend placement of the lumbar pedicle screws into the anterior subchondral bone and slight penetration of the anterior sacral cortex with the sacral pedicle screws, particularly in the osteoporotic spine. It is important to align all screws in the longitudinal and horizontal axes to avoid screw torque or bending at the time of plate placement, thereby avoiding the potential for implant or pedicular failure and screw migration in the future (Fig. 12.9) (55). Hsu (19a) noted significant leg pain in eight of his first 30 patients in which he performed distraction on the

implanted pedicular screw for alignment purposes. He noted that such a constant eccentric pressure to the pedicle wall may lead to significant bony necrosis with collapse of the adjacent neuroforamina from overdistraction at the operative level (Fig. 12.10). The pedicle screws are placed until the large cancellous threads are buried into the depth of the pedicle.

Sacral pedicular screws are placed last. If only one sacral level screw is instrumented, the screws are usually placed in the S1 pedicle located just caudal to the superior sacral facet. A second sacral screw can be placed at the level of the second pedicle 45° lateral into the sacral alae (38). If there appears to be tenuous fixation secondary to osteopenic bone, anterior purchase of the cortex is recommended. The use of methylmethacrylate is rarely necessary. Once the screws are placed, a malleable aluminum template is fashioned to the sagittal contour of the spine, and any osteophytes and remaining fusion mass, as well as the posterior aspect of the superior facet are removed to allow a flat surface for plate placement. Impingement of the inferior facet of the noninstrumented segment above the fixation should be avoided (50). The appropriate-sized plate spacer washers (flat or tapered) are placed over the screw, allowing a flat surface for placement of the plate, thereby decreasing the potential for unwanted screw torque.

Bone is now placed over the exposed bony surfaces

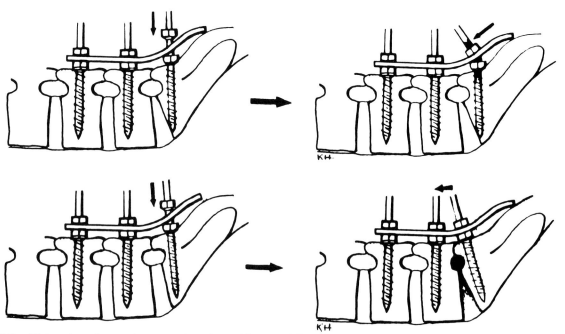

Figure 12.9. Tightening of nuts when screw is set in position varying from 90° in relationship to the plate results in unidirectional torque, which may result in screw weakening and delayed pedicle erosion or fracture. (From Zucherman J, Hsu K, White A, Wynne G: Early results of spinal fusion using variable spine plating techniques. Spine 1988;13:570.)

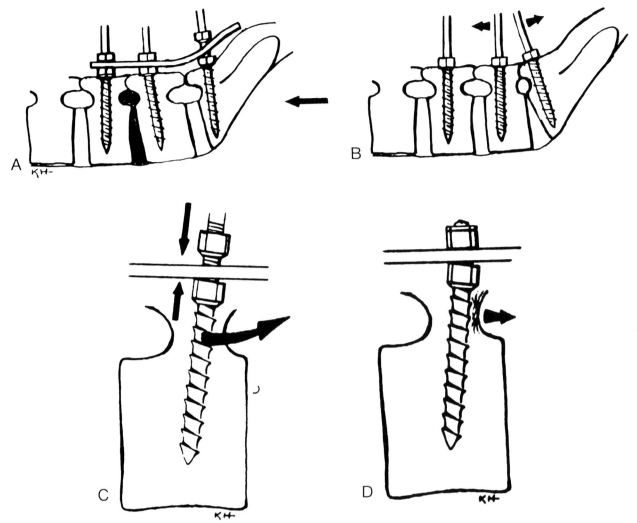

Figure 12.10. When excessive distraction is applied at one segment, the adjacent segment may become compressed, causing disc narrowing and/or foraminal stenosis. (From White AH, Rothman RH, Ray CD: Lumbar spine surgery techniques and complications. St. Louis: CV Mosby 1987:322–338.)

(posterolateral fusion) prior to plate placement. The contoured slotted plate is fitted over the pedicular screws, and a tapered hex nut with the tapered end toward the plate is screwed down firmly, followed by the flat hex nut used to lock the entire construct. The VSP 45° open-ended hex nut wrench should be used in holding or adjusting the lower taper nut, while the upper hex nut is tightened. It is important not to strip the threads of the screws when placing the plate (55). Therefore, to assist in aligning the screws, one may use the VSP screw alignment bar or rod with careful consideration to the possibility of pedicular fracturing, loosing, or migration. Once the plates are in place, additional bone graft is added, and the canal, nerve roots, and foramen are once again inspected prior to closure. A bolt cutter is used to

cut the end of the protruding screws even with the locking nut. Case examples are shown in Figures 12.11–12.13.

Postoperative Immobilization

The issue of postoperative immobilization after the use of VSP instrumentation is unsettled (1,32,38,55). Due to the rigidity of the system and demonstrated lack of translation at instrumented segments on lateral flexion and extension views (32), many surgeons believe postoperative immobilization is unnecessary. It is the authors' belief that when the VSP instrumentation is used alone with a posterolateral fusion in the setting of anterior middle column disruption from trauma, some form of immobilization is needed until a solid fusion mass develops in order to prevent late collapse.

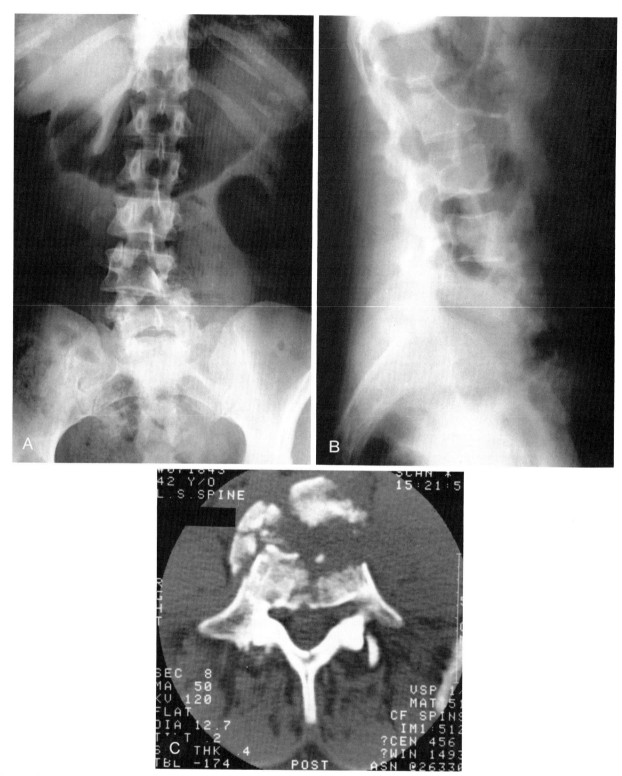

Figure 12.11. *A* and *B*, AP and lateral plain roentgenograms reveal a comminuted burst fracture of L5 in a 42-year-old fe-male; *C*, An axial CT image of L5 reveals vertebral body comminution without canal compromise.

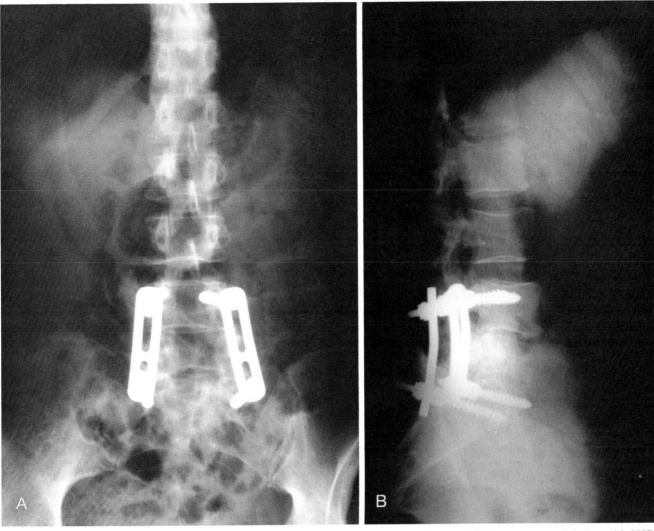

Figure 12.12. *A* and *B*, Postoperative AP and lateral plain roentgenograms, revealing an L4-S1 posterolateral fusion with VSP plating of the L5 burst fracture.

BIOMECHANICS

To understand the true value and clinical fortitude of transpedicular fixation, the surgeon should have a basic understanding of the implant's biomechanics or behavior in certain clinical situations. An average adult spine experiences around 400 newtons of axial force during quiet standing and up to 7000 N of force during heavy lifting (35). For forces of this magnitude, a spinal surgical implant with considerable strength and endurance is needed in a setting of moderate to severe ligamentous or bony instability of the spine. Although the optimum spinal fixation device has not been developed, many surgeons believe that transpedicular fixation offers rigid, segmental fixation over a limited number of spinal segments, offering excellent posterior fixation with added middle and

anterior column stabilization through screw penetration into the anteriorly situated vertebral body.

The characteristics of pedicular screw fixation have been thoroughly investigated by such investigators as Krag (23), Zindrick (54), Ruland (34), Goel (14), Halvorson (17), and others (3,16,53). Zindrick (54) studied different pedicular screw fixation systems in fresh cadaveric spines and found that: (*a*) the pedicle screws with the largest diameter threads had the best pullout fixation strength overall; (*b*) screws that penetrated the anterior cortex of the vertebral body had much greater fixation than screws that coursed any distance through the vertebral body up to and including the subchondral bone; (*c*) screws with continuous threading throughout their length had greater fixation strength than screws threaded solely within the vertebral body; and (*d*) the force to

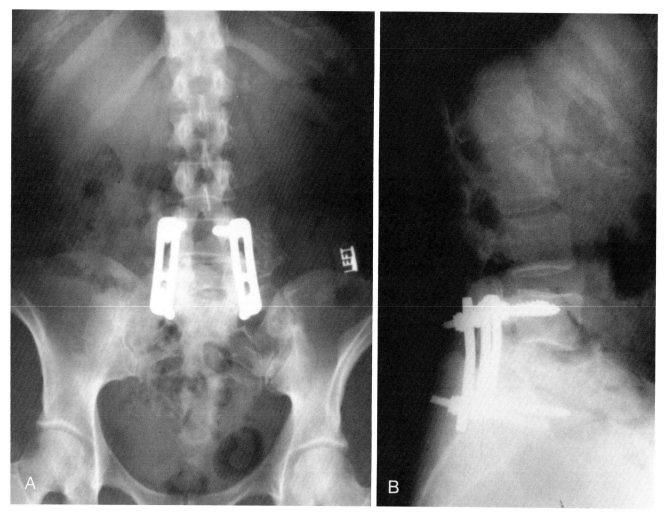

Figure 12.13. *A* and *B*, AP and lateral plain roentgenograms at 8 months follow-up, revealing a mature posterolateral fusion with excellent fracture alignment without collapse.

failure was inversely proportional to the degree of vertebral osteoporosis. Zindrick also noted that pressurized methylmethacrylate placed in the pedicle could double the original pullout strength of a failed pedicular screw.

Krag (23) noted optimum screw fixation with pedicular screw depths greater than 50% of the depth of the vertebral body. Halvorson (17) compared the differences in actual pullout strengths of pedicular screws in osteoporotic vs. normal spine and found significant differences in fixation stability. In normal spines with vertebral bone density averaging 1.17 g/cm², the average pullout strength of the pedicle screw was 1530 ± 369 newtons, while in osteoporotic spines with vertebral bone densities averaging 0.819 g/cm², the average pullout strength was 210 ± newtons.

Ruland et al. (34) also found a strong linear correlation between bone mineral density measured with dual pho-

ton absorptiometry and load to failure in his human cadaveric study comparing tensile loads to failure of five spinal implants (C-D laminar hook, single C-D, Steffee pedicular screw, triangulated C-D, and triangulated Steffee pedicular screw). In this study, Ruland et al. found that triangulated pedicular screw systems (transverse plate placed prior to attachment of longitudinal rod or plate) exhibited greater fixation than the conventional pedicular screw or laminar hook system (p < 0.05) (34). An interesting and promising finding was that in those triangulated systems that illustrated metal failure, the location of breakage was removed from the metal-bone interface seen with the conventional pedicular screw system.

The importance of implant fatigue and its clinical relevance has recently been studied by McAfee et al. (27) in a survivorship analysis of 100 consecutive patients who were treated with VSP instrumentation with a 2-year follow-up period. At 2 years, there was a 6% incidence of metal failure and a 3% incidence of radiographic pseudarthrosis. Survivorship analysis of the data revealed a 70% implant survival rate at 10 years, with a predicted fusion survival of 90%. This means that long-term implant fatigue may not correlate with a poor clinical outcome as long as the rigidity of the system allows for optimum fusion mass maturation prior to instrument failure.

Goel et al. (14) completed an interesting three-dimensional nonlinear finite element model of the intact L4-L5 one-motion segment/two vertebrae and L3-L5 two-motion segment/three vertebrae. Using CT-computed reformatted signals in the setting of a simulated bilateral decompression spinal procedure stabilized with VSP plates and an interbody fusion, they found that cancellous bone beneath the pedicle screws was shielded by the screw plate system. There was greater measured load transferred to the internal fixation devices than to the posterior elements. They also noted increased localized stress in the cortical shell of the pedicle in all loading modes (compression, flexion, extension), supporting the possibility of future screw loosening and breakage.

Yoganandan et al. (53) studied human cadaveric lumbar spines in an effort to quantify the biomechanical characteristics of VSP stabilization of the injured lumbar spine under increasing compression/flexion forces. He found that the VSP-instrumented lumbar spines with compromise to the anterior vertebral spinal canal responded with increased energy absorption. Therefore, carrying capacity compared to the injured spine without instrumentation, although the fixated construct was never as strong as the uninjured intact spine. He also noted that although the initial stiffness of the fixated injured spine (82.3 ± 12.9 N/mm) was superior to the unfixated injured spine (45.6 ± 8.3 N/mm), both exhibited a similar final stiffness (300.5 ± 52.4 vs. 295.2 ± 43.1 N/mm) far less than the uninjured intact spine (490.0 ± 84.7 N/mm). Thus, it seems that beyond a certain level of stress, the VSP-instrumented spine responds in a sim-

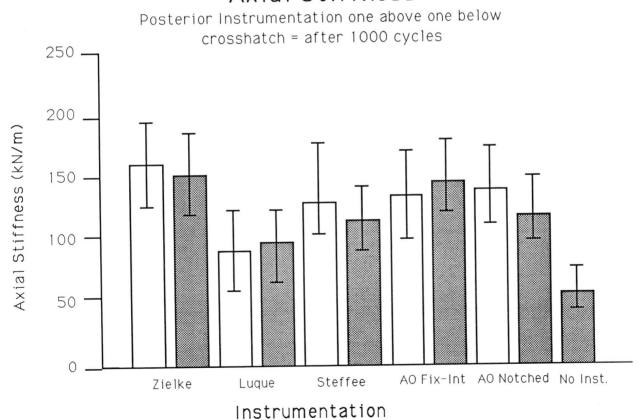

Figure 12.14. Comparison of axial stiffnesses measured on constructs of different instrumentations. (From Ashman RB, Gaypin RD, Corin JD, et al: Biomechanical analysis of pedicle screw instrumentation systems in a corpectomy model. Spine 1989;14:1398.)

ilar manner as an unfixated injured spine. These findings imply the need for additional stability, possibly through an anterior stabilization procedure.

Recently, there have been two good human cadaver and calf spine studies in the literature, making direct biomechanical comparisons of different pedicular screw constructs. Ashman et al. (3), in a one-above/one-below fresh human L1 corpectomized spine model, compared a number of different pedicular systems (Zielke, VSP/Steffee, AO fixateur interne, Luque plate, and AO notched plate) under a low-level axial load, testing stiffness and torque strength of all implants. They found that the AO notched plate, Luque plate, Steffee plates, and AO fixateur interne had similar axial stiffnesses (121 kn/m, 100 kn/m, 108 kn/m ± 42 kn/m respectively; Fig. 12.14) and that the tensile strength measured in the body of the implant that loads up to 450 N all were below the endurance level of 316 L stainless steel (310 MPa) (Fig. 12.15). An interesting finding in their study was that those systems with more rigid plate screw interfaces (i.e., Steffee, fixateur interne) yielded pedicle screw shank tensile strengths, measured at relatively low loads (175–270 N), below the endurance level of 316 L stainless steel (Fig. 12.16).

Therefore, even though these more rigid systems illustrated a greater correction force than the more unconstrained Luque/AO notched plate systems, these systems are more prone to implant fatigue and loosening.

In a calf lumbar spine model corpectomized at L3, Gurr (16) compared the biomechanics of various lumbar posterior fixation systems with cyclic nondestructive loading in axial compression, flexion, and rotation. They found that the C-D pedicle screw and Steffee systems were able to restore the torsional stiffness to that of the original intact spinal segments (fixation L1-L5 vertebrae). In addition, both systems were able to reduce the intervertebral displacement between the 2nd and 4th lumbar levels to a range recorded for the intact lumbar spine, unlike the Harrington distraction rod and Luque rectangular rod with sublaminar wire system.

Clinical Follow-up

To date, the number of clinical follow-up studies on VSP plating of the spine has been limited and short follow-up lacking a suitable control to infer the efficacy and clinical applicability of the implant systems for various

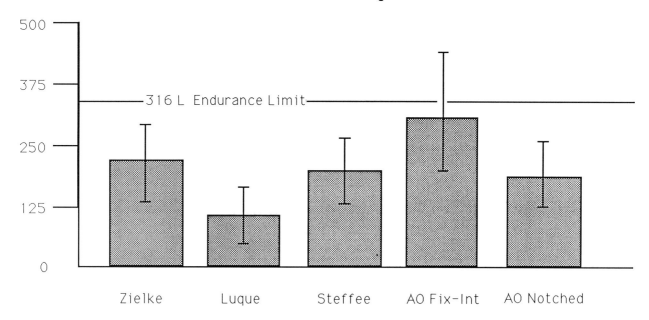

Figure 12.15. Tensile stress in body of the implant measured at an axial load of 450 newtons. (From Ashman RB, Gaypin RD, Corin JD, et al: Biomechanical analysis of pedicle screw instrumentation systems in a corpectomy model. Spine 1989; 14:1398.)

Measured Stress v. Axial Load

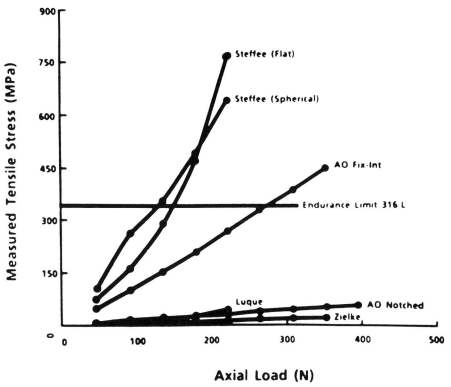

Figure 12.16. Measured stress vs. axial load for each of the systems tested. The endurance limit (310 MPa) of 316 L stainless steel is indicated. (From Ashman RB, Gaypin RD, Corin JD, et al: Biomechanical analysis of pedicle screw instrumentation systems in a corpectomy model. Spine 1989;14:1398.)

spinal disorders. As mentioned previously, a number of clinical settings in which VSP instrumentation has been utilized included spinal instability secondary to trauma, degenerative and herniated disc disease, spondylolisthesis, and the failed back with deficiency of the posterior elements. Traditional surgical attempts at posterior spinal fusion for these problems revealed an average pseudarthrosis rate by plain radiographic evaluation (8,29,43, 44,50,51) of 5% to greater than 20% for one- to two-level fusions, with the highest rate of pseudarthrosis being at the L4-L5 level.

Schwaegler (36) compared the efficacy of single-level fusion with VSP instrumentation (39 patients) with no instrumentation (29 patients) in comparable cases of single-level disease failing conservative treatment. Patients fused with VSP instrumentation experienced no evidence of pseudarthrosis, while those fused without instrumentation had a pseudarthrosis rate of 21% in an average follow-up of 2 years. There were no instrumentation failures. Dietz (10) followed 151 patients treated with VSP plates for an average of 30 months and found a fusion rate of 84%. Kabins et al. (20), in an unpublished retrospective review of 39 patients who underwent single-level L4, L5 fusions with bilateral VSP plates and mostly interbody grafting, recorded only one patient with documented pseudarthrosis after an average of 12 months follow-up. Grubb (15) in a 2-year follow-up compared three similar groups of patients (total 45) undergoing one- or two-level fusions with VSP instrumentation vs. those patients who underwent posterolateral fusion without instrumentation and those who underwent posterolateral fusion with compression U rod instrumentation. The patients in the VSP-instrumented group experienced no evidence of pseudarthrosis compared with 30% (one-level), with 40% (two-level), and 0% (one-level), with 80% (two-level) pseudarthrosis rates in the posterolateral fusion without instrumentation and the compression U rod instrumented groups, respectively. Another large series of VSP instrumentation with allograft vs. autograft bone grafting recorded pseudarthrosis rates in the range of 8–66% (39,47,55).

The comparison of autogenous vs. allograft iliac bone

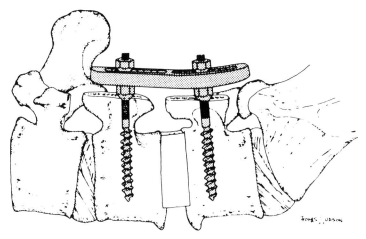

Figure 12.17. Interbody graft and immediate stability are achieved with application of VSP spine plates. (From Steffee AD, Sitkowski DJ: Posterior lumbar interbody fusion and plates. Clin Orthop 1988;227:99.)

grafting in VSP-plated patients was illustrated by West et al. (47), who experienced a 66% pseudarthrosis rate in 21 patients undergoing primary fusion with Red Cross freeze-dried allograft and local bone graft vs. a 9% pseudarthrosis rate in 41 similar patients undergoing fusion with autogenous iliac bone graft. In an unpublished study, Kabins (20) experienced an 83% pseudarthrosis rate in patients undergoing unilateral VSP plating with allograft, compared with a 3% pseudarthrosis rate when autograft was used. The merits of autogenous bone grafting have been widely supported by other authors in the spine literature.

Posterior Lumbar Interbody Fusion

Posterior lumbar interbody fusion (PLIF) has been performed by some surgeons in degenerative disc disease and spondylolisthesis cases. The enthusiasm for PLIF is best expressed by Cloward (6,7,40) who reviewed 45 years of experience with the procedure and believed it should be applied routinely in all lumbar disc surgery. He emphasized his concern that decompressive spinal surgery may relieve the sciatic portion of the patient's symptoms, but too often the inciting cause of the low back pain, i.e., the disc and innervated surrounding tissues, is not addressed. Only with removal of the offending tissues with foraminal distraction and bone grafting can patients be truly rendered asymptomatic. A proponent of the use of VSP instrumentation in association with PLIF surgery is Steffee, who routinely performs the procedure during lumbar surgery any time a disc space is elevated (39). In a recent review of his cascading spine series (39), Steffee found a 91% fusion rate with the VSP and PLIF group. He also noted minimal complications with no evidence of pseudarthrosis in another group of 67 pa-

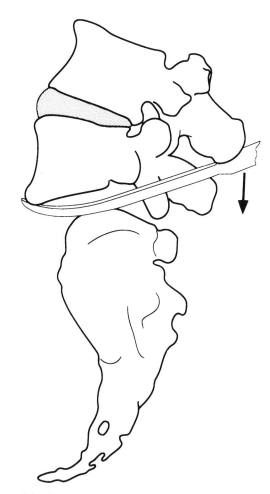

Figure 12.18. Illustration of lever stretching soft tissues in L5, S1 disc space. (From Steffee AD, Sitkowski DJ: Reduction and stabilization of grade IV spondylolisthesis. Clin Orthop 1988;227:89.)

tients undergoing VSP and PLIF, with 36 patients of that group being followed for 6 months–1 year (40). Steffee's indications for VSP and PLIF include instability associated with herniated and degenerative disc disease, spondylolisthesis, and the failed back syndrome. Recently, Chapman (5) reviewed 89 patients who underwent VSP and PLIF with morselized cancellous bone graft through a limited annulotomy with a 1–2-year follow-up. He reported a complication of eight durotomies, four transient nerve impairments, four screw failures, and an improvement in pain scores (1–4) from 3.9 preoperatively to 1.8 postoperatively. Although it is beyond the scope of this chapter to review the indications, shortcomings, and controversies of PLIF, the use of VSP transpedicular instrumentation may aid spinal stability during PLIF maturation (Fig. 12.17).

Spondylolisthesis

Recently, many surgeons have begun using internal fixation in adult patients with degenerative spondylolisthesis as a means of preventing further slippage. Kabins (20), in unpublished data, reviewed 15 patients with degenerative spondylolisthesis and four patients with retrolisthesis who underwent VSP posterolateral fusion, and compared them with 53 patients with degenerative spondylolisthesis treated by Herkowitz (19), whose patients underwent decompression and fusion without instrumentation or decompression alone. No patients in Kabins' study at follow-up demonstrated further slip as compared with 22% of Herkowitz's patients in the de-

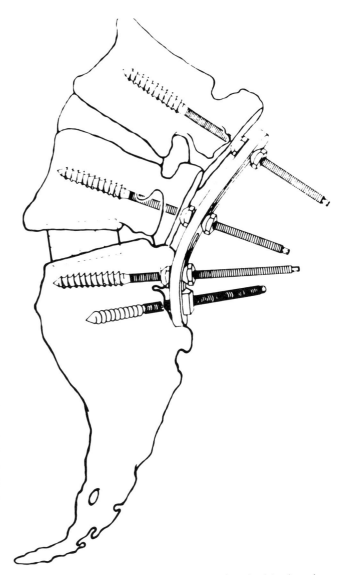

Figure 12.20. L5-S1 displacement reduced with plates bent for "new lordosis." Two points of fixation above and below the interbody fusion are in place. (From Steffee AD, Sitkowski DJ: Reduction and stabilization of grade IV spondylolisthesis. Clin Orthop 1988;227:89.)

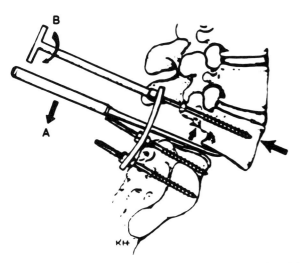

Figure 12.19. *A*, Grade IV displacement being reduced by traction by L5 screw. *B*, Bone from rounded end and of sacrum and/or inferior endplate of L5 may also have to be removed. (From Steffee AD, Sitkowski DJ: Reduction and stabilization of grade IV spondylolisthesis. Clin Orthop 1988;227:89.)

compression fusion group and 65% of patients in the decompression alone group.

The operative reduction of high-grade spondylolisthesis is considered today to be one of the most controversial issues in spine surgery (42). Steffee, the proponent of the procedure, cites the inability of a fusion in situ to relieve stretch or pinch on a nerve root from a drastically anterior slipped vertebra (40). To date, Steffee has been able to achieve 100% fusion success rate with no significant complications using VSP plate instrumentation with PLIF in his reduction of high-grade slips (39). His methods of reduction and stabilization involve initial stretching of soft tissues prior to the elevation and translation of the involved vertebral body (41). The structures cited as being hindrances to reduction include the annulus and posterolateral longitudinal ligament, the pseudarthrosis of the pars, and the anterior iliolumbar ligament.

To begin stretching of the responsible tissues, a lever is used to elevate the L5 body (L5, S1 slip) into proper position, normalizing the displacement angle (Fig. 12.18). During such reduction, it is prudent to utilize dermatosensory evoked potentials to monitor for any possible neurologic trauma from nerve stretch or impingement. Once the L5 vertebra is in proper alignment, pedicle screws are placed with the intended plate fixation spanning two motion segments above and below for severe slips and one segment above and below for minor

slips. Bilateral VSP plates are placed next with subsequent tightening of both L5 pedicular screws simultaneously (Fig. 12.19). Following this, one plate is removed at a time and contoured to the lumbar spine for the appropriate lordosis (Fig. 12.20). The plates are placed over a prepared posterolateral bone grafting, and attention may then be directed to the performance of an interbody fusion, if warranted. Case examples of spondylolithesis are shown in Figures 12.21–12.24.

Trauma

A short rigid fixation system such as VSP instrumentation may be used for thoracolumbar injuries, especially low lumbar burst fractures. It was believed that flexion com-

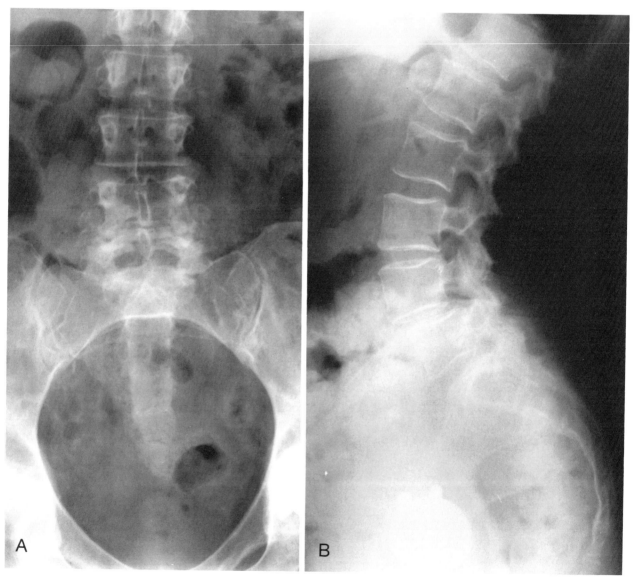

Figure 12.21. *A* and *B*, AP and lateral plain roentgenograms reveal a grade 1 L5-L6 (extra lumbar vertebra) degenerative spondylolisthesis in a 71-year-old female.

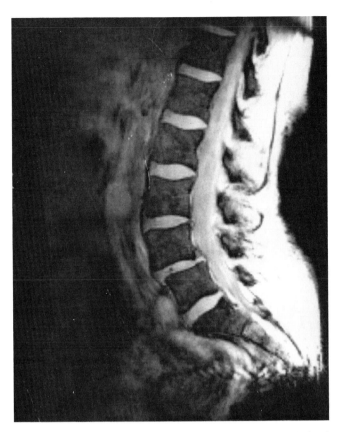

Figure 12.22. MRI reveals minimal to moderate ventral dural impingement from the L5-L6 degenerative spondylolisthesis.

pression injuries to the spine with disruption of the anterior and middle columns can be treated with VSP instrumentation with posterolateral bone grafting alone without the need for postoperative bracing. Only now, with more recent available biomechanical cadaver and clinical survivor analysis, surgeons are realizing that posterior stabilization alone in the above clinical setting may not be enough when using the VSP system in spinal trauma.

Schwaegler et al. (37) reviewed 20 patients with thoracolumbar burst fractures and fractures of the lumbosacral junction treated with VSP instrumentation and posterolateral bone grafting with two patients undergoing a second anterior procedure. They reported a successful fusion in 19 of 20 patients with no evidence of pseudarthrosis and an average loss of lordosis of 9°. Three screws (all less than 7 mm in diameter) broke with no resultant effect on the fusion maturation, and two screws pulled out secondary to osteoporosis. Although Schwaegler's study and a few in the literature (9,12) attest to the successful stabilization of flexion compression spine injuries with short rigid posterior fixation devices, more recent studies cite significant problems due to the lack of anterior column support (11,50). Ebelke et al. (11) re-

viewed 21 burst fractures treated with two motion segment VSP instrumentation and fusion with a follow-up of 6–33 months. Of the eight patients who also underwent anterior bone graft augmentation, all patients after survivor analysis had 100% implant survival through 27 months. Of the 13 patients with posterior fixation and fusion only, only 49% implant survival was calculated at 18 months and longer. Whitecloud (50) documented poor results in four out of five patients with thoracolumbar fractures treated with VSP plating and bone grafting, citing screw breakage and recurrence of deformity as a primary mode of failure. Both authors cite the need for anterior bone grafting in situations of anterior column disruption. An et al. (2) reviewed the treatment of lower lumbar burst fractures treated with body cast alone, posterior spinal fusions with Harrington rod instrumentation, Luque rod instrumentation, and Steffee plates, and found that Steffee plating was best in restoring and maintaining lumbar lordosis. Harrington rod instrumentation increased vertebral height, but produced loss of lumbar lordosis. Luque rod instrumentation was moderately effective in restoring lumbar lordosis, but was found not to restore vertebral height. Therefore, Steffee plating seems to be effective in stabilizing burst fractures of the lumbar spine, but postoperative body cast or brace should be used, unless an additional anterior procedure has been performed.

Unilateral VSP Instrumentation

In light of the potential adverse side effects from the rigidity of bilateral VSP systems (i.e., osteoporosis secondary to stress shielding, instability or degenerative changes above or below the instrumented levels) the use of unilateral VSP placement is being considered to replace bilateral placement in certain clinical situations. Kabins et al. (20) undertook a retrospective review of isolated L4-L5 floating fusions in 41 consecutive patients with an average follow-up of 23.5 months. Patients treated with unilateral procedures (18 patients) had a greater number of previous spinal surgical procedures and a greater number of spinal segments operated on than those who were treated with bilateral VSP placement (23 patients), making the surgical time and estimated blood loss equal in both groups. Overall, the unilateral and bilateral VSP groups experienced similar L4-L5 fusion rates (94% bilateral groups; 100% unilateral group). There was no increased evidence of metal failure in the unilateral group as one might expect.

The authors concluded that unilateral VSP placement may be just as effective as bilateral placement, but with less morbidity. They recommended bilateral VSP placement in patients with significant osteoporosis, patients with suboptimal unilateral pedicular fixation, patients re-

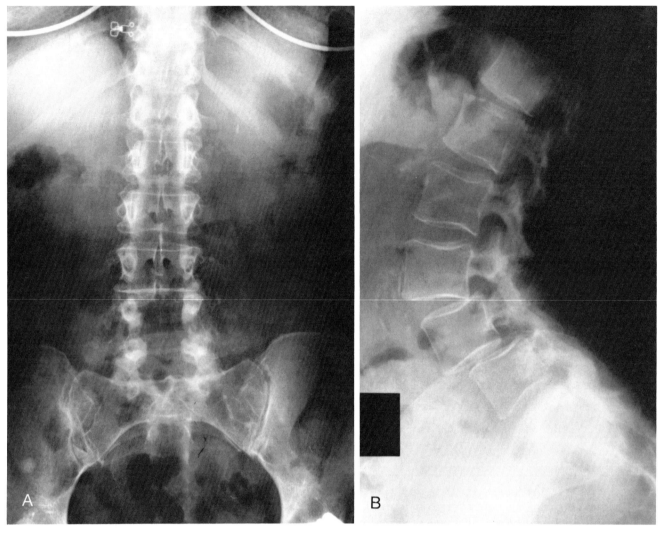

Figure 12.23. *A* and *B*, AP and lateral plain roentgenograms revealing significant grade L4-L5 and L5-L6 degenerative spondylolisthesis.

quiring multilevel fixation, and those cases of reconstruction following burst fractures or tumor resections.

Complications

Clinical studies are now beginning to substantiate the potential morbidity expected with short rigid internal fixation and constructs. These include: (*a*) increased instability and degenerative changes in the motion segments above and below the VSP plate (55); (*b*) fatigue failure at the screw plate interface; (*c*) screw loosening or migration from excessive torque at the pedicle interface from inability to achieve a perpendicular pedicle screw/pedicle fit (48); (*d*) the entrapment of neuroforaminal contents in adjacent spinal segments from overdistraction at the instrumented sites; (*e*) an increased incidence of infection (55) secondary to increased operative time and

construct size; and (*f*) the potential for recurrence of deformity after lumbar burst fractures from lack of anterior support.

Whitecloud et al. (50) specifically looked at the rate of complications of VSP instrumentation in 40 patients with an average follow-up of 20 months operated on for a myriad of spinal problems. These problems included iatrogenic posterior spinal instability, spinal stenosis, spondylolisthesis, thoracolumbar spine fractures, and pseudarthrosis. The overall complication rate in this series was 46%, although most of these complications were minor. In patients undergoing previous posterior spinal procedures, the overall complication rate was 63%. Forty out of 45 patients with thoracic spine fractures had breakage of hardware with recurrence of deformity; six patients had increased nerve root irritation from improper screw placement; and overall, seven patients with older screw

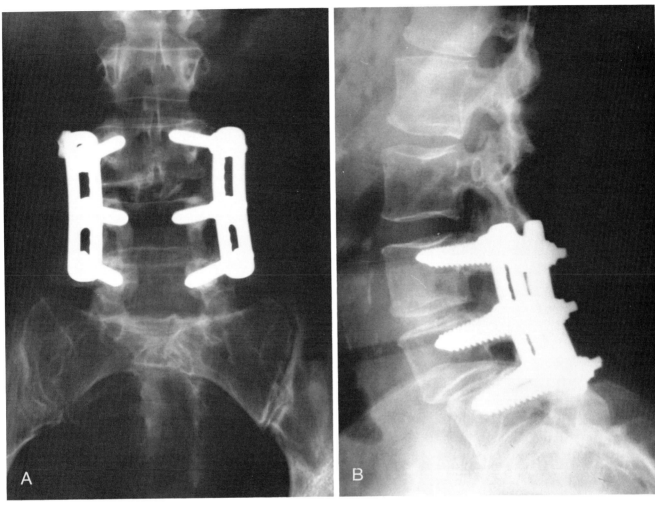

Figure 12.24. *A* and *B*, Postoperative AP and lateral plain roentgenograms revealing L4-L6 posterior lateral fusion with VSP instrumentation and L4-L5 posterolateral interbody fusion with good clinical result.

designs had screw breakage. In Steffee's original article (38) on VSP instrumentation of 120 patients, he reported 17 wound infections, two nerve root compression injuries, and eight spine plate problems including loosening, migration, or breakage. Many authors have documented the potential for facet disruption due to plate rigidity and application method of the lowest unfused segment above the instrumentation.

The clinical incidence of VSP screw breakage ranges from 0–25% in the literature (46,50). With the new 4th-generation screw and plate implants, the incidence of metal fatigue and failure has decreased substantially in recent years.

CONCLUSION

As surgeons become more experienced with the technical skills of VSP instrumentation and better long-term randomized prospective clinical studies are performed, the

indications, potential complications, and advantages of the VSP system will be more clearly defined. We can conclude that the VSP system is a short, rigid segmental spinal construct system that allows excellent posterior spinal fixation, preserving the maximal number of motion segments possible. The incidence of metal fatigue and failure, screw loosening, and instrument migration is lessened with newer metallic constructs and a better understanding of the biomechanics of transpedicular fixation systems.

VSP instrumentation can be a technically difficult and time-consuming procedure associated with significant minor and major complications if strict details are not adhered to in its clinical application and technical insertion. The system appears ideal where rigid immobilization for bone fusion enhancement is needed, especially in cases of pseudarthrosis. The system also appears efficacious for short segment instability such as spondylolisthesis with or without the need for reduction and in cases of lumbar burst fractures. Its routine use for stabilization of decompressive procedures for degenerative disc disease, herniated disc disease, or spinal stenosis with or without PLIF is not widely accepted and is in need of further study. It seems that if significant anterior column disruption is associated with posterior ligamentous instability, then an additional anterior stabilization procedure with VSP instrumentation may be needed. Alternatively, postoperative bracing or casting should be strictly adhered to prevent late anterior collapse.

REFERENCES

1. Allison RE, Amundson G: Spinal fixation using the Steffee pedicle screw and plate system. AORN J 1989;49:1016.
2. An HS, Vaccaro AR, Cotler JM, et al: Burst fractures of low lumbar spine: Comparison between body cast, Harrington rod, Luque rod and Steffee plate. Spine (in press).
3. Ashman RB, Gaypin RD, Corin JD, et al: Biomechanical analysis of pedicle screw instrumentation systems in a corpectomy model. Spine 1989;14:1398.
4. Boucher HH. A method of spinal fusion. J Bone Joint Surg 1959;41B:248.
5. Chapman TM, Phillips E, Cheaning SJ, et al: Use of autogenous morselized cancellous bone PLIF with VSP system and posterior fusion. Poster presentation NASS, Monterey, CA, 1990.
6. Cloward RB: Posterior lumbar interbody fusion updated. Clin Orthop 1985;193:16.
7. Cloward RB: The treatment of ruptured lumbar intervertebral discs by vertebral body fusion. I. Indications, operative technique, after care. J Neurosurg 1953;10:154.
8. DePalma AF, Rothman RG: The nature of pseudarthrosis. Clin Orthop 1968;59:113.
9. Dick W: The "Fixateur Interne" as a versatile implant for spine surgery. Spine 1987;12:882.
10. Dietz JW, Leung KYK, Lingbloom HL: Steffee plate lumbar fusions. Presented at AAOS meeting, Anaheim, CA 1991.
11. Ebelke DK, Asher MA, Neff JR, et al: Survivorship analysis of VSP spine instrumentation in the treatment of thoracolumbar burst fractures. Presented at SRS meeting, Honolulu, HI, 1990.
12. Esses SI: The AO spinal internal fixator. Spine 1989;14:37.
13. Field BT, Wiltse LL, Zindrick MR, et al: The Long Beach Spinal Fixation System. Proc Second Annual Meeting North Amer Lumbar Spine Assoc. Laguna Niguel, CA, 1985.
14. Goel VK, Kim YE, Lim TH, et al: An analytical investigation of the mechanics of spinal instrumentation. Spine 1988;13:1003.
15. Grubb SA, Lipscomb HJ, Derian TC: Results of one and two level lumbar fusions with Steffee plate instrumentation—two year follow-up. Poster presentation NASS meeting, Monterey, CA, 1990.
16. Gurr KR, McAfee PC, Shih CM: Biomechanical analyses of anterior and posterior instrumentation systems following corpectomy: A calf spine model. J Bone Joint Surg 1988;70A:1182.
17. Halvorson TL, Cook SD, Kelley LA, et al: Effects of bone mineral density on pedicle screw pull-out strength. Presented at AAOS meeting, Anaheim, CA, 1991.
18. Harrington PR, Dickson JH: Spinal instrumentation in the treatment of severe progressive spondylolisthesis. Clin Orthop 1976; 117:157.
19. Herkowitz HN, Kurz LT: Degenerative spondylolisthesis; prospective study comparing decompression versus decompression with fusion. Presented at the ISSLS meeting, Boston, MA, 1990.
19a. Hsu K, Zucherman JF, White AH, et al: Internal fixation with pedicle screws. In: White AH, Rothman RH, Ray CD, ed. Lumbar spine surgery. St. Louis: CV Mosby; 1987;322–338.
20. Kabins MB, Weinstein JN, Found EM, et al: Isolated L4-L5 floating fusions using the variable screw placement system: Unilateral vs bilateral. Presented at Resident AOA Conference, Kansas City, MO, 1991.
21. King D: Internal fixation for lumbo-sacral fusion. Am J Surg 1944;66:357.
22. Kostuik JP, Errico TJ, Gleason TF: Techniques for internal fixation for degenerative conditions of the spine. Clin Orthop 1986;203:219.
23. Krag MH, Beynnon BD, Pope MH, et al: Depth of insertion of transpedicular vertebral screws into vertebra: Effect upon screw-vertebrae interface strength. J Spinal Disorders 1989;1:287.
24. Krag MH, Beynnon BD, Pope MH, et al: An internal fixator for posterior application to short segments of the thoracic, lumbar, or lumbosacral spine: design and testing. Clin Orthop 1985;203:75.
25. Louis R: Posterior vertebral bone plates, surgical technique. Paris: Howmedica, CEPRIME Publisher, 1982.
26. Magerl FP: Stabilization of the lower thoracic and lumbar spine with external skeletal fixation. Clin Orthop 1984;189:125.
27. McAfee PC, Weiland DJ: Survival analysis of pedicular fixation systems. Presented at SRS meeting, Honolulu, HI, 1990.
28. Mirkovic S, Abitboll JJ, Steinmann J, et al: Anatomic considerations for sacral screw placement. Presented at NASS meeting, Monterey, CA, 1990.
29. Prothero SR, Parker JC, Stinchfield FE: Complications after low-back fusion in 2000 patients. J Bone Joint Surg 1966;48A:57.
30. Rodegerdts V: Spondylolisthesis reduction [Abstract]. Proc ISSLS, Sydney, Australia, April, 1985.
31. Roy-Camille R, Saillant G, Berteaux D, et al: Early management of spinal injuries. In: McKibbin B, ed. Recent advances in orthopaedics. New York: Churchill-Livingstone, 1979.
32. Roy-Camille R, Saillant G, Mazel C: Internal fixation of the lumbar spine with pedicle screw plating. Clin Orthop 1986;203:7.
33. Roy-Camille R, Saillant G, Mazel C: Plating of thoracic, thoracolumbar and lumbar injuries with pedicle screw plates. Orthop Clin North Amer 1986;17:147.
34. Ruland CM, McAfee PC, Warden KE, et al: Triangulation of pedicle instrumentation systems: A biomechanical analysis. Presented at AAOS meeting, Anaheim, CA, 1991.
35. Schultz AB: Loads on the lumbar spine. In: Yayson MIV, ed. The lumbar spine and back pain. New York: Churchill-Livingstone, 1987;204–214.
36. Schwaegler P, Cram R, Lorenz M, et al: A comparison of single level fusions with and without hardware. Presented at NASS meeting, Monterey, CA, 1990.
37. Schwaegler PE, Lroenz MA, Vrbos L, et al: Treatment of spine fractures with pedicle screws and plates. Presented at AAOS meeting, Anaheim, CA, 1991.
38. Steffee AD, Discup RS, Sitkowski DJ: Segmented spine plate with pedicle screw fixation: A new internal fixation device for disorders of the lumbar and thoracolumbar spine. Clin Orthop 1986;203:45.
39. Steffee AH: Personal communication.
40. Steffee AD, Sitkowsi DJ: Posterior lumbar interbody fusion and plates. Clin Orthop 1988;227:99.

41. Steffee AD, Sitkowski DJ: Reduction and stabilization of grade IV spondylolisthesis. Clin Orthop 1988;227:89.

42. Steffee AD: The reduction of high-grade slips with VSP instrumentation: Reporting on a series of 40 cases. Presented at NASS meeting, Monterey, CA, 1990.

43. Truchly G, Thompson WAL: Posterolateral fusion of the lumbosacral spine. J Bone Joint Surg 1962;442:505.

44. Watkins MB: Posterolateral fusion in pseudarthroses and posterior element defects of the lumbosacral spine. Clin Orthop 1964;35:80.

45. Weiland DJ, McAfee PC: The use of pedicle screws for posterior spine instability: One hundred consecutive patients. Presented at NASS meeting, Monterey, CA, 1990.

46. West JL, Bradford DS, Ogilvie JW: Complications in Steffee plate pedicle screw fixation. Presented at NASS meeting, Quebec, Canada, 1989.

47. West JL, Ogilvie JW, Bradford DS: Use of allograft bone with pedicle screw plate fixation. Presented at AAOS, Anaheim, CA, March, 1991.

48. White AH, Rothman RH, Ray CD: Lumbar spine surgery techniques and complications. St. Louis: CV Mosby, 1987:322–338.

49. White AH, Zucherman JF, Hsu KY: Lumbosacral fusions with Harrington rods and intersegmented wiring. Clin Orthop 1986; 203:185.

50. Whitecloud TS III, Butler JC, Cohen JL, et al: Complications with the variable spinal plating system. Spine 1989;14:472.

51. Wiltse LL, Bateman JG, Hutchinson RH, et al: The paraspinal sacrospinalis-splitting approach to the lumbar spine. J Bone Joint Surg 1968;50A:919.

52. Yamamoto H, Yamashita H: Pedicular screw and spinal plate for reduction and fusion of spondylolisthesis in aged patients [Abstract]. Internat Soc Study Lumbar Spine 1985; Sydney, Australia.

53. Yoganandan N, Larson SJ, Pintar F, et al: Biomechanics of lumbar pedicle screw/plate fixation in trauma. Neurosurgery 1990; 27:873.

54. Zindrick MR, Wiltse LL, Widell EH, et al: A biomechanical study of intrapedicular screw fixation in the lumbosacral spine. Clin Orthop 1986;203:99.

55. Zucherman J, Hsu K, White A, et al: Early results of spinal fusion using variable spine plating techniques. Spine 1988;13: 570.

Luque Semirigid Segmental Spinal Instrumentation of the Lumbar Spine

Eduardo R. Luque

INTRODUCTION

Segmental spinal instrumentation of the lumbar spine has evolved with the development of research and technology in the last decade. Double L rods have been transformed into a semirigid screw and plate-fixation system (1,2, 8,9,12,13,15,17,20), then to a rigid, semirigid system with the possibility of using hooks, pedicle screws, and a bar instead of a plate.

The technique described in this chapter is based on anatomy, patient history, and indications. The instrumentation of the lumbar spine has two objectives: to correct deformity and to enhance the possibilities of arthrodesis (16,19).

Indications for fixation of the lumbar spine may include instability of any one or multiple segments due to spondylolisthesis, spinal stenosis, fractures, tumors, deformities, and infections (Fig. 13.1). Other indications may be painful disc syndrome, retrolisthesis, vertebral translation, lumbar scoliosis, degenerative disc disease, and correction of pseudarthrosis.

The anatomy of the pedicle has been amply described. It is well known that the best bone in the lumbosacral vertebra is the lamina (Table 13.1). The facets produce sclerotic bone, especially in degenerative diseases. The sacrum is the poorest bone stock for fixation, although it has good bone around the facet, and at the lamina. The anterior cortex is thin, and the cancellous bone is poor for screw fixation in the sacrum. Enhanced fixation may be achieved by anterior cortical purchase or screw insertion beneath the endplate in the sacrum. The cortices of the ilium consist of good quality bone (2), but not in the osteoporotic spine.

HISTORY OF SEGMENTAL FIXATION OF THE LUMBAR SPINE

The use of segmental spinal instrumentation (SSI) began in the 1970s, with the purpose of enhancing the possibilities of arthrodesis over more than two lumbar spaces, where the rate of pseudarthrosis was 20–35% (2).

The original technique used two L rods and sublaminar wires, and no effort was made to provide lordosis or to produce correction.

The fixation to the sacrum was particularly difficult because of anatomic variations and the lack of spaces in the sacral sac. A substantial improvement was achieved in the rate of pseudarthrosis, but neurologic complications at the level of S1 were reported by some authors. A more rigid construct was described by Armstrong and popularized by Zimmer, Inc. as the Luque rectangle, and later by Dove as the Hartshill rectangle (1). Ashman and Wenger at the Scottish Rite Hospital, and Gaines at the University of Missouri, came out with some concrete conclusions by testing the instrumentation in the biomechanical laboratory (8,9,23).

First, rigid crosslinking would load the system evenly and make it more rigid. Sublaminar wires were good for correcting lateral and axial deformity, but were inefficient in the correction of rotation (3). Wire fixation of the pedicle after laminectomy and sacral fixation with wire were difficult and inefficient. The anatomy and the deformity of the spine were tridimensional, and included axial curves as well as rotational deformities.

Dr. King from Stanford University in 1947 was the first American on the West Coast to use intrapedicular screws crossing the facet of L5-S1 into the pedicle of S1,

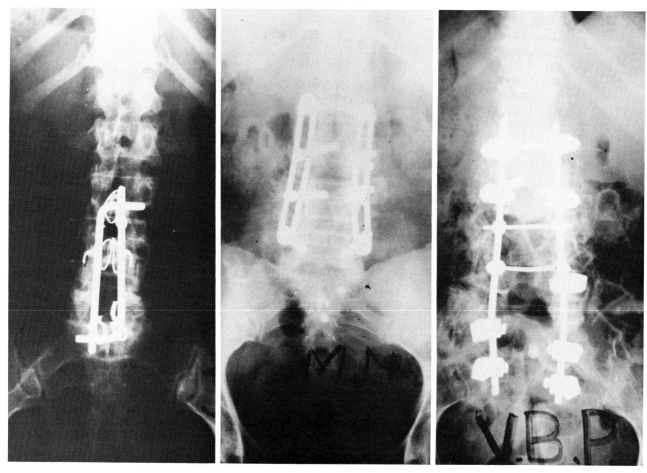

Figure 13.1. *A*, AP 1976. Narrow canal posterior decompression; double L bar; sublaminar wires L2-S1; poor immobilization S1 (facet fusion). *B*, AP 1986. Narrow canal total posterior decompression L3-L5. Interpedicular spine fixation with plates provides good triangulation (posterolateral fusion).

C, AP 1990. Narrow neural canal L2-S1—complete posterior decompression. Claw hooks in sacrum distraction; sublaminar hook in L4 rigid interpeduncular screws L2 and L1—double crosslink and share loading (posterolateral fusion).

to obtain an L5-S1 fusion. Nonetheless, the technique did not have wide acceptance. In the 1970s, European authors used screws successfully through the lateral mass in the cervical spine. In the lumbar region, the need to correct the rotational deformities in degenerative diseases, the need to increase stability in cases where extensive

Table 13.1.
CT Study Showing Bone Density and Cortical Thickness of One Lumbosacral Junction.

	Bone Density (Hounsfield Units)				Average Cortical Thickness (mm)		
	L5	S1	S2		L5	S1	S2
Vertebral body	347	236	189	Pedicle	3	2.2	2.8
Pedicle	331	141	101	Neural canal	4.3	3.7	3.9
Lamina	930	503	503				

laminectomies had to be performed, and the need to obtain a rigid tridimensional fixation of the lumbosacral junction led to the use of interpedicular screws.

We selected a semirigid system on the basis of the findings of Hatcher from Stanford, who noted the lack of callous formation in long bone by stress shielding, caused by rigid plate and screw fixation.

The alignment of several screws was made technically easier and more anatomic. The Luque II plate provided many of these characteristics, but lacked a good sacral fixation, and it was necessary to avoid the most cephalad joint in the instrumentation. It was also somewhat cumbersome because of the amount of metal implanted in relation to the space for the bone graft (Fig. 13.2).

The idea of using hooks came about as an alternative in the fixation of the sacrum. Sublaminar claw hooks and miniplates offer some advantages in the treatment of

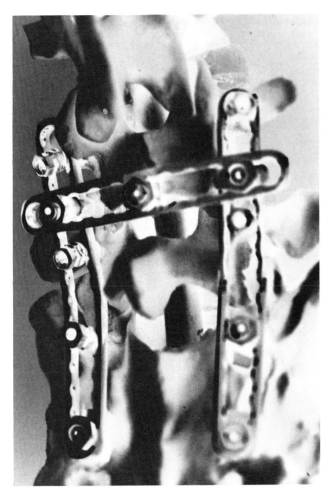

Figure 13.2. Luque II SSI immobilization (semirigid) claw hooks at S1-S2 level, interpedicular screws L5-L4 crosslink L4-L5 with distraction sublaminar L4 hook and share loading the entire system. A lot of metal; technically demanding.

certain pathologies such as burst fractures, extreme instability of one or two segments, especially in the osteoporotic patient. This makes the instrumentation easier to use, more versatile, and safer, and provides us with several options. We eliminate a great deal of metal for the single large plate by using an axial rod with the offset screw lock of the miniplates to the rod. This instrumentation is versatile in that instrumentation is obtained by the screw that can engage the plate with 15% tolerance circumferentially. At the same time, the miniplate can rotate around the rod before it is definitely set (Fig. 13.3).

The development of single hook to the miniplate and the double claw hooks permits us to use the best bone available, the lamina and the facets. The use of hooks either as a rigid claw around the facet of S1 (20), or as a claw fashion into the pedicle of S1 and S2, again simplifies the procedure and produces a good sacral fixation.

In the upper lumbar area, a rigid central bar with rigid laminar hooks above and below enhances the use of triangulated interpeduncular screw to lock rotation (Fig. 13.4 and 13.5).

Adding the rigid sublaminar claw hooks gives total rigidity in flexion extension and permits a greater degree of correction of deformity, without approaching the endurance level of 316 stainless steel, and still keeps some of the micromovement in the semirigid pedicle screws.

BIOMECHANICS

Rigid pedicle screw systems have certain disadvantages. They are difficult to align; thus it may overstress and break the screws (up to 20% breakage) (4,6,10,21,23–25) (Fig. 13.6). Also, they may produce stress shielding and inhibit bone formation due to overstiffness. Also, there is a greater tendency to cut out in soft or osteoporotic bone, which may produce neurologic deficits. Rigid sys-

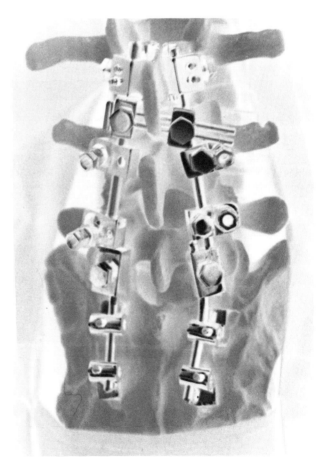

Figure 13.3. The new multiple-use segmental instrumentation. Note claw hooks in S1 and S2 bilaterally. Interpedicular screws at L5-L4 level; a crosslink and sublaminar claw hooks in L3; crosslink at L3-L4.

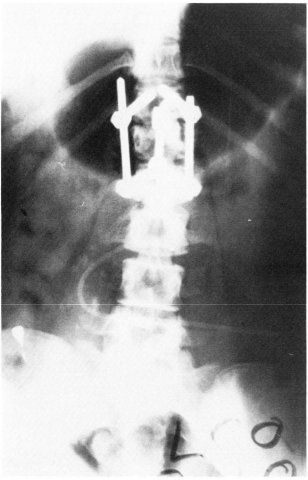

Figure 13.4. Rigid interpedicular screws one above and one below with sublaminar claw hooks in the middle line.

to the strength of the metal and the bone it is introduced into (6,25). In rigid systems, the most common problem is that of metal breakage; in semirigid systems, there is a loss of correction.

TECHNIQUE

All patients must have AP and lateral x-rays. Instability is most obvious on dynamic lateral x-rays, which should also be obtained (6,7,19,22). A standing lateral x-ray gives the normal lordosis for that particular patient, which should be duplicated as close as possible at the time of surgery.

All necessary procedures to secure an accurate diagnosis should also be done as indicated. These may include myelography, CT scan, MRI, CT myelogram, IV-enhanced CT, gadolinium-enhanced MRI, discography, techne-

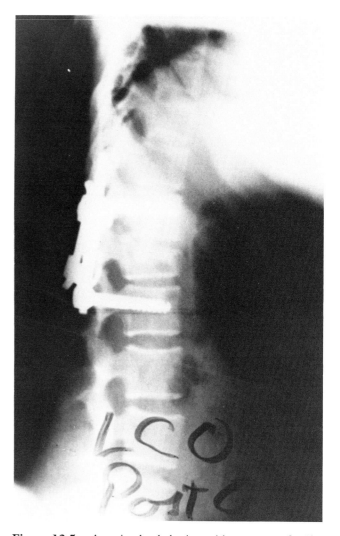

Figure 13.5. Anterior load sharing with a strut graft. Claw hook configuration protecting stress against the screws.

tems have their great virtue in their ability to correct and maintain deformity as long as the metal or the bone do not fail. Their loading is in cantilever, and correspondingly, their weakest point is at the screw (rod)-plate junction.

The semirigid systems depend more on their pullout power and will correspondingly rely more on thread design and quality of bone to maintain correction.

Some authors recommend rigid fixation without reduction of deformity. While this relieves some stress from the screw plate rod angle, it would only be satisfactory in a limited number of cases.

It appears that the introduction of sublaminar hooks into the system would be necessary to enhance instrumentation by holding on to the best bone available at each vertebra segmentally (8).

Load sharing with the anterior and middle columns is the clue to all instability of the spine, as whatever instrumentation used posteriorly is only a tension band limited

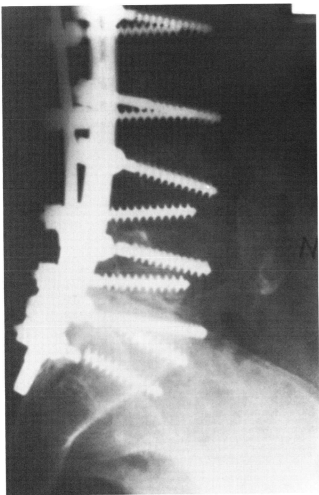

Figure 13.6. Patient with instrumentation from L2 to S1 with a rigid system. Notice the multiple failure of the implant as it was overstressed on application.

prevent penetration of the cortex of the pedicle. With a wire holder it is easy to feel one's way through the spongy core of the pedicle and into the body with the K-wire. Once all guide pins are in position in the pedicles, AP and lateral x-rays are taken. This makes it possible to determine the exact position of the guide pins and the length of the screw needed for fixation. It is important to try to introduce the largest screw possible.

With the K-wires in place, tap the pedicle with a sharp cannulated tap. This avoids the possibility of going outside the pedicles and the need to use an image intensifier in surgery. Taps should be used only in one surgical procedure and discarded. While tapping, care should be taken not to push the K-wire through the vertebral body (Fig. 13.8).

At this stage, a plate or combination of miniplates is selected according to the biomechanical needs of each

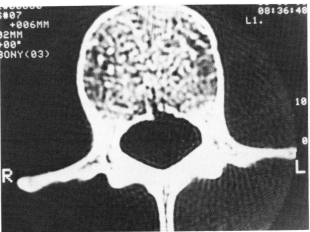

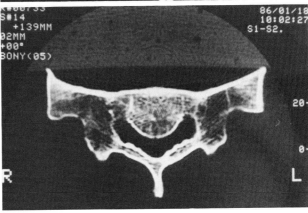

Figure 13.7. Computerized axial tomography of L1 vertebra (*top*) showing size of pedicle, bone density in the pedicle, and vertebral body and thickness of the different cortices (*bottom*) S1, S2 showing best bone available at the posterior cortex and poor bony stock between it and the anterior cortex.

tium/indium/gallium scanning, electrodiagnostic procedures, injection studies, and personality psychological evaluation studies.

All levels to be instrumented with interpedicular screws should have an axial CT or MRI to determine the placement, size, and quality of bone in the pedicles (Fig. 13.7).

After a routine midline exposure, dissection is carried out laterally enough to see the tips of the transverse process of all vertebrae to be instrumented.

To find the pedicle through a posterior approach, we use a line of intersection between the midline of the transverse process and the facet. At this point of entry, a curette is used to locate the inside of the pedicle, and to identify proper position, a blunt K-wire is then used to go through the vertebra. The use of the blunt K-wire helps

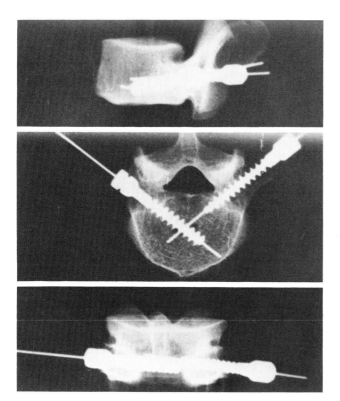

Figure 13.8. K-wire in place, triangulating the forces and avoiding the most cephalad facet to be instrumented. The tap that should be inserted only the length of the pedicle is to the right in the AP picture. On the opposite side, a screw is already in place.

case. The screws are placed through the plates and introduced halfway, and K-wires are removed, achieving proper alignment of the spine. If bars and miniplates have been used, the bars are connected to the miniplates after the correct amount of lordosis has been introduced into the system (5,13,18,19). The system should always be crosslinked, and it must be done at this stage. If hooks are to be used, they are introduced at the same time as the K-wires, and are engaged onto the plates or bar as the screws are introduced into the pedicles.

This would include sacral fixation, sublaminar claw hook, fixation of the most cephalad vertebra, or any other hook used in correction of fixation of a particular pathology. The flexibility of screw plate angulation of this system permits manipulation of the screws into alignment by connecting to the screwdriver, which in turn serves as a "joystick," allowing correction of pathology in a tridimensional manner before engagement of the head of the screw or hook into the plate. A list of different forces applicable when using this method would include derotation of vertebra upon vertebra, distraction bilaterally, or distraction on one side and compression on the other, production of correction of lordosis of kyphosis, and correction of degenerative listhesis.

It is important to seat the plate on the cephalad vertebra in such a way that the joint is not included into the area of immobilization. If this rule is not followed, the plate will produce facet impingement and pain. Several sizes of plates and a multiplicity of screw sizes and widths are necessary to accommodate the different sizes of pedicles and vertebral bodies. To derotate vertebra upon vertebra, total facetectomies are necessary. Posterior lateral arthrodesis should accompany pedicular segmental fixation. This is accomplished with local and bank bone, but occasionally, in severe deformities or larger deformities, it is necessary to harvest bone either from the iliac crest or from adjacent ribs. Decortication of all bone posteriorly and laterally underneath the plate before it is set down by the screws gives a good bed of living raw bone. This way, by compressing the graft, good contact is assured with the cancellous decorticated live bone in an ideal position for arthrodesis. Following surgery, patients are kept at bed rest and log-rolled for 1 to 2 days. They are then allowed to stand up, some with a back support. They are never permitted to resume normal activities before 6 months postoperatively, and manual workers are protected longer.

CASE MATERIAL AND RESULTS

In Mexico, the total number of patients treated with this instrumentation is 4,051 at the time of writing. The number of cases performed in the United States is 3,398, and the number of cases performed overseas is 653.

No major complications have been reported in cases done in 1990. In a personal series, all with a follow-up of more than 3 years, 57 cases had the following diagnoses:

- Multiple operated patients in 24;
- Degenerative spondylolisthesis in 4;
- Degenerative scoliosis in 3; and
- Stenosis of the neural canal in 26 patients.

Age ranged from 20–86 years with an average of 66 years. There were 20 males and 27 females. Pain was the most important presenting symptom, from 7–10, average 8.6 (on a scale of 1–10). Postoperative score averages were 3.2. Follow-up average was 3.6 years, ranging between 3–4 years. Correction achieved ranged from 20–100% with an average value of 73%. The number of spaces instrumented was 2–5. All patients had a posterolateral fusion along with interpedicular screw and plate fixation.

COMPLICATIONS

There was one loose screw and one broken screw. There were two wound infections. One had a drop foot, which recovered at 1 year. Pseudarthrosis was apparent in

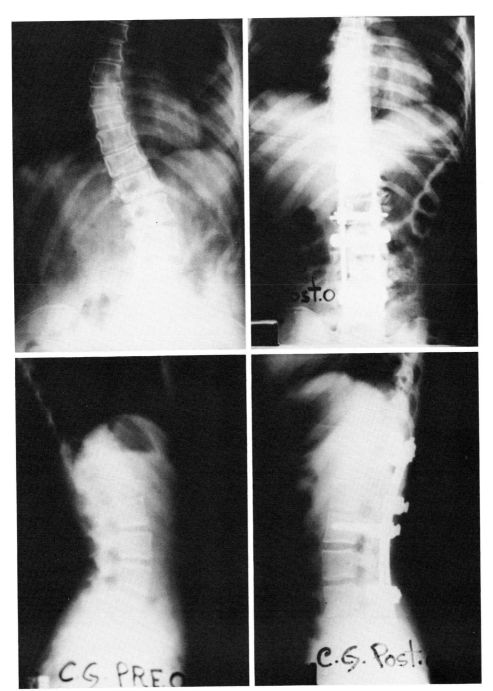

Figure 13.9. Upper left AP of a 14-year-old with idiopathic lumbar scoliosis, neutral vertebra T10 and L5. Upper right, sublaminar claw hooks at T11-L4, interpedicular screws at L1 derotating and aligning the spine crosslink at L2 lower left lateral preoperatively. Lower right lateral, postoperatively with good lordosis conserved.

most recent patients. At follow-up, four patients were reoperated; one to remove a loose screw, one to remove instrumentation for drop foot, two for ensuing pseudarthrosis. All four improved. All infections cleared up. There were four transient urinary tract infections. Pain was relieved from an average of 8.6–3.1 at follow-up. Thirty-two patients considered themselves cured.

Seventeen patients were happy with their results but still had discomfort. Eight patients felt disabled, and their surgeries were considered failures.

DISCUSSION

In the last 4 years, the evaluation of interpedicular segmental instrumentation with semirigid systems has changed significantly. Safety, both in technique and in postoperative maintenance of correction, has been stressed. In this system, safety margin may be increased by using x-rays for screw insertion. Fusion rate may improve by complementing the posterior tension band with compression hooks, occasionally using bony struts or PLIFs in the anterior vertebral column, sharing compression anteriorly and tension posteriorly. It is also felt that postoperative immobilization should be used until a fusion is solid. Any metallic fixation device will break if a solid fusion is not obtained, although the author's new semirigid system seems to avoid this problem for a much longer period of time. Following these principles, shorter areas of arthrodesis are possible to solve segmental pathology. Intersegmental correction of rotation can be accomplished by the use of instrumentation as well as the correction of coronal and sagittal curves (Fig. 13.9).

Taps may be broken at the time of surgery if one puts too much leverage in solid bone. Breakage of taps and screws can be avoided by handling them gently, and also by the use of segmental addition of distraction and compression hooks and external immobilization postoperatively. The use of screws through the pedicle can achieve correction and fixation, which is impossible with other methods. This is especially true in patients with short segmental pathology or with absence of posterior spinal elements. Any semirigid system can act only as a tension band, and anterior load sharing by the vertebral column is necessary. It is important to recognize that the instrumentation is only a temporary internal immobilization while solid bony arthrodesis takes place. In cases of fractures or tumors, a cast is recommended until solid union is obtained—a minimum of 3 months.

In the lumbar pathology group, some cases, like the elderly obese female, were not treated with external immobilization, but with major restrictions of their usual activities.

Some important contraindications to the use of this technique include gross infection of soft tissue, morbid obesity, highly osteoporotic bone absence of pedicles, and tumors where no screw purchase is possible.

REFERENCES

1. Allen BL Jr, Ferguson RL: The Galveston technique and pelvic fixation for use with L-rod instrumentation. Orthop Trans 1984;8:170.
2. Armstrong GWP: In: Luque ER ed. Application of SSI to the lumbosacral spine. Segmental spinal instrumentation. Slack Thorofare, N.J., 1984;235–254.
3. Ashman RB, Birch JG, Bone LB, et al: Mechanical testing of spinal instrumentation. Clin Orthop 1983;227:113–125.
4. Ashman RB, Galpin RD, Corin JD, et al: Biomechanical analysis of pedicle screw instrumentation systems in a corpectomy model. Spine 1989;14:1398–1405.
5. Carson E: Three Dimensional Evolution of Spine Annual Scoliosis Research Society British Scoliosis Conference 1986.
6. Denis F: Spinal instability as defined by the three column spine concept in acute spinal trauma. Clin Orthop 1984;189:65–76.
7. Denis F: Pathomechanics of acute thoracol and lumbar fractures. In: Segmental Spinal Instrumentation (Luque ER, ed.). Slack, Thorofare, N.J., 1984;255–285.
8. Gaines R: Personal communication share loading in IPFS Sept. 1988.
9. Gaines R: Three dimension evaluation of the spine. Personal communication.
10. Galping RD, Covin SD, Johnston CE II, et al: Biomechanical testing of pedicle screw instrumentation systems in a burst fracture model. Presented at Scoliosis Research Society meeting, Vancouver, British Colombia, Canada, 1987.
11. Heining C: Personal communication.
12. Luque ER: The anatomic basis and development of segmental spinal instrumentation. Spine 1982;7:256–259.
13. Luque ER: The correction of postural curves of the spine. Spine 1982;7:270–275.
14. Luque ER: Segmental spinal instrumentation of the lumbar spine. Clin Orthop 1986;203:126–134.
15. Luque ER: Development of interpeduncular fixation for thoracolumbar fractures. Presented at American Spinal Injury Association meeting. San Diego, California, 1988.
16. Luque ER: Interpeduncular segmental fixation. Presented at the American Academy of Orthopaedic Surgeons. New Orleans, Louisiana, 1986.
17. Luque ER: The evolution of segmental spinal instrumentation. Presented at the American Academy of Orthopaedic Surgeons. Las Vegas, Nevada, 1989.
18. Luque ER: Interpedicular segmental fixation. Clin Orthop 1986;203:54–57.
19. Luque ER, Rapp GF: A new semirigid method of interpeduncular fixation of the spine. Orthopaedics 1988;11:1445–1450.
20. Picaso R, Luque ER: The sacrum: A new internal fixation device. Submitted for presentation at the Scoliosis Research Society meeting, Baltimore, Maryland, 1988.
21. Steffee AD, Biscup RS, Sitkowski DJ: Segmental spine plates with pedicle screw fixation: a new internal fixation device for disorders of the lumbar and thoracolumbar spine. Clin Orthop 1986; 203:45–53.
22. Trammell TR, Rapp G, Maxwell KM, et al: Luque interpedicular segmental fixation of the lumbo sacral spine. Orthop Review, Vol xx, No. 1. 1991;57–63.
23. Wenger DR, Carollo JJ, Wilkerson JA Jr, et al: Laboratory testing of segmental spinal instrumentation versus traditional Harrington instrumentation for scoliosis treatment. Spine 1982;7:265–269.
24. Wittenberg RH, Coffee MS, Swarts DE, et al: Fatigue failure characteristics of cyclical loaded spine implants 36th. Annual meeting Orthopaedic Research Society, New Orleans, Louisiana, 1990.
25. Zindrik MR, Wiltse LL, Widell EH, et al: A biomechanical study of intrapeduncular screw fixation in the lumbosacral spine. Clin Orthop 1986;203:99–112.

FOURTEEN

The Wiltse System

Richard D. Peek, Leon L. Wiltse, and Mark F. Hambly

INTRODUCTION

The initial use of the Wiltse system in humans started on May 24, 1984 at the Long Beach Memorial Hospital. Twenty other centers in the United States have since started using this system, and as of this writing, we are awaiting final approval in the United States by the Food and Drug Administration (FDA).

We allowed some flexibility in the system to protect the screws and rods from breaking and to prevent stress shielding. The connecting rods were given about the same strength as the screws. The size of the screw is limited by the size of the pedicles, and there seemed no reason for the connecting rods to be stronger than the screws.

Pedicle screw fixation has provided the spine surgeon with a powerful and versatile new tool. Rates of pseudarthrosis in the lumbosacral spine continue to be high, particularly when there has been surgical removal of all or part of the facet joints. Wiltse pedicle internal fixation reestablishes the continuity of the facet joints. The fusion has been increased to 91.7% in the Phase II FDA study.

The Wiltse pedicle system offers a reliable point of fixation to the vertebra. Pedicle screw fixation does not rely upon distraction, compression, or the presence of the posterior elements for fixation. By using some special instruments, pedicle screws allow the surgeon to exert some distraction or compression forces as needed.

The pedicle screw system we describe here allows the surgeon to place the pedicle screws in the most appropriate position and then interconnect the screws by a malleable stainless steel rod and a unique saddle-clamp assembly. In order to create a template, an aluminum, hand-malleable mastering rod is used to create a model (Fig. 14.1). Using this master, an exact stainless steel duplicate can be fabricated. For this, a variety of bending instruments have been developed. In the case of particularly severe deformity over many levels, a major bending system is available that allows one to accurately contour the necessary rods. These stainless steel rods are placed into the saddle-clamp assembly. A unique lock washer attached to the top saddle prevents loosening and allows the surgeon to use a single nut, thereby lowering the profile of the assembly. In the case of a simple bend, it is not necessary to use an aluminum mastering rod. It is generally possible to create the necessary bends free-hand, using only the hand-held bending device and various bending irons.

TECHNIQUE

At least for the beginner, fluoroscopic guidance is strongly suggested whenever inserting pedicle screws. Only the lateral image, however, is necessary, unless the patient has undergone prior fusion attempts that have obliterated the normal bony architecture. In these cases, AP imaging may be helpful in finding the pedicle.

POSITIONING

When it is anticipated that only the lateral image will be necessary, the patient is placed in a kneeling position on the Andrews or a similar frame. If both the AP and lateral images are necessary, the patient is placed on his abdomen on a radiolucent table. We use a frame designed by Homer Pheasant, but several others are available. However, the kneeling position is generally preferred because it decreases bleeding and makes sufficient lumbar lordosis easily obtainable.

SURGICAL APPROACH

A midline approach is used when a central decompression is necessary (Fig. 14.2*A*). Otherwise, we usually prefer a paraspinal approach, particularly below L3 in obese or very heavily muscled patients. In fact, Magerl has recommended that in these patients, lateral stab wounds be made when using a midline approach to direct the screws medially. The paraspinal approach presents the surgeon with a direct view to the pedicles and to the bony surfaces

Figure 14.1. Screws are in place. Soft aluminum rod has been molded so that it fits the saddles on the screws. This aluminum rod will be used as a "master" from which to bend the stainless steel rod.

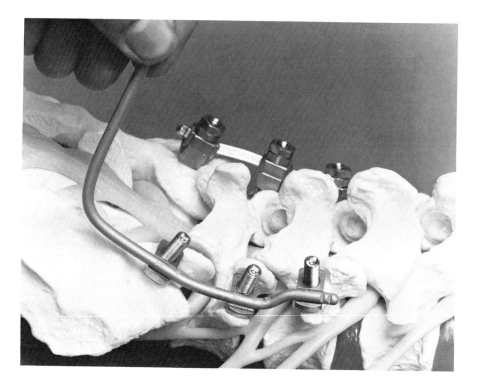

without overly aggressive retraction (Fig. 14.2*B*). Decompression of the lateral recesses and foramina can be performed easily through the paraspinal approach.

PEDICLE LOCALIZATION

The pedicle is localized using standard landmarks. A long-handled awl, which allows the operator to keep his hand out of the x-ray beam, is often used with the fluoroscopic image (Fig. 14.3*A*). Once properly aligned, the awl is used to perforate the cortical bone overlying the pedicle. A probe designed by Steffee is used to cannulate the medullary canal of the pedicle (Fig. 14.3*B*). As mentioned previously, an attempt is made to medially angulate the screws, except at S2, where the screws are laterally directed. The pedicle is probed more deeply with the blunt end of a small K-wire. Once the location of the wire has been verified fluoroscopically, the hole is tapped. In young patients with normally hard bone, the screws need not penetrate to great depth, but in osteoporotic patients, the anterior cortex of the vertebral body should be engaged. A nerve hook with a small tip that will not damage the tapped bony threads is used at 12, 3, 6, and 9 o'clock positions to verify that the cortex of the pedicle has not been violated at these positions (Fig. 14.4). Feeler screw length is determined by using a K-wire that is advanced within the vertebra until it reaches the desired

depth. We make a special point of engaging the anterior cortex of S1 (2).

HARDWARE AND APPLICATION

Our screws are available in five diameters: 5.0 mm and 5.8 mm for use in the lower thoracic and proximal lumbar vertebrae; 6.5 mm and 7.5 mm for use in the lower lumbar 8 vertebrae and sacrum. A full range of screw lengths is available. The serrated rod is 4.75 mm in diameter and is cut to proper length as desired by the surgeon. Spacers that elevate the rod saddle assembly off the bone to allow for the packing of a minimal amount of bone graft under the implant (Fig. 14.5) are available.

When the screw is seated, a saddle is placed on the screw. A single or double saddle may be used, depending upon whether one or two rods are to be inserted (Fig. 14.6). The saddle will not rotate on the screw because the screw shank is flat on one side. The saddle can be medially or laterally directed, at the preference of the surgeon. The saddles are generally placed in the direction that allows for placement of a maximum amount of bone graft and also to avoid impingement upon the cephalad facet joint. The rods and saddles have longitudinal serrations that interlock, preventing rotation of the rod within the saddle. Finally, the single jam nut is tightened onto the saddle-clamp assembly with the T-handle socket

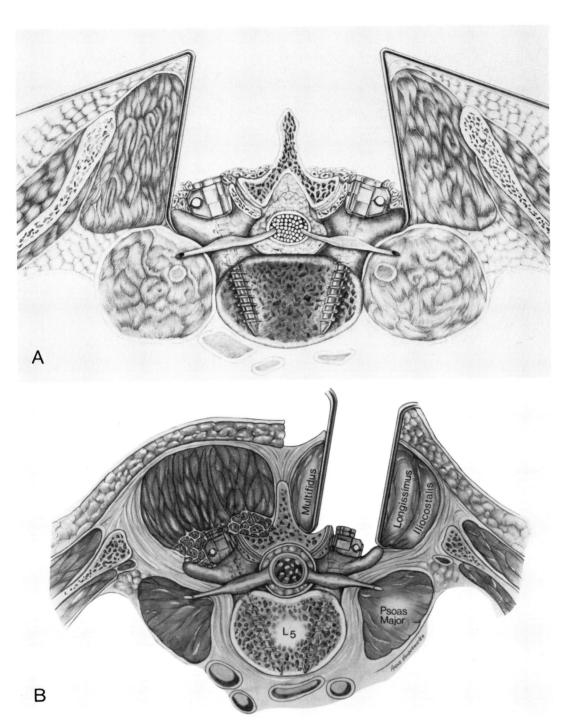

Figure 14.2. *A*, Midline approach with pedicle screws in place. It is easy to see why angulating the screws medially can be difficult in a large person. A stab wound can be made out laterally, and a special tube is available to put through the stab wound and pass through the muscles down to the starting point on the bone. *B*, The paraspinal approach allows the screws to be placed in direct line with the pedicles, allowing ideal medial placement. The fusion is easily performed without disturbing the midline ligamentous structures. Note angulation of screws. (From Guyer DW, Wiltse LL: The Wiltse pedicle screw system. Orthopaedics 1988;10:1458.)

Figure 14.3. *A*, Long-handled pyramid-tipped awl allows the surgeon to locate the pedicle fluoroscopically without exposing the surgeon's hand to the beam. Once localized, the awl is impacted with a mallet to perforate the cortex. The long handle in the picture above is disassembled to allow for sterilization. (From Rinner JA: Wiltse pedicle screw fixation systems, Fig. 7). *B*, The Steffee probe used for finding the medullary canal of the pedicle. The snap on handle has been removed. One snap on handle serves several different tools in the set.

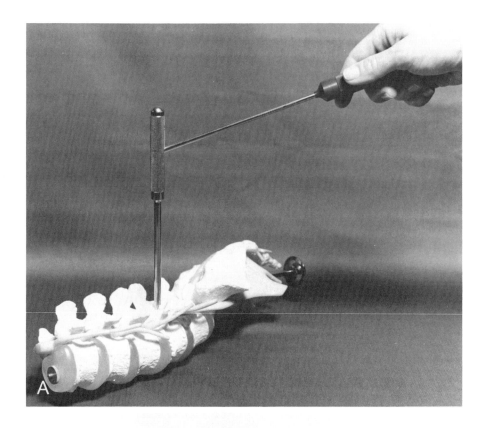

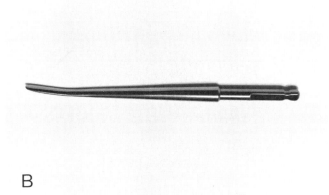

B

wrench and the nut locking mechanism bent up onto the sides of the nut, thus securing the rod to the screw (Fig. 14.7).

ROD BENDING AND PLACEMENT

Once the screws and saddles are appropriately placed, a hand-malleable aluminum mastering rod is bent to match the contour of the screw heads on each side. These aluminum rods are the same diameter as the stainless steel rods and serve as a template. The aluminum mastering rod is usually placed in the middle saddle clamp first, and a nut tightened over it, then contoured to fit the remaining saddles proximally and distally. It is important to mark the position of the saddle on the aluminum rod with a small chisel prior to removing it from the saddles in order to create a point of reference for bending the steel replica.

If the necessary bend is particularly simple, the rod can be "eyeballed" and bent using a hand-held bending device in combination with a French bender or bending irons. However, for more complex bends, a table-mounted vice

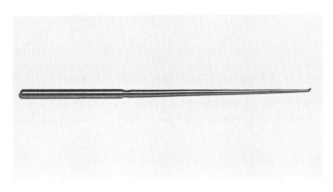

Figure 14.4. Short-tipped pedicle nerve hook, used as a "feeler." The pedicle, once cannulated, is probed at the 12, 3, 6, and 9 o'clock positions to ensure that the cortical confines of the pedicle have not been violated. The short tip prevents destruction of the tapped bony threads.

is used that allows the master rod to be placed directly next to the stainless steel rod to be used (Fig. 14.8). Using a combination of bending irons and by visualizing the rods in both the AP and lateral planes, the rod can be bent accurately.

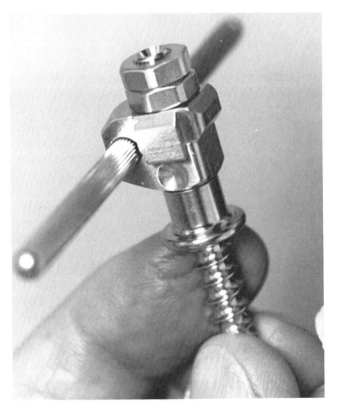

Figure 14.5. Composite picture of fixation components. These consist of the pedicle screw, clamp, saddle, nuts, and a 4.75-mm serrated stainless steel rod. (From Rinner JA: Wiltse pedicle screw fixation systems, Fig. 24.)

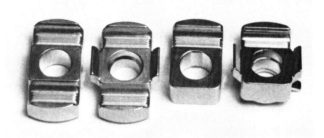

Figure 14.6. Saddle clamps. On the left are double saddles that accommodate two rods, and on the right, a single saddle. Note the serrated edges that prevent rod rotation once tightened.

For extremely complex bends, the "major bending apparatus" is used (Fig. 14.9). When using this, the appropriately bent aluminum template is first placed into the center tower and the other towers adjusted to fit the contour of the rod. The template is then removed and the steel rod contoured to fit into each tower. Surgeons who have had considerable experience with the system seldom find it necessary to use the major bender. It is best if the fusion bed is prepared by the surgeon while the rods are being bent by the assistant. The bone graft is harvested from the posterior superior iliac spine through the same incision, regardless of whether a paraspinal or midline approach has been used. Some of the bone graft is placed around the screws prior to insertion of the rods to ensure that all available bony surface area is included in the fusion bed. As mentioned previously, a spacer is generally placed under each saddle.

At this point, the stainless steel rods are placed into the saddles (Figs. 14.10 and 14.11), and the saddle clamps are tightened, using a socket wrench on the nut and the crow's foot wrench on the saddle to prevent it from rotating when tightening the jam nut (Fig. 14.12). The locking mechanism is crimped (Fig. 14.13) and the re-

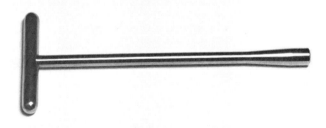

Figure 14.7. T-handle socket wrench used for final tightening of jam nuts.

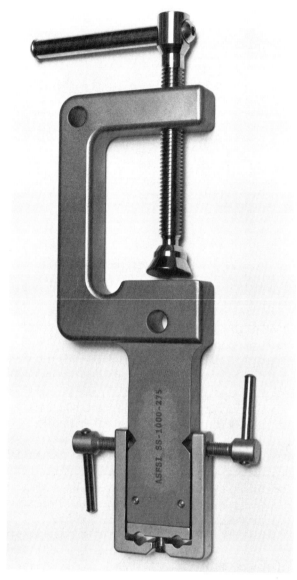

Figure 14.8. Table-mounted bending vice. This is fastened to a sterile table, and the aluminum template rod is placed on one side and the rod to be contoured, opposite the template rod.

mainder of the bone graft is packed around the construct. The wound is carefully irrigated. Drains are routinely used. The wound is closed in the usual fashion.

POSTOPERATIVE TREATMENT

Postoperatively, the patient is mobilized as quickly as possible. He is trained to get out of bed with minimal trunk rotation. The use of an overhead trapeze is dis-

couraged. A corset may be used solely to limit the extremes of bending.

PREVENTION OF INFECTION

Great attention must be paid to the maintenance of sterile technique throughout the entire surgical procedure. Infection can be a serious problem, particularly in revision cases. The following recommendations are made to minimize the chances of infection.

1. Use perioperative antibiotics.
2. Drain the wound.
3. Use the double-glove technique.
4. Use the laminar flow operating room.
5. Use the largest operating room available so that equipment can be moved easily about without contaminating the surgical field.
6. Limit the number of operating room personnel entering and leaving the room throughout the procedure.
7. Be careful when draping the patient and the C-arm.
8. Delay opening the special instrument set until the last possible moment. Usually do any necessary decompression first.

If infection is suspected in the postoperative period, we immediately take a smear of the wound as well as a culture. If the smear is positive for organisms, we usually take the patient back to the operating room immediately, not waiting for the culture results. This decision, of course, is also based on clinical signs. If the smear is negative, we await culture results before beginning surgery. If it is necessary to reoperate, we carefully open the wound in layers, looking for the source of infection. If it is superficial to the fascia, we do not open the fascial closure. If the infection is deep to the fascia, it is opened and irrigated copiously. If a paraspinal approach has been made, more often than not, only one side is infected, and the other need not be opened. To determine if one side is free of infection, we go to the other side and insert a long, 16-gauge needle more or less horizontally from far out laterally in normal skin area and aspirate a little blood from the bone graft area. This is smeared immediately, and if negative for bacteria, that side is not opened.

In a fair percent of cases, only the bone graft site at the ilium is infected, and with care, only this area needs be opened, keeping the recipient areas clean. While doing debridement, the bone graft is left in place, but a careful removal of the infected soft tissue with copious irrigation is done. We then insert inflow-outflow tubes (ones that reverse direction), and close the wound tightly with stan-

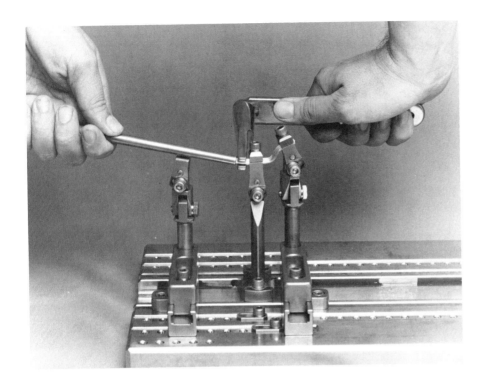

Figure 14.9. This is called the "major bender" and is used in cases where several levels are to be fixed and the bending procedure is very complicated. (From Rinner JA: Wiltse pedicle screw fixation systems, Fig. 22.)

dard and also retention sutures, usually for 4 days' duration. We have had extremely good success using this technique in the relatively few cases of infection that we have had. If this routine fails to stop the infection, we would again drain, debride, and leave the wound open and close secondarily.

DISCUSSION

Pedicle screw fixation systems that utilize a screw plate assembly allow for correction and immobilization of a deformity only in the sagittal plane and require that any deformity in the coronal plane be brought in line with the plate. In other words, the deformity must accommodate the fixation system. The Wiltse system allows the surgeon to create a construct that accommodates to the deformity; thus, no manipulation of the vertebrae is necessary. Yet, the system allows for correction or reduction of deformity if desired.

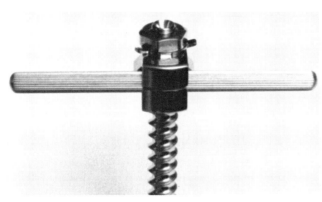

Figure 14.10. Shows the low-profile single rod with one nut and the little "ears" on the saddle that can be bent up to stop the nut from loosening.

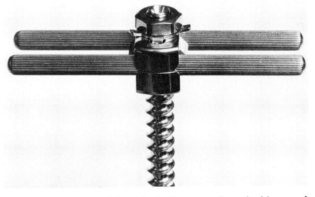

Figure 14.11. Double-rod, single nut, and nut-locking mechanism. The crimper is used to bend the small "ears" up against the nut. This prevents the nut from loosening. This small lock washer is part of the clamp and is not actually a separate washer.

Figure 14.12. The crow's foot wrench is used to maintain final saddle position while tightening jam nuts. (From Rinner JA: Wiltse pedicle screw fixation systems, Fig. 25.)

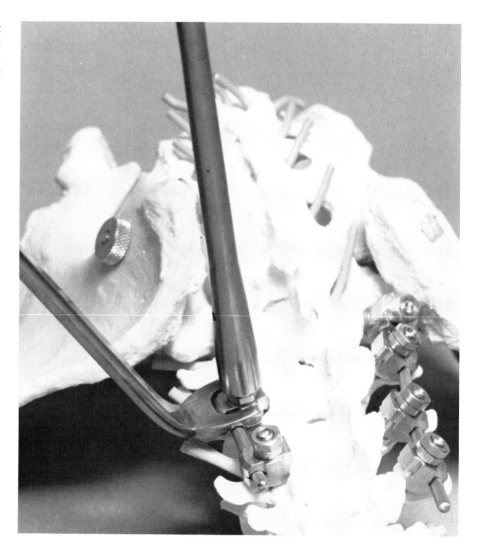

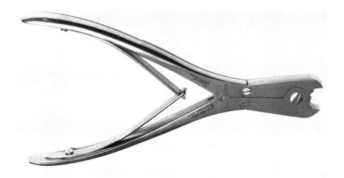

Figure 14.13. Lock washer crimper. This is used to crimp the small "ears" in the lock washer up against the nut to prevent loosening of the nut.

Our system has a number of other distinct advantages. The unique saddle-screw-rod junction provides uniform and equal transfer of load to each point of fixation, thereby decreasing the likelihood of loosening or hardware fatigue failure. The orientation and small size of the saddle-rod assembly prevents any impingement upon the facet joints cephalad or caudad to the fusion. The system allows the surgeon the freedom of reducing a displaced vertebra, as in the case of a degenerative or high-grade spondylolisthesis. By using "joysticks," which can be attached to the implanted screws, the degree of lordosis or kyphosis can be adjusted as necessary. Often, simply spreading or compressing the screw heads will serve to produce the correct degree of lordosis.

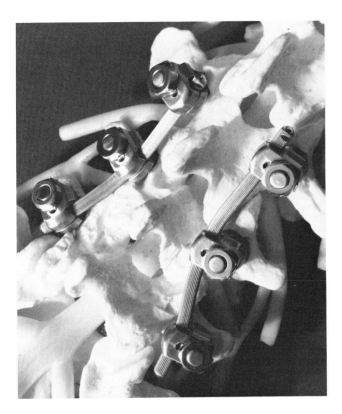

Figure 14.14. Single-rod and double-rod constructs are shown on a model.

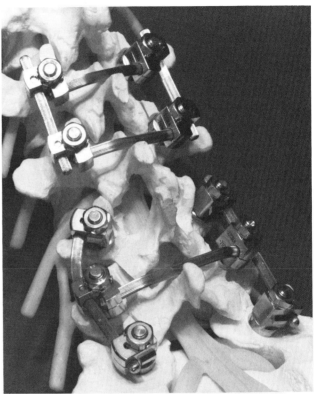

Figure 14.15. H construct. Pedicle screws are in L4 and S1 bilaterally with a cross-brace at L5. Note medial placement of rods.

By using a double saddle assembly, one can use two rods on each side of the vertebrae, effectively doubling the strength of the construct. This may be necessary when a level has been bridged, since jumping across a vertebra leaves a long lever arm acting on the rods (Fig. 14.14). This may be necessary when treating burst fractures or after a vertebrectomy with anterior strut grafting.

In cases of severe instability, as after vertebrectomy or severe fracture dislocation, cross-braces are necessary. One might say that constructs spanning more than one level or that skip a pedicle for any reason should be cross-braced at least at one location. Medially angulating the pedicle screws greatly diminishes the tendency for one vertebra to laterally translate on the one below. Adding a cross-brace markedly decreases this tendency.

Some other situations in which cross-bracing is important are where there is a distraction force placed on the vertebra or when there has been anterior bone loss with an anterior strut graft. There are several cross-bracing configurations that are appropriate for various situations. Figure 14.15 demonstrates cross-bracing in the center of the rods (mid-cross-bracing) and also cross-bracing at the ends of the rods (end-cross-bracing). In these cases, if only one end is cross-braced, a "V" is formed; if both ends are cross-braced, a rectangle is formed. A construct with both ends cross-braced and with the pedicle screws angulated medially is a very strong one.

ACKNOWLEDGMENT

The research for this fixation device was done at the Long Beach Memorial Medical Center with financial aid from a research grant from the research foundation of that institution.

REFERENCES

1. Wiltse LL, Bateman JG, Hutchinson RN, et al.: The paraspinal sacrospinalis-splitting approach to the lumbar spine. J Bone Joint Surg 1968;50A:919.
2. Zindrick MR, Wiltse LL, Widell EH, et al.: A biomechanical study of intrapeduncular screw fixation in the lumbosacral spine. Clin Orthop 1986;203:99.

FIFTEEN

The Vermont Spinal Fixator

Martin H. Krag

INTRODUCTION

The use of the pedicle as a method for spinal implant attachment became a major advance in spine surgery. It provides a grip on the vertebra that resists loads of any type. Placement of a truly transpedicular screw was first reported in 1969 by Harrington and Tullos (14), but was really first developed as a practical method by Roy-Camille. It was the author's experience with the Roy-Camille system in 1981 that led to the idea of the internal fixation device, which later came to be called the Vermont spinal fixator (VSF). This was further stimulated by a meeting in 1981 with Magerl and Schläpfer concerning their work on an external spinal fixator (33,34,46,47). At that time, there were no published descriptions of any other transpedicular system, not to mention the basic anatomic and biomechanical research. This led to a series of anatomic and biomechanical studies which led to exact specifications for the VSF and clinical use in July, 1986 (Figs. 15.1 and 15.2). Presented here is a summary of those studies as well as a summary of clinical experience thus far. Further details and a more thorough review are published elsewhere (21–23).

DESIGN RATIONALE AND RELATED TESTING

Screw Design

At the time that decisions were needed for screw lengths and diameters for the VSF, the only morphometric data available were those of Saillant (44), which provided only average values. Thus, new data were collected (26,28). Subsequently, other related studies have been described (1,2,8,36,37,54). Figure 15.3 shows the "chord length" or length of screw shaft that can be inserted without penetration of the anterior cortex. Note the relative constancy in length for different vertebral levels. In contrast, the pedicle diameter (Fig. 15.4 and Table 15.1) is more

variable. Between vertebral levels, the diameter doubles in size between L1-L5, although it is approximately constant from T9-L1. Variability also occurs between specimens at a single level, as shown in Table 15.1. For example, at L1, 9% of pedicles have a diameter ≤3.9 mm, and 27% (9 + 18%) have a diameter ≤5.9 mm. Because of this variability, careful preoperative assessment, such as by CT scanning, is important. Based upon these data, the VSF screw major diameters were chosen to be 5.0, 6.0, and 7.0 mm.

On the topic of thread design, no studies were available that independently varied pitch (distance between threads), tooth profile (buttress vs. "V") and minor diameter (which determines tooth height). Thus, a study was undertaken (28) comparing eight different designs (all combinations of: 2-mm or 3-mm pitch, buttress or "V" tooth profile, and 3.8-mm or 5.0-mm minor diameter), all of which had a major diameter of 6.0 mm. This study, which used pullout testing from fresh frozen-thawed human cadaveric vertebrae, showed that: (*a*) tooth profile was unimportant; (*b*) 2-mm pitch threads were slightly stronger than those with 3-mm pitch; and (*c*) the 3.8-minor diameter screws were somewhat stronger (19%–26%, depending upon subgroup) than the 5-mm diameter screws for pullout, but this was offset by a reduction to less than half ([3.8/5] = 44%) for flexural rigidity (3). It seemed fairly clear to us that bending loads were probably more important than axial pullout loads. Thus, based upon these results, we selected a buttress profile, a 2-mm pitch, and a minor diameter 1 mm less than the major diameter for the VSF screws.

Articulation

The basic design concept for the VSF is for it to have a simple, compact, low "fiddle-factor" articulation that allows three-dimensional (3-D) positional adjustability and 3-D positional control between a transpedicular screw

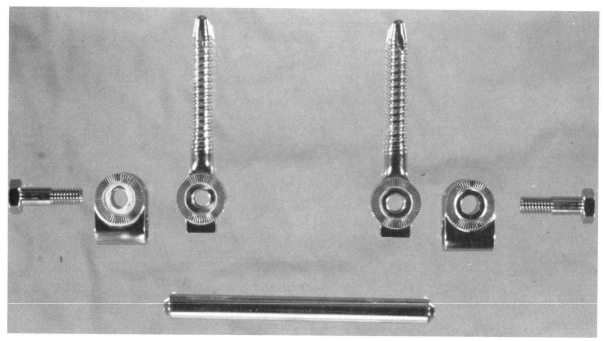

Figure 15.1. Components of Vermont Spinal Fixator (VSF) consists of screw, clamp, rod, and locking bolt. 3-D positioned adjustability is allowed: flexion-extension occurs across the toothed interface between screw and clamp; distraction-compression and axial rotation occur between the clamp and rod. 3-D positional control is produced by tightening of the bolt, which locks both interfaces. (Reprinted with permission from Reference 21.)

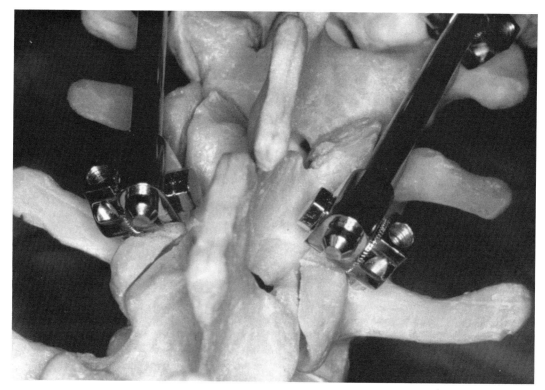

Figure 15.2. VSF implanted on plastic spine model. Note absence of interference with facet joints and of bone graft bed. Also note absence of contact of laminae by rod, which is not needed, since screw-rod articulation provides 3-D positional control. (Reprinted with permission from Reference 21.)

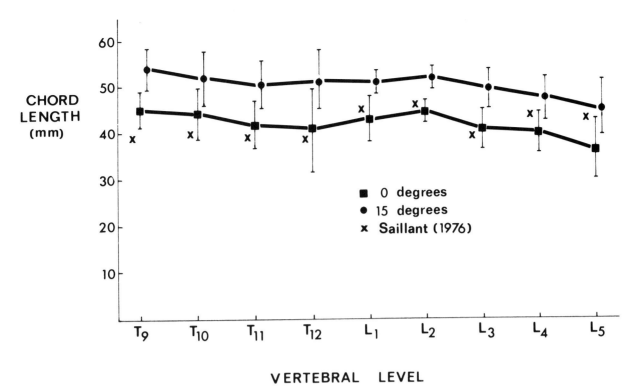

Figure 15.3. Screw-path length (chord length) measured along a line at 0° and 15° relative to the sagittal plane, and compared to means ("x") from Saillant (1976). (Reprinted with permission from Reference 28.)

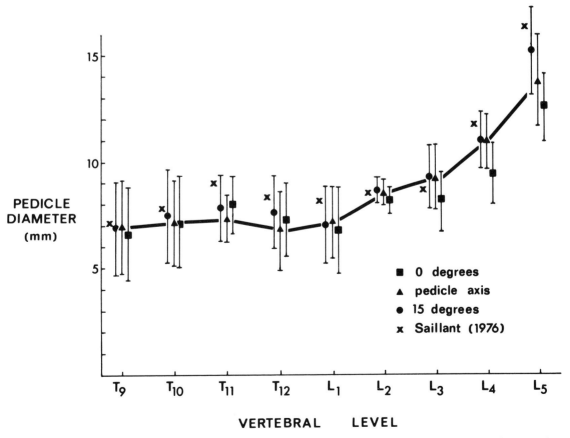

Figure 15.4. Pedicle diameter means ±1 S.D. for each vertebral level, measured three different ways and compared to means ("x") from Saillant (1976). (Reprinted with permission from Reference 28.)

239

Table 15.1.
Pedicle Diameter and Distribution by Size

Level	Mean	SD	#	3–3.9 mm	4–4.9 mm	5–5.9 mm	6–6.9 mm	7–7.9 mm	8–19.4 mm
T_9	6.88	2.23	14	14%	7%	14%	21%	7%	35%
T_{10}	7.47	2.24	18	11		11	39		39
T_{11}	7.83	1.56	22			14	18	14	55
T_{12}	7.63	1.79	24			21	21	12	46
L_1	7.01	1.84	22	9		18	18	14	41
L_2	8.67	0.64	14					7	92
L_3	9.30	1.51	24				8	12	79
L_4	11.03	1.36	24						100
L_5	15.15	1.97	20						100

and a longitudinal linking element. The rationale for 3-D adjustability is to allow optimal screw placement based upon only anatomic constraints, and not constraints imposed by the implant (e.g., the position of a hole in a plate).

The rationale for 3-D positional control is to provide resistance to all types of motions and forces, not to just a few specific types: it is this feature that makes an implant truly a "fixator." In addition, this feature allows the load resistance to be larger in magnitude. An example is shown in Figure 15.5 from the work of Carlson et al. (5), who compared two types of articulations for attachment to

transpedicle screws placed into the sacrum: a fully constrained linkage (Fig. 15.5A), exemplified the VSF, and a hinged or semiconstrained linkage (Fig. 15.5B), exemplified by a screw free to toggle relative to the plate through which it passes. The constrained linkage was shown to be significantly stronger, due to its greater ability to spread out the applied force along the screw length, and reduce force concentration on the dorsal cortex.

The design used for the VSF is shown in Figures 15.1 and 15.2. The transpedicular screw articulates by means of a "face gear" with the side of a clamp, which in turn fits around the smooth longitudinal rod. Both the screw-clamp and clamp-rod interfaces are secured with a simple locking bolt that passes through the clamp and threads into the head of the screw. The locking bolt has a spiralock thread pattern, which is primarily used in aircraft and other critical high-vibration applications, and prevents the need for a separate locking nut. The face gear has 60 radially-arranged teeth, which allow angular adjustability of ±3°. The smooth finish of the rod allows infinite adjustability, as well as maximal contact area between clamp and rod, thus maintaining high strength (approximately 1000 lbf to push the clamp along the rod) and fatigue resistance (no loosening at 1×10^6 cycles of flexion/extension load) (27).

Longitudinal Component

A rod was selected because it is simple in form, it has the same bending strength in flexion/extension as in lateral bending, and it allows the use of the articulation described above. Although the VSF design could use almost any rod diameter, we presently use 6 mm. This was chosen for two reasons. First, the largest VSF screw (7-mm major diameter) has a 6-mm minor diameter, and thus the rod is no weaker in bending strength than the strongest screw. Second, 6 mm is almost exactly the diameter of Harrington distraction rods, which rarely become bent in vivo. Thus far, no VSF rods have bent or broken.

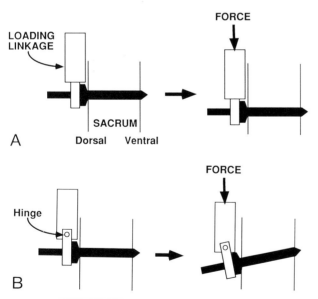

Figure 15.5. Two types of articulations tested on sacral transpedicular screws by Carlson et al. A, Constrained articulation provides 3-D positional control, as exemplified by the VSF. B, Semiconstrained articulation allows flexion-extension; exemplified by screw-plate systems in which screw toggle is allowed. (Reprinted with permission from Reference 5.)

Whether this rod diameter provides the optimal stiffness remains to be established. McAfee et al. (35) showed in animal experiments that stiffer implants, although they produced greater local osteopenia, also produced a higher fusion rate. Another consideration in trauma management is that too small a rod would allow excessive flexibility and undesired motion of bone fragments. A third issue is degeneration at the disc adjacent to the fusion. Hsu et al. (15,16) have conjectured that a high implant stiffness may cause more rapid degeneration of adjacent discs (compared to bone grafting with no implant). An alternative hypothesis, however, is that a greater amount of surgical dissection for the implant cases is the cause of the accelerated degeneration. In addition, it can be surmised (Fig. 15.6) that the bone graft (Fig. 15.6B) produces the dominant "motion concentration" on the adjacent discs and that the additional effect of an implant is relatively small, whether it is flexible (Fig. 15.6C) or stiff (Fig. 15.6D).

Transverse Connectors

The importance of transverse connectors is not yet clear. For axial pullout, Wörsdörfer (53) reported no strengthening effect from a transverse connector: two transversely-connected screws (Fig. 15.7C) were no more than twice as strong as single screws (Figs. 15.7A or 15.7B). Kling et al. (18) did find some strengthening, but it was only 31% for 4-mm Schanz screws and only 16% for 5-mm Schanz screws. For torsion or axial compression, Gurr et al. (12) found that the connector provided no increase in stiffness of the Cotrel-Dubousset implant. Fi-

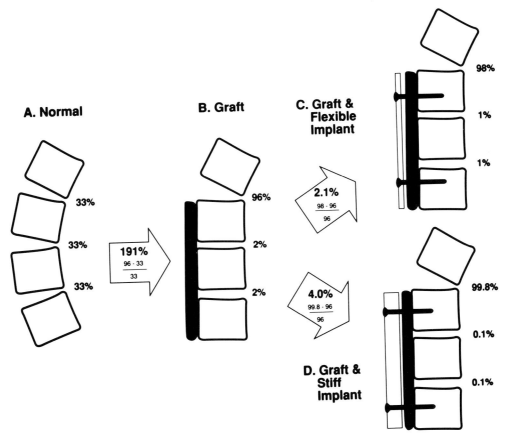

Figure 15.6. Effect of posterior bone graft and implant (flexible or stiff on "motion concentration" at the motion segment (MS) immediately above the fusion). *A*, Normal. Motion evenly distributed across all three MS (33%, 33%, 33%). *B*, Graft. For the same total motion, motion at the two lower MS is reduced to 2% each, "concentrating" 96% of the motion at the upper MS. Compared with *A*, this is equivalent to a 191% increase at the upper MS. *C*, Graft and flexible implant. Motion at the two lower MS is reduced to 1% each. Upper MS motion is increased to 98%. However, compared with *B*, this is equivalent to only a 2.1% increase in motion concentration at the upper MS. *D*, Graft and stiff implant. A very stiff implant reduces motion at lower two MS to 0.1%. Compared with *B*, this still is equivalent to only a 4.0% increase in motion concentration. (Reprinted with permission from Herndon C, 1991.)

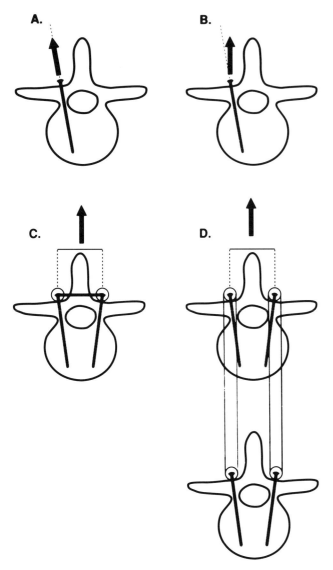

nally, for loads that tend to produce lateral translation (shifting), Carson et al. (6) found that connectors produced little reduction in the strain on implanted screws, provided the screws were oriented 15° or more away from the sagittal plane.

The reason so little strengthening was produced by the implanted connector in the work of Gurr et al. (12) and Carson (6) may be that the lower vertebral body to which the longitudinal rods attach (Fig. 15.7D) functions as an "intrinsic transverse connector." Provided the screws are obliquely oriented (i.e., not parallel to each other), this intrinsic connector is capable of strengthening screw resistance to pullout, lateral shifting, and axial rotation. Thus, an implanted connector would have little additional strengthening effect.

If all the screws are parallel (e.g., when the pedicle axis orientation is 0° relative to the sagittal plane), and a very high level of spinal trauma is present, a transverse connector may be useful. The VSF design allows easy addition of a smaller rod clamped obliquely between the two longitudinal rods.

SURGICAL METHOD AND RELATED TESTING

Presented here is the technique that has evolved since 1986 for implantation of the VSF, the rationale for it, and the results of related studies performed here and elsewhere.

Entry Point and Orientation

The method popularized by Roy-Camille et al. (42,43) is to orient the screw "straight ahead," namely, parallel both to the sagittal plane and to the transverse plane through the vertebral endplate (Fig. 15.8, *left*). Although this has the advantage of simplicity, it has also yielded a high rate of screw penetration out of the pedicle. Even if accurately performed, this method positions the upper screw shaft immediately below the inferior articular process of an uninstrumented mobile vertebra. To a large extent, avoidance of this facet joint impingement is provided by the "inward" method popularized (Fig. 15.8, *middle*) by Magerl (33,34), and even more so by orienting the screws "up and in" (Fig. 15.8, *right*) (23). The oblique orientation also provides a longer screw path length, which may allow a stronger "grip" by the screw on the vertebra. Finally, the oblique orientation allows the intrinsic transverse connector role of the vertebrae to come into play, as illustrated in Fig. 15.9. The straight-ahead screws resist lateral shifting only by screw-bone friction, which is small. The up and in screws resist lateral shifting by means of the compressive strength of bone. The differences between the straight ahead and

Figure 15.7. Screw pullout test methods and effect of transverse connector. *A,* Pullout along the axis of the screw. This is probably not a load type commonly seen in vivo. *B,* Pullout parallel to the sagittal plane. An isolated anteriorly directed pull on the vertebrae is probably uncommon in vivo. Nonetheless, this is more accurately modeled by screw pullout shown here than by that shown in Figure 15.7A. The transverse connector effect of the lower vertebra (shown in Fig. 15.7D), however, is still missing. *C,* Transverse connector. The pullout load should be attached to the screws as shown, not to the middle of the connector, to duplicate the in vivo situation and to avoid bending the connector. The transverse connector effect of the lower vertebra (as shown in *D*), however, is missing here as well. *D,* Transverse connector effect of the lower vertebra. The lower vertebra ties together the lower screws, which are attached by way of the longitudinal rods to the upper screws. The lower vertebra thereby strengthens the grip of the upper screw on the upper vertebra. This should be taken in account in measuring the effect of any implanted transverse connector. (Reprinted with permission from Herndon C, 1991.)

STRAIGHT AHEAD   INWARD   UP & IN

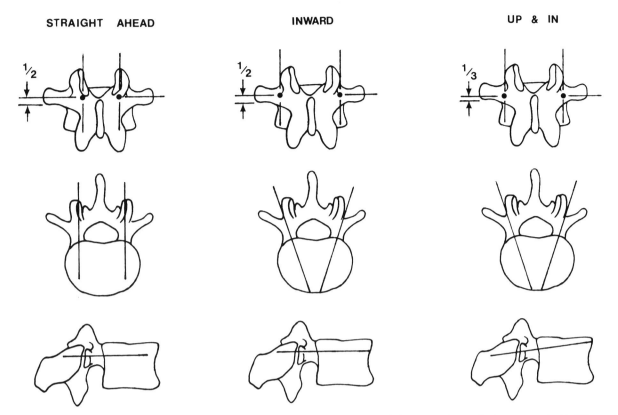

Figure 15.8. Entry point and orientation alternatives for transpedicle screws. *A*, "Straight ahead." The entry point is the intersection of a line that bisects the transverse process and a line that bisects the facet joint. Orientation is parallel to the sagittal plane and parallel to the endplates. *B*, "Inward." The entry point is more lateral, and the orientation is anteromedial along the pedicle. The longitudinal line is along the lateral aspect of the facet joint (superior articular process). *C*, "Up and in." The entry point is more lateral and lower (more caudad). The transverse line divides the upper and lower thirds of the transverse process. The orientation is still anteromedial but also anterocephalad (up and in), although not enough to intersect the superior endplate. (Reprinted with permission from Reference 23.)

the up and in approaches are summarized in Figure 15.10. Pedicle axis angle relative to sagittal plane varies at each level (Fig. 15.11).

The optimal method to surgically implant a transpedicle screw, in the author's opinion, is to use radiography to align a drill bit or probe even before entry into bone. This may be done easily using an oblique ("coaxial") view along the axis of the pedicle, as shown in Figure 15.12. A simple technique is to first position a C-arm image intensifier so its central beam is parallel to the pedicle axis. This axis varies both between vertebral levels and between individuals (Fig. 15.13). Positioning of the C-arm can be done based on preoperative CT scans, or by adjustment until the pedicle cortex is clearly seen "end-on," is somewhat medial to the lateral cortex of the vertebral body, and is between the upper and lower endplates. Next, the drill bit or probe is centered over the pedicle, and the shaft angulated 30–45° out of the way of the central beam, to allow easy visualization of the tip

STRAIGHT AHEAD   UP & IN

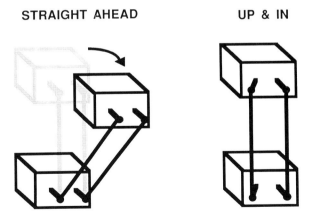

Figure 15.9. Straight-ahead orientation of the screws causes them to be parallel, and thus lateral shifting meets with little resistance (friction between screw and bone). Up-and-in orientation causes an interlocking or toenailing effect, which resists this lateral shifting. (Reprinted with permission from Reference 23.)

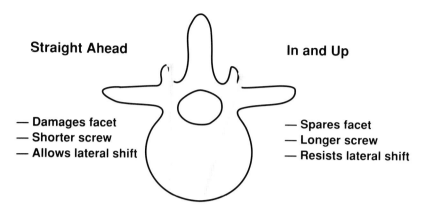

Figure 15.10.   Straight-ahead compared with in-and-up screw placement. (Reprinted with permission from Herndon C, 1991.)

and the pedicle. Finally, the instrument shaft is then rotated up to be parallel to the central beam. A drill bit so positioned appears as a spot, shown in Figure 15.11 held by a Kelly clamp. This technique allows the surgeon to be sure that correct alignment is obtained before, rather than after, "commitment" is made. This is contrary to the situation with an AP x-ray view, as shown in Figure 15.13, and as demonstrated in the careful and useful cadaveric work of Weinstein et al. (52).

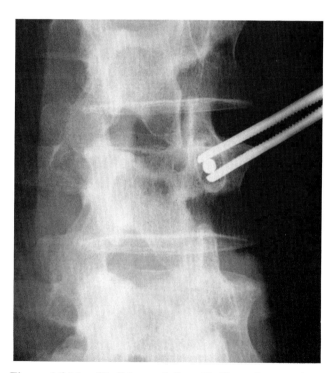

Figure 15.11.   "Pedicle coaxial" or "bull's eye" x-ray view, along the pedicle axis, oblique to the sagittal plane. Drill bit is seen end-on as a spot, held by a surgical clamp, along central beam of image intensifier. Correct entry point and orientation are seen even before drill insertion is performed. (Reprinted with permission from Reference 23.)

Drill insertion can then be accomplished. Use of a power driver with variable speed allows a great degree of control. After the drill is inserted to the desired depth, measure the length of it that protrudes: this subtracted from the total length is equal to the length of the screw to be used. Next, the driver is used to insert a 6–10-cm Kirschner wire oriented parallel to the drill bit into a nearby spinous process. This is used as a visual guide to the pilot hole orientation; vertebral cancellous bone may not be sufficiently strong for the screw to "follow" the hole, especially if the surgeon experiences any difficulty in retracting soft tissue laterally.

The special anatomy of the sacrum provides an alternative to the anteromedial orientation, namely the anterolateral orientation, shown in Figure 15.14 as the "promontory" and the "alar" orientations, respectively. There are proponents for each of these approaches, and recommendations differ significantly between authors concerning details (Table 15.2), but facts on this subject are few.

Anatomic data (1,8) and screw pullout data (56,57) have been reported, but the latter involved no right-left comparison and high interspecimen variability. Thus, we (8,21) compared right vs. left testing of these two screw orientations using flexion loading (probably more clinically relevant than axial pullout), and showed the promontory screws to provide as strong or stronger fixation than the alar screws. Because of this greater strength, and because by intraoperative radiography the promontory can be seen more easily than the anterior-most portion of the ala, the author continues to prefer anteromedial placement of sacral screw, into the anterior-most portion of the promontory near the midline.

Hole Preparation Method

Various methods have been recommended to form a pilot hole: drill bit (23,24,33,34,42), curette (9,30), curved

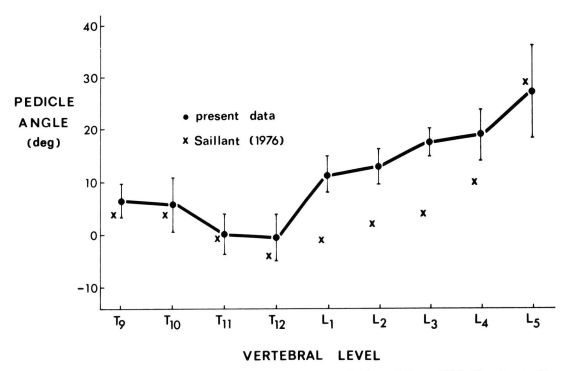

Figure 15.12. Pedicle axis angle relative to sagittal plane for each vertebral level. Means ±1 S.D. are shown, compared to means ("x") from Saillant, 1976. (Reprinted with permission from Reference 28.)

flat probe (13,48), and straight probe (11,39). Despite this variety, only two studies have been performed that compare methods. Moran et al. (37) compared a curved probe to a drill bit. Our reanalysis of their data (11,21) showed no significant difference between these methods. There is also no difference between a conical-tipped straight probe and a drill bit (11). Thus, there appears not to be mechanical grounds for selecting between these methods. In the author's experience, the use of a drill bit inserted as described below has been very safe, and provides a method that does not involve a "learning curve" to provide a dependably neat cylindrical pilot hole for screw placement.

Although tapping is advised by some authors, the evidence seems to be against it. Zindrick et al. (57) tested cadaveric vertebrae and found little difference overall, but found weakening of some specimens with tapping. This is similar to data from other cancellous bone sites (20, 38,49).

To repair or prevent stripout of screws, polymethylmethacrylate (PMM) can be used (17,55), but extrusion against cord or roots, infection, and difficulty of removal should be kept in mind. We (40) investigated the use of morselized cadaveric corticocancellous bone graft as an alternative and compared this to PMM. The latter was clearly superior: it provided a "repaired" pullout strength greater than the initial strength. However, the probably

safer technique of bone grafting produced a strength that was still 70% of the initial strength. Whether the superior strength of PMM is worth the potential complications remains to be established.

Depth of Insertion

A variety of clinically based recommendations have been made, ranging from screw placement just deep enough to reach into the vertebral body (42) to screw tip placement at the anterior cortex of the body (7,24,26,33,34). However, the biomechanical data show that a significant improvement in strength is obtained by an increase in screw penetration depth (25,30,56), as shown in Figure 15.15.

To reduce the risk of anterior cortex penetration by drill bit or probe, the author uses the following technique. By means of a power driver, the drill bit is inserted ⅔–¾ of the maximum depth under C-arm x-ray control. A "near approach" or "off-lateral" view is used, as shown in Figure 15.16. This view is tangential to the anterior cortex of the body at the location at which penetration would occur if the drill were inserted too far. With this view, the drill bit tip appears most nearly to approach the anterior cortex. This same method has been applied to the knee (10) and hip (4,31,41,45,50,51). While this view is used, the drill bit is advanced to the anterior cortex

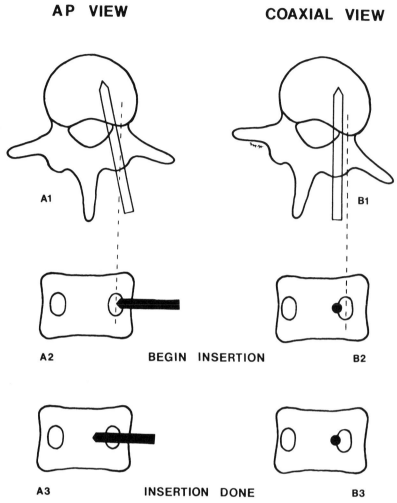

Figure 15.13. Anteroposterior (AP) vs. pedicle coaxial view for accuracy in visualizing breakout of screw through medial cortex of pedicle. *A*, AP view before beginning of drill insertion (A2) shows drill bit tip to appear centered over pedicle. It is not apparent that breakout has occurred. *B*, With the pedicle coaxial view, before beginning of drill insertion (B2), breakout can be anticipated. After insertion (B3), breakout can be seen no less well. (Reprinted with permission from Reference 21.)

by tapping on it with a mallet. In addition to watching the x-ray appearance, one can both hear a sound change and feel an increase in vibration of the drill bit shaft as it makes contact with the anterior cortex.

In the authors' experience, this "triple monitoring" technique provides a very low probability of anterior cortex penetration, and yet allows maximal screw-bone interface strength.

Device Removal

Should these implants be routinely removed, or only if specific clinical conditions so require? A consensus has by no means been reached. Most authors have made no mention of this topic, although concern has been raised about a number of issues that retained implants present, such as: (*a*) impaired assessment of fusion solidity (3, 32); (*b*) impaired visualization by diagnostic radiographic techniques; (*c*) accelerated degeneration or altered function at adjacent motion segments (15,16); (*d*) prolonged stress shielding of the fusion mass; (*e*) irritation to overlying tissue, (*f*) possibility of its being a

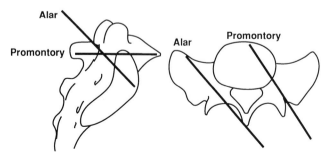

Figure 15.14. Two commonly used sacral screw placements: anterolaterally into the ala and anteromedially into the promontory. (Reprinted with permission from Reference 22.)

Table 15.2.
Methods for Sacral Screw Placement

Author	Level	Entry Site	Transverse Plane Angle[a]	Sagittal Plane Angle[b]	Depth
Cotrel et al. (6a)	S1	Midpoint between L5-S1 facet and S1 foramen	30° lateral	?	?
Edwards et al. (9)	S1	Base of L5-S1 facet	From inferodorsal corner of L5 spinous process to entry site		Through anterior cortex
Guyer et al. (13)	S1	Caudal and just lateral to S1 superior articular process	25° medial	?	To anterior cortex
Krag (23)	S1	Center of S1 pedicle seen by x-ray oriented along S1 pedicular axis	Towards midline (from preop CT)	Towards promontory	To anterior cortex
Louis (32)	S1	Lateral to L5-S1 facet and S1 foramen	35–45° lat	35–45° caud	?
Magerl (33)	S1	Intersection of lines along lateral and inferior edges of S1 superior articular process	15–20° med	Towards promontory	To anterior cortex
Roy-Camille et al. (42)	S1	?	30° lat	?	?
Steffee et al. (48)	S1	Just below S1 superior articular process	0°	0°	To anterior cortex
Guyer et al. (13)	S2	Midway between 1st and 2nd dorsal foramina	40–50° lat	10–15° ceph	?
Steffee et al. (48)	S2	?	45° lat	?	?

[a] "lat" means anterolateral; "med" means anteromedial orientation.
[b] "ceph" means anterocephalad; "caud" means anterocaudal orientation.

site for hematogenous spread of infection; (*g*) altered local damage in the event of future regional trauma, and (*h*) long-term metal toxicity. Ölerud (39) does not remove his device before at least 1 year has passed. Dick (7) and Kinnard (19) recommend routine removal if discs are spanned that have not also been grafted. The author recommends its routine removal, as for most other metallic hardware. Only the long-term results will establish which approach provides the best balance between the risks and costs of an additional surgical procedure for device removal, and the functional benefits thereby achieved.

Clinical Experience

A program of VSF human implantation between July, 1986, and August, 1988, involved 54 patients and one surgeon (the author). The major objectives for these implantations were to obtain:

1. A bone fusion spanning only the abnormal motion segments, using instrumentation that does not extend beyond the fusion;
2. A satisfactory or better alignment across the grafted vertebrae; and
3. An acceptably small incidence of device-related complications.

The major indication for entry into the study was the presence of mechanical insufficiency suspected to be the cause of debilitating back pain or of significant risk to neural elements. The diagnoses of the 54 patients are shown in Table 15.3.

The treatment and follow-up program were as follows. A bivalved thoracolumbar orthosis (no thigh extension) was worn for 6 months (during recumbency for at least the first 6 weeks). Mobilization was done as rapidly as tolerated by symptoms (usually 2–3 days postoperatively), and activities gradually progressed to normal at 6 months. Follow-up clinically and radiographically was done at 1 week, 6 weeks, 3 months, 6 months, 9 months, and 12 months. The implant was then removed (in 29 of 54 cases), typically at 12 months, and follow-up continued until at least 6 weeks postremoval. Those cases in which removal did not occur were generally followed until at least 24 months postimplantation.

Radiographic assessment early in the series included lateral x-rays obtained with the patient both supine and upright. Since no difference in kyphosis angle was seen between these films on any patients, this was discontinued. Lateral x-rays in the upright posture were subsequently obtained at 1 week, 6 weeks, and 3 months. Flexion/extension laterals were obtained at 6 months, 9 months, 12 months, and after removal. CT scans were

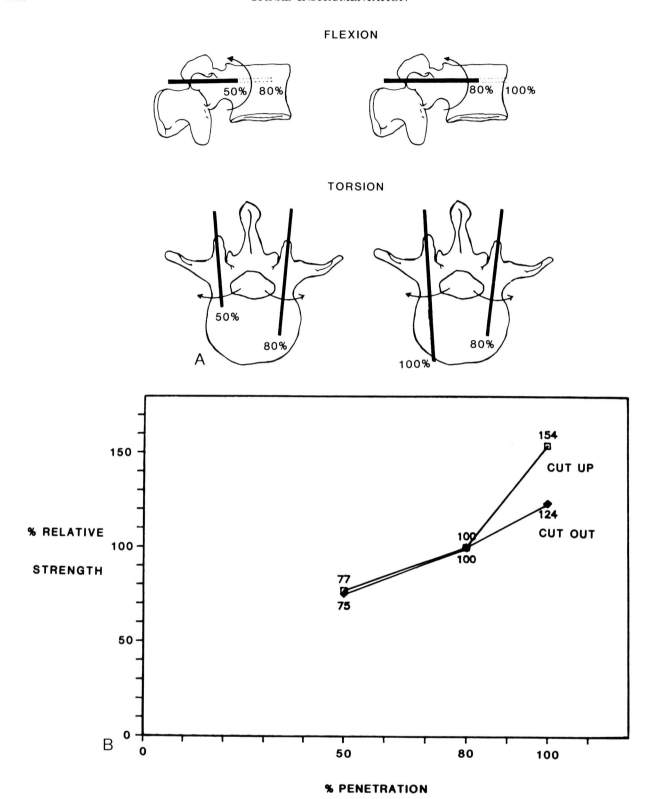

Figure 15.15. *A*, Experimental design. Opposite pedicles of each vertebra had screws implanted to different depths; 50 and 80% depth in half of the specimens; 80 and 100% (to cortex) in the other half. One each of two bending moments were then sequentially applied to opposite screws in each vertebra: "torsion," tending to move the screw tip laterally; and "flexion," tending to move the screw tip cephalad. (Reprinted with permission from Reference 25.) *B*, Strength (relative to that of the 80% depth screw) versus depth of penetration. This relationship is approximately linear. (Reprinted with permission from Reference 22.)

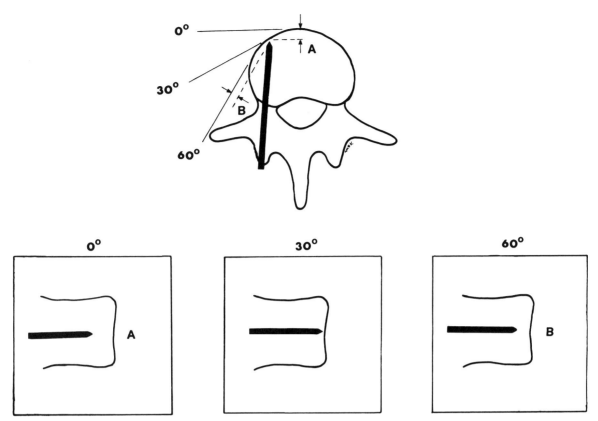

Figure 15.16. "Near approach" x-ray view to decrease likelihood of anterior penetration. When drill (or screw or probe) tip is actually at the anterior cortex, the lateral view (0°) misleadingly shows the tip to still be some distance A away from the cortex. At too oblique an angle of view (60°), the tip again misleadingly appears to be some distance B away from the cortex. Only when the view is tangent to the point of penetration (30° in this case) does the tip appear most nearly to approach actual breakthrough. (Reprinted with permission from Reference 21.)

Table 15.3.
A Series of Patients Who Underwent Applications of VSF

Diagnosis	
Trauma	
Burst	15
Fracture/Dislocation	3
Other	2
	20
Pseudarthrosis	
Degeneration	7
Spondylolisthesis	8
	15
Spondylolisthesis	
Isthmic (Grade 1)	5
Degeneration	3
	8
Degeneration	9
Tumor	1
Infection	1
Total	54

obtained before implantation on all patients, and after implantation on most of those whose VSF was removed.

The vertebral levels into which screws were placed for these 54 patients are shown in Table 15.4. Implantations have been as high up as T9 and as low down as the sacrum, the latter of which were all into the promontory through the S1 pedicle. Note that most of the trauma implantations occurred in the thoracolumbar region, and most of the nontrauma implantations were in the lumbosacral region.

The number of vertebrae spanned by the VSF and bone graft are shown in Table 15.5. This shows the short-length vertebral segment instrumented by the VSF. Only one normal vertebra above and one normal vertebra below the abnormal vertebra(e) are involved. Thus, for example, the 10 cases of two-vertebrae fusions include single-level pseudarthroses or disc degenerations. As another example, the 18 trauma cases with three vertebrae include burst fractures that extend into the inferior endplate of the injured vertebra, and cases of two-level pseudarthroses.

Table 15.4.
Distribution of Screw Placement By Vertebral Level

Vertebra	Trauma Upper	Trauma Lower	All Upper	All Lower
T9	1	0	2	0
T10	2	0	2	0
T11	4	0	4	0
T12	9	1	9	2
L1	2	6	3	6
L2	1	9	3	9
L3	1	2	7	2
L4	0	1	21	5
L5	0	1	3	11
S1	0	0	0	19
Total	20	20	54	54

Table 15.5.
Number of Vertebrae Spanned by VSF (1–54)

Levels	Trauma	All
2	0	10
3	18	39
4	1	3
5	1	2

To illustrate the overall experience, a few representative cases will be described.

Case 1. Fracture-Dislocation Reduction (Fig. 15.17).

This 23-year-old male sustained a T12-L1 bilateral facet fracture-dislocation and complete T12 paraplegia. He was medically stabilized and at 8 days after

injury, realignment, VSF placement from T12 to L2, and line grafting from T12 to L2 were performed. He was mobilized in a wheelchair within a few days thereafter in a bivalved body jacket.

Case 2. Fusion in Situ to the Sacrum (Fig. 15.18).

This 24-year-old 220-lb. professional hockey player previously underwent bone grafting from L4-S1 for treatment of back and leg pain produced by L5 spondylolisthesis, and developed a pseudarthrosis. For treatment of his persistent, debilitating back pain, he underwent repeat autogenous bone grafting and VSF placement from L4-S1. No effort was made to achieve reduction of the spon-

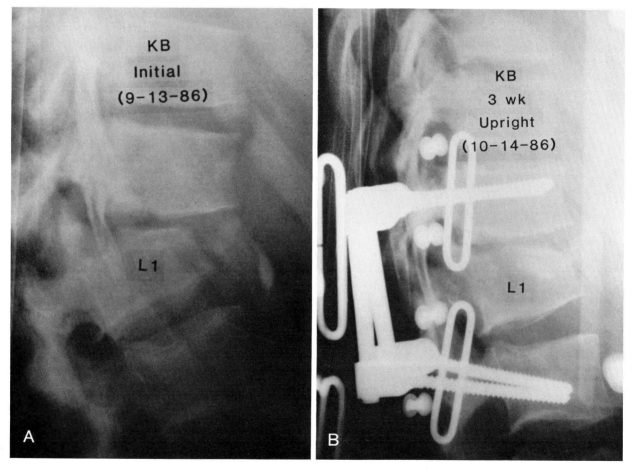

Figure 15.17. Clinical case #1. Fracture-dislocation at T12-L1. *A*, Initial. *B*, After realignment and VSF placement.

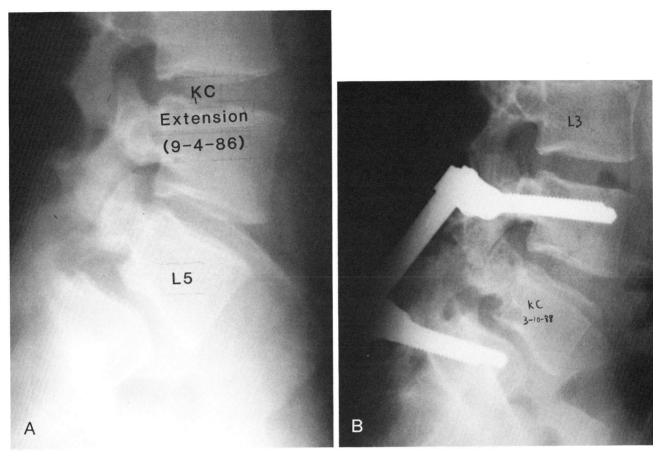

Figure 15.18. Clinical case #2. Fusion in situ from L4-S1. *A*, Flexion-extension views show pseudarthrosis at L4-L5 and L5-S1, from previous attempt at fusion. *B*, 18 months after VSF placement and new bone graft placement. No motion seen on flexion-extension. (Reprinted with permission from Krag

MH: Internal fixation of the lumbosacral spine: experience with the Vermont Spinal Fixator. In: Lin PM, Gill K (eds), Lumbar Interbody Fusion, Chapter 22, p 257, Figures 22-5B, Aspen Publishers.)

dylolisthesis. He gradually progressed in his activities in a plastic lumbosacral orthosis over the subsequent 6 months, at which time he resumed competitive training. Follow-up to 18 months showed apparently solid fusion, and no implant changes. Device removal has not yet occurred.

Case 3. "Short Segment" Fusion (Fig. 15.19). This 35-year-old large-animal veterinarian had single-level disc and facet joint degeneration develop at L4-L5 that caused sufficient back and leg symptoms to prevent him from pursuing his profession. He underwent decompression and autologous iliac crest bone grafting at L4-L5, and device removal 12 months later. A solid fusion was seen to be present at removal and on subsequent flexion-extension x-rays. He has returned full time to his career without residual symptoms.

Case 4. "Long Segment" Fusion (Fig. 15.20). This 21-year-old physical therapy student was noted, post-

partum, to have a large retroperitoneal ganglioneuroma which extended into virtually all the L2, L3, and L4 vertebral bodies and encroached into the spinal canal at these levels. She underwent simultaneous anterior and posterior resection of tumor, and placement of VSF from L1-L5 (S1 was fully lumbarized). Bone graft was placed only posteriorly and included autogenous iliac crest and cadaveric tibia. A bivalved orthosis was worn for 6 months. Hardware was removed 23 months later, and a solid graft was noted, both intraoperatively and on subsequent flexion-extension x-rays.

The results in terms of fusion rate have been as follows. In the 34 cases in which device removal was undertaken, 29 had a solid fusion, and five were found to have a nonunion. These consisted of: two female cigarette smokers with previous pseudarthroses whose freeze-dried corticocancellous cadaveric graft pieces were embedded in a fibrous matrix with no bony consolidation, one male patient with diabetic nephropathy on renal dialysis

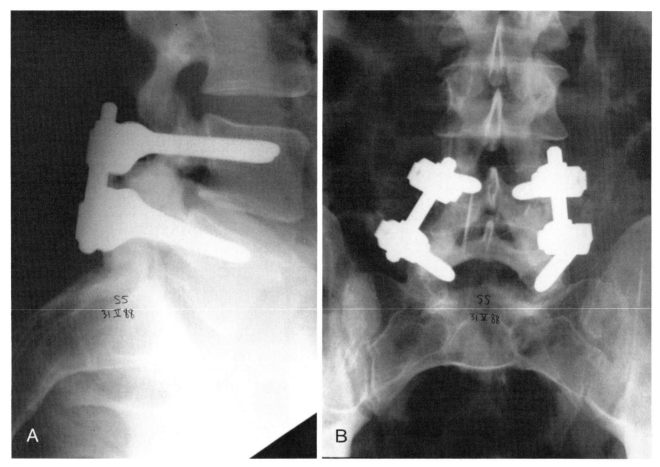

Figure 15.19. Clinical case #3. Short segment fusion from L4-L5. Compact design of VSF readily allows such single mo- tion segment implantations. *A*, Lateral view. *B*, Lateral view. (Reprinted with permission from Reference 22.)

who developed a linear transverse pseudarthrosis, and two otherwise-healthy male patients (one trauma, one non-trauma) who also developed linear transverse pseud-arthroses. These five cases were all regrafted. Four of them had the VSF removed 1 year subsequently, and solid fusion was seen. One of the five (the patient on renal dialysis) has not yet had the VSF removed, although there is no radiographic or clinical evidence for nonunion. Of the 20 cases in which device removal has not been attempted, there is also no radiographic or clinical evi-dence for nonunion (this includes flexion/extension lat-eral x-rays). Thus, the known number of nonunions is $5/54 = 9.3\%$ for all patients. For the trauma subgroup, it is $2/20 = 10\%$.

The complications have been as follows: In one patient, one of the L4 transverse processes split during screw placement ($1/216$ screws $= 0.46\%$), as a result of which the screw was placed into the next vertebra (L3). One patient had one screw at L3 ($1/216$ screws $= 0.46\%$), causing radicular dysesthesia that resolved after device

removal. One patient had one screw placed through the medial cortex of the S1 pedicle ($1/216$ screws $= 0.46\%$), causing dysesthesia and motor weakness, which have only partially resolved after device removal. There has been one infection after device placement ($1/54$ patients $= 1.8\%$) and one infection after device removal ($1/29$ patients $= 3.4\%$).

CONCLUSION

The VSF provides a means to achieve spinal fusion in a way that minimizes the number of vertebrae involved. It does this by involving only those vertebrae affected by the structural abnormality for which the fusion is per-formed. The mechanics of the VSF do not require "extra" vertebrae to be instrumented, in contrast to the mechan-ics, for example, of Harrington distraction rods.

This improvement in fusion length is accomplished without any increase in complication rates. As shown here, the rates for the VSF are at least as good as those

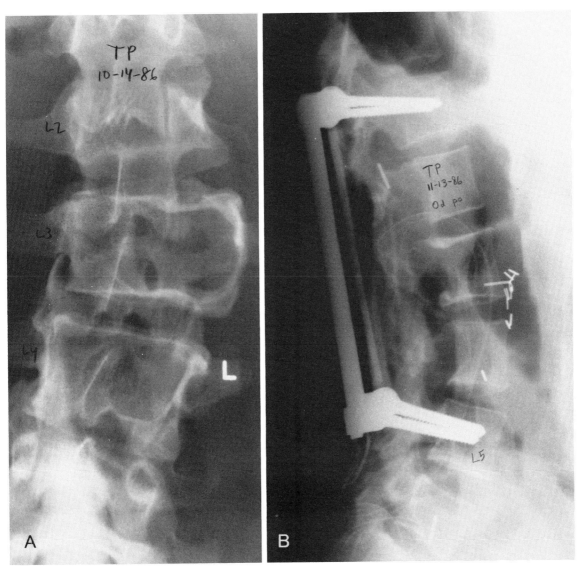

Figure 15.20. Clinical case #4. Long segment fusion from L1 to L5 for ganglioneuroma of L2-L4. Note full lumbarization of S1. Screws placed only into L1 and L5. *A*, Preoperative AP view. *B*, Postoperative lateral view. (Reprinted with permission from Reference 21.)

for other devices that typically involve substantially longer spinal segments. The functional implications of this reduction in fusion length remain to be determined exactly, but there are many indications that the shorter the fused segment, the better the functional result.

These results have encouraged a multicenter prospective research project for the VSF, now under way.

REFERENCES

1. Asher MA, Strippgen WE: Anthropometric studies of the human sacrum relating to dorsal transsacral implant designs. Clin Orthop 1986;203:58–62.
2. Banta CJ, King AG, Dobezies EJ, et al: Measurement of effective pedicle diameter in the human spine. Orthopaedics 1989;12:939–942.
3. Blauth M, Tscherne H, Haas N: Therapeutic concept and results of operative treatment in acute trauma of the thoracic and lumbar spine: the Hanover experience. J Orthop Trauma 1987;1:240–252.
4. Brodsky JW, Barnes DA, Tullos HS: Unrecognized pin penetration of the hip joint. Contemp Orthop 1984;9:13–20.
5. Carlson GD, Abitbol JJ, Anderson DR, et al: Screw fixation in the human sacrum: an in vitro study of the biomechanics of fixation (8208.212) (Journal submission), 1991.
6. Carson WL, Duffield RC, Arendt M, et al: Internal forces and moments on transpedicular spine instrumentation: the effect of pedicle screw angle and transfixation: the 4R-4 bar linkage concept. Spine 1990;15:893–901.
6a. Cotrel Y, Dubousset J: Nouvelle technique d'osteosynthese rach-

idienne segmentarie par voie posterieure. Rev Chir Orthop 1984;70:489–494.

7. Dick W: The "fixateur interne" as a versatile implant for spine surgery. Spine 1987;12:882–900.

8. Dohring EJ, Krag MH, Johnson CC: Sacral screw fixation: a morphologic, anatomic and mechanical study. (Abstract) Proc North Amer Spine Soc Annual Meeting, Monterey, California, 1990;174.

9. Edwards CC: Spinal screw fixation of the lumbar and sacral spine: Early results treating the first 50 cases. (Abstract) Proc 21st Annual Meeting Scoliosis Res Soc, 1986;99.

10. El-Khoury GY, McWilliams FE: A simple radiological aid in the diagnosis of small avulsion fractures of the knee. J Trauma 1978;18:275–277.

11. George DC, Krag MH, Johnson CC, et al: Hole preparation techniques (drill versus probe) for transpedicular screws: effect upon pullout strength from human cadaveric vertebrae. Spine (In press, 1981).

12. Gurr KR, McAfee PC: Cotrel-Dubousset instrumentation in adults: a preliminary report. Spine 1988;13:510–520.

13. Guyer DW, Wiltse LL, Peek RD: The Wiltse pedicle screw fixation system. Orthopaedics 1988;11:1455–1460.

14. Harrington PR, Tullos HS: Reduction of severe spondylolisthesis in children. South Med J 1969;62:1–7.

15. Hsu KY, Zucherman J, White A, et al: Deterioration of motion segments adjacent to lumbar spine fusions. (Abstract) Proc North Amer Spine Soc, Colorado Springs, Colorado, 1988;113–114.

16. Hsu K, Zucherman JF, White AH, et al: Internal fixation with pedicle screws. In: White AH, Rothman RH, Ray CD, eds. Lumbar spine surgery: techniques and complications. St. Louis: CV Mosby, 1987;322–338.

17. Kleeman BC, Gerhart TN, Hayes WC: Augmenting screw fixation in osteopenic trabecular bone. Proc Soc Biomaterials Annual Meeting, 1987.

18. Kling TF Jr, Vanderby R Jr, Belloli DM, et al: Cross-linked pedicle screw fixation in the same vertebral body: a biomechanical study. Proc Scoliosis Res Soc, 1986.

19. Kinnard P, Ghibely A, Gordon D, et al: Roy-Camille plates in unstable spinal conditions: a preliminary report. Spine 1986; 11:131–135.

20. Koranyi E, Bowman CE, Knecht CD, et al: Holding power of orthopaedic screws in bone. Clin Orthop 1970;72:283–286.

21. Krag MH: Biomechanics of thoracolumbar spinal fixation: A review. Spine 1991a;16:87–89.

22. Krag MH: Spine fusion: Overview of options and posterior internal fixation devices. In: Frymoyer JW, ed. The adult spine: Principles and practice. New York: Raven Press, 1991b;1919–1945.

23. Krag MH: Biomechanics of transpedicle spinal fixation. In: Weinstein JN, Wiesel S, eds. The lumbar spine. Philadelphia: WB Saunders, 1990;916–940.

24. Krag MH, Van Hal ME, Beynnon BD: Placement of transpedicular vertebral screws close to anterior vertebral cortex: description of methods. Spine 1989;14:879–883.

25. Krag MH, Beynnon BD, DeCoster TA, et al: Depth of insertion of transpedicular vertebral screws into human vertebrae: effect upon screw-vertebra interface strength. J Spinal Dis 1988a; 1:287–294.

26. Krag MH, Weaver DL, Beynnon BD, et al: Morphometry of the thoracic and lumbar spine related to transpedicular screw placement for surgical spinal fixation. Spine 1988b;13:27–32.

27. Krag MH, Beynnon BD, Frymoyer JW, et al: Fatigue testing of an internal fixator for posterior spinal stabilization. Proc American Academy of Orthopaedic Surgeons 54th Annual meeting, San Francisco, CA, 1987.

28. Krag MH, Beynnon BD, Pope MH, et al: An internal fixator for posterior application to short segments of the thoracic, lumbar, or lumbosacral spine: design and tesing. Clin Orthop 1986;203:75–98.

29. Lavaste F: Biomechanique du rachis dorso-lombaire. Deuxieme Journees d'Orthopedie de la Pitie 1980;19–23.

30. Lavaste F: Etude des implants rachidiens. Mémoire de biomechanique. Thesis "Ingeneur" Ecole Natl Supér des Arts et Metiers à Paris, 1977.

31. Lehman WB, Grant A, Rose D, et al: A method of evaluating possible pin penetration in slipped capital femoral epiphysis using a cannulated internal fixation device. Clin Orthop 1984;186:65–70.

32. Louis R: Fusion of the lumbar and sacral spine by internal fixation with screw plates. Clin Orthop 1986;203:18–33.

33. Magerl FP: Stabilization of the lower thoracic and lumbar spine with external skeletal fixation. Clin Orthop 1984;189:125–141.

34. Magerl F: External skeletal fixation of the lower thoracic and the lumbar spine. In: Uhthoff HK, Stahl E, eds. Current concepts of external fixation of fractures. New York: Springer-Verlag, 1982; 353–366.

35. McAfee PC, Farey ID, Sutterlin CE, et al: Device-related osteoporosis with spinal instrumentation. Spine 1989;14:919–926.

36. Misenhimer GR, Peek RD, Wiltse LL, et al: Anatomic analysis of pedicle cortical and cancellous diameter as related to screw site. Spine 1989;14:367–372.

37. Moran JM, Berg WS, Berry JL, et al: Transpedicular screw fixation. J Orthop Res 1989;7:107–114.

38. Nunamaker DM, Perren SM: Force measurements in screw fixation. J Biomech 1976;9:669–675.

39. Ölerud S, Karlström G, Sjöström L: Transpedicular fixation of thoracolumbar vertebral fractures. Clin Orthop 1988;227:44–51.

40. Pfeifer BA, Krag MH, Johnson CC: Repair of failed pedicle screw fixation: A biomechanical study comparing polymethylmethacrylate, morselized bone, and matchstick bone reconstruction (submitted 1/91 to Spine for publication).

41. Rooks MD, Schmitt EW, Drvaric DM: Unrecognized pin penetration in slipped capital femoral epiphysis. Clin Orthop 1988;34:82–89.

42. Roy-Camille R, Saillant G, Mazel C: Internal fixation of the lumbar spine with pedicle screw plating. Clin Orthop 1986;203:7–17.

43. Roy-Camille R, Demeulenaere C: Ostéosynthèse du rachis dorsal, lombaire et lombo-sacré par plaque métalliques vissées dans les pédicules vertébraux et les apophyses articulaires. Presse Méd 1970;78:1447–1448.

44. Saillant G: Etude anatomique des pédicules vertébraux: application chirurgicale. Revue de Chirurgie Orthopedique 1976;62 (2):151–160.

45. Shaw JA: Preventing unrecognized pin penetration into hip joint. Orthop Rev 1984;13:142–152.

46. Schläpfer F, Magerl F, Jacobs R, et al: In vivo measurements of loads on an external fixation device for human lumbar spine fractures. Institute of Mechanical Engineers. 1980;31/80:59–64.

47. Schläpfer F, Wörsdörfer O, Magerl F, et al: Stabilization of the lower thoracic and lumbar spine: comparative in vitro investigation of an external skeletal and various internal fixation devices. In: Uhthoff HK, Stahl E, eds. Current concepts of external fixation of fractures. New York: Springer-Verlag, 1982;367–380.

48. Steffee AD, Biscup RS, Sitkowski DJ: Segmental spine plates with pedicle screw fixation: a new internal fixation device for disorders

of lumbar and thoracolumbar spine. Clin Orthop 1986;203:45–53.

49. Vangsness CT, Carter DR, Frankel VH: In vitro evaluation of the loosening characteristics of self-tapped and non-self-tapped cortical bone screws. Clin Orthop 1981;157:279–286.

50. Volz RG, Martin MD: Illusory biplane radiographic images. Radiology 1977;122:695–697.

51. Walters R, Simon SR: Joint destruction: A sequel of unrecognized pin penetration in patients with slipped capital femoral epiphysis. Proc Eighth Open Scientific Meeting of the Hip Society. St. Louis: CV Mosby, 1980;145–164.

52. Weinstein JN, Spratt KF, Spengler D, et al: Spinal pedicle fixation: Reliability and validity of roentgenogram-based assessment and surgical factors on successful screw placement. Spine 1988;13:1012–1018.

53. Wörsdörfer O: Operative stabilisierung der thorakolumbalen und lumbalen wirbelsäule: Vergleichende biomechanische Untersu-chungen zur stabilität und steifigkeit verschiedener dorsaler fixations-systems. Thesis, Medizinisch-Naturwissenschaftliche Hochschule der Universität Ulm, 1981.

54. Zindrick MR, Wiltse LL, Doornik A, et al: Analysis of the morphometric characteristics of the thoracic and lumbar pedicles. Spine 1987;12:160–166.

55. Zindrick MR, Patwardhan A, Lorenz M: Effect of methylmethacrylate augmentation upon pedicle screw fixation in the spine. Proc International Society for the Study of the Lumbar Spine, Dallas, Texas, 1986a.

56. Zindrick MR, Wiltse LL, Widell EH, et al: Biomechanical study of interpedicular screw fixation in the lumbosacral spine. Clin Orthop 1986b;203:99–111.

57. Zindrick MR, Wiltse LL, Holland WR, et al: Biomechanical study of intrapedicular screw fixation in the lumbosacral spine. Proc International Society for Study of the Lumbar Spine Annual Meeting, Sydney, Australia, 1985.

Transpedicular Fixation with AO Dynamic Compression Plates

Rick C. Sasso, Howard B. Cotler, and John S. Thalgott

INTRODUCTION

The use of the narrow, dynamic compression plate (DCP) in the treatment of thoracic and lumbar spine fractures was briefly described by the AO group in their Manual of Internal Fixation (21). They cited the technique of Roy-Camille for performing internal fixation with pedicle screw plating (28,29). Instead of using his round hole plates, however, they advocated narrow DCPs, which allow the screws to be angled through the holes in any direction.

The DCP was developed by the AO group in 1965. They touted the DCP as representing an improvement on the traditional round hole plate because of the special geometry of the screw holes that allows for two unique advantages. The first is that axial compression may be achieved without the use of a tension device if a special offset drill guide is used. The second is that it is possible to angle the screws through the holes in any direction desired. The first advantage is not applicable to the posterior transpedicular placement of these plates, but is useful for compression of the bone graft after an anterior corpectomy and instrumentation with the broad 4.5-mm DCP. The second advantage is very significant for posterior plating since the screws may be angled in an unlimited direction in order to properly enter the vertebral pedicles. The magnitude of the angulation is 25° longitudinally in each direction parallel to the plate axis and 7° sideways, perpendicular to the long axis (Fig. 16.1).

A plate may be named by its anatomic and biomechanical characteristics. The anatomic properties of a plate are described by its material configuration, such as a T, round hole, or slotted plate. The biomechanical characteristics are determined by the functional manner in which the plate is operating, such as a compression, tension band, or neutralization plate. The function of a specific plate is not necessarily governed by its anatomic configuration. For example, a round hole plate can biomechanically function as a static compression, tension band, or neutralization plate, depending upon the manner in which it is employed. Unfortunately, the DCP is named by one of its possible biomechanical functions rather than by its anatomic characteristics. It is thus sometimes confusing when describing the use of this plate. Even if the screw is placed centrally rather than eccentrically through the plate hole, thereby not utilizing the self-compressing function, the plate is called a dynamic compression plate. A more appropriate name would identify the plate by its semicylindrical screw holes, which anatomically distinguish this plate from the others (Fig. 16.1).

The major advantage of the DCP for the spine surgeon is that the screw does not have to be inserted at right angles to the axis of the plate, but can be inserted obliquely. Because of the semicylindrical configuration of the screw holes and the hemispherical characteristic of the screw heads, the screw can be angled through the hole in all directions (Fig. 16.1B). In a round hole configuration, the head is seated in the hole when the screw is perpendicular to the axis of the plate (Fig. 16.2). If the screw is inserted obliquely, a torsional force occurs at the head as it engages the hole, attempting to fully seat the head in its perpendicular position. This torsional force is transmitted as a moment to the screw threads, causing asymmetric forces at the thread-bone interface (Fig. 16.2B). These asymmetric forces increase as the moment arm (screw length) increases and may lead to stress risers. The advantage of placing cancellous screws oblique to the axis of the plate is important when the hole does not lie exactly over the center of the pedicle. In a fixed hole system, this will occasionally occur (Fig. 16.2C and D). Oblique orientation of the screw through the plate hole into the pedicle without a concomitant torsional moment

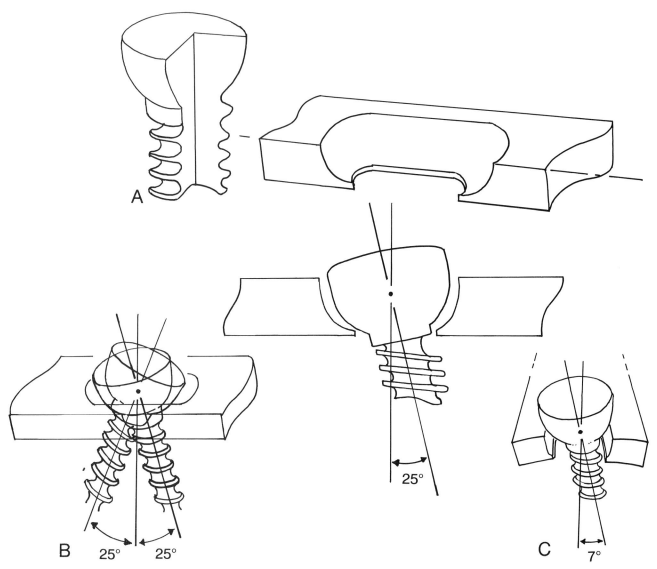

Figure 16.1. The DCP screw hole. *A*, The semicylindrical hole and corresponding hemispherical screw head allow the screw to be angled through the plate in any direction. The hemispherical screw head can be fully seated in the DCP hole despite oblique insertion. *B*, In the long axis of the plate, the screw can be angled 25°. This allows *C* a 50° arc. *C*, In the plane perpendicular to the long axis of the plate, the screw can be angled 7° (a 14°-arc).

experienced by the screw tip in the vertebral body is optimal (Fig. 16.3).

The DCPs are named for the diameter of the outer thread of the cortical screw that corresponds to that particular plate. The 4.5-mm cortical screw has an 8.0-mm head that interfaces with the 4.5-mm DCP screw hole. The 6.5-mm cancellous screw also has an 8.0-mm head and is used with the 4.5-mm DCP. The 4.5-mm DCP is made in a broad and narrow fashion. The broad 4.5-mm DCP has the holes staggered about the long axis of the plate in order to avoid placing the screws in the same plane. This is advantageous in a long bone and the an-

terior vertebral body because the chance of fracture occurring through the plane of the screws is decreased. The narrow DCP is characterized by all of the holes being in line with the long axis of the plate and is the type applicable to pedicle screw plating (Fig. 16.4). The screws are named by the outside diameter of their thread. The 6.5-mm cancellous screw has a 3.0-mm core, and a 2.75-mm pitch (Fig. 16.5). It is imperative that when using the 6.5-mm cancellous screw, the fully threaded modification be used. This provides thread fixation in the pedicle, which is the strongest region for fixation of the vertebral complex (29). These full-thread cancellous

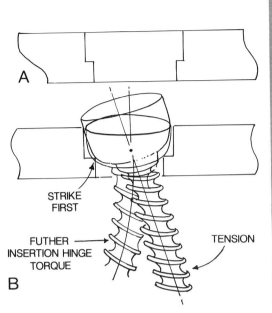

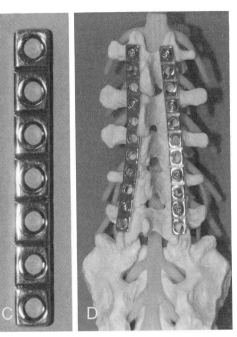

Figure 16.2. A round screw hole. *A*, A longitudinal section through a round screw hole. *B*, A screw inserted obliquely through this hole. The head is not fully seated as it first impacts the plate. Further insertion causes a bending moment at the threads as the head attempts to orient perpendicular to the plate. *C*, Round hole plate. *D*, Round hole plate used for a spinal internal fixation.

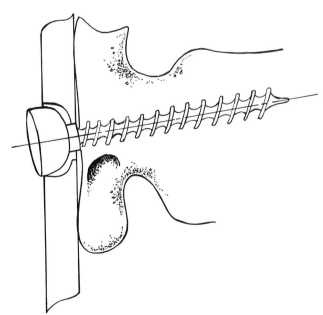

Figure 16.3. The hole is not exactly centered over the pedicle; however, the DCP screw hole allows oblique orientation of the screw so that it can be directed through the pedicle and into the vertebral body.

screw modifications are generally not included in the standard large fragment set and must be ordered separately.

The bending strength of a screw is proportional to its core diameter, while the pullout strength is proportional to the effective thread diameter (21). The effective thread diameter is equal to the outside thread diameter minus the core diameter. The 4.5-mm cortical screw is fully threaded and has a core diameter of 3.0 mm and a 1.75-mm pitch. Both screws have a head diameter of 8.0 mm which takes the 3.5-mm hexagonal screwdriver. The 3.2-mm drill bit corresponds to both the 4.5-mm cortical and 6.5-mm cancellous screws, since the core diameters are equal. The two screws have equal bending strength, but the 6.5-mm cancellous has a stronger pullout strength.

INDICATIONS

Pedicle screw plating with DC plates and 6.5-mm fully threaded cancellous or 4.5-mm cortical screws has been used to treat fractures, tumors, and degenerative conditions of the thoracic and lumbar spine. The principles of anatomic reduction with rigid internal fixation have been outlined by the AO group for the past three decades. These principles apply in the axial skeleton as well as the extremities. The advantages of internal fixation in the long bones for management of fractures, pseudarthrosis,

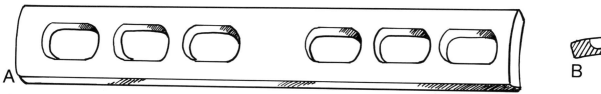

Figure 16.4. 4.5-mm narrow DCP. *A,* Top and *B,* end-on views. All screw holes are in line with the long axis of the plate.

The holes accommodate 8.0-mm hemispherical screw heads as possessed by the 6.5-mm cancellous and 4.5-mm cortical screws.

and osseous deformities have been clearly established (21). The same type of problems are encountered in the osseous portion of the spinal column and it is, thus, consistent that they be successfully managed with the use of internal fixation.

Thalgott (31,32) reported on a series of North American patients with lumbar degenerative disease reconstructed with internal fixation using AO DCPs, resulting in a high fusion rate. In the patient with longstanding, painful, degenerative lumbar disease, stable fixation with 4.5-mm narrow DCPs and pedicle screws, as an addition

to arthrodesis of the painful spinal segment, allows for faster rehabilitation when compared to patients with uninstrumented or less rigidly fixed fusions. It has been shown by Ransom (25) that the use of narrow DCPs and arthrodesis of the lumbar spine provide a higher and faster fusion rate compared with uninstrumented or Luque wire-rod combinations. This is clearly a significant advantage of transpedicular fixation in fusion of degenerative lumbar spines.

The AO group has championed a philosophy of rigid internal fixation for fractures with early rehabilitation of the injured extremity or joint. The use of internal fixation allows faster rehabilitation of the muscles, periarticular structures, and joint cartilages to avoid fracture disease. Fracture disease is a well-recognized atrophy of the soft tissues with progressive loss of function, joint stiffness, and demineralization of the immobilized bone (21). These concepts also apply with regard to spinal column fractures. If the spinal column can be anatomically reduced with segmental transpedicular fixation, mobilization of the patient is more rapid, and total body fracture disease is prevented.

The goals of fracture treatment of the limbs and the spine are the same: the restoration of normal anatomy and pain-free function. This is facilitated by anatomic reduction, optimal stabilization, and early mobilization. A specific goal for spine fractures is to allow the return of as much function as possible of injured neural elements by anatomic reduction and stable fixation in order to prevent further neurologic damage and provide for an optimal milieu for neurologic return. Operative stabilization of spinal injuries can bring about anatomic reduction, facilitate nursing care, and shorten the period of rehabilitation (10,11,15). Fractures of the thoracic and lumbar spine were treated with DCP pedicle screw plating and reported by Sasso and Cotler (28).

Limitation to pedicle screw plating in the thoracic spine is related to the size of the pedicles. This should be evaluated preoperatively. The plain AP radiograph may be used to roughly evaluate the diameter of the pedicle. If only the sclerotic cortical margins of the pedicle are seen on an AP film and no cancellous bone is evident within the pedicular confines, it is unlikely that the pedicle is suitable for screw insertion. A preoperative computed

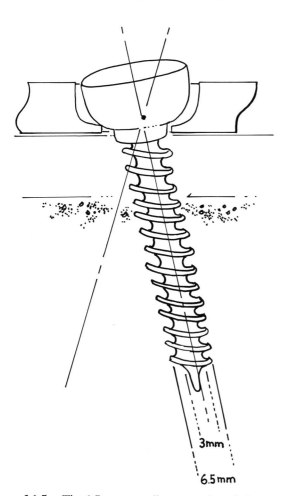

Figure 16.5. The 6.5-mm cancellous screw has a 3.0-mm core and a 6.5-mm outer thread diameter.

tomography (CT) scan is the optimal study because it allows for measurement of the pedicle diameter. Banta and King have coined the term "effective pedicle diameter" (4), which is the maximal cancellous diameter available for the screw. This concept is useful during the preoperative planning stage when deciding whether or not a cylindrical screw of a specific diameter will fit into an oblong, and sometimes asymmetric pedicle.

The DC plate and screws may also be used to stabilize metastatic spinal tumors. Hall and Webb have had wide experience with this technique (14) of anterior plate fixation after vertebrectomy and decompression. They conclude that these standard 4.5-mm broad (femoral) DC plates provide adequate stabilization. Also, this anterior plating system has been used after decompression of thoracolumbar spine fractures. Haas, Blauth, and Tscherne (13) have described a technique that uses two plates in the lateral and anterolateral positions to stabilize the vertebrae and tricortical iliac crest graft. They believe that anterior implants should exert a compressive force on the graft to inhibit graft dislocation and support healing. Furthermore, they believe its application should be easy and safe, and should have a low profile to reduce the chance of erosive bleeding. They contend that these re-

quirements are best fulfilled by the AO plates. Tension and shear forces cannot be completely neutralized by a single anterior plate in the lumbar spine, according to Haas, et al. (13). They describe the first plate positioned laterally and the second anterolaterally with the two plates as close to a 90° angle as possible. The dynamic compression plate will allow for up to 1.8 mm compression on the bone graft. The 6.5-mm cancellous screws are placed close to the endplate of the vertebral body for enhanced fixation.

SURGICAL TECHNIQUE

The surgical technique has undergone changes over the years. Also, the technique differs slightly for a traumatic injury, decompression, or fusion for degenerative spondylosis.

Initially, the European technique was used, which entails predrilling the pedicular cortex with a 3.2-mm drill bit under image intensification and placing 2-mm Kirschner wires (K-wires) into the pedicles (Fig. 16.6A and B). The Kirschner wire placement is verified with AP and lateral images (Fig. 16.7A and B). The 4.5-mm narrow AO DCP is bent to conform to the desired configuration

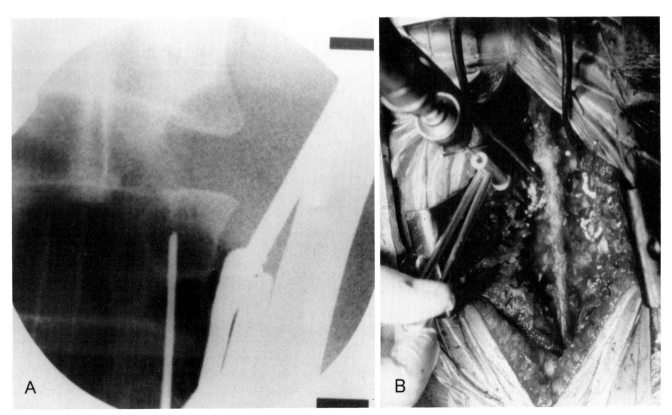

Figure 16.6. *A*, AP view under image intensification of the pedicle. *B*, Using the AO-stopped drill guide and standard length AO 2.0-mm guide pins, these are drilled into the instrumented pedicles to a depth of 35 mm.

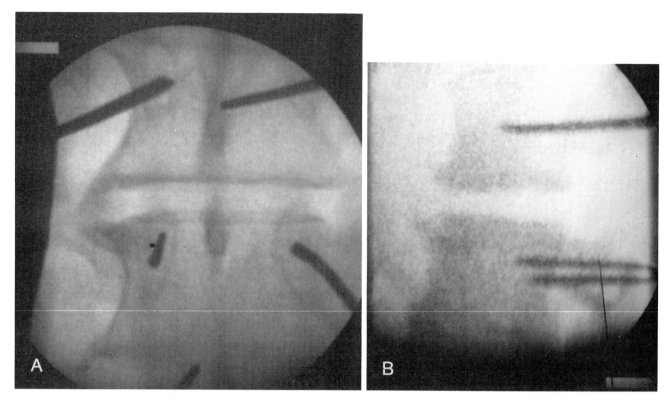

Figure 16.7. *A,* AP and *B,* lateral images document wire position.

and placed over the K-wires. The wires are sequentially removed, and 3.2-mm drill holes are drilled into the pedicle. A depth gauge is inserted into the holes to confirm that none of the pedicular cortices is violated. More recently, with greater experience in finding the pedicle, a rongeur is used to remove the cortex over the pedicle and a pedicular probe (AcroMed, Cleveland, Ohio) is placed into the pedicle and the vertebral body without the use of image intensification. The depth gauge is similarly used to confirm that none of the pedicular cortices is violated. The first few millimeters of the pedicle may be tapped; however, little overall difference has been found in the strength of screws through tapped specimens (17). The 4.5-mm narrow AO DCP is bent to conform to the desired configuration, and the 6.5-mm screws are inserted through the plate holes and into the pedicles.

The landmarks of transpedicular fixation have been well described by other authors (2,26). The posterior entrance to the pedicle is a line that bisects the long axis of the transverse process and crosses the laminar edge at the level of the facet. The angle of insertion should be parallel to the endplates and angled 10–20° toward the midline to ensure that they do not penetrate the lateral wall of the vertebral body. The length of the screws may be measured directly by inserting the depth gauge about 80% into the body as seen on the lateral image. However,

the length is usually 45 mm at L3, L4, and L5 in males; and 40 mm at L3, L4, and L5 in females (Fig. 16.8*A* and *B*). Krag (17) has championed a slightly different orientation for the pedicle screws. His entry site is slightly lower, at the interval between the lower one-third and upper two-thirds of the transverse process. The screw is then not only angulated medially (along the pedicle axis), but also inclined cephalad toward the superior endplate. This allows the entry site, and thus the dorsally protruding screw head, to be farther away from the facet joint. Theoretically, this may decrease the incidence of degeneration of this facet. Also, the path is longer, thus, screw length is greater, which increases the bone-screw interface area.

If fixation to the sacrum is required, S1 pedicle screws or sacral alar screws can be used. The entry point for the S1 pedicle is located at the intersection of a vertical line tangential to the lateral border of the S1 facet and a horizontal line tangential to its inferior border. The screws converge toward the midline and aim toward the anterior corner of the promontory (Fig. 16.9). The length of the 6.5-mm full-threaded cancellous screw in the S1 pedicle is standardized in most patients. Females generally accommodate a 30–35 mm length and males a 35–40 mm length. It is not necessary to engage the anterior cortex.

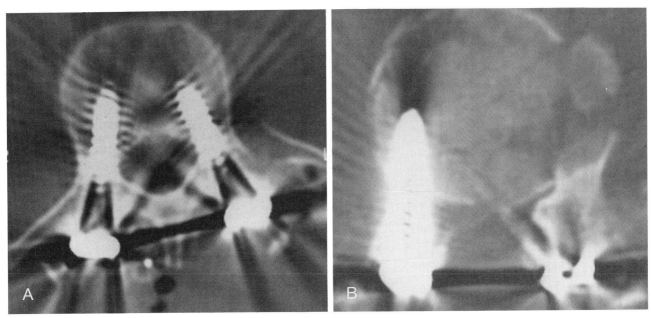

Figure 16.8. Postoperative CT scans demonstrating the depth of penetration in a degenerative case (*A*) and a trauma case (*B*).

An alternative in sacral fixation is to insert the screws into the sacral ala, parallel to the surface of the sacroiliac joint. The entry point shifts slightly medial as the screw direction diverges lateral. These screws inserted parallel to the sacroiliac joint aim toward the anterior superior angle of the lateral mass of the sacrum. Multiple-point sacral fixation is optimal (1). Combinations of pedicular (S1 and S2) and alar screws are used to achieve this goal (Fig. 16.10). Alar screws have been found to be much easier to introduce than S1 pedicular screws, and recent data have demonstrated almost equal pullout strength for the alar vs. the S1 pedicular screws (34). The DCP is bent to the proper lordosis and twisted externally approximately 30° to allow two screws to be placed into the sacral ala (Fig. 16.11). The 3.2-mm drill bit is used to pierce the cortex under the most caudal two plate holes. The drill is angled 30° caudally and 30° laterally. A 35-mm screw is usually satisfactory for the second to last hole, while the most caudal hole usually takes a 25-mm screw.

If a fracture requires reduction, either open manipulation of the spine or indirect reduction techniques using 5.0-mm pedicular Schanz screws and two femoral distractors are used (Fig. 16.12*A–E*). The rationale for the number of levels instrumented is similar to that of Roy-Camille (27). Burst fractures are instrumented two vertebra above and two below the fracture (Fig. 16.13*A–D*). Fracture-dislocations are instrumented one motion level above and one motion level below the injured interval (Fig. 16.14*A–C*). These guidelines are followed for ideal cases; however, at times, instrumentation levels

require modification due to contiguous vertebral fractures.

The DCP has a center hole interval of 16 mm and a center hole distance across the fracture blank of 25 mm. The average vertical distance between two adjacent pedicles (27) is 26 mm. Every other hole is, thus, usually used for adjacent vertebrae. At the fracture blank, consecutive holes are usually appropriate.

Image intensification or biplane roentgenograms are used to reconfirm placement of all screws. Posterior iliac crest bone graft is then placed over the transverse processes and facet joints after decortication has been performed. Postoperatively, a thoracolumbar-sacral orthosis (TLSO) is applied, and progressive sitting to 90° with the brace in place is allowed. A lateral roentgenogram is taken of the spine, and after confirmation of satisfactory alignment, the patient is allowed out of bed and progressive physical therapy is begun.

The technique for decompression and fusion for degenerative spondylosis is slightly different. Decompression and placement of the posterolateral bone graft is completed prior to beginning internal fixation. Wide exposure is completed by defining the lateral edge of the transverse processes and the lateral margins of the sacral ala. Large self-retaining retractors are imperative for good visualization of the posterior structures. The technique for decompression begins with partial resection of the inferior facets at the instrumented level with a gouge bilaterally (Fig. 16.15). The lamina, spinous processes, and interspinous ligaments are left intact. The ligamen-

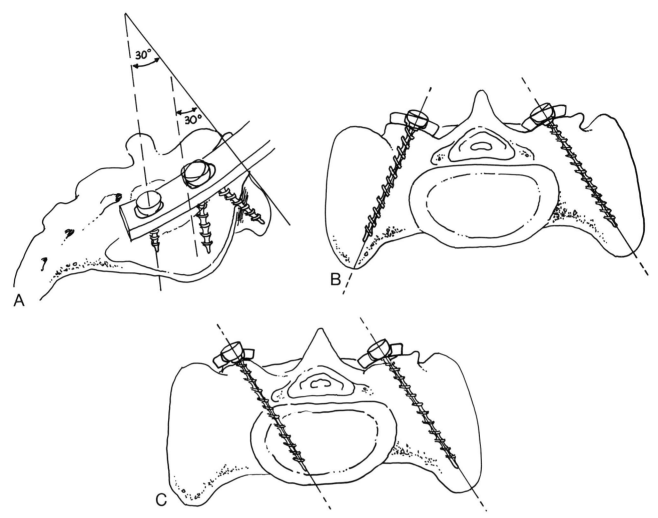

Figure 16.9. Sacral screw fixation. *A*, Lateral view of the S1 pedicle and alar screws. The cephalad hole depicts the difference between the S1 pedicle screw aiming toward the anterior corner of the promontory and the alar screw angled 30° caudad, parallel to the sacroiliac joint. The last hole is also fixed with a sacral alar screw. *B*, Top view of sacral alar screws aiming toward the anterior superior angle of the lateral mass of the sacrum. *C*, Top view of a sacral alar screw and an S1 pedicle screw. Note that the entry point of the alar screw is slightly medial to that of the pedicle screw.

tum flavum is then resected, permitting not only access to the spinal canal, neuroforamen, and intervertebral disc, but also direct visualization of the pedicle. A curved beaded probe may be easily passed cranially, caudally, and medially around the pedicles to give the surgeon a three-dimensional appreciation of that structure. Subsequent drilling and instrumentation of the pedicle can then be done under direct visualization. The cranial most segment is instrumented by using traditional landmarks, i.e., the line bisecting the transverse process and the laminar edge. Great care is taken to maintain the mechanical integrity of the apophyseal joint and capsule of the superior segment during plate and screw insertion.

Once the decompression is accomplished, the graft is harvested and placed on the transverse processes along the laminar edge of the segments to be instrumented. It is imperative that a meticulous fusion technique be used to ensure a rapid arthrodesis. Fresh frozen cortical cancellous allograft is also used to augment the fusion mass.

When the exposure, decompression, and arthrodesis have been completed, the osteosynthesis phase begins by unilateral cannulation of the pedicles with 2-mm guide pins. The depth of insertion is controlled by the Synthes drill guide with an adjustable stop. Radiographs are taken in the AP and lateral planes to check guide pin positions. Small corrections can be made when the pedicle is overdrilled with a 3.2-mm drill bit inserted through the stopped drill guide. The drilled pedicle is then checked

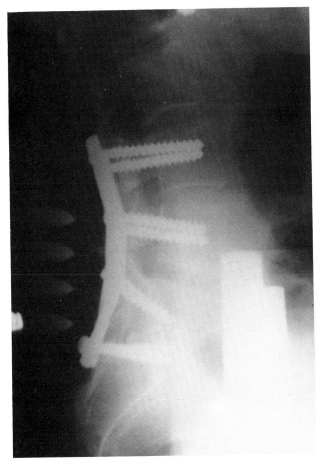

Figure 16.10. Lateral radiograph after placement of a narrow DC plate using Daneck-Rush modified screws in the instrumented pedicles. The narrow DC plates are targeted laterally, and the adjuvant sacral alar screws are placed at a 45° angle into the sacral ala.

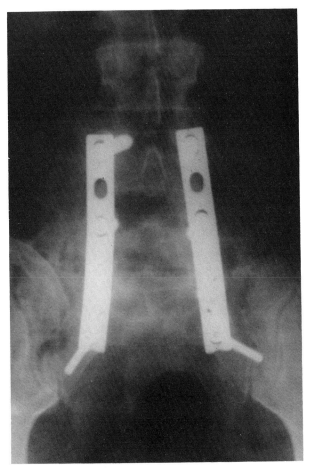

Figure 16.11. AP radiograph of an L4-sacrum fusion for a failed lumbar laminectomy syndrome. Note the orientation and position of the sacral alar screws.

with the AO large fragment depth gauge to ensure that there has been no violation of the pedicular cortical walls. The next step is plate selection and contouring. Generally, a 5-hole DCP is used for L4 to sacrum fusion and a 7-hole DCP for fusing L3 to the sacrum. The 2-mm guide pins are placed back in the 3.2-mm holes, and the appropriate length DCP is selected. The plate is then placed over the guide pins in the instrumented pedicles. The plate is contoured to fit the spine. This is done by using a Synthes plate bender and hand held bending irons for the DCPs. The goal is to fit the plates as closely as possible to the sagittal curvature of the spine in order to minimize stresses placed on the plate screw interface. Once the plate is appropriately contoured, the screws are inserted into the pedicles (Fig. 16.16*A* and *B*).

Sacral fixation is achieved as discussed above with alar and/or pedicle screws. If S1 pedicle fixation is desired, the S1 nerve root is found. This is quite easily seen after

the facets and the ligamentum flavum have been resected. The beaded probe is used to define the cranial and medial border of the first sacral pedicle. This is drilled with a 3.2-mm bit to a depth of approximately 25 mm. The appropriate-length 6.5-mm screw is snugly tightened into the S1 pedicle after the cranial segments are instrumented. A second method of achieving sacral fixation is with an S2 pedicle screw. This 6.5-mm cancellous screw is usually 25 mm long. The third manner of obtaining sacral purchase is by alar screws. One or two screws can be used by bending the caudal end of the plate 30° externally (laterally), as described above. These techniques allow multiple-point sacral fixation, which has been shown by Aebi to be superior to single-point, sacral fixation (1).

The careful, judicious use of methylmethacrylate to augment screw fixation in vertebral bodies and sacral pedicles can be safe if meticulous surgical technique is used (Fig. 16.17*A–C*). Once the plate and screws have been

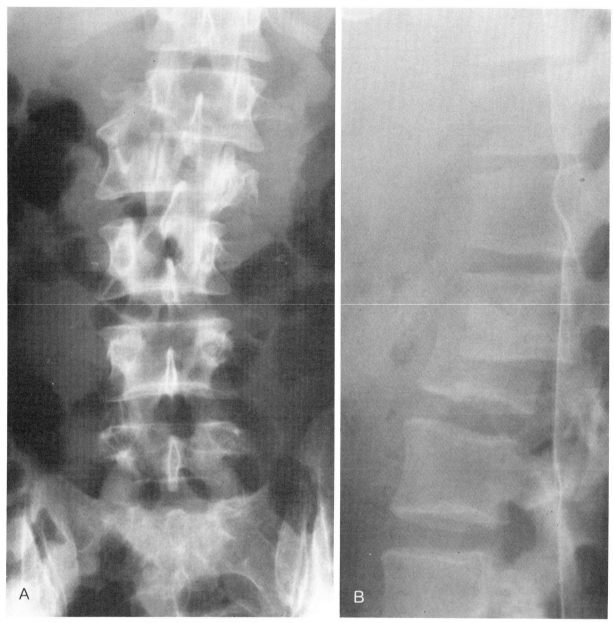

Figure 16.12. *A*, AP and *B*, lateral radiographs of an L1-L2 fracture dislocation. Using 5-mm pedicular Schanz screws and two femoral distractors an indirect reduction was performed

(*C*). *D*, AP and *E*, lateral radiographs showing the reduction and internal fixation.

applied to the spine and it is determined that a screw fixation is unsatisfactory, the undesirable screw may be removed singly, maintaining fixation in the other segments. The pedicle in question is then surrounded by pledgets and carefully probed with the AO depth gauge to ensure there are no violations of the pedicle's cortex. If there are no perforations found, the methylmethacrylate at 1-minute postmixing is loaded in a 5.0-ml syringe with an IV extension tubing cut obliquely. This is then

placed into the vertebral body past the pedicles, and the liquid cement is injected into the cancellous bone of the vertebral body and brought out through the pedicle. The screws are placed through the plate into the pedicle with careful observation that there has not been any violation of the methylmethacrylate into the spinal canal.

The final radiograph is taken after placement of the plates and screws. Prior to closure, the wound is irrigated with pulsed jet lavage. Drains are laid both deeply and

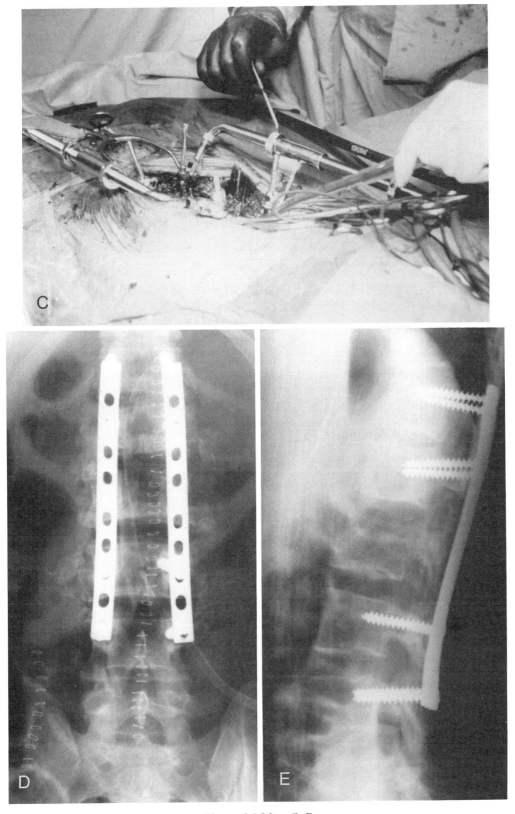

Figure 16.12. *C–E*

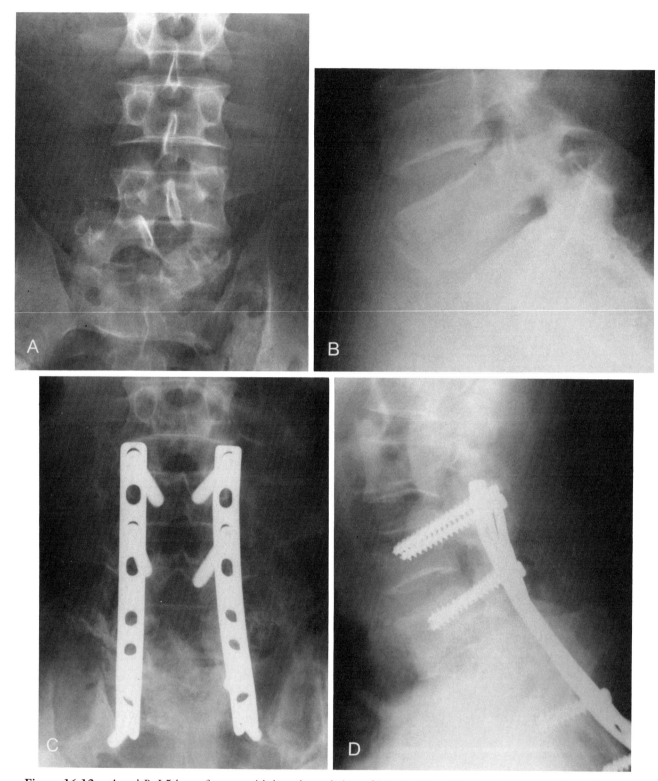

Figure 16.13. *A* and *B*, L5 burst fracture with lateral translation of L4. *C*, AP and *D*, lateral postoperative radiographs.

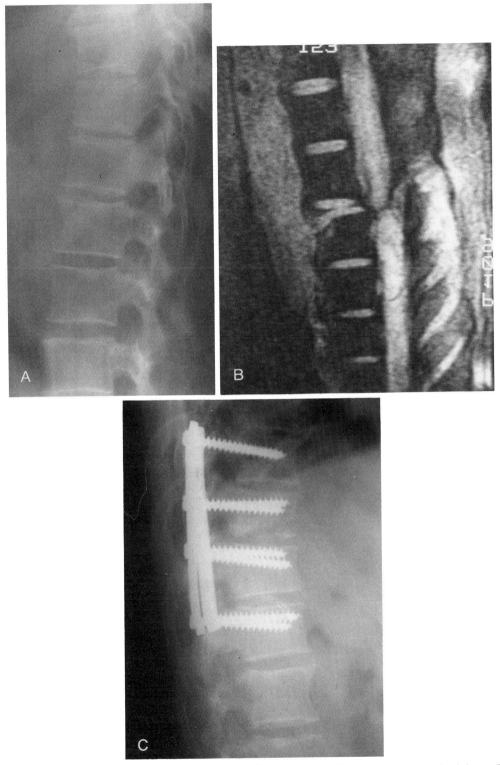

Figure 16.14. *A*, Lateral radiograph of a T11-T12 fracture-dislocation. *B*, MRI demonstrating the injury. *C*, Postoperative lateral radiograph.

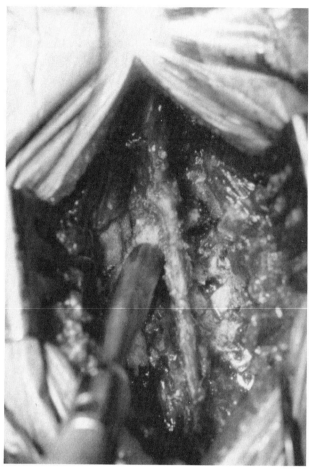

Figure 16.15. After a wide exposure is completed, the facets of the instrumented levels are amputated with a gouge. This allows access to the ligamentum flavum, pedicles, and lateral gutters of the instrumented segments.

subcutaneously. Prophylactic antibiotics are given immediately preoperatively and for 48 hours postoperatively. The patient is mobilized the first or second postoperative day in a lumbosacral orthosis. The brace is worn for at least 3 months, but the patient is allowed cautious exercise during this period. Rehabilitation is started with swimming pool exercises at 4–6 weeks and advanced to resistive exercises at 3 months. Bracing is terminated with radiographic evidence of union.

TREATMENT OF METASTATIC TUMORS

Surgical management of metastatic tumors of the spinal column has become more common with increased survivorship in this patient population. The advent of successful chemotherapy and radiotherapy has provided patients with metastatic disease a longer life span. These patients may have had unstable spines from erosion of the anterior and middle spinal columns from metastatic

disease. They are at risk for severe neurologic injury and intractable pain secondary to their instability. Many of these patients present with profound neurologic deficits and may be significantly helped with appropriate neurologic decompression and restoration of the load-bearing capability of the spinal column as well as reduction of their spinal deformity. Common locations for metastatic tumors to the spine are the anterior and middle columns of the vertebral body. These cannot be approached by classic laminectomy. This posterior approach for an anterior problem merely accentuates the instability and does not relieve the anterior compressive forces on the neural elements. The posterior approach alone allows the spine to further collapse into kyphosis, causing further anterior cord compression and worsening of the neurologic deficit. The anterior deformity and neural compression may be addressed by an anterior decompression, and restoration of the spinal column load-bearing capacity with a DCP methylmethacrylate construct. The tumor may be directly removed from the neural structures and the collapsed vertebral segments resected (Fig. 16.18A–C). The reconstruction is accomplished with a combination of methylmethacrylate and AO DC plates (23). The "rebar effect" may be obtained by the narrow DC plates, and the "mass effect" by methylmethacrylate across the defect.

The twin I-beam construct is obtained by placing a smaller plate across the defect anteriorly as far to the contralateral side as possible. A secondary larger plate is fixed to the structurally sound vertebral bodies above and below the defect. This essentially puts two plates in parallel across the segmental defect. These plates are then crosslinked with screws between the plates, and the outer plate is secured to the vertebral body above and below with 6.5-mm cancellous screws. Once this construct is completed, it is encased in polymethylmethacrylate. Care should be taken to protect the dural contents from methylmethacrylate while it is polymerizing. The heat of the polymerization process is not dangerous to the neural structures; however, a mass effect by leakage of the methylmethacrylate around the spinal cord may cause neural compression. This may be prevented by using a removable plastic sheet across the exposed neural structures. This rigid fixation construct allows immediate mobilization of the patient without any external braces.

Posterior instability and neural compression may also be symptomatic in this patient population. The posterior tumors may be addressed with radical posterior debridement of the tumor. A simultaneous posterior transpedicular spinal stabilization with narrow AO DC plates may be accomplished. This construct is then augmented with methylmethacrylate if stability is not optimal. This is a safe, rigid construct that also allows immediate mobilization of the patient without external support.

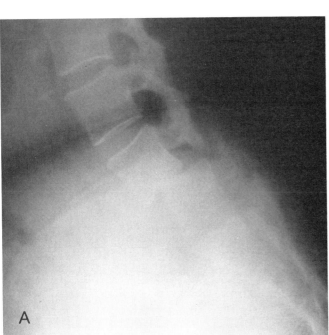
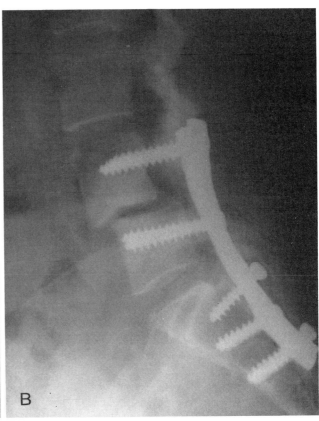

Figure 16.16. *A*, Preoperative lateral radiograph of a post-laminectomy intragenic grade II spondylolisthesis. *B*, Postoperative lateral radiograph demonstrating the partial reduction just from the internal fixation.

TREATMENT OF TRAUMATIC INJURIES

Acute fractures of the thoracic and lumbar spine treated with DCPs were evaluated in a prospective investigation (28). The indications for the procedure were unstable fracture dislocations below the 8th thoracic vertebra or low lumbar fractures that would be difficult to treat with conventional spinal implants. The patients were discharged home or to the regional spinal cord injury rehabilitation unit at an average of 12 days postoperatively. The mean number of levels instrumented was 3.3, and the mean number of levels fused was 3.3. The average operative time was 4.5 hours, and the average blood loss per procedure was 2,275 cc. There was no increase in neurologic deficit in any patient in this series. The Frankel functional classification showed nine patients had improved and 14 patients remained the same. The Lucas and Ducker Motor Index increased from a mean of 79.4% preoperatively to 85.5% at the most recent follow-up.

One patient developed an asymptomatic pseudarthrosis demonstrated by breakage of both plates through unfilled screw holes at the corresponding segment. The remainder of the patients developed solid fusion. One hundred and twenty pedicle screws were implanted in this series, and one screw failed. A total of 26 alar screws were placed, and one fractured. Both of these failures occurred in the asymptomatic pseudarthrosis prior to plate breakage. Other complications included one wound infection, one case of arachnoiditis after an intradural bone fragment was excised, and a dural tear created by a K-wire, which did not result in neurologic deficit or CSF leak.

Significant sagittal angular change occurred postoperatively to lessen the relative kyphosis (increased lordosis in the lumbar spine). At the 3-month follow-up measurements, however, the angles were not significantly different from their preoperative values. The reason for the return to the relative kyphotic deformity is likely due to the screw being able to toggle at the screw plate junction. The ramifications of a nonrigid screw plate interface will be reviewed in the discussion section.

TREATMENT OF DEGENERATIVE DISEASE

Thalgott, et al. reviewed a series of 46 North American patients who underwent reconstruction of the lumbar spine using the DCP and pedicle screws as augmentation

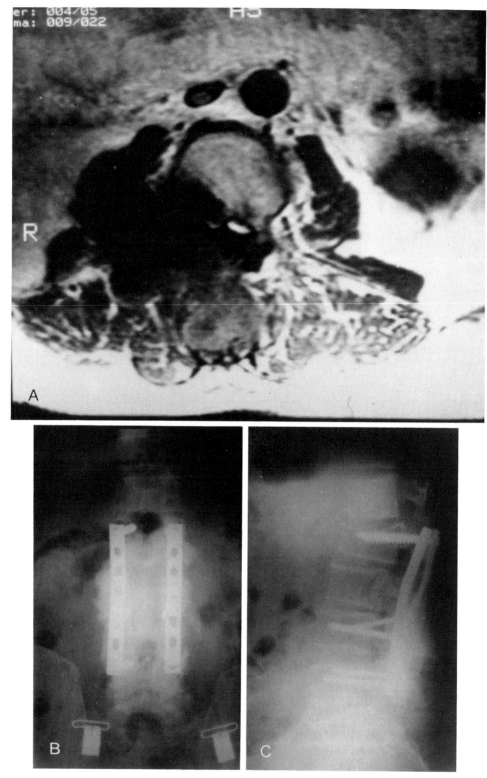

Figure 16.17. *A*, Sagittal MRI demonstrating posterolateral involvement with metastatic melanoma. *B*, AP and *C*, lateral radiographs after posterolateral decompression and stabilization with AO plates to the lumbar spine. The patient survived 8 months postoperatively, had excellent relief of his pain, and remained neurologically intact.

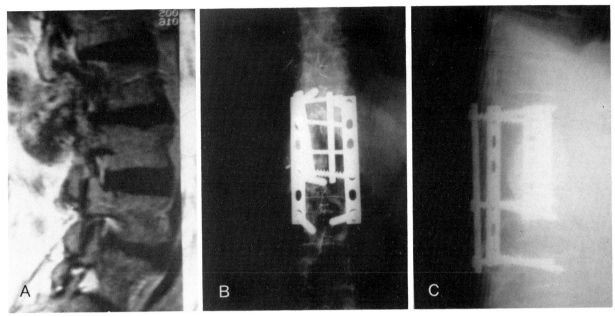

Figure 16.18. *A*, MRI demonstrating anterior and posterior involvement from metastatic renal cell carcinoma. The patient presented with a large back mass and profoundly paraparetic. *B*, AP and *C*, lateral radiographs after simultaneous anterior and posterior decompression and stabilization with AO plates and methylmethacrylate. The patient survived 6 months, neurologically improved, and had excellent relief of his pain.

of the lumbar fusion (31). The mean follow-up was 1.25 years. Thirty-one of the 46 patients had a prior lumbar spine surgery with poor outcomes, and 15 had no prior surgery. All were treated surgically for lumbar degenerative disease with decompression, internal fixation with AO plates, and fusion with autologous bone grafting posterolaterally. The results of surgery in 17 patients with failed interbody fusion included good to excellent pain relief in 59%, and solid fusion in 76%. In 14 patients with failed posterior surgery, the good to excellent pain relief rate was 79%, and the fusion rate was 86%. In 15 patients undergoing primary surgery, there was 89% good to excellent pain relief, and a solid fusion rate of 87%. The benefits resulting from augmentation of the fusion from internal fixation using DCPs were concluded to be positive.

Complications in this series included two early and one delayed wound infection, five cases of screw loosening, three cases of screw breakage (Fig. 16.19*A–B*), and three cases of screw impingement upon a nerve root (Fig. 16.20). The implant failure rate was calculated to be approximately 9%.

COMPLICATIONS

Complications encountered in using this device have been significantly reduced in subsequent series when compared with the early experience. This indicates the existence of a "learning curve" effect. The major disadvantages of any plate-screw system are its limited reduction capabilities, risk of vascular and neural injury, and reported high incidence of infection. The combined degenerative and traumatic series in these studies demonstrated an infection rate of 5.8%. This is in accordance with recent studies of pedicle screw plate fixation that report approximately a 6% incidence of postoperative infection (18,27,31,35). With the advent of modern instrumentation, the postoperative infection rate in spinal surgery has increased (19) and a rational method of treating postoperative infection after spinal instrumentation is necessary.

The principle of maintaining internal fixation in the face of sepsis has been well recognized for three decades. Moe (20) has upheld this concept in spinal surgery by showing that the maintenance of instrumentation and bone grafts in the presence of postoperative infection had no deleterious effect on the eventual outcome. It is recommended that the infection be managed without their removal. Thalgott, et al. (33), in a multicenter study that analyzed postoperative infections in spinal implants, found that the type of infection and the host defense mechanisms were both important in determining the clinical outcome. Their data demonstrated that single organism infections could generally be dealt with by a single irrigation and debridement, and closure over suction

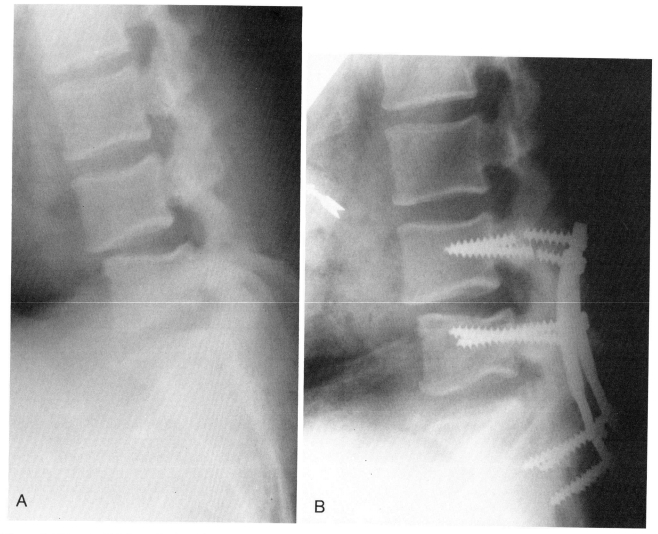

Figure 16.19. *A,* 300-lb professional body builder with an L4-L5 grade 1 spondylolisthesis. *B,* Postoperative lateral radiograph demonstrates screw breakage and eventual nonunion.

drainage tubes without the use of an inflow irrigation system. Multiple organism infections were found to require an average of three irrigation debridements. They had a higher percentage of successful closures with closed inflow-outflow suction irrigation systems when compared with simple suction drainage systems without constant inflow irrigation. Multiple organism infections with myonecrosis were exceedingly difficult to manage and resulted in poor outcomes. Patients without normal host defenses were found to be at high risk for developing postoperative wound infections. Specifically, cigarette smoking was found to be a significant factor.

Other complications included impingement of a nerve root secondary to a pedicle screw. This occurred in three out of 46 cases in the degenerative series. No vascular injuries occurred in either of the above traumatic or de-

generative series. One dural tear was created by a K-wire in the traumatic series. K-wires are no longer utilized in the delineation of the pedicle, and a pedicle finder is now routinely used. Krag has reviewed the pertinent literature (17) and does not believe a difference exists in pullout strengths of screws placed in holes prepared by a drill or a probe.

Radiographic evaluation of fusion in these patients is sometimes difficult because the fusion tends to occur under the plate, and resorption of the bone graft occurs laterally. However, many of these patients have been explored who have significant resorption and were found to have a solid arthrodesis below the plate (Fig. 16.21). Conversely, patients who were thought to have a solid fusion and were found to have a pseudarthrosis have been explored for other reasons. Great care must be taken when

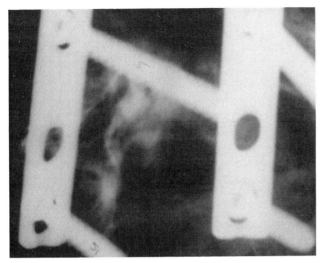

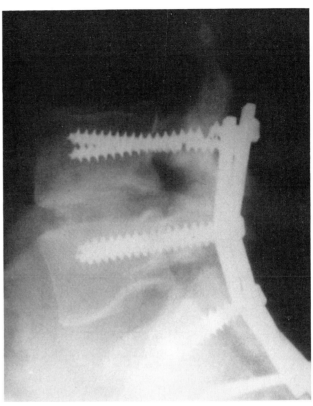

Figure 16.20. This is a selective nerve root block demonstrating screw violation of the L5 nerve root in a patient who had new L5 symptoms postoperatively. The patient's symptoms resolved after percutaneous removal of the L5 screw.

Figure 16.22. A 45-year-old businessman who underwent L4 to the sacrum fusion for grade 1 spondylolisthesis at L5-S1. The patient was quite active postoperatively and suffered broken screws at L4-L5 and underwent anterior interbody fusion at L4-L5 with excellent relief of his symptoms. This case clearly demonstrates the use of anterior interbody fusion in salvage of failed posterior fusions or instrumentation failure.

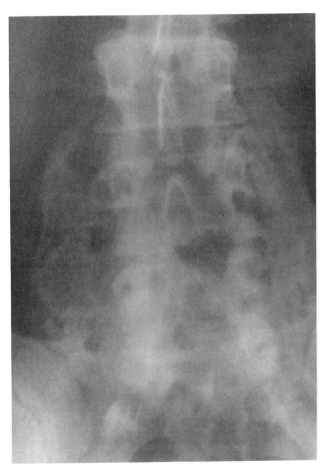

evaluating any reported fusion rate in the presence of transpedicular fixation. Anterior interbody fusions have been used successfully for salvage of pseudarthrosis of this transpedicular fixation (Fig. 16.22). A recent review of the DC plate in reconstruction of failed lumbar surgery (32) shows that three-level fusions require anterior interbody fusion (Fig. 16.23 *A* and *B*) secondary to graft resorption or implant failure in one-third of the cases. We are currently advocating for three-level fusions an anterior and posterior fusion as described by Kozak and O'Brien (16).

DISCUSSION

The advantages of this method include immediate stabilization of the lumbar spinal segments and the probability of a better mechanical milieu for arthrodesis. This method does not require the presence of lamina for fix-

Figure 16.21. The patient (see Fig. 16.11) is now 4 years postsurgery, plates removed, with excellent relief of his back and leg pain, and a solid fusion.

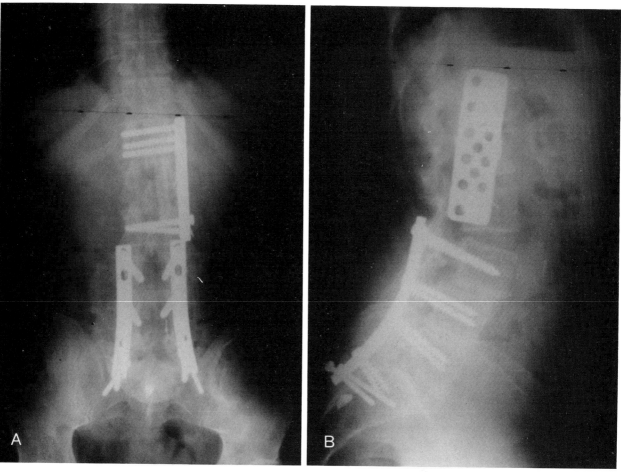

Figure 16.23. *A*, AP and *B*, lateral radiographs of a 46-year-old with a failed laminectomy syndrome that had a global fusion anteriorly and posteriorly 2 years before. The patient had excellent relief of his back pain, but still had some residual leg pain. The patient then lost control of his bowel and bladder approximately a year later, and was found to have a large herniated disc at T12-L1 with caudal migration along the L1 vertebral body. The patient underwent resection of the L1 vertebral body, decompression of his cauda equina, with excellent return of his bowel and bladder control.

ation nor does it necessarily violate the spinal canal. The fixation achieved by spinal plates is far more rigid than that provided by the traditional hook-rod systems of Harrington. AO 6.5-mm full-threaded cancellous screws provide good fixation in the pedicle, as demonstrated by Zindrick, et al. (34). Their study showed pullout strength is greater in fully threaded, as opposed to partially threaded screws, and that 6.5-mm screws are significantly stronger than 4.5-mm screws. With regard to sacral screw placement, Zindrick, et al. also found that bone-screw interface strengths of alar screws are greater than that of S1 pedicle (promontory) screws (34). Although conceptually the fixation of the spine with this device is in a neutralization mode that neutralizes torsional, shear, and bending forces, in reality, the posterior plate fixation acts similar to the mechanics of a long bone fracture with an "incomplete tension band." The spine clearly has a compression side and a tension side in the erect loaded

spinal column. The compression side of the spine is a composite structure that has an elastic disc component, and a compressed anterior body if a fracture complicates the picture. Implants placed across the intact disc space posteriorly behave similarly to a long bone fracture plated on the tension side without continuity of the compression side. This loads the plate-screw construct with a flexion moment. This is less stable than a construct loaded in tension with a stable compression side (21). These principles are time-honored mechanical constructs that were used and developed by the AO Group (21). It is based on an engineering principle first applied surgically by Pauwels (24). Theoretically, any posterior spinal plating with intact discs will always have a bending moment at the screw-plate interface. The "spinal-tension-band" (21, 31) can be completed only by the use of an anterior or posterior interbody fusion (Fig. 16.24*A–C*). This significantly increases the rigidity of the construct.

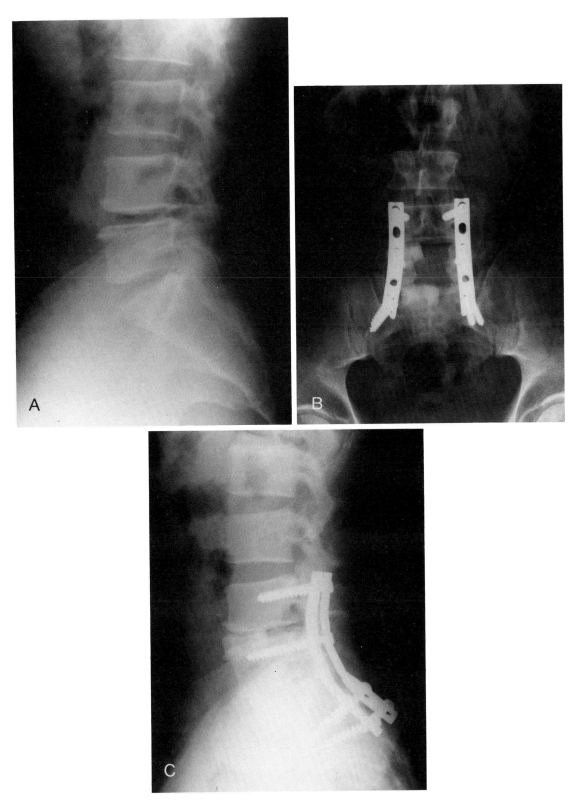

Figure 16.24. *A*, Lateral radiograph of a postlaminectomy failed back syndrome with back and leg pain. Note the L4-L5, L5-S1 disc space narrowing, L4-L5 traction spurs, and L4-L5 retrolisthesis. *B*, AP and *C*, lateral radiographs after a 360° decompression and fusion with the use of AO DC plates.

While performing anterior interbody fusions in patients with solid posterior fusions and intact instrumentation, there often is a great deal of motion in the disc space at the instrumented level. This confirms clinically that posterior immobilization, even with a solid arthrodesis radiographically, does not immobilize the disc space and therefore places flexion stresses across the posterior plate-screw implants. Kozak and O'Brien have found that simultaneous combined anterior and posterior fusion result in a higher fusion rate and recommend it for multilevel lumbar fusions and in the postlaminectomy patient (16).

Plate fixation has two basic types of mechanical design. The first is a cantilever loaded system in which the screw is rigidly fixed to the plate. This rigid type system was developed by Dr. Arthur Steffee of the United States. The second type is a nonrigid plate-screw interface (noncantilever loaded), pioneered by Roy-Camille and Louis with fixed interval hole plates. This has been modified by Dr. Eduardo Luque with a slotted plate. Both of these systems allow semirigid immobilization of the spine. The narrow tibial DC plate is well suited for transpedicular fixation of the spine using either cancellous or cortical screws. This is a noncantilever loaded construct that is clearly modeled after the Roy-Camille system. The AO system is one of the nonrigid type, and allows micromotion at the plate-screw junction. Biomechanically, it has been shown that the cantilever loaded systems are significantly more rigid than the noncantilever implants (21). The appropriate stiffness for facilitating optimal bony union, however, is unknown. Stiffer implants produce greater stress shielding and greater related osteopenia. Theoretically, the osteopenia will gradually remodel as resorption around the screws causes load shifting back to the bone graft mass (17). Stiffer implants also tolerate fewer load cycles before failure. The cantilever loaded systems have a reportedly high percentage of screw breakage (30).

Associated interbody fusions may be done simultaneously or at a second stage if the lateral fusion is unsatisfactory or if the fixation is deteriorating, as indicated by screw breakage, loosening, or other evidence of failure. Posterior plating may also be done to salvage pseudarthrosis of interbody fusion attempts by completing the tension band and providing a more stable, mechanical construct for fusion to occur.

In injuries that sustain significant compression of the anterior vertebral body, a void remains after posterior reduction and internal fixation due to compressed cancellous bone, as occurs in the metaphysis of the tibial plateau and in pilon fractures. The posterior fixation device thus acts as a tension band. However, since the compression side is not structurally intact, the device is loaded with significant bending forces. Since the screw is allowed to toggle within the limits of the screw hole, slow loss of initial postoperative correction may occur as the patient assumes a vertical posture, thereby loading the tension band device. The importance of these phenomena is uncertain, but initial results are encouraging, with a greater than 95% arthrodesis rate using DCPs and pedicle screws in low thoracic and lumbar fractures. The long-term effect of increased relative kyphosis (decreased lordosis) in the lumbar spine may prove to cause increased incidence of degenerative spondylosis in the future. The advantage of pedicle screw plating is particularly significant in the lower lumbar spine where restoration of lordosis is necessary and preservation of motion is optimal. The advantages of plate-screw fixation (Fig. 16.25) over Harrington rod or Harri-Luque (Fig. 16.26) fixation are that it provides a more rigid construction, does not require the presence of lamina, does not violate the spinal canal, and requires only light postoperative brace immobilization. The DCPs are better able to restore lumbar lordosis and maintain the lordosis postoperatively.

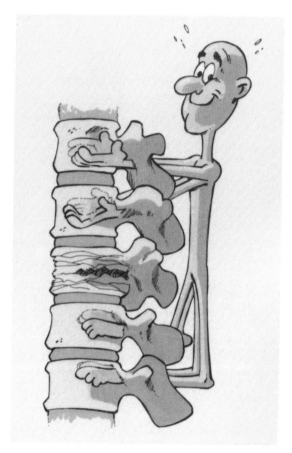

Figure 16.25. Screw-plate fixation demonstrating biomechanical advantages.

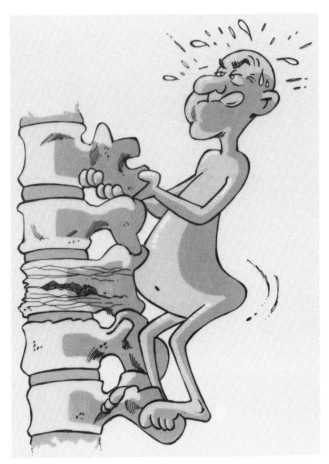

Figure 16.26. Harrington rod fixation demonstrating biomechanical disadvantages.

This technique will not reduce a retropulsed fragment of a burst fracture. If the patient has a complete neurologic deficit, then this is inconsequential, and the fixation is done only for restoration of the spinal column anatomy and stability. In neurologically intact patients, no problems with progression of neurologic deficit using this technique have been encountered. In a patient with a burst fracture and a partial neurologic deficit, an anterior decompression and strut graft may be performed if this technique is employed posteriorly. Anterior stabilization can be obtained with the broad (femoral) DCP. Bone (6) reported this technique to have a low screw breakage and plate failure rate.

SUMMARY

The AO instrumentation described has proven to be a valuable adjunct in attaining fusion of the lumbar spine. The implants are readily available in all centers equipped with AO large fragment sets. This is an extremely demanding procedure, however, and if used, must be lim-

ited to those surgeons who have specific training in transpedicular fixation along with extensive experience in spinal surgery.

REFERENCES

1. Aebi M, Etter C, Schläpfer F, et al: Biomechanical evaluation of a modified internal fixator for the lumbosacral junction. AO Grant Paper. 35th Annual Meeting of Orthopaedic Research Society, Las Vegas, Nevada, February 6–9, 1989.
2. Aebi M, Etter C, Kehl T, et al: Stabilization of the lower thoracic and lumbar spine with the internal spinal skeletal fixation system. Spine 1987;12:544–551.
3. Ashman RB, Calpin RD, Corin JD, et al: Biomechanical analysis of pedicle screw instrumentation systems in a corpectomy model. Spine 1989;14:1398.
4. Banta CJ, King AG, Dabezies EJ, et al: Measurement of effective pedicle diameter in the human spine. Orthopaedics 1989;12:939–942.
5. Blauth M, Tscherne H: Therapeutic concept and results of operative treatment in acute trauma of the thoracic and lumbar spine. The Hanover experience. J Orthop Trauma 1987;1:240–252.
6. Bone LB, Johnston CE, Ashman RB, et al: Mechanical comparison of anterior spinal instrumentation in a burst fracture model. J Orthop Trauma 1988;3:362; J Orthop Trauma 2:195–201.
7. Boucher HH: A method of spinal fusion. J Bone Joint Surg 1959;41B:248–259.
8. Daniaux H, Seykora P, Genelin A, et al: Application of posterior plating and modifications in thoracolumbar spine injuries. Indications, techniques, and results. Spine 1991;16:S125–S133.
9. Denis F: Spinal instability as defined by a three-column spine conception in acute spinal trauma. Clin Orthop 1984;189:65–76.
10. Dickson JH, Harrington PR, Erwin WD: Results of reduction and stabilization of the severely fractured thoracic and lumbar spine. J Bone Joint Surg 1978;60A:799–805.
11. Flesch JR, Leider LL, Erickson DL, et al: Harrington instrumentation and spine fusion for unstable fractures and fracture-dislocations of the thoracic and lumbar spine. J Bone Joint Surg 1977;59A:143–153.
12. Goel VK, Lim TH, Gwon J, et al: Effects of rigidity of an internal fixation device. A comprehensive biomechanical investigation. Spine 1991;16:S155–S161.
13. Haas N, Blauth M, Tscherne H: Anterior plating in thoracolumbar spine injuries. Indications, technique, and results. Spine 1991;16:S100–S111.
14. Hall DJ, Webb JK: Anterior plate fixation in spine tumor surgery. Indications, technique, and results. Spine 1991;16:580–583.
15. Jacobs RR, Asher MA, Snider RK: Thoracolumbar spinal injuries: a comparative study of recumbent and operative treatment in 100 patients. Spine 1980;5:463–477.
16. Kozak JA, O'Brien JP: Simultaneous combined anterior and posterior fusion: an independent analysis of a treatment for the disabled low back pain patient. Spine 1990;15:322–328.
17. Krag MH: Biomechanics of thoracolumbar spinal fixation. A review. Spine 1991;16:584–597.
18. Louis R: Fusion of the lumbar and sacral spine by internal fixation. Clin Orthop 1986;203:18–33.
19. Micheli LJ, Hall JE: Complications in the management of adult spinal deformities. In: Epps CH Jr, ed. Complications in orthopaedic surgery. 2nd ed., vol 2. Philadelphia: JB Lippincott 1986;1227–1229.
20. Moe JH: Complications of scoliosis treatment. Clin Orthop 1967;53:21–30.

21. Muller ME, Allgower M, Schneider R, et al: Manual of internal fixation. 3rd ed. Berlin: Springer-Verlag, 1991;627–682.

22. O'Brien JP, Dawson HO, Heard W, et al: Simultaneous combined anterior and posterior fusion. A surgical solution for failed spinal surgery with brief review of the first 150 patients. Clin Orthop 1986;203:191–195.

23. O'Neill J, Gardner V, Armstrong G: Treatment of tumors of the thoracic and lumbar spine column. Clin Orthop 1988;227:103–112.

24. Pauwels F: Der schenkelhalsbruch, em mechanisches problem, 25, Enke, Stuttgart, 1935.

25. Ransom N, LaRocca HS, Thalgott JS: Comparative results of three posterolateral lumbosacral arthrodesis techniques: no instrumentation, sublaminar wiring and AO intrapedicular screw-plate fixation. Paper Presentation, Amer Academy Orthop Surg, New Orleans, 1990.

26. Roy-Camille R, Salliant G, Berteaux D, et al: Osteosynthesis and thoracolumbar spine fractures. Metal plates screwed through the vertebral pedicles. Reconst Surg Traumatol 1976;15:2–16.

27. Roy-Camille R, Salliant G, Mazel C: Internal fixation of the lumbar spine with pedicle screw plating. Clin Orthop 1986;203:7–27.

28. Sasso RC, Cotler HB, Reuben JD: Posterior fixation of thoracic and lumbar spine fractures using DC plates and pedicle screws. Spine 1991;16:5134–5139.

29. Schläpfer F, Wörsdörfer O, Magerl F, et al: Stabilization of the lower thoracic and lumbar spine: comparative invitro investigation of external skeletal and various internal fixation systems. In: Uhthoff HK, ed. Current concepts of external fixation of fractures. Berlin: Springer-Verlag 1982;367–380.

30. Steffee AD, Biscup RS, Sitakowski DJ: Segmental spine plates with pedicle screw fixation. A new internal fixation device for disorders of the lumbar and thoracolumbar spine. Clin Orthop 1986;203:45–53.

31. Thalgott JS, LaRocca HS, Aebi M, et al: Reconstruction of the lumbar spine using AO DCP plate internal fixation. Spine 1989;14:91–95.

32. Thalgott JS, LaRocca HS, Gardner V, et al: Reconstruction of failed lumbar surgery using narrow AO DCP plates for spinal arthrodesis. Spine 1991;16:S170–S175.

33. Thalgott JS, Cotler HB, Sasso RC, et al: Postoperative infections in spinal implants: classification and analysis; A multicenter study. Spine (In press), 1991.

34. Zindrick MR, Wiltse LL, Widell EH, et al: A biomechanical study of intrapedicular screw fixation of the lumbosacral spine. Clin Orthop 1986;203:99–112.

35. Zuchermann J, Hsu K, White A, et al: Early results of spinal fusion using variable spine plating system. Spine 1988;13:570–579.

SEVENTEEN

The Puno-Winter-Byrd (PWB) Spinal System for Transpedicular Fixation of the Lumbar Spine

Rolando M. Puno and J. Abbott Byrd, III

INTRODUCTION

Providing stability to the spine by achieving arthrodesis has been practiced since the turn of the century. Hibbs (31) and Albee (2) in separate publications in 1911 described the technique for surgical fusion as a treatment for tuberculosis involving the spine. Since then, other fusion methods have been developed and used for the treatment of a wide variety of spinal disorders (10,12,14,16,17,23,24,27,32,34,42,55,73,78–81,86–89,95), including those of the lumbar and lumbosacral area. However, a high incidence of nonunion following an attempted lumbar and lumbosacral arthrodesis remains a major problem (1,13,18,33,82). Factors that contribute to the development of pseudarthrosis include the presence of spondylolisthesis (23,78,83), fusion involving two or more motion segments (72,78,79,83,87,96), a history of previous laminectomy (1,72,78), the presence of an existing pseudarthrosis (72), cigarette smoking (11), and the absence of a suitable internal fixation (71).

It is a well-known fact that immobilization has a positive effect on bone healing and is based on the extensive experience of orthopaedic surgeons in the treatment of extremity fractures. It is reasonable then to apply the same principles to the spine. Spinal immobilization may be achieved by external immobilization, internal fixation, or both. Unfortunately, external immobilization is somewhat ineffective in providing stability to the spine, especially at the lumbosacral junction. Surgeons have attempted to address this problem by developing methods of internal fixation of the spine (43). Increased interest in internal fixation of the spine has led to the development of a wide variety of devices. Implant configurations have included screw fixation of the facet joints and/or lamina (24,35,36,38,59,84), rod and hook systems (7,21,28,29,37,70,75,85,91,97), springs (6,77,

90), spinous process plates (15,63,74,90,93,94), and segmental fixation by either sublaminar wires (46–48) or spinous process wires (19,20). Segmental fixation using sublaminar wires has been shown to provide a higher degree of stability when compared with previously described hook and rod systems (25,38,46,61). However, this technique is dependent upon the presence of the lamina for fixation and therefore not applicable for laminectomized patients who often require fusion of the lumbar or lumbosacral spine. Attempts to develop segmental instrumentation for the laminectomized spine led to the development of transpedicular fixation because it is not dependent on the presence of the posterior neural arch. Although the ilium has been used for added fixation, it has the disadvantage of crossing the sacroiliac joint (3,25,48).

Although popular in Europe for many years, a wave of enthusiasm for transpedicular fixation of the spine swept through North America during the 1980s. While technically demanding, the advantages of pedicle screw fixation have become readily apparent to a growing number of surgeons. It is a technique that allows the surgeon to thoroughly decompress the neural elements by the removal of the spinous processes, lamina, and even facet joints and pars interarticularis, if necessary. At the same time, immediate stability to the spine via transpedicular screw fixation is provided (25). The earlier transpedicular fixation systems are primarily of the plate type (30,44, 45,64–68) and are satisfactory for some patients. However, difficulty is encountered if contouring is required to accommodate both sagittal (lordosis) and coronal (scoliosis) curvatures. In addition, the transverse dimension of the available plates limits the space available for the application of bone graft. Transpedicular external fixation has been also designed and used for fractures (50) and for temporary fixation as a diagnostic test for lumbosacral instability (57). However, the problems of protrusion of the device, pin tract infection, and potential for accidental penetration of the screw through the anterior cortex of the vertebral body make the device very unappealing (41).

The problems described led us, in 1984, to begin the development of a new pedicle screw system. The Puno-Winter-Byrd (PWB) pedicle screw system is a rod and screw transpedicular fixation device designed to provide immediate mechanical stability to the instrumented spinal segments while bony fusion is taking place. Like any spinal instrumentation system, it is used as an adjunct to the surgical fusion technique. It must be remembered that the primary goal of surgery is to produce a solid fusion, and the device should not be used as a substitute for meticulous technique in the arthrodesis procedure.

RATIONALE FOR THE PWB SYSTEM

We believe that the following criteria should be met to constitute an ideal spinal implant. First, the implant should be applicable to patients with spinal abnormalities in both the sagittal and coronal planes. Second, the implant should provide a reasonable degree of stability to the spine, yet have features that act to decrease the stress at the bone-implant interface, which theoretically should prevent stress shielding. Third, the device should be small enough to allow adequate room for placement of bone graft material. Finally, the method of implantation should be simple, thereby minimizing the risk to the patient.

The need for the preservation of normal lumbar lordosis demands that a spinal implant be contoured in the sagittal plane. However, the presence of degenerative scoliosis or degenerative lateral translation at the lumbar area often requires that the device be contoured in the coronal plane as well. Recognizing the difficulty of contouring a plate system in two planes led us to the use of a screw-rod system to address both the sagittal and coronal plane requirements of instrumenting the lumbar spine.

The purpose of all spinal fixation systems is to provide an optimum degree of stability to the instrumented spine to enhance the success rate for obtaining a solid fusion. However, there are no data available to prove exactly what is the optimum degree of rigidity. Historically, spinal fixation systems have had as their goal total rigidity with the thought that this would best enhance solid fusion. On the other hand, it is known from experience with long bone fractures that rigidly fixed fractures often produce less abundant callous than those fractures treated in a cast, which allows some degree of fracture motion. This would suggest that totally rigid spinal fixation may not be necessary to provide the optimum milieu for a solid fusion (56). In addition, totally rigid pedicle screw fixation of the lumbar spine can create potential problems

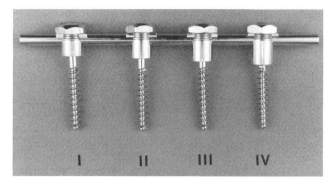

Figure 17.1. Final implant design (PWB II). The seats come in four heights (Types I–IV, from left to right).

such as a loosening at the bone-screw interface, especially in osteopenic bone (49), screw breakage (92), and stress shielding (53,76). With these problems in mind, the PWB pedicle screw system was developed to allow for micromotion between the screw and the rod via the use of a special coupling device. The micromotion produces a "shock absorber" effect to decrease the stress concentration at both the bone-screw interface and screw-rod interface, which then enhances load sharing between the device and the bone.

Finally, the PWB pedicle screw system was designed to simplify implantation. The system has only six components. It also utilizes standard implantation techniques, which will be described in full detail later in the chapter.

As the PWB transpedicular system evolved, several design changes were made in an attempt to satisfy the aforementioned criteria. The final implant system (Fig. 17.1) resulted from five prototype designs (Figs. 17.2 and 17.3).

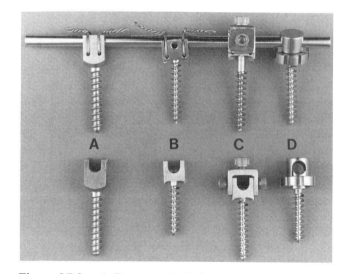

Figure 17.2. *A,* Prototype 1. *B,* Prototype 2. *C,* Prototype 3. *D,* Prototype 4.

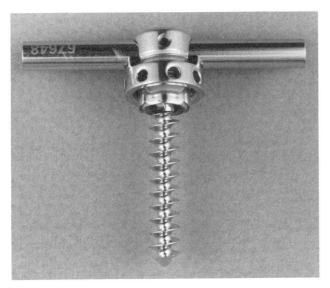

Figure 17.3. Streamlined version of Prototype 4 (PWB I).

BIOMECHANICAL STUDIES

The biomechanical study (62) was initiated for the purpose of testing the mechanical properties of a new transpedicular instrumentation for the lumbar and lumbosacral spine. During the course of the study, different designs were studied and compared with other implants available (i.e., Luque ring, Luque-Galveston, and Steffee plate). Mechanical testing was performed using a universal testing machine (MTS) with axial and torsional capabilities to produce test loads on the specimen. The maximum loads and moments used in the testing were determined through a pilot test using formalin-fixed spines. Additional information was also obtained in the evaluation of different testing techniques. The specimens were tested in axial load, flexion, lateral bending, extension, and torsion. The maximum loads

(axial load: 450 N, bending moment: 31.2 Nm, torque: 11.2 Nm) were considered nondestructive. The tests were initially done using plastic spine models to provide anatomic simulation for fixation attachment. These models also allowed the investigators to compare different implant configurations using specimens of essentially the same mechanical characteristics, thereby minimizing interspecimen variability.

Tests were also performed using fresh cadaver spines. Biomechanical testing was initially performed only on uninstrumented specimens. The specimens were then instrumented and tested with the devices implanted, using the same test regimen as previously described for the plastic models. In an effort to offset interspecimen variability, the rigidity of its implant configuration was calculated based on the percentage change in the amount of energy absorbed from the results gathered from uninstrumented intact spines.

Prior to testing the plastic models and fresh cadaver specimens, the stiffness of the plate and rod were compared by performing a three-point bending test, resulting in some estimates on how the working portions of the instrumentation compared mechanically. The test showed that the Steffee plate was 230% stiffer than the 0.25″ rod in the sagittal plane and 700% stiffer in the coronal plane. When used to instrument the model spines, there appeared to be corresponding differences in the rigidity between the plate and rod-based implants (Table 17.1). The Steffee plate with S2 fixation was the most rigid system (with the least amount of energy absorbed), while the Luque-Galveston was the most flexible. However, a dramatic decrease in rigidity with the plate system was noted when the S2 fixation was removed.

The rigidity exhibited by the new device (Fig. 17.2C: Prototype 3) was intermediate between the wired implants and the plate. Neither approached the rigidity of the Steffee plate with S2 fixation, but both were more

Table 17.1.
Energy Absorbed in Model Spines[a]

	Axial (Nn × 100)	Flexion (Nm × deg.)	Lat. Flex. (Nm × deg.)[b]	Extension (Nm × deg.)	Torsion[c] (Nm × deg.)
Luq-Gal	67.8	264.5	*	**	107.8
Luque Ring	60.3	171.1	294.1	326.0	40.5
Prototype 1	70.6	193.0	***	303.4	70.6
Prototype 2	38.1	111.8	157.7	122.7	24.8
Steffee w/ S2	28.3	110.8	58.5	120.8	13.1
Steffee w/o S2	45.2	337.5	120.5	127.3	17.5

[a]Reprinted with modification from Puno RM, Bechtold JE, Byrd JA, et al: Biomechanical analysis of transpedicular rod systems. A preliminary report. Spine, In press.
[b]* means unable to sustain moments greater than 2.64 Nm; ** means unable to sustain moments greater than 12.97 Nm; *** means unable to sustain moments greater than 10.81 Nm.
[c]Values recorded represent energy absorbed (area under the curve) by the system at set maximum loads or moments (Axial load = 450; Bending = 31.2 Nm; Torque = 11.2 Nm).

rigid than the Steffee plate without S2 fixation in compression and anterior bending. The wired implant (Fig. 17.2B: Prototype 2) exhibited less rigidity with greater energy absorbed by the system on practically all the test modes when compared with its clamped counterpart (Fig. 17.2C: Prototype 3).

When comparing cadaveric and plastic spines, similar trends in mean absorbed energy were seen. However, the observed differences in the mean values for the five implant configurations (Luque ring, Luque-Galveston, Steffee plate with and without S2 fixation, and Prototype 4) tested were not statistically significant ($p > 0.05$) for compression and bending test modes. In contrast, under torsional loading, the Luque-Galveston was significantly less rigid than the Luque ring ($p < 0.05$) and both of these wired implants were significantly less rigid ($p < 0.05$) than the pedicle screw systems (Prototype 4 and Steffee plate). The PWB 1 (Fig. 17.3) is a streamlined version of Prototype 4 and was used in patients as part of a prospective clinical trial. During the course of the study, the design was revised to the current design configuration (Fig. 17.1), where the tightening nut is applied from the top of the rod rather than below for easier application during surgery. However, the mode of clamping was not altered, making the first and second versions of the final implant mechanically equivalent.

Crosslinking two longitudinal spinal rods has been shown to increase torsional stiffness (5). In a previous study on anterior spinal fixation (60) by one of the authors (RMP), instrumented plastic models showed increased torsional stiffness to 255% when one crossbar was used and 318% with two crossbars. Testing of the crosslink device in fresh cadaveric spine specimens showed a commensurate increase in torsional stiffness to 150% and 195% with one and two crossbars, respectively.

INDICATIONS

The PWB pedicle screw system was developed for internal fixation of the lumbar and lumbosacral spine in order to provide stability while fusion is taking place. The principal indications for its use include those situations requiring surgery from instability or potential instability of the lumbar and lumbosacral spine. Controversy still exists regarding the definition of instability as well as the identification of patients who will or will not benefit from lumbar spinal surgery. Specific indications for implantation of the PWB pedicle screw system include spondylolisthesis, potential instability following lumbar decompression, degenerative lumbar scoliosis, degenerative disc disease, pseudarthrosis from previous failed sur-

gery, as well as fractures and tumors of the lumbar spine requiring surgical treatment for stabilization.

There are no contraindications specific to the PWB pedicle screw system, though there are certain relative contraindications specific to the use of pedicle fixation. These include a history of recent spine infection, severe osteopenia or bony abnormalities preventing secure screw purchase, metal sensitivity, or where fusion is expected to successfully occur without internal fixation. However, as in all surgical procedures, the final decision regarding the use of pedicle screw fixation rests with the surgeon.

MORPHOMETRY OF THE PEDICLE

The introduction of newer technology in the treatment of patients has led surgeons to continually add new techniques to their armamentarium. Transpedicular instrumentation of the spine is an example and has proven to be of value, as evidenced by the increasing acceptance of this type of fixation in North America and the rest of the world. However, experience has shown that this technique is a demanding procedure because of the low tolerance for error when placing the screws in the pedicle.

This section will deal with the important anatomic and technical considerations related to this new technique of fixation. Several authors have addressed this issue (8,9,40,58,69,99). Salliant (69) in 1976 reported some of the first data regarding different dimensions of pedicle anatomy as they relate to its use in transpedicular screw fixation. His reports consisted of mean values of both transverse and sagittal diameters, pedicle direction in relation to the sagittal plane, and distance between the entry point of the screw (posterior aspect of the laminar cortex) and the anterior cortex of the vertebral body. The latter was based on screws directed ("straight-ahead" insertion) parallel to the sagittal plane, not necessarily following the axis of the pedicle. This technique has the disadvantage of having a shorter length for screw purchase and at the same time provides a smaller effective diameter if the direction of the screw is not in line with the axis of the pedicle.

Krag et al. (40) gave a more detailed description of the morphometry of the vertebral anatomy for use in transpedicular fixation between T9 and L5. Their study showed a good correlation between measurements obtained by CT scan and the ones by direct caliper measurements of the specimens. Their findings were similar to that of Salliant (69), except for the amount of angulation of the pedicles. They attributed this to the fact that the measurement of the pedicle angle was a less explicitly defined measurement in their study. They found that screws of 5–7 mm are compatible with the anatomic constraints, especially of the lower lumbar area. They also found that the transverse diameter of the pedicle is not significantly affected by the direction of the screw insertion. However, other factors such as length of acceptable penetration and mechanical characteristics of the bone-screw interface are affected by the direction of screw insertion. This will be discussed in more detail later.

Zindrick et al. (99) have extended the previous study, and their analysis includes all of the thoracic and lumbar spine. Their data are in close agreement with other published data (9,40,69).

Olsewski et al. (58) has taken it one step further and compared pedicle dimensions between males and females and found a substantial difference. Their measurements are compared with previously published reports and are exhibited in Figures 17.4–17.8. As shown, there is a stepwise increase in size from the 1st through the 5th lumbar vertebrae, but the mean transverse and sagittal diameters for males in their study were consistently larger in the earlier studies where males and females were combined in the analysis. The transverse and sagittal angles in their study were quite similar for both sexes. This means that the pedicle architecture between males and females is essentially the same. Clinically, this means that the technique of implantation for males and females is

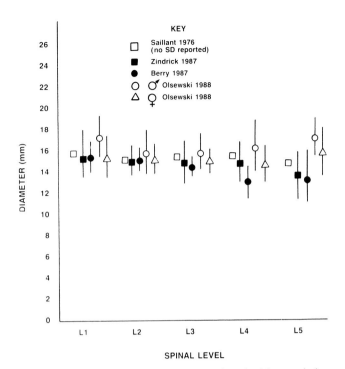

Figure 17.5. Sagittal diameters. (Reprinted with permission from Olsewski JM, Simmons EH, Kallen FC, et al: Morphometry of the lumbar spine: Anatomical perspectives related to transpedicular fixation. J Bone Joint Surg 1990;72:541–549.)

essentially the same, but attention should be directed to the differences in their sizes.

All the aforementioned studies dealt with the measurement of the outside diameter of the pedicle. Banta et al. (8) stressed the importance of the effective pedicle diameter (EPD), which they defined as the maximal cancellous diameter available for screw placement within the pedicle without the risk of blowout fracture or cutting through the cortex. They measured 16 cadaveric spines from T6-L5 and found a graduated mean increase in the EPD ranging from 4.8 mm at T6 to 5.9 mm at L5. These measurements were found to be significantly smaller than previously reported (9,40,69,99) outside diameters of the pedicles. They report that the best possible fixation can be achieved by the largest fully threaded screw which fits the pedicle entirely, thus making the effective pedicle diameter of considerable importance when choosing the screw. This is supported by other studies showing that the major factors in screw design affecting pull-out strength are the major diameter of the screw, with the larger diameter screw achieving better fixation (45,66,98), and fully threading the screws (98). In theory, it would be ideal to have the screw occupy the entirety of the EPD to maximize fixation. However, this would mean that each particular pedicle would have to

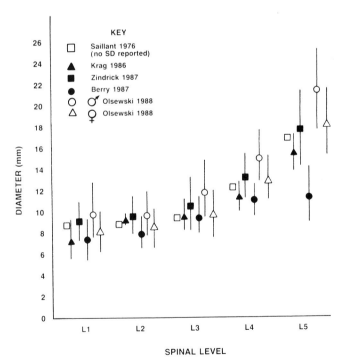

Figure 17.4. Transverse diameters. (Reprinted from Olsewski JM, Simmons EH, Kallen FC, Mendel FC, Severin CM, Berens DL: Morphometry of the lumbar spine: Anatomical perspectives related to transpedicular fixation. J Bone Joint Surg 1990;72:541–549.)

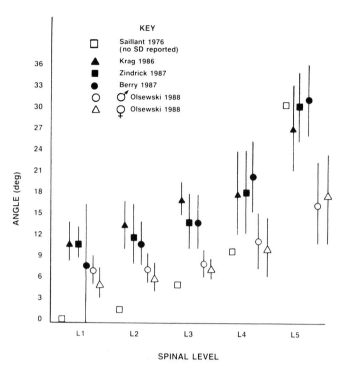

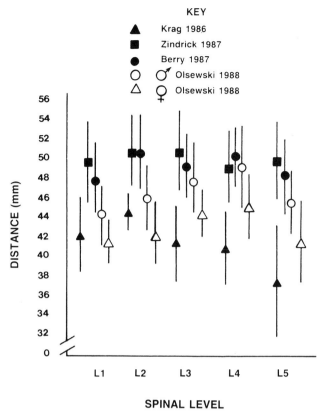

Figure 17.6. Transverse angles. (Reprinted with permission from Olsewski JM, Simmons EH, Kallen FC, et al: Morphometry of the lumbar spine: Anatomical perspectives related to transpedicular fixation. J Bone Joint Surg 1990;72:541–549.)

Figure 17.8. Distance from the posterior aspect of the laminar cortex to the anterior cortex of the vertebral body along the pedicle axis. (Reprinted with permission from Olsewski JM, Simmons EH, Kallen FC, et al: Morphometry of the lumbar spine: Anatomical perspectives related to transpedicular fixation. J Bone Joint Surg 1990;72:541–549.)

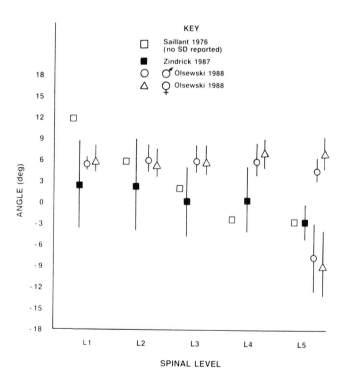

Figure 17.7. Sagittal angles. (Reprinted with permission from Olsewski JM, Simmons EH, Kallen FC, et al: Morphometry of the lumbar spine: Anatomical perspectives related to transpedicular fixation. J Bone Joint Surg 1990;72:541–549.)

have a specific size screw. In practice, it would be difficult to carry out. In our experience, a screw with an outside diameter of 6.5 mm is adequate for most adult lumbar pedicles.

As discussed in this section, the most important dimensions for pedicle fixation are those of the pedicle diameter, the amount of bony purchase, and the degree of angulation by which the screw was inserted. Pedicle diameter is important because it limits the screw diameter, consequently limiting the inherent strength of the screw (40). In addition to the quality of the host bone, the diameter and length of the screw determine the strength of the bone-screw interface. As substantiated in laboratory testing (39,98), screws inserted deeper and at an angle in relation to the sagittal plane performed better in static pullout testing and cyclic loading. In surgery, medially directed screws have the added advantage of decreasing the blind spot (distance between the screw tip and the anterior cortex) encountered on lateral radiography during screw insertion (99). It should be noted, however, that, although this is true for most of the thoracic and lumbar vertebrae, the 11th thoracic through the 1st lumbar vertebrae are exceptions, since their pedicles are mostly parallel to the sagittal plane. In this situation, extreme care should be taken because a standard lateral radiograph can give the surgeon an illusion that the screw is still within the bony confines when, in fact, it has penetrated the anterolateral aspect of the vertebral body.

Important potential complications secondary to screw cutout include injury to the great vessels anterior to the lumbar spine and injury to the nearby nerve roots. Although it has been shown that purchase of the anterior cortex of the vertebral body significantly increases the pullout strength of the screw, the danger of a potentially devastating injury to the great vessels outweighs the increased mechanical advantage. The authors strongly urge the surgeon not to penetrate the anterior cortex of the vertebral body. The neural elements also must be considered. The nerve roots are very close to the medial and inferior walls of the pedicles. It is for this reason that violation of the walls of the pedicles should be avoided, especially at the described areas.

Sacral fixation differs from that of the lumbar spine because of the differences in their anatomic configurations. There are three possible pathways for screw fixation in the sacrum. The first pathway inserts the screw from lateral to medial through the sacral pedicle to the sacral promontory. The second pathway inserts the screw through the alae in a directly anterior fashion. The third pathway directs the screw from medial to lateral to the alae without violating the sacroiliac joint. A study performed by Asher and Strippgen (4) helped to develop a sacral implant and to identify optimum transsacral fixation sites. They showed that the longest purchase for screw fixation in the first sacral vertebra is one that is directed medially through the pedicle into the vertebral body. Zindrick's (98) published biomechanical data support that screws directed towards the vertebral body and those inserted at 45° toward the alae showed the highest pullout force. Merkovic et al. (54) provided evidence that there are a number of significant anatomic structures that can be damaged by screws placed too long through the anterior cortex of the sacrum. The internal iliac vein and artery and the L4 and L5 nerve roots are most commonly at risk of injury from a protruding sacral screw. The screws placed through the pedicle are least likely to injure the neurovascular bundle. In a separate study, Esses et al. (22) arrived at the same conclusion that safe screw implantation in the sacrum could be assured only by directing the screw medially toward the promontory. They also advocated placing the sacral screw superior to the first sacral foramen and parallel to the lumbosacral disc. We agree with the above data and recommend screw fixation to the sacrum be directed medially towards the promontory.

Mastery of the anatomy of the pedicle is absolutely necessary for surgeons performing pedicle fixation to minimize the complications related to this procedure. Radiologic guidance intraoperatively is a very useful adjunct, and is highly recommended.

COMPONENTS OF THE PWB PEDICLE SCREW SYSTEM

The PWB pedicle screw system is composed of five basic components, each manufactured from 316 LVM stainless steel. The basic components are the pedicle screws, seat, rod, cap, and nut (Fig. 17.9). The pedicle screws are 6.5-mm diameter cancellous screws that are offered in lengths from 25–55 mm in 5-mm increments and de-

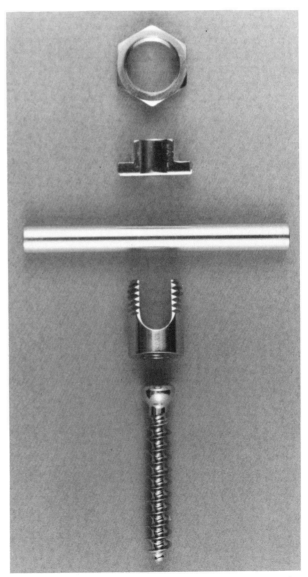

Figure 17.9. Exploded view of PWB II. (From top to bottom: Nut, cap, rod, seat, and pedicle screw).

signed to provide maximum purchase in the cancellous bone of the pedicle and vertebral body. The PWB seats are the receptacle for the rod and are secured to the spine by pedicle screws that pass through the seat and into the pedicle and vertebral body. The conical shape of the underside of the screw head and the countersink at the bottom of the seat allows the screw to be inserted at any angle necessary while maintaining alignment of the seats, which facilitates rod contouring and placement. The seats are provided in four different heights to accommodate for the normal lumbar lordosis with minimal rod contouring. The seat heights are as follows: Type I, 1.68 cm; type II, 1.83 cm; type III, 1.98 cm; type IV, 2.13 cm. Washers are provided if additional height is required. The rods are 0.25″ in diameter, smooth, and are provided in multiple lengths. In addition, the rods may be cut to specific length as necessary if the standard lengths do not suffice. The caps and nuts are all of one standard size. Tightening of the nut applies pressure to the cap which securely holds the rod in the seat.

The instruments for implantation of the system include a pedicle awl, graduated pedicle probe, depth gauge, seat reamer, screwdriver, seat holder, rod holder, cap and nut alignment guide, torque socket wrench, and a set of in-situ benders (Fig. 17.10). A distractor and compressor are also provided.

SURGICAL TECHNIQUE

The patient is positioned prone on rolled sheets to pad the chest and iliac crests or, if available, on frames designed for this purpose. The abdomen should be kept free from external compression to decrease the likelihood of excessive intraoperative bleeding secondary to vena cava compression. Patient positioning should allow for satisfactory intraoperative lateral and PA radiographs.

The surgical exposure is done through a longitudinal midline posterior incision made down to the tips of the spinous processes. The posterior elements are exposed to the tips of the transverse processes using subperiosteal dissection. Facet joint capsules and facet articular surfaces are removed in preparation for arthrodesis of the spine. Care should be taken to preserve the interspinous ligament and integrity of the facet joints between the instrumented and noninstrumented spine. When indicated, surgical decompression of the involved neural elements is performed prior to spinal instrumentation and fusion.

The most demanding aspect of the surgical procedure is the accurate location of the pedicle canal, as discussed previously. Once the spine is exposed, the pedicle canal is located using the transverse process and superior articular facet as anatomic landmarks. The entrance to the pedicle canal in the lumbar spine is located at the inter-

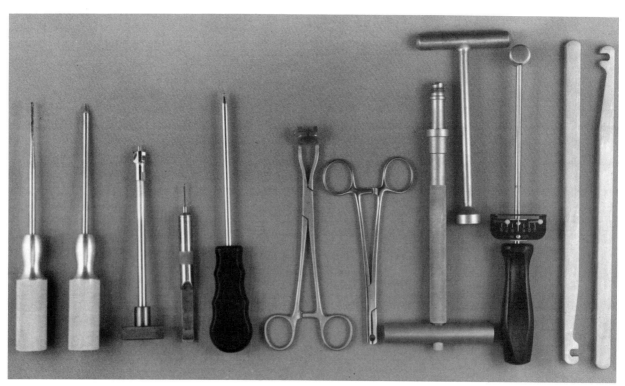

Figure 17.10. Instruments for implantation. (From left to right: awl, pedicle probe, seat reamer, depth gauge, screwdriver, seat holder, rod holder, nut and cap alignment guide, socket wrench, torque wrench, in-situ benders).

section of a line drawn transversely through the mid-portion of the transverse process and a second line drawn vertically through the lateral margin of the superior articular facet (Fig. 17.11). Before making any pedicle holes, the surgeon should inspect the exposed spine and visualize where each of the holes will be placed in the coronal plane. It is possible to vary the entrance site to the pedicle canal by a few millimeters either medially or laterally, and the surgeon should take advantage of this to enhance pedicle hole alignment in the coronal plane. Usually, it is not difficult to align the pedicle holes in a spine that has no coronal plane deformity. However, instrumenting a spine with scoliosis or vertebral translation is somewhat more difficult. If possible, the surgeon should place the pedicle holes so that they define a smooth curve, as this will facilitate rod placement. Prior to creating a hole in the pedicle canal, it is helpful to remove the posterior cortical bone at the selected entrance site. This will expose an underlying "red dot" or cancellous bone and indicates that the proper location has been selected. The pedicle awl is then used to make a starting hole approximately 4 mm deep at the intersection of these lines. It is important for the surgeon to remember that the shape, size, and direction of the pedicle canal changes as one advances down the lumbar spine.

As a general rule, the first lumbar pedicle canal is almost parallel to the sagittal plane (0°). The more caudal lumbar pedicles are more medially directed, with the angle between the axis of the pedicle and the sagittal plane increasing by approximately 5° at each level caudal to L1 (i.e., L1, 0°; L2, 5°; L3, 10°; L4, 15°; and L5, 20°). The pedicle probe is then inserted in the started hole and appropriately angled towards the midline, depending upon the level being instrumented. The pedicle probe is then advanced through the cancellous bone of the pedicle canal into the cancellous bone of the vertebral body. This is done using a controlled downward force in combination with a rotational motion over an arc of 90°, taking care to feel the cancellous bone as the pedicle probe is advanced. The pedicle probe should not be rotated more than 90°, as this will create a hole that is too large for the pedicle screw. The prepared pedicle canal hole should penetrate at least 50–60% of the vertebral body, and in no instance should it extend anterior to the vertebral body margin.

The method of inserting pedicle screws into the sacrum is somewhat different from the lumbar spine because of its size and configuration. In general, the cancellous bone of the sacrum provides little screw purchase, and, because of this, it is recommended that the anterior cortex of the sacrum be engaged by the pedicle screw. At the S1 level, the entrance to the pedicle canal is just caudal and lateral to the superior articular process. The pedicle awl is used to make the initial starting hole at this location, followed by the pedicle probe which is angled 20–30° medially towards the S1 vertebral body and advanced to the anterior cortex. The pedicle probe is then carefully advanced through the anterior cortex by lightly tapping it with a mallet, listening for a sound change indicating that the anterior has been perforated. Directing the S1 pedicle hole medially avoids damage to the vascular and neural structures that cross the sacral ala more laterally, as well as prevents violation of the sacroiliac joint (22,54).

Once the pedicle canal hole is prepared, its depth is then measured using either the depth scale on the pedicle probe or the depth gauge. The length of screw necessary will be 5 mm longer than that measured to compensate for the thickness of the screwhead and seat that are to be placed. The depth gauge is also used to palpate the walls and bottom of the pedicle hole to make sure that the pedicle hole is entirely within bone. As shown in Figure 17.8, the length of screws needed for the lumbar spine is relatively constant. A screw length of between 40–50 mm is usually sufficient to provide the desired penetration of the vertebral body without going beyond the anterior cortex.

Use of radiographic assistance to monitor the insertion of the pedicle probe and pedicle screws is highly recommended. One technique is to use a C-arm in the PA and lateral projections to guide the placement of the pedicle probe. Another option is to use the PA and lateral radiographs taken with seat trials in the prepared pedicle holes to make certain that the holes are within the bone prior to screw placement.

The contour of the spine to be instrumented is observed. If well placed, the pedicle holes will be aligned in the sagittal plane either in a straight line or a smooth curve. However, because of lumbar lordosis, kyphosis, or spondylolisthesis, the holes are frequently not aligned

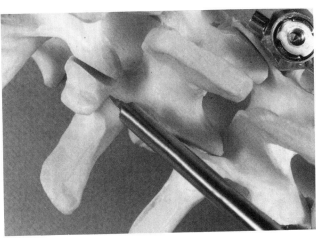

Figure 17.11. Entrance of the pedicle screw.

in the sagittal plane. To compensate for this, the rod seats come in four heights, as previously mentioned. This facilitates seat alignment in the sagittal plane, making contouring and placement of the rod easier.

The most posterior or prominent level is instrumented first. By using this segment as a reference point and placing the shortest seat (type I seat) in this location, the instrumentation is kept as close as possible to the spine, thereby providing a lower profile while increasing the mechanical stability. Usually, in a short segment fusion to the sacrum, the most prominent segment is S1 and is instrumented first. Once this segment has been selected, the bone about the pedicle hole is flattened using the seat reamer on an air powered drill with a cylindrical bit (Fig. 17.12). This step is extremely important because the orientation of the seats is determined by how they lay on the underlying bone. The goal is to place the seats as parallel as possible to the sagittal and transverse plane. Once the bony bed is prepared, appropriately sized trial seats are temporarily implanted. Radiographs are taken at this point to verify the placement. This also enables the surgeon to select the appropriate size seats that best align with the sagittal plane. The permanent seats are then placed with the appropriate length screws. The screw is tightened with the screwdriver at the same time using the seat holder to properly align the seats in a longitudinal direction (Fig. 17.13).

Once all of the pedicle screws and seats are placed on one side of the spine, the proper length rod is selected. The selected rod should allow 5–6 mm extension beyond the inferior and superior most seats. The rod is then contoured with a French-type rod bender to fit the seats. The rod holder is then used to introduce the rod into the pedicle seats. The caps and nuts are then placed at

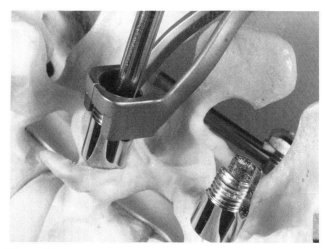

Figure 17.13.   Insertion of the pedicle screw with the use of the screwdriver and seat holder.

each level using a special alignment guide designed specifically for this purpose (Fig. 17.14). This instrument assures that the nut is applied in good alignment with the threaded portion of the seat and prevents cross-threading. The nut is then turned clockwise slowly with the socket wrench incorporated in the alignment guide. If properly threaded, the nuts will advance quite smoothly. At this point, the threaded pin that holds the cap should be loosened slowly while the socket wrench is further turned to further thread the nut in place.

Once the rod is secured and all the caps and nuts are in place at each level, the torque socket wrench is used to sequentially tighten the nuts until the rod is fully seated in each of the pedicle seats. This should be done gradually, taking several passes up and down the row of nuts, as this will facilitate proper seating of the rod. It is necessary

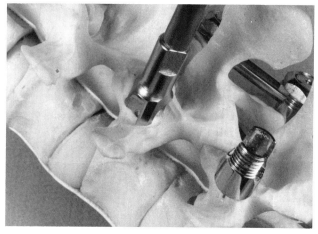

Figure 17.12.   The recipient bone is flattened using a hand reamer or a power drill with a cylindrical bit.

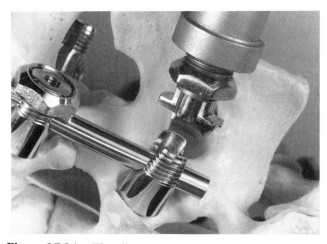

Figure 17.14.   The alignment guide holds both the cap and nut. The instrument enables the surgeon to place the cap easily and guide and thread the nut easily onto the seat.

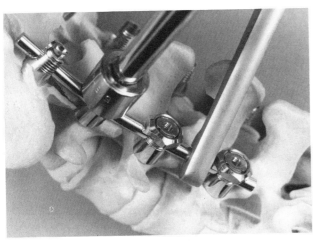

Figure 17.15. The torque wrench is used to tighten the nuts to the desired amount of torque.

to hold the rod with an in-situ bender while tightening the nuts to avoid applying undue torque to the instrumentation system (Fig. 17.15). A torque of at least 120 inch-lbs is delivered on each nut to provide adequate limiting friction between the rod and seat. Radiographs are taken to verify the final screw placements as well as the final sagittal and coronal lumbar curvatures (Fig. 17.16).

Compression and/or distraction of the spine may be accomplished with the socket wrench in place over the nut. Once the nut is loosened, the distractor or compressor is applied to the wrench. After manipulation, the nut is retightened. This sequence may be repeated as necessary to produce the desired correction. After the instrumentation is secured on one side of the spine, the contralateral side is instrumented.

The last step is the application of the crosslink mechanism (Fig. 17.17). Whenever possible, two crosslinks should be used. It is applied initially by securing the side

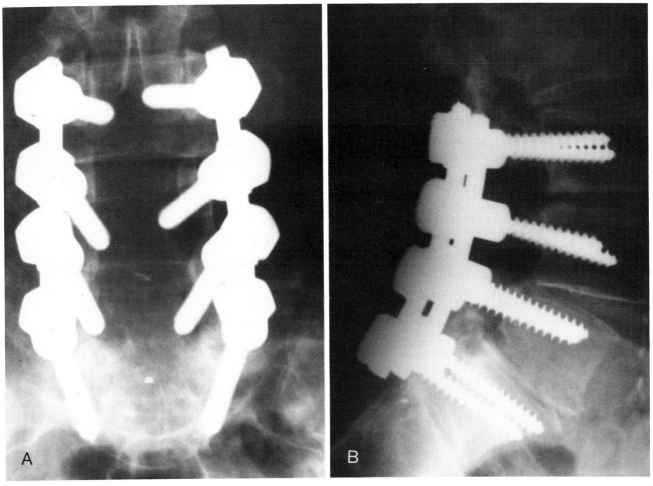

Figure 17.16. *A* and *B*, Radiographs to verify the final screw placements as well as the final sagittal and coronal curvature of the spine.

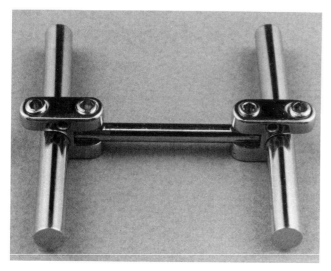

Figure 17.17. From left to right: Side clamp, crosslink pin, side clamp.

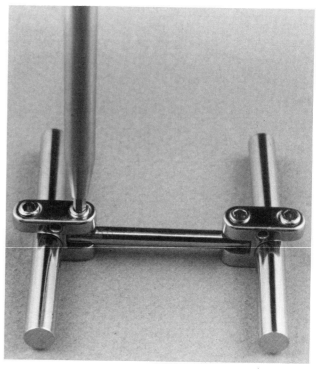

Figure 17.19. Application of the 4-mm crosslink pin in between the two side clamps while the set screws are tightened.

clamps on to the longitudinal rods (Fig. 17.18). This is followed by placing the appropriate length pin (4 mm diameter) to bridge the two side clamps (Fig. 17.19) and tightening the set screws. The pin can be cut intraoperatively to the appropriate length if the available size does not fit the space between the side clamps.

Once the instrumentation is in place, the arthrodesis procedure is performed by meticulous decortication and bone grafting. Bone is packed in the facet joints, around the seats, and underneath the rods. It is sometimes preferable to decorticate the transverse processes and place the bone graft in the lateral gutter prior to rod placement. This makes visualization of the graft bed easier. The wound is closed in the usual fashion.

CLINICAL DATA

The initial pilot study was started in March, 1988, with the implantation of the first version of the Puno-Winter-Byrd (PWB I) system in 47 patients. Twenty-three males and 24 females with an average age of 57 years comprised the study group. The preoperative diagnoses included spondylolisthesis, degenerative disc disease, failed back syndrome, and a combination of any of the above. While the majority of the patients in this group has not reached a 2-year follow-up, the preliminary results appear to be promising.

During implantation on the first few patients, the surgeons encountered certain difficulties. Intraoperatively, stripping of the screw threads was noted in two patients, while there was application of an excessively long screw in another patient. The patient with the long screw was brought back to the operating room, and the screw was

replaced with a shorter one. There were three broken screws and slippage in four rods noted out of 204 screws and seats implanted. Other complications unrelated to the instrumentation included neurologic deficit in one

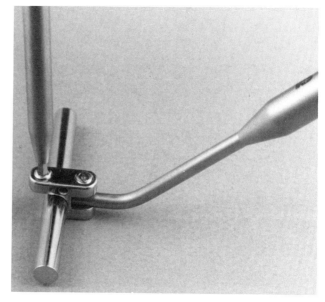

Figure 17.18. Application of the side clamp with a side clamp holder.

patient, wound infection in one, seroma formation in two, ileus in one, hematoma in one, and pulmonary embolism in one.

There were several things learned during the pilot phase of this study. The surgeons found that implantation of the first version (Fig. 17.3: PWB I) was somewhat tedious because of the implant design. It was technically difficult to position the wrench when the nut was tightened, since it required that the nut be advanced from under the rod. Although it provided satisfactory fixation of the rod, the design was not "user friendly." A design improvement was in order and led to the development of the PWB II (Fig. 17.1), where the nut is applied from the top of the rod. Mechanical testing performed by the manufacturer indicated that the clamping mechanisms of the two versions are substantially equivalent in both static and fatigue loading situations.

With the final implant in hand, the second phase of the clinical trials started. Between November, 1989, and November, 1990, there were 75 patients who were enrolled in the study and who underwent spine fusion with instrumentation using the PWB II device. This group consisted of 31 males and 44 females, with an average age of 50 years. The preoperative diagnoses included spondylolisthesis in 30 patients, degenerative disc disease in 14, failed back syndrome in 12, spinal stenosis in 6, and combined diagnoses in 12. There was one patient for whom a diagnosis was not reported. Instrumentation failures were noted in four out of the 396 screws, and seats implanted. These included one screw pullout and three instances of rod slippage. There had been no report of screw breakage with the new version. Other complications that were not directly related to the instrumentation included neurologic deficit in two, wound infection in one, pneumonia in one, and mental status change in one.

COMPLICATIONS

Complications of lumbar pedicle fixation generally fall into three categories. The first category is concerned with the placement of the screws; the second deals with failure of the instrumentation; and the third results from the adverse effects the instrumentation has on the vertebrae above and below the instrumented segment.

As with all pedicle fixation systems, the most significant complications from the use of the PWB transpedicular fixation system arise from misplacement of the pedicle screws. The lumbar roots are in close proximity to the medial and inferior borders of the pedicle and are at significant risk of injury if the pedicle screw exits in these directions. While there is more room for error superiorly and laterally, it is still possible to injure the next cephalad

nerve root. The great vessels anterior to the spine are always in danger of injury if the screws penetrate the anterior cortex of the vertebral body. Adequate exposure of the landmarks, radiographic monitoring, and a thorough knowledge of the anatomy should help minimize the above complications.

Device-related complications noted from the use of the PWB transpedicular spine fixation system included rod slippage in four patients, which has been attributed to one of two causes. Either the nut was not fully tightened by the surgeon at the time of surgery or the nut was cross-threaded, preventing full tightening of the nut. Both of these can leave the rod unsecured in the seat. In an attempt to prevent this occurrence, the surgeon should carefully thread and fully tighten the nuts. A nut alignment guide (Fig. 17.14) aids the surgeon in the placement of the nut without cross-threading while a torque wrench assures the surgeon that he is delivering the appropriate amount of torque to each nut. The security of the nut can be evaluated using a spreader to make sure that the rod does not slip with respect to the seats.

The possibility of pedicle screw breakage also exists. This has occurred on three occasions using the first version (PWB I), while it has not occurred with the final implant (PWB II). It is hoped that the micromotion occurring between the screw and the seat will act as a "shock-absorber" and prevent this from occurring to any significant degree. Likewise, the possibility of rod breakage exists, though this has not been observed to date. It is believed that this will be an unlikely occurrence because of the rod size and the micromotion considerations.

Complications may also occur as a result of interference by the instrumentation with the vertebrae above and below the instrumented segment. This is most likely to happen superiorly where there is close proximity between the pedicle and the first unfused facet joint above the instrumentation. The PWB system allows the surgeon to insert the screw at an angle and in a more lateral position so as to prevent this interference from happening. In addition, care must be taken when instrumenting the superior-most segment to minimize damage to the uninvolved facet joint, which is best accomplished by placing the entrance to the pedicle canal as inferiorly as possible and also by removing as little bone as possible when preparing the seat site. By following these steps, encroachment upon the uninvolved facet joint will be kept to a minimum. Although possible, it is much less likely that the instrumentation will interfere with the caudal vertebra. If it does occur, interference is usually in the extremely lordotic spine where there is a short pars interarticularis and little distance between the instrumented pedicle and the uninvolved facet joint. In this situation, the entrance to the pedicle canal should be made as superiorly and laterally as possible. Also, seat site flattening should be kept to a minimum. If too much bone is removed, it is possible to cut into the pars interarticularis, thereby predisposing it to fracture.

DISCUSSION

Transpedicular instrumentation has greatly increased the surgeon's ability to segmentally stabilize the lumbar spine. This ability to securely fix short segments of the lumbar spine has advanced transpedicular fixation beyond the capabilities for previously used lumbar instrumentation such as hooks, rods, and wires. In general, the use of transpedicular fixation is indicated in addressing the problem of existing or potential lumbar instability. More specifically, this would include spondylolisthesis, scoliosis, fracture, tumors, degenerative disc disease, lumbar instability associated with destabilizing decompression, and repair of pseudarthrosis.

While there are several transpedicular systems available, they generally fall into two broad categories. They are either of the screw and plate design or the screw and rod design. In our opinion, the screw and rod design is preferable, as it allows contouring in both sagittal and coronal plane curvatures. There are, however, unique design features of the PWB transpedicular spinal system further enhancing its function. Foremost of these is the fact that the screw and seat are two separate pieces, providing the micromotion necessary to decrease stress concentration at the screw-seat junction and thereby minimizing failure. In addition, the surgeon is able to compensate for the various small differences in pedicle direction from segment to segment without sacrificing seat alignment. This facilitates the ease of rod placement. The availability of four seat sizes allows careful tailoring of the instrumentation construct for each individual case despite the natural variations occurring from patient to patient. The PWB transpedicular system is readily and easily implantable and provides the meticulous surgeon a new pedicle screw system that securely immobilizes the spine.

Our results are very preliminary, as the follow-up period has not been long enough to allow the authors to provide any meaningful comment regarding fusion rates and eventual functional results. However, the early results appear quite promising.

REFERENCES

1. Adkins EWO: Lumbosacral arthrodesis after laminectomy. J Bone Joint Surg 1955;37:208–223.
2. Albee FH: Transplantation of a portion of the tibia into the spine for Pott's disease. JAMA 1911;57:885–886.
3. Allen BL, Ferguson RL: The Galveston technique for L rod instrumentation of the scoliotic spine. Spine 1982;7:276–284.
4. Asher MA, Strippgen WE: Anthropometric study of the human sacrum relating to dorsal transsacral implant design. Clin Orthop 1986;203:58–62.
5. Asher M, Carson W, Heinig C: A modular spinal rod linkage system to provide rotational stability. Spine 1988;3:272–277.
6. Attenborough CG, Reynolds MT: Lumbo-sacral fusion with spring fixation. J Bone Joint Surg 1975;57B:283–288.
7. August AC, Tencer AF, Mooney V: A biomechanical comparison of the methods of posterior fixation in lumbosacral spine fusion. Proc of the Orthop Res Soc Annual Meeting, Las Vegas, Nevada, 1985.
8. Banta CJ, King AG, Dabezies EJ, et al: Measurement of the effective pedicle diameter in the human spine. Orthopedicds 1989;12:939–942.
9. Berry JL, Moran JM, Berg WS, et al: A morphometric study of human lumbar and selected thoracic vertebrae. Spine 1987; 12:362–367.
10. Bradford DS: Treatment of severe spondylolisthesis—A combined approach for reduction and stabilization. Spine 1979;4:423–429.
11. Brown CW, Orme TJ, Richardson HD: The rate of pseudoarthrosis (surgical nonunion) in patients who are smokers and patients who are nonsmokers: A comparison study. Spine 1986;11:942–943.
12. Chow SP, Leong JCY, Yau AC: Anterior spinal fusion for deranged lumbar intervertebral disc. Spine 1980;5:452–458.
13. Cleveland M, Bosworth DM, Thompson FR: Pseudoarthrosis in the lumbar spine. J Bone Joint Surg 1948;30A:302–312.
14. Cloward RB: Treatment of ruptured intervertebral disc by vertebral body fusion—indication, operative technique, and after care. J Neurosurg 1953;10:154–168.
15. Cobey MC: The value of the Wilson plate in spinal fusion. Clin Orthop 1971;76:138–140.
16. Curran JP, McGaw WH: Posterolateral spinal fusion with pedicle grafts. Clin Orthop 1968;59:125–129.
17. De Palma AF, Prabhakar M: Posterior-posterobilateral fusion of the lumbosacral spine. Clin Orthop 1966;47:165–171.
18. De Palma AF, Rothman RH: The nature of pseudoarthrosis. Clin Orthop 1968;59:113–118.
19. Drummond DW, Narechania R, Wenger D, et al: Wisconsin segmental spinal instrumentation. Proc Sco Res Soc Annual Meeting, Montreal, Quebec, 1981.
20. Drummond DW, Guadagni J, Keene JS, et al: Interspinous process segmental spinal instrumentation. J Pediatr Orthop 1984;4:397–404.
21. Edwards CC: Sacral fixation device—Design and preliminary results. Proc Sco Res Soc Annual Meeting. Orlando, Florida, 1984.
22. Esses SI, Botsford DJ, Huler RJ, Rausching W: Surgical anatomy of the sacrum—A guide to rational screw fixation. Proc N Amer Spine Soc Annual Meeting, Monterey, California, 1990.
23. Freebody D, Bendall R, Taylor RD: Anterior transperitoneal lumbar fusion. J Bone Joint Surg 1971;53B:617–627.
24. Graham CE: Lumbosacral fusion using internal fixation with a spinous process for the graft. Clin Orthop 1979;140:72–77.
25. Gurr KR, McAfee PC, Shih CM: Biomechanical analysis of posterior instrumentation systems after decompressive laminectomy. J Bone Joint Surg 1988;70A:680–691.
26. Guyer DW, Yuan HA, Werner FW, Frederickson BE, Murphy D: Biomechanical comparison of seven internal fixation devices for the lumbosacral junction. Spine 1987;12:569–573.
27. Harmon PH: End results from lower lumbar-spine vertebral body fusions for the disc syndromes, carried out by an abdominal extraperitoneal approach. J Bone Joint Surg 1959;41A:1355–1356.
28. Harrington PR: Treatment of scoliosis. Correction and internal fixation by spine instrumentation. J Bone Joint Surg 1962; 44A:591–610.
29. Harrington PR, Dickson JH: Spinal instrumentation in the treat-

ment of severe progressive spondylolisthesis. Clin Orthop 1976; 117:157–163.

30. Herrmann HD: Transarticular (Transpedicular) metal plate fixation for stabilization of the lumbar and thoracic spine. Acta Neurochir 1979;48:101–110.

31. Hibbs RA: An operation for progressive spinal deformities. NY J Med 1911;93:1013–1016.

32. Hodgson AR, Wong SK: A description of a technic and evaluation of results in anterior spinal fusion for deranged intervertebral disc and spondylolisthesis. Clin Orthop 1968;56:133–162.

33. Howorth MB: Evolution of spinal fusion. Ann Surg 1943; 117:278–289.

34. Inoue SI, Watanabe T, Hirose A, et al: Anterior discectomy and interbody fusion for lumbar disc herniation. Clin Orthop 1984; 183:22–31.

35. King D: Internal fixation for lumbosacral fusion. Am J Surg 1944;66:357–361.

36. King D: Internal fixation for lumbosacral fusion. J Bone Joint Surg 1948;30A:560–565.

37. Knodt H, Larrick RB: Distraction fusion of the spine. Ohio State Med J 1964;60:1140–1142.

38. Kornblatt MD, Casey MP, Jacobs RR: Internal fixation in lumbosacral spine fusion—A biomechanical and clinical study. Clin Orthop 1986;203:141–150.

39. Krag MH, Beynon BD, Pope MH, Frymoyer JW, Haugh LD, Weaver DL: An internal fixator for posterior application to short segments of the thoracic, lumbar, or lumbosacral spine—Design and testing. Clin Orthop 1986;203:75–98.

40. Krag MH, Weaver DL, Beynon BD, Haugh LD: Morphometry of the thoracic and lumbar spine related to transpedicular screw placement for surgical spinal fixation. Spine 1988;13:27–32.

41. Krag MH, Fredrickson BE, Yuan HA: Spinal instrumentation. In: Weinstein JN, Wiesel SW, eds. The lumbar spine. Philadelphia: WB Saunders 1990;916–940.

42. Lane JD, Moore ES: Transperitoneal approach to the intervertebral disc in the lumbar area. Ann Surg 1948;127:537–551.

43. Lange F: Support of the spondylitic spine by means of buried steel bars attached to the vertebrae. Am J Orthop Surg 1910;8:344–361.

44. Lesoin F, Bouasakao N, Cama A, Lozes G, Combelles G, Jomin M: Posttraumatic fixation of the thoracolumbar spine using Roy-Camille plates. Surg Neuro 1982;18:167–173.

45. Louis R: Fusion of the lumbar and sacral spine by internal fixation with screw plates. Clin Orthop 1986;203:18–33.

46. Luque ER: The anatomic basis and development of segmental spinal instrumentation. Spine 1982;7:256–259.

47. Luque ER, Casis N, Ramirez-Wiella G: Segmental spinal instrumentation in the treatment of fractures of the thoracolumbar spine. Spine 1982;7:312–317.

48. Luque ER: Segmental spinal instrumentation of the lumbar spine. Clin Orthop 1986;203:126–134.

49. Luque ER, Rapp GF: A new semirigid method for interpedicular fixation of the spine. Orthopaedics 1988;11:1445–1450.

50. Magerl FP: Stabilization of the lower thoracic and lumbar spine with external fixation. Clin Orthop 1984;189:125–141.

51. Matthiass HH, Heine J: The surgical reduction of spondylolisthesis. Clin Orthop 1986;203:34–44.

52. McAfee PC, Werner FW, Glisson RR: A biomechanical analysis of spinal instrumentation systems in thoracolumbar fractures—Comparison of traditional Harrington distraction instrumentation with segmental spinal instrumentation. Spine 1985;10:204–217.

53. McAfee PC, Farey ID, Sutterlin CE, Gurr KR, Warden KE, Cunningham BW: Device related osteoporosis with spinal instrumentation. Spine 1989;14:919–926.

54. Mirkovic S, Arbitbol JJ, Steinmann J, Edwards CC, Garfin SR: Anatomic consideration for sacral screw fixation. Proc N Amer Spine Soc Annual Meeting, Monterey, California, 1990.

55. O'Brien JP, Dawson MHO, Heard CW, Momberger G, Speck G, Weatherly CR: Simultaneous combined anterior and posterior fusion. Clin Orthop 1986;203:191–195.

56. Ogilvie JW, Bradford DS: Lumbar and lumbosacral fusion with segmental fixation. Proc Sco Res Soc Annual Meeting, Orlando, Florida, 1984.

57. Ölerud S, Sjöström L, Karlström G, Hamberg M: Spontaneous effect of increased stability of the lower lumbar spine in cases of severe chronic back pain—The answer of an external transpeduncular fixation test. Clin Orthop 1986;203:67–74.

58. Olsewski JM, Simmons EH, Kallen FC, Mendel FC, Severin CM, Berens DL: Morphometry of the lumbar spine: Anatomical perspectives related to transpedicular fixation. J Bone Joint Surg 1990;72:541–549.

59. Pennal GL, McDonald GA, Dale GG: A method of spinal fusion using internal fixation. Clin Orthop 1964;35:86–94.

60. Puno RM, Bechtold JE, Kim AB, Sun BN, Bradford DS: Anterior spinal fixation—Clinical and biomechanical analysis. Proc Ortho Res Soc Annual Meeting, New Orleans, Louisiana, 1986.

61. Puno RM, Hartjen CA, von Fraunhofer JA, Holt RT, Johnson JR: Biomechanical analysis of the Cotrel-Dubousset spine instrumentation system. Proc Orthop Res Soc Annual Meeting, San Francisco, California, 1987.

62. Puno RM, Bechtold JE, Byrd JA, Winter RB, Ogilvie JW, Bradford DS: Biomechanical analysis of transpedicular rod systems—A preliminary report. Spine 1991; 16:973–980.

63. Reimers C: Die Dorsale Spannverstrebung von Wirbelsäulenabschnitten mittels innerer Schienung. Chirurgie 1956;17:10.

64. Roy-Camille R, Roy-Camille M, Demeulenaere C: Ostéosynthése du rachis dorsal, lombaire et lombo-sacré. La Presse Medicale 1970; 78:1447–1448.

65. Roy-Camille R, Saillant G, Berteaux D, Salgado V. Osteosynthesis of the thoraco-lumbar spine fractures with metal plates screwed through the vertebral pedicles. Reconst Surg Traumat 1976;15:2–16.

66. Roy-Camille R, Berteaux D, Saillant J: Synthése du rachis dorsolombaire traumatique pars plaquées vissées dans les pédicules vertébraux. Revue de Chirurgie Orthopédique 1977;63:452–456.

67. Roy-Camille R, Saillant G, Marie-Anne S, Mamoudy P: Behandlung von Wirbelkfrakturen und-laxationen am thorako-lumbalen Übergang. Orthopäde 1980;9:63–68.

68. Roy-Camille R, Saillant G, Mazel C: Internal fixation of the lumbar spine with pedicle screw plating. Clin Orthop 1986;203:7–17.

69. Saillant G: Étude anatomique des pédicules vertébraux. Reveu de Chirurgie Orthopédique 1976;62:151–160.

70. Scaglietti O, Frontino G, Bartolozzi P: Technique of anatomical reduction of lumbar spondylolisthesis and the surgical stabilization. Clin Orthop 1976;117:164–175.

71. Schwaegler P, Cram R, Lorenz M, Zindrick M, Collatz M, Behal R. A comparison of single level fusions with and without hardware. Proc N Amer Spine Soc Annual Meeting, Monterey, California, 1990.

72. Selby D: Internal fixation with Knodt's rods. Clin Orthop 1986; 203:179–184.

73. Shaw EG, Taylor JG: The results of lumbosacral fusion for low back pain. J Bone Joint Surg 1956;38B:485–497.

74. Sicard A, Menegaux J: L'abord anterieur de l'articulation sacroiliaque. J Chir 1959;77:29.

75. Sijbrandij S: A new technique for the reduction and stabilisation of severe spondylolisthesis—A report of two cases. J Bone Joint Surg 1981;63B:266–271.

76. Smith KR, Hunt TR, Asher MA, Anderson HC: The effect of a stiff spinal implant on the lumbar spine in dogs. J Bone Joint Surg 1991;73A:115–123.

77. Stanger JK. Fracture-dislocation of the thoracolumbar spine. With reference to reduction by open and closed operation. J Bone Joint Surg 1947;29A:107–118.

78. Stauffer RN, Coventry MB: Posterolateral lumbar spine fusion. J Bone Joint Surg 1972;54A:1195–1204.

79. Stauffer RN, Coventry MB: Anterior interbody lumbar spine fusion. J Bone Joint Surg 1972;54A:756–768.

80. Takeda M: A newly devised "three-one" method for the surgical treatment of spondylolysis and spondylolisthesis. Clin Orthop 1980;147:228–233.

81. Tanturi T, Kataja M, Keski-Nisula L, et al: Posterior fusion of the lumbosacral spine. Acta Orthop Scand 1979;50:415–425.

82. Thompson WAL, Ralston EL: Pseudoarthrosis following spine fusion. J Bone Joint Surg 1949;31A:400–405.

83. Thompson WAL, Gristina AG, Healy WA: Lumbosacral spine fusion—a method of bilateral posterolateral fusion combined with a Hibb's fusion. J Bone Joint Surg 1974;56A:1643–1647.

84. Toumey JW: Internal fixation in fusion of the lumbosacral joints. Lahey Clin Bull 1943;3:188–191.

85. Vidal J, Fassio B, Buscayret C, Allieu Y: Surgical reduction of spondylolisthesis using a posterior approach. Clin Orthop 1981;154:156–165.

86. Watkins MB: Posterolateral fusion of the lumbar and lumbosacral spine. J Bone Joint Surg 1953;35A:1014–1018.

87. Watkins MB, Bragg C: Lumbosacral fusion results with early ambulation. Surg Gynecol Obstet 1956;102:604–606.

88. Watkins MB: Posterolateral bone-grafting for fusion of the lumbar and the lumbosacral spine. J Bone Joint Surg 1959;41A:388–396.

89. Watkins MB: Posterolateral fusion in pseudoarthrosis and posterior element defects of the lumbosacral spine. Clin Orthop 1964;35:80–85.

90. Weiss M: Dynamic spine alloplasty (spring-loading corrective devices) after fracture and spinal cord injuries. Clin Orthop 1975;112:150–158.

91. White AH, Wynne G, Taylor LW: Knodt rod distraction lumbar fusion. Spine 1983;8:434–437.

92. Whitecloud TS, Butler JC, Cohen JL, Candelora PD: Complications with the Variable Spinal Plating system. Spine 1989;14:472–476.

93. Williams EWM: Traumatic paraplegia. In: Matthews DN, ed. Recent advances in surgery of trauma. London, Churchill Livingstone, 1963;171–186.

94. Wilson PD, Straub LR: Lumbosacral fixation with metallic-plate fixation. AAOS Instruct Course Lect 1952;9:53–57.

95. Wiltse LL, Bateman JG, Hutchinson RH, Nelson WE: The parapsinal sacrospinalis-splitting approach to the lumbar spine. J Bone Joint Surg 1968;50A:919–926.

96. Wiltse LL: Proceedings: Lumbar spine—posterolateral fusion. J Bone Joint Surg 1975;57B:261.

97. Zielke K, Strempel AV: Posterior lateral distraction spondylodesis using the twofold sacral bar. Clin Orthop 1986;203:151–158.

98. Zindrick MR, Wiltse LL, Widell EH, et al: A biomechanical study of the intrapeduncular screw fixation in the lumbosacral spine. Clin Orthop 1986;203:99–112.

99. Zindrick MR, Wiltse LL, Doornik A, et al: Analysis of the morphometric characteristics of the thoracic and lumbar pedicles. Spine 1987;12:160–166.

EIGHTEEN

AO Internal Fixator

Pablo Vazquez-Seoane, Stanley D. Gertzbein, and Hansen A. Yuan

INTRODUCTION

The surgical treatment of spinal fractures has gained much attention during the last two decades (8,11). Unstable fractures in the thoracolumbar region have been a therapeutic challenge. There has been intense debate regarding the appropriateness of surgical intervention in these cases (6). Various methods of nonsurgical and surgical techniques have been described. Treatments include bed rest, postural reduction with body cast, and surgical stabilization depending on fracture types, neurologic status, and patient factors. Nonetheless, controversy still exists concerning specific indications and exact surgical techniques.

According to Gertzbein and Eismont, goals in the treatment of thoracolumbar spinal injuries are: (*a*) restoration of alignment and stabilization of the spinal column; (*b*) improvement in neurologic status; and (*c*) early mobilization and rehabilitation of the patient (15). Even today, opinions regarding the implementation of these goals are divided. There are proponents for the nonsurgical treatment (18,26), and proponents for surgical stabilization (7,8,11). Neurologic compromise is a strong indication for surgical intervention. In the neurologically intact patient, controversy between conservative vs. surgical approach still exists. Some authors suggest that a kyphotic deformity of greater than 30° and 50% of canal compromise are structural indications for surgery (4,27). Denis et al. believe that unstable fractures are better managed surgically to provide early rehabilitation and to avoid late complications of pain and progressive deformity (7).

Another controversial subject is the surgical approach between anterior versus posterior approach in treating unstable fractures. Each approach has its own advantages. The anterior retroperitoneal approach to the spine has the advantage of a direct visualization of the anterior and middle column of the spine (12,17,28). Decompression

under direct visualization is more complete and safer in terms of protecting the spinal cord. Reduction of deformity is also possible by postural manipulation and direct distraction of the vertebral bodies. Bone graft with or without metal implant is then utilized to obtain stability and to achieve a solid fusion. Currently, there are several systems in use for anterior fixation, such as the Kaneda device and the Syracuse I plate. The anterior approach has not gained overwhelming popularity in part because of the technically demanding nature of the procedure. Potential complications involving the retroperitoneal approach have been described. Injury to the great vessels, graft complications, and failure of hardware are potential problems facing surgeons (5). Unfamiliarity with the anterior approach is another reason many surgeons prefer posterior techniques.

The posterior approach to the spine is widely utilized, and is a more familiar technique to surgeons. The familiarity with this approach has inspired multiple techniques for posterior spine fixation. The posterior or posterolateral approach has some drawbacks. Decompression of the canal is difficult and often incomplete. If the reduction is attempted indirectly by distraction, failure of adequate decompression is frequent, particularly in late cases.

Harrington rods have been used for many years for treatment of burst fractures. The use of Harrington rods for trauma evolved since its introduction in 1949 for postpolio spinal deformity and scoliosis. Historically, this was the first effective surgical treatment modality for spine fractures, and rapidly gained acceptance. The principle of Harrington rods is based on distraction forces utilizing laminar hooks as the way to gain purchase to the posterior elements of the spine. With time, it became apparent that distraction rods had a number of shortcomings. Utilizing distraction forces alone along a straight rod produced a loss of lumbar lordosis (3). Using Harrington rod fixation for fractures generally requires the fusion levels to extend two to three levels above and two levels below the injury. This long fusion mass over five motion segments (16) may limit motion unnecessarily and may compromise function, particularly in the low lumbar region. These long fusions have also been implicated in the facet and disc degeneration of the levels below the fusion (22). Modification of Harrington system such as rod contouring, square-ended Moe rod, and segmental wiring have been used to improve lumbar lordosis and to enhance stability.

The advent of Edwards rod sleeves offered another dimension to rod fixation. With the sleeves, a lordotic vector was applied to the lumbar spine through a polyethylene spacer between the rod and the posterior elements (13).

Ideally, an effective system would combine the ease of the posterior approach, decompression and reduction achieved by the anterior approach, and fusion of a short segment. Research in this area has lead to pedicular segmental fixation. With pedicle screw fixation, the goal is to restore the anatomy of the burst vertebra and to limit the number of fused levels. Pedicle screw-plate systems have been used successfully in the degenerative disorders of the lumbar spine (24,25). However, these plate systems do not permit significant reduction of the fractured spine. Instrumentation was then developed that would allow distraction and restoration of lordosis, while fusing only one level above and one below the fracture. This is an exciting concept, and currently, there are a number of systems that offer this capability (10,23). Successful results have been reported, and more research and clinical trials are ongoing.

AO FIXATEUR INTERNE (DICK)

The development of the "fixateur interne" has its origins in the developments by Friedrich P. Magerl (20). Since 1977, Magerl has been working on the applications of the external spinal skeletal fixator (ESSF). The ESSF system consists of obtaining segmental spinal fixation through posteriorly placed pedicle screws held rigidly fixated by an external apparatus. He utilizes 5-mm Schanz screws placed into the pedicles through either an open or closed technique. Magerl and the Swiss Research Institute Laboratory for Experimental Surgery in Davos developed a connecting device to obtain rigid external fixation of the screws. Magerl reported using the ESSF for fractures and infections. His results were very encouraging, but it was inconvenient for the patient to have an external fixation apparatus for weeks at a time.

With the ESSF, Magerl launched a new dimension in spinal instrumentation. His ideas regarding reduction and restoration of anatomy while fusing only a limited number of segments have great potential. Also, he tried to achieve optimal stability for immediate mobilization with minimal external support.

Based on these ideas, W. Dick modified the ESSF (10). The fixatuer interne (FI), as developed by Dick, consists of long 5-mm Schanz screws that are inserted posteriorly through the pedicles into the vertebral bodies. The connector is a 7-mm threaded longitudinal rod with flat sides and clamps that are mobile in every direction, and it is completely implanted using the posterior approach. The clamps hold the Schanz screw; the threaded rod permits distraction (or compression). Through the long lever arm of the Schanz screws and movable clamps it is possible the application of lordotic (or kyphotic) forces. The configuration can then be fixed in the desired position with nuts.

Biomechanical testing of the FI was done by Dick on human cadaveric spines (9). Comparison was then made among Harrington rods, Jacobs rods, and the Roy-Camille plate. The spines were mounted on a universal testing machine (Rumul Mikroton 654) and submitted to pure bending moments. Their results showed that the Harrington rods disengaged at an average of 6–10 N (9). The strongest construct was the FI implant and could sustain significant higher forces. Mean angulation with anterior bending moment of 5 N was 1°, with 10 N was 2.9°, with 15 N, 6.1°, and with 20 N was 6.6°. This testing was done on old osteoporotic spines with an average age of 78 years. On one young patient who died from a pulmonary embolus 17 days after surgery, biomechanical testing was performed. The results were very different from those in the older bone. Angulation deformation reached .9° with 10 N of anterior bending, 1.1° with 15 N, 1.4°, with 20 N and 2.4° with 47 N. No loosening occurred, and no residual deformity was defected. After the removal of the device, the spine was completely disrupted at an anterior bending moment of 9 N (9).

SURGICAL INDICATIONS

Presently, the indication for the use of the FI is generally limited to the treatment of fractures. It is indicated for unstable burst fractures from T11-L5 with or without neurologic compromise. The use of the FI is limited by the size of the pedicles. Dick has found it possible to use the FI in levels as high as T8. In our experience, pedicle dimensions in the thoracic spine are smaller than in the lumbar spine, and careful measurements must be taken prior to pedicle screw insertion. The FI instrumentation can be applied in Chance fractures, burst fractures, fracture dislocations, and pure dislocations. The FI is a versatile instrument for various fracture patterns.

PATIENT EVALUATION

Each patient has to be evaluated carefully and treated appropriately. Spine fractures are frequently present in the multiply injured patient, and complete trauma evaluation is needed. A thorough and carefully documented neurologic examination must be performed. Furthermore, frequent repeat examinations should be performed to detect any changes in the neurologic status. Radiologic evaluation of the fracture should include plain x-rays and CT scans. The CT scan is very valuable in evaluating the type of fracture and the degree of canal compromise. An MRI scan could also be of value in identifying suspected hematomas or associated disc injuries.

Once the evaluation is complete and the fracture requires surgical intervention, it is our feeling that surgery should be performed as soon as possible, usually within the first 24 hours. Early fixation of spine fractures has been found extremely helpful in early mobilization of the patient and therefore reducing respiratory complications, decubiti, and thromboembolic phenomenon. Another important advantage with early surgery is the ease of indirect decompression and reduction of deformity.

SURGICAL TECHNIQUE

We recommend spinal cord monitoring on patients who remain neurologically intact or who show an incomplete lesion. Under general anesthesia, the patient is turned on the prone position over a fluoroscopically compatible table. A standard midline posterior approach is used. The paravertebral musculature is then stripped subperiosteally. Complete exposure is done to the tips of the transverse processes at the level of the fracture and at the segment above and below the fracture. Caution is taken not to disrupt the intertransverse process ligament.

The lamina and facet joints are prepared and carefully stripped from all soft tissues. The joint capsule and articular cartilage are also removed to enhance fusion. Laminectomy is performed only in rare circumstances and should not be done routinely. Anatomic landmarks of the pedicles onto the posterior elements are carefully established on the vertebrae above and just below the level of the injury. With some experience, the entry point for the Schanz screw is easily identified. The usual point is found at the level of the midtransverse process line and just lateral and caudal to the border of the upper articular process. This position is then confirmed with the use of the image intensifier. The high-speed burr is then used to mark the entry point and to perforate the posterior cortical bone. Utilizing a blunt pedicle finder, the pedicle is then identified and the blunt probe is advanced into the pedicle and vertebral body. The image intensifier is utilized during this procedure to identify the correct sagittal angle and depth. The correct position is parallel or slightly convergent to the superior endplate and with 10–15° angulation towards the midline. The pedicle finder is then removed and the Schanz screw advanced without tapping. The position and angle are then verified using the image intensifier. The screw is then carefully advanced by hand. The appropriate length is determined by the image intensifier. The tip of the screw should not perforate the anterior cortex in order to avoid injury to the great vessels.

The rods are then connected to the screws. The first step in reducing the fracture involves the application of distraction. Distraction is applied through the distracting nuts. The dorsal vertebral body height is then restored and is visualized with the image intensifier. The next step is restoration of lordosis. This is achieved by forcefully compressing the long dorsal Schanz screw. This can be done by a loop of wire near the end of the screw and by carefully tightening the wire with a jet twister. This maneuver is visualized with the image intensifier. It is most important that the distraction and restoration of body height is done prior to any attempts in restoring lordosis. Without distraction, creating lordosis may produce cord impingement with possible catastrophic neurological damage.

Once the reduction is complete, all the nuts are tightened, and a stable construct is obtained. The long end of the Schanz screw is then cut with a special device that produces a flush and smooth surface. A standard posterior-lateral fusion is performed with iliac crest bone graft. Only one level above and one below of the fracture are fused (two motion segments).

CLINICAL RESULTS

There are now numerous reports in the literature of very encouraging results utilizing the FI (1,2,10,14,19,21). The largest series are from Dick in Switzerland (10). His technique does not include posterolateral fusion, but involves transpedicular insertion of the iliac crest. Lindsey and Dick reported good results in 80 fractures with neurologic deficit (19). The mean wedge angle of the fracture was corrected from 17.4° to 7.9°, and maintained at 8.4° after 1 year. On the other hand, the kyphosis angle measured by the Cobb technique showed a loss of 5° after removal of the device. They recommended posterolateral fusion or transpedicular interbody fusion to limit this loss of correction.

In 1987, Aebi et al. also reported good results with FI. Average anterior body height after the injury was 57.2%, which changed to 91.7% postoperatively (1). This was maintained at 87.5% after 1 year. The posterior vertebral body height after the injury was 88.4%, which improved to 103.2% postoperatively, to 97% after 1 year. Loss of angular correction was noted to be 4° at 1 year after surgery (1). Overall fusion rates have been very high with only sporadic reports of nonunion (1,10,14,19).

Esses et al. reported excellent results with the FI in a multicenter study (14). In 89 cases, they report no nonunions, an average improvement of kyphotic deformity of 14° and of 30% mean improvement in canal compromise. They also report only two cases of loss of some reduction, which was attributed to nut loosening. Other authors have reported the use of the FI for nontraumatic indications with good results (21). At this time, these reports are limited with small numbers. Currently, most centers are using the FI for the unstable spine fracture, as described above.

Complications with the FI can be divided in two groups: complications of pedicle screw placement and complications of implant failure. Pedicle screw placement is crucial to the success of the FI. Nerve damage is possible and has been reported in the literature (14). Great vessel damage from screws penetrating anterior cortex of the vertebral body is also possible. Surgeons planning to use segmental pedicular fixation should have a very clear knowledge of the anatomy prior to performing these types of operations. Anatomic insertion of the pedicle screw should always be verified with radiologic imaging. The most common form of implant failure has been the screw fracture (14). In most cases, the broken screw has not produced significantly symptomatology for the patient.

CONCLUSIONS

Each fracture and each patient should be evaluated and treated individually. Utilizing careful planning and judgment, effective treatment plans can be formulated to treat these complicated fractures.

The use of the FI currently offers a safe and effective method of treatment for unstable spine fractures. The FI will allow the surgeon to fuse only two motion segments, to reduce kyphotic deformities, and to improve canal space. The fusion rate is high, and a slight loss of correction and occasional screw fracture can be expected, but overall preservation of the reduction is expected.

REFERENCES

1. Aebi M, Etter C, Kehl T, et al: Stabilization of the lower thoracic and lumbar spine with the internal spinal skeletal fixation system. Spine 1987;12:544–555.
2. Aebi M, Etter C, Kehl T, et al: The internal fixation system: a new treatment for thoracolumbar fractures and other spinal disorders. Clin Orthop 1988;227:30–43.
3. Balderston R, Winter R, Moe J: Fusion to the sacrum for non-paralytic scoliosis in the adult. Orthop Trans 1984;8:170.
4. Bradford D: Instrumentation of the lumbar spine—An overview. Clin Orthop Rel Res 1986;203:209–218.
5. Brown LP, Bidwell KH, Holt RJ, et al: Aortic erosions and lacerations associated with the Dunn anterior spinal instrumentation. Scoliosis Research Society, 1985.
6. Denis F: The three column spine and its significance in the classification of acute thoracolumbar spine injuries. Spine 1983; 8:817–831.
7. Denis F, Armstrong G, Searls K, et al: Acute thoracolumbar burst fractures in the absence of neurological deficit (a comparison between operative and nonoperative treatment). Clin Orthop 1984;189:142–149.
8. Dewald RL: Burst fractures of the thoracic and lumbar spine. Clin Orthop Rel Res 1984;189:150–161.
9. Dick W, Woersdoerfer O, Magerl F: Mechanical properties of a new device for internal fixation of spine fractures: "the fixateur interne." In: Perren SM, Scneider E., eds. Biomechanics: current interdisciplinary research. Martinus Nijhoff, 1985.
10. Dick W: The "fixateur interne" as a versatile implant for spine surgery. Spine 1987;12:882–899.
11. Dickson JH, Harrington PR, Erwin WD: Results of reduction and stabilization in the severely fractured thoracic and lumbar spine. JBJS 1978;60A:799–806.
12. Dunn HK: Anterior stabilization of thoracolumbar injuries. Clin Orthop Rel Res 1984;189:116–124.
13. Edwards C, Simmons S, Levine A, et al: Primary rigid fixation of 135 thoracolumbar injuries: analysis of results using the rod sleeve method. Orthop Trans 1985;9:479.
14. Esses SI, Botsford DJ, Wright T, et al: Operative treatment of spinal fractures with the AO internal fixator. Spine 16:s146–s150.
15. Gertzbein S, Eismont F: Trauma of the lumbar spine: classification and treatment. In: Weinstein J, Wiesel S, eds. Philadelphia: WB Saunders, 1990.
16. Jodoin A, Dupuis P, Fraser M, et al: Unstable fractures of the thoracolumbar spine: A 10-year experience at Sacre-Coeur Hospital. J Trauma 1985;25:197–202.
17. Kaneda K, Abumi K, Fujiya M: Burst fractures with neurologic deficits of the thoracolumbar spine: results of anterior decompression and stabilization with anterior instrumentation. Spine 1984;9:788–795.
18. Krompinger WJ, Fredrickson BE, Mino DE, et al: Conservative treatment of fractures of the thoracic and lumbar spine. Orthop Clin North Am 1980;17:161–170.
19. Lindsey R, Dick W: The fixateur interne in the reduction and stabilization of thoracolumbar spine fractures in patients with neurological deficit. Spine 16:s140–s145.
20. Magerl F: Stabilization of the lower thoracic and lumbar spine with external skeletal fixation. Clin Orthop 1984;189:125–141.
21. Marchesi D, Thalgott J, Aebi M: Application and results of the AO internal fixation system in nontraumatic conditions. Spine 16:s162–s169.
22. Michel CR, Lalain JJ: Late results of Harrington's operation: Long-term evaluation of the lumbar spine below the fused segments. Spine 1985;10:414–420.
23. Olerud S, Karlstrom G, Sjostrom L: Transpedicular fixation of thoracolumbar vertebral fractures. Clin Orthop 1988;227:44–51.
24. Roy-Camille R, Saillant G, Mazel C: Internal fixation of the lumbar spine with pedicle screw plating. Clin Orthop Rel Res 1986; 203:7–17.
25. Steffe AD, Biscup RS, Sitakowski DJ: Segmental spine plates with

pedicle fixation: A new internal fixation device for disorders of the lumbar and thoracolumbar spine. Clin Orthop Rel Res 1986;203:43–53.

26. Weinstein J, Collalto P, Lehmann T: Thoracolumbar "burst" fractures treated conservatively: a long-term follow-up. Spine 1988; 13:33–38.

27. Willen J, Lindahl S, Nordwall A: Unstable thoracolumbar fractures—A comparative clinical study of conservative treatment and Harrington instrumentation. Spine 1985;10:111–122.

28. Yuan HA, Mann KA, Found EM, et al: Early clinical experience with the Syracuse I-plate: an anterior spinal fixation device. Spine 1988;13:278–285.

NINETEEN

Edwards Instrumentation: A Modular Spinal System

Charles C. Edwards

INTRODUCTION

System Evolution

The Edwards Modular System has evolved from a 12-year effort to sequentially overcome the problems and limitations faced by surgeons who seek to reconstruct the deformed or unstable spine. It combines the contributions of Paul Harrington (axial control and versatility) and Ramon Roy-Camille (segmental screw fixation) and adds the concept of adjustable transverse control in all dimensions.

In the late 1970s, the author concentrated on the surgical reconstruction of the injured spine. From this experience, it became apparent that for optimal results a surgeon should first determine the primary vector(s) of injury from radiographs and then use instrumentation to directly counteract these deforming forces (19,21). Since most thoracolumbar fractures were caused by compression, flexion, and rotational forces, instrumentation was needed that could generate distraction, extension (lordosis), and provide rotational control. Harrington rods contributed the necessary distraction, but, even when contoured, provided only minimal extension and virtually no rotational control resulting in frequent hook dislodgement. To provide the necessary active lordosis and rotational control, rod-sleeve spacers and the Rod-Sleeve Method were developed to improve reduction and provide "indirect decompression" of flexion-compression injuries (between 1979–1981) (6). The Rod-Sleeve Method consistently yielded anatomic alignment, but laminar edge resorption with occasional hook dislodgement still occurred. These hook interface problems led to the design of an L-shaped anatomic hook in 1982 (30). The L design increased hook-laminar contact area over C-shaped hooks to reduce laminar resorption and hook dislodgement (19,30).

The next problem confronted was the inability to anchor rods directly to the sacrum so as to apply compression or distraction forces across the lumbosacral junction. The Sacral Fixation Device was developed in 1983 to overcome this limitation (7,9). It combined spinal screws designed for sacral alar or lumbar pedicle fixation, with rods that could be ratcheted in either compression or distraction and anatomic hooks in three sizes, which served as linkages between the rods and screws (Fig. 19.1). The Sacral Fixation Device introduced two new capabilities: (1) the ability to attach spinal rods directly to the sacrum with screws; and (2) the ability to attach to proximal vertebrae with either laminar hooks or pedicle screws (11).

The capability of secure fixation in compression across the lumbosacral junction improved our in situ fusion union rate and effectiveness in treating low lumbar nonunions (27). However, we still lacked the versatility needed to correct most lumbar deformities without anterior or transspinal releases and forced manipulation. In an effort to achieve more correction of deformity with less surgery, the author sought to incorporate intraoperative stress-relaxation. However, this required instrumentation with adjustability in *all* planes of motion. This requirement was fulfilled with the development of adjustable pedicle connectors in 1985 (10,22). Connectors served as linkages between spinal screws and rods. They could be shortened or lengthened and positioned to translate individual vertebra in any direction. Combining adjustable connectors with bidirectional ratcheting rods made it possible to gradually apply corrective forces and maintain stable fixation in all dimensions.

During the past 5 years, the author and associates have focused on the development of surgical procedures that incorporate stress-relaxation to improve correction of kyphosis (19,26), spondylolisthesis (13), scoliosis, and

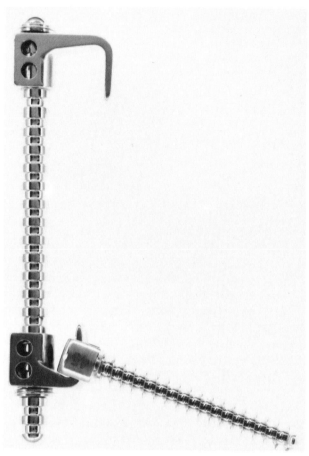

Figure 19.1. Sacral Fixation Device. Sacral fixation is provided by a spinal screw directed from the base of the L5-S1 facet across the sacral ala. The screw is attached to a ratcheted Universal spinal rod with an Anatomic hook linkage and held in place with a C-washer.

The six components or "modules" described above can be assembled into a variety of "constructs," depending on the biomechanical needs of each case. For example, the Compression construct is designed to provide both stabilization and physiologic axial loading to promote bony union. Other constructs are designed to apply optimum corrective forces over time for greater reduction of deformity with less invasive surgery than required in the past. These include the Rod-sleeve construct for thoracolumbar fractures, the Distraction-Lordosis (D-L) construct for lower lumbar fractures and degenerative listhesis, the Kyphoreduction construct, Spondylo construct, and various Scoliosis constructs. Extensive studies of these constructs have demonstrated improved clinical results. More importantly, we have learned that instrumentation to adjustably control the position of individual vertebrae in all planes of motion opens the door to a wide range of new surgical techniques and treatment possibilities.

In order to transfer these new capabilities to other surgeons and generate a clinical database for the continued evolution of new surgical procedures, the Spinal Fixation Study Group was formed in 1986. It is supported by the Spinal Research Foundation and Scientific Spinal, Ltd. The program has been limited to carefully selected spinal surgeons who regularly attend workshops and forward radiographs and clinical data to the Spine Documentation Center at the University of Maryland. Through quarterly workshop seminars and the ongoing analysis of the over 3000 cases presently in our documentation center, we are able to refine the new surgical procedures, define their indications, and further advance our reconstructive capabilities.

other thoracic and lumbar deformities. As the scope of our surgery expanded, we saw the need to enhance the overall stiffness of the final construct in selected cases. This need was met with the recent addition of adjustable rod crosslinks.

Over the past decade, Edwards modular instrumentation has become a comprehensive posterior spinal system composed of six basic components:

1. Anatomic hooks for attachment to thoracic or lumbar lamina;
2. Screws for secure fixation to the sacrum or lumbar pedicles;
3. Bidirectional ratcheted universal rods for axial control;
4. Various-sized rod-sleeves as fixed transverse spacers;
5. Pedicle connectors for adjustable transverse control in all directions; and
6. Adjustable rod crosslinks for control of relative rod position and instrumentation stiffness.

Biomechanical Principles

The author's surgical philosophy is based on first identifying the forces of deformation and resulting planes of instability and then applying corrective forces in the opposite directions (11,19,21). To carry out this philosophy and achieve biocompatible fixation, the Edwards Modular System incorporates five mechanical principles:

1. *Versatility of Attachment.* Linkages (i.e., hooks or adjustable connectors) between the screws and rods permit placement of screws in the most advantageous position and orientation for each vertebra. This versatility facilitates segmental fixation of even the most complex deformities, allows the surgeon to direct each screw through the strongest bone stock available, and avoids any impingement of adjacent unfused facets.

2. *Three-Dimensional Control.* Axial control (segmental compression and/or distraction) is provided by ratcheted spinal rods. Independent control of vertebral translation

in the coronal, sagittal, and rotational planes is achieved using sleeves (spacers), adjustable pedicle connectors, and rod crosslinks. The ability to control the position of individual vertebrae in all planes of motion makes it possible to apply all necessary corrective forces via the implants themselves. Hence, there is rarely need for external outriggers, bulky instruments, manual manipulations, or extensive releases.

3. *Stress Relaxation.* Independent axial and transverse adjustability makes it possible to slowly move individual vertebrae in any direction. The ability to apply corrective forces in small gradations over time allows the surgeon to slowly stretch out contracted tissues even after many years of deformity (13,19,26). By utilizing intraoperative viscoelastic stress-relaxation, we are less dependent on anterior or transcanal resections (Fig. 19.2).

4. *Dynamic Loading.* After reduction, most deformities remain unstable in the same planes as the initial deformity. Hence, instrumentation should exert forces in the opposite directions until fusion. This is accomplished by loading the rods within their elastic range. We select sleeves of the appropriate thickness or adjust pedicle connectors to slightly bow the spinal rods in order to generate continuing lordosis or other corrective forces (19). The result is improved late maintenance of correction (25).

5. *Load Sharing.* The constructs are designed to apply

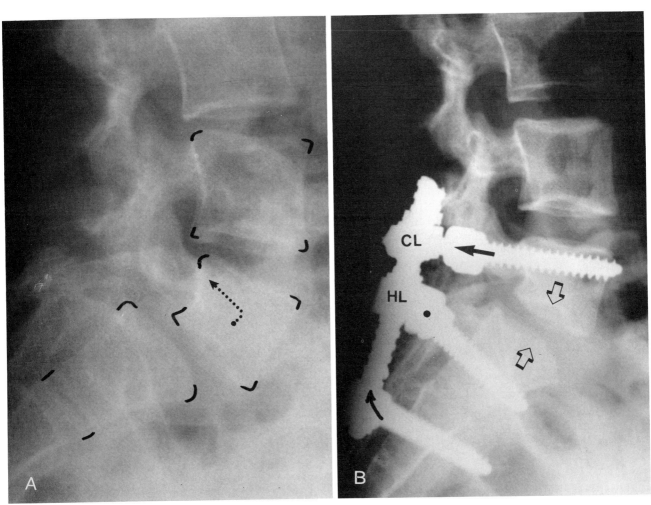

Figure 19.2. Reduction/Fixation of Spondylolisthesis. *A*, Midgrade L5-S1 spondylolisthesis in a 16-year-old female. Reduction requires distraction for restoration of height, combined with posterior translation of the lumbar spine. *B*, Correction of deformity using the Spondylo Construct. Hook (HL) and connector linkages (CL) provide sufficient versatility to attach and reduce spondylolisthesis and other spinal deformities. Axial control with ratcheted Universal rods combined with transverse control with the threaded connectors makes it possible to control the position of every vertebra in all three dimensions. Fine, axial and transverse adjustability permit very slow application of corrective forces in order to fully utilize stress relaxation. Following reduction, the instrumentation facilitates physiologic axial loading to promote union.

only the forces needed to correct deformity or instability without unnecessary residual restraints which could stress-shield bone and interfere with healing. For example, several constructs incorporate distraction and bending forces to correct deformity, but then permit unrestricted physiologic axial loading across the instrumented vertebrae. After reduction, the instrumentation works in conjunction with the vertebrae and ligaments to form a stable construct with a composite modulus (stiffness) sufficient to stop unwanted gross motion, but not so rigid as to stress-shield the developing fusion or overly stiffen the instrumented spine. The resulting semirigid fixation appears to promote union and lessen subsequent breakdown of the adjacent motion segments. Hence, the instrumentation is biuocompatible, and late removal is usually unnecessary (25).

Description of System Components

1. *Anatomic Hooks.* The L-shaped hooks (manufactured by Scientific Spinal, Ltd., Baltimore, Maryland and protected under U.S. Patents 4,369,769, 4,567,884, 4,569,338 and foreign patents covering Great Britain, Europe and Japan with other patents pending) make contact with both the edge and undersurface of proximal lamina. This improves stress distribution to minimize resorption, loosening, and dislodgement. Seating for distal hooks is improved by a round, rather than square body and tapered, rather than rectangular shoe (11,19,30).

The hooks are also designed to minimize canal protrusion so they can be safely placed around either the inferior or superior laminar edge. The portion of the hook between the body and shoe has a straight incline that directs the flat hook shoe against the undersurface of the lamina. The hooks are available in three heights (low, medium, and high) to ensure a snug fit about the lamina and low profile for spinal rods.

Anatomic hooks also provide a linkage between spinal screws and rods to permit variable screw orientation. When used with Universal rods, they can be ratcheted either proximally or distally on the same rod. They can also be used with older Harrington or Reverse Ratchet rods for unidirectional ratcheting (Fig. 19.1).

2. *Spinal/Sacral Screws.* To minimize risk of infection, the Edwards screw has self-tapping, recessed flutes so that there is no need to use a sharp tap prior to screw insertion. The tip of the screw is a hemispheric ball to guide the screw down a predrilled hole and push away, rather than penetrate, any soft tissues encountered should the screw exit the anterior cortex. Screws are provided in various lengths, from 30–50 mm. Adjustment in length between the 5-mm screw increments is accomplished with a seat-

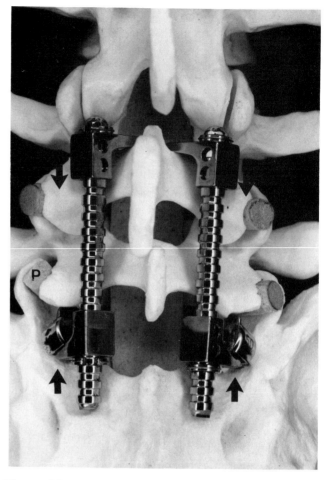

Figure 19.3. Instrumentation assembled for segmental compression. Spinal screws for sacral or lumbar pedicle fixation have blunt tips for safe insertion and a proximally tapered minor diameter to enhance fatigue strength. Anatomic hooks for either laminar attachment or as a fixed linkage between the screws and rod are available in three sizes (low, medium, and high). Universal rods allow bidirectional ratcheting for segmental compression or distraction. Adjustable connectors between the midposition screws and rods can be lengthened or shortened as needed to reduce deformity or increase the rigidity of fixation.

ing reamer. This makes it possible to secure bicortical sacral ala fixation without the risks of excess penetration.

For optimum strength of fixation, screws are fully threaded. The threads are relatively deep to grip more bone so as to prevent loosening or pullout. To maximize near-cortex fixation, proximal screw threads taper slightly to create a wedge effect. This offsets the near-cortex expansion that occurs with insertion of all bone screws (Fig. 19.3).

Several design features that reduce the incidence of screw breakage were first introduced by the Edwards spinal screw. These include a tapered proximal minor diameter to eliminate the stress riser effect at the shank:head junction (22), a screw seating reamer to provide lateral head support (22), and the use of a hook or connector linkage between the screw and rod to absorb peak impact loading (7). Despite frequent use of spinal screws for complex deformities, the incidence of screw breakage remains well below 1%.

Spinal screws are available in four head configurations. The *standard* screw has a double-bevel opening to accommodate the shoe of an Anatomic hook or adjustable connector. Its geometry facilitates insertion of the hook linkages, but then locks the lumbosacral angle during the application of compression. The *distraction* screw head has a fixed angle slot that preserves lumbosacral lordosis during distraction. *Angled* and *straight-hole* screws articulate directly with the spinal rods for low-profile instrumentation to either the sacrum or anterolateral vertebral bodies.

3. *Universal Rods.* Universal rods were initially designed to combine the best of Harrington rods for distraction, Edwards Reverse Ratchet rods for compression and Moe rods for rotational control. They were refined between 1985–1989 to enhance their versatility (22). The present fully ratcheted Universal rod permits ratcheting in both directions for segmental compression, distraction, or neutralization (17). Ratchets permit fine (1/16″) gradations for axial control with both wide and narrow C-washers to maintain precise hook or connector position. The rods have an octagon at one end that provides rotational control in 45° increments for contouring or derotational maneuvers. They have the same 1/4″ outside diameter as earlier rods; however, their larger minor diameter and the lack of a discrete stress-riser make the Edwards Universal rod less susceptible to fatigue failure. Accordingly, rod breakage rates remain well below 1%. Grooves at both ends of the rod and terminal lock washers prevent hook:rod disengagement (Fig. 19.3).

4. *Spinal Rod-Sleeves.* Polyethylene rod-sleeve spacers provide translational and rotational control by wedging between the rod, facets, and spinous processes (19). They are available in four sizes to accommodate thoracic, thoracolumbar, lumbar, and low lumbar spine anatomy. The polyethylene contains sulfate for x-ray visualization. The ability to select sleeves of different sizes and sculpt them with a burr makes it possible to vary the lordotic or translational force applied by the rod and sleeve(s) during spinal reconstruction.

5. *Adjustable Connectors.* Connectors between the rods and spinal screws act as universal joints to facilitate fixation of malpositioned vertebrae. By extending or shortening the connectors, it is then possible to gradually reduce kyphosis, lateral, retro, or spondylolisthesis and

actively derotate scoliotic vertebrae. After reduction, connectors are locked to fix the rod-screw position and stabilize the spine. Two types of connectors are available. Ring connectors are placed during rod assembly and can be ratcheted up or down the rod to facilitate reduction of complex deformities (Fig. 19.3). Snap connectors can be added following rod assembly.

6. *Rod Crosslinks.* Adjustable rod crosslinks connect the right and left Universal rods in selected constructs. They serve to improve the reduction of coronal plane deformity and to enhance construct stability (2,4,5,35,36). Rod crosslinks are added to long constructs or those left in distraction to raise construct stiffness to optimal levels.

Construct Selection

The first step in planning spinal reconstruction is construct selection. The six components of the Edwards Modular System are assembled to form various "constructs" (22), depending on the biomechanical needs of the case at hand. The Compression construct is used in cases with intact facets when the goal of fixation is to promote fusion. When disrupted facets preclude compression, the simple Neutralization construct is substituted. The Rod-Sleeve construct provides anatomic reduction with relatively short instrumentation for thoracolumbar fractures. The D-L construct uses pedicle screws to effect short segment distraction and lordosis for reduction of low lumbar fractures or degenerative listhesis.

Chronic deformities are addressed with the Kyphoreduction, Spondylo, and Scoliosis constructs. They apply corrective forces very gradually to facilitate stress-relaxation and reduce the need for anterior or transcanal release procedures. The Kyphoreduction construct provides three-point loading followed by posterior column shortening for chronic posttraumatic or other kyphotic deformities. The Spondylo construct achieves full reduction of spondylolisthesis and spondyloptosis. Optimum treatment of scoliosis, especially with secondary listhesis, requires careful preoperative planning and selection of the appropriate Scoliosis construct for each case.

Preoperative Planning

Before embarking on a reconstructive spinal procedure, the author recommends the following planning sequence:

1. Analyze standing and bending films as well as contrast studies to determine the direction of forces causing spinal deformity and/or instability, sites of neural impingement, and the presence of anterior bony bridges

or posterior blocks to reduction which must be resected before spinal instrumentation.

2. Diagram the necessary corrective forces on preoperative AP and lateral films with a wax pencil.

3. Select or design the construct to apply the needed corrective forces.

4. Decide the most proximal and distal vertebrae that must be instrumented to maintain stable fixation without excessive length of instrumentation and select sites for laminar hook, spinal screw, or sleeve attachment.

5. Select the optimum type, size, and orientation of hook or connector linkages between spinal screws and the Universal rods. In general, hooks are safer and more efficient in the thoracic spine, while screws are safer and more effective in the low lumbar and sacral spine.

6. Determine the order of reduction when treating deformities. For most translational deformities first distract, then translate, and finally compress. For angular deformities, apply 3-point loading then compress or distract.

7. Mark the location of crosslinks to enhance the stability of long constructs or those to be left in net distraction.

THE COMPRESSION CONSTRUCT

The compression construct provides in-situ fixation in compression across the facets of just one or multiple motion segments. Hook linkages between the rod and spine permit physiologic axial loading through the posterior bony elements, yet block tension and shear (27). This creates an ideal environment for bony union in the treatment of nonunions and for primary fusions with intact facets (27,42). It provides an active extension moment for stable fixation after reduction of dislocations or chance fractures (11,14,20,31).

Technique

Anatomic hooks are used for attachment in the thoracic spine or for proximal attachment in the lumbar spine for cases with no central stenosis. To insert proximal hooks, resect the overhanging distal edge of the adjacent cephalad lamina and detach the ligamentum flavum. Notch the cephalad edge of the lamina to be instrumented about 5 mm to the ridge formed by the distal insertion of the ligamentum flavum. Feel around the lamina with a #3 Penfield dissector. Load a high Anatomic hook on the Anatomic hook holder. Lower the hook into the laminotomy while holding the tip of the hook shoe against the edge and undersurface of the lamina. If there is more than 3 mm space between the hook body and lamina, convert to a shorter medium Anatomic hook (Fig. 19.4).

In cases with borderline canal stenosis, use spinal screws for proximal attachment to avoid further canal

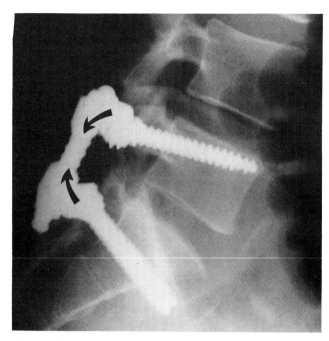

Figure 19.4. Hook-to-Screw L4-S1 Compression Construct. Dowel-shaped iliac bone plugs (P) in the facets promote fusion and maintain foraminal height. High Anatomic hooks over the notched L4 lamina provide proximal fixation. Sacral screws inserted across the ala are attached to the Universal rods with low hook linkages. The application of compression with a spreader blocks flexion and rotation and facilitates unrestricted axial loading to promote union.

compromise. For lumbar pedicle fixation, the posterior cortex over the pedicle is removed with a burr. A probe is used to locate the center of the pedicle, and 2-mm bits are inserted. After correct orientation is confirmed radiographically, the hole is expanded to 3.5 mm in 1-cm increments. All four quadrants of the hole are palpated with a depth gauge to ensure that there is no pedicle cortex penetration after each increment and prior to screw insertion (22). In most cases, a screw length is selected that will approach, but not penetrate, the anterior vertebral body cortex. The seating reamer is used to prepare a bed prior to inserting screws with a standard hex screwdriver. Finally, screw portion is confirmed radiographically (Fig. 19.5).

For sacral fixation, the author described bicortical screw placement across the lateral sacral ala in 1984 (7,17), a location that both simplifies insertion and improves the strength of fixation (46). First, a 2-mm drill bit enters the sacrum in the dimple found at the base of the L5-S1 facet. It is directed approximately 35° lateral and 25° caudal to parallel the superior endplate of S1 (Figs. 19.4 and 19.5). The bit is manually pushed to contact the anterior cortex of the sacrum, where an AP

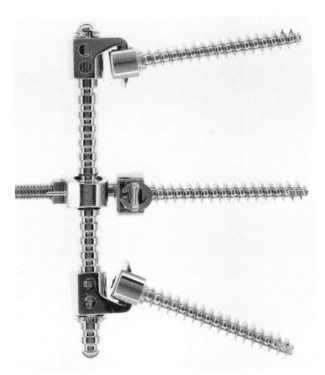

Figure 19.5. Screw-to-Screw Compression Construct. Proximal screw fixation is used in cases with laminectomy or stenosis.

balancing the compressive loads between both rods, stop washers are applied, and any excess rod is cut off (14,17,20).

When pedicle screws are used for proximal fixation, the rod is reversed. The octagonal end of a straight rod is directed distally through a low hook linkage and held in place with a narrow washer. Another low Anatomic hook is placed over the proximal end of the rod and inserted into the screw slots. The spreader is then placed adjacent to the proximal hook to apply compression.

For optimal results when treating multiple nonunions, we recommend screw fixation on both sides of each nonunion. Midposition vertebrae are attached to the rods with pedicle connectors. During the application of compression, the midposition connectors are shortened to prevent excess lordosis and to provide considerable rotational stability (16) (Fig. 19.6).

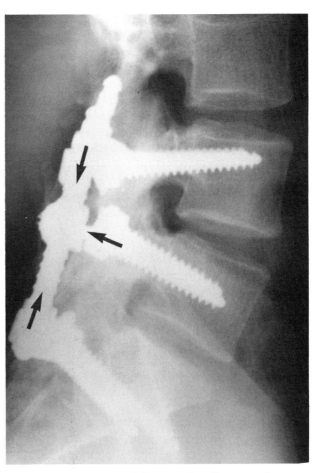

Figure 19.6. Segmental Compression Construct. Instrumentation as assembled in Figure 19.3 is used for the treatment of multiple nonunions. Segmental screw fixation offers both considerable rigidity and the physiologic advantages of dynamic axial loading.

radiographic image should show the tip of the bit 1–2 cm from the anterior sacroiliac joint. The hole is expanded with a 3.5-mm bit. The drill should just penetrate the anterior alar cortex, but remain within the anterior reflection of the sacroiliac ligament. A depth gauge is used to carefully feel around the medial edge of the anterior alar hole in order to select the correct length screw. When medial sacral screw orientation is preferred, the sacral screw is inserted just lateral to the L5-S1 facet, directed 25° medial through the S1 pedicle toward the junction of the anterior cortex and the S1 endplate in the midline.

After placing hooks and/or screws we recommend lateral decortication and insertion of a bone plug across each facet joint (Fig. 19.4). Some surgeons find lateral graft placement easier before instrumentation. Universal rods of the appropriate length are selected and contoured when crossing the lumbosacral junction. If hooks are used for proximal fixation, the octagonal end of the Universal rod is passed cephalad through the body of the proximal hook. A narrow washer is crimped in the groove at the end of the rod to fix it to the hook. A second hook is placed over the distal end of the rod and inserted into either the distal screw slot or about the distal lamina. After assembling both rods, a spreader is used on the distal end of the lower hook to apply compression. After

Results

The Compression construct is one of the most frequently used constructs in the Edwards Modular System. The Spinal Fixation Study Group series includes 882 cases treated with the Compression construct including 354 with lumbar pseudoarthrosis, 52 with dislocations, and 448 with spondylosis or instability. Surgeons have found the construct easy to master and associated with an 85% probability of fusion and a very low incidence of complications. Detailed reports are published on the treatment of lumbar nonunions and thoracolumbar dislocations. In 1989, Edwards and Weigel presented 56 nonunions between L3 and the sacrum occurring in 33 patients. All were treated with the Compression construct, iliac grafting, and postoperative bracing. Edwards sacral screws were used for distal attachment. Proximal attachment was with either Anatomic laminar hooks or pedicle screws. Postoperatively, patients required much less analgesia than prior in situ fusion controls. Complications were limited to one infection in a diabetic, transient radiculopathy in two with associated decompressions, and asymptomatic breakage of three early design screws.

Patients were followed for 2 years; union was assessed with quantitative flexion-extension films. Overall, 86% of the pseudoarthroses were successfully repaired after one operation with repair of all one to three nonunions in 82% of the patients (28); a considerable improvement over the results expected for in situ fusion alone. A similar study was conducted on 42 patients by McCutcheon and Cohen. They experienced a comparable fusion success rate of 86%; complications were confined to transient radiculopathy in one patient, infection in one, and late breakage in three (42).

Dislocations tested with a short segment Compression construct fixation have been reviewed by several authors (31,38). Levine and Edwards noted that the Compression construct maintained excellent reduction and promoted early union in all cases. However, late reduction of dislocation or excessive compression without use of facet bone plugs was found to accentuate bulging of the disrupted disc (39).

NEUTRALIZATION CONSTRUCT

The posterior Neutralization construct combines proximal angled hole screws, distal straight-hole screws, and Universal rods for short segment in situ fixation. It is useful in primary fusions when facets have been resected and compression cannot be applied.

When treating chronic spondylolysis, a hybrid construct is used to resist anterior slippage. Angle hole screws proximally are connected to standard screws with low or medium hook linkages distally. Slight compression is then applied to create a posteroinferiorly directed force to compress the defect and help prevent anterior slippage (16).

For anterior vertebral body neutralization, one or two Universal rods are used in conjunction with straight-hole screws. Bicortical screws are placed laterally in the vertebral body and the Universal rod(s) inserted. Distraction is applied to eliminate any kyphosis and facilitate placement of a large anterior graft. Gentle compression is then applied with the same rod(s) across the graft using a spreader on the outside of the distal screws (16). Postoperative bracing is recommended. Experience with anterior fixation is limited, and long-term results are not yet available.

ROD-SLEEVE CONSTRUCT

Indications

The Rod-sleeve construct (Fig. 19.7) combines Anatomic laminar hooks with straight Universal rods and polyethylene sleeves. The Rod-Sleeve Method is used in the treatment of T8-L3 thoracolumbar burst fractures and fracture-dislocations with an intact anterior ligament. When surgery is performed within several days of injury, it is usually possible to *in*directly decompress retropulsed fragments via ligamentotaxis and hyperlordosis (6,19).

Biomechanics

Polyethylene sleeves are centered directly over the superior facets of the fractured vertebrae, where they span the spinous processes above and below the traumatic disruption. In the sagittal plane, the sleeves wedge between the rods and facets to restore maximum lordosis. By articulating with the posterior elements above and below the injury, the rod-sleeves automatically correct anteroposterior translational deformity as well. In the coronal plane, sleeves wedge between the facets and spinous processes to correct medial-lateral translation. The sagittal plus coronal wedge effect yields rotational alignment and stability as well (6,17,19,44). The result is anatomic alignment for most thoracic or lumbar injuries (Fig. 19.8).

Other features of the Rod-Sleeve construct are responsible for better late maintenance of alignment than previously reported for alternative techniques (19,25,33). The L-shaped Anatomic hooks have a much greater laminar contact area than the former C-shaped hooks for less laminar resorption and hook loosening. Also, resorption between the rod and midposition lamina is eliminated by

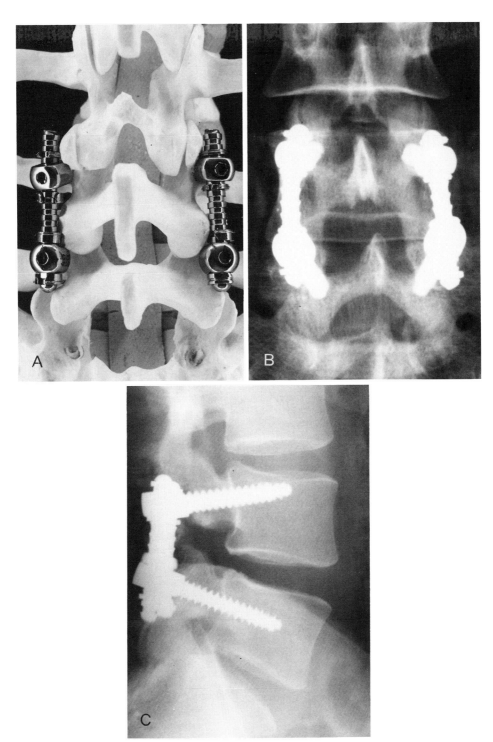

Figure 19.7. Posterior Neutralization Construct. *A*, Angle-hole screws are used proximally and straight-hole screws distally. Wide or narrow washer fixation adjacent to the screw heads maintains screw to screw distance for semirigid fixation. *B* and *C*, Postoperative radiographs of patient with prior surgical re-section of left L4-L5 facet. Note the medial-cephalad orientation of proximal screws to avoid the adjacent facets and the low profile of the instrumentation. (Case courtesy of Dr. David Wong, Denver, CO).

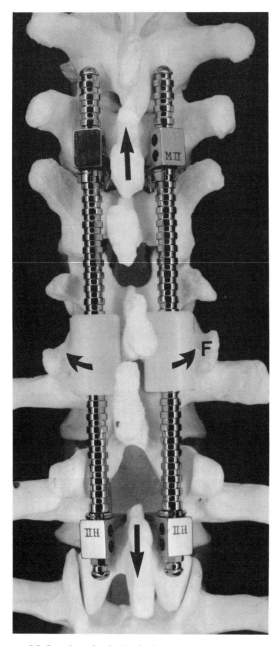

Figure 19.8. Standard Rod-Sleeve Construct. The Rod-Sleeve Construct provides both distraction and lordosis. Sleeves wedged between the superior facets of the fractured vertebra (F) and spinous processes on either side of the injury correct translational displacement and provide rotational stability. In this model, proximal fixation is achieved with medium Anatomic hooks placed at the junction of the facets and lamina. Distal fixation is with high Anatomic hooks placed under the lamina. Distraction is provided with Universal rods and maintained with wide washers proximally and narrow washers distally.

the broad contact surface and compatible low modulus of elasticity between the sleeve and laminar bone (19, 30). Finally, the appropriate size sleeves will bow the rods within their elastic range. This provides a dynamic lordotic force that compensates for anterior ligament stress-relaxation to maintain full lordosis and stable fixation until fusion (17,19).

Because the Rod-Sleeve Method generates considerable corrective force, length of instrumentation can be much shorter than with previous rod techniques. The Standard Sleeve construct spans only three interspaces for lumbar injuries and four interspaces for thoracic fractures.

Standard Sleeve Technique

The Standard Sleeve construct is selected when the preoperative CT scan demonstrates a "stable posterior arch," such that anterior pressure against the superior facet will be transmitted through the pedicles to major vertebral body fragments (17,19).

At surgery, the patient is placed over two transverse rolls to facilitate postural reduction. After posterior dissection, the surgeon selects the largest sleeve that will fit comfortably between the superior facet of the fractured vertebrae and the adjacent spinous processes. Generally, small (2-mm) sleeves are used for thoracic constructs, medium (4 mm) for thoracolumbar, large (6 mm) for upper lumbar, and elliptical (8 mm) for midlumbar placement. Bony prominences and/or sleeves are trimmed with a burr as needed to provide a snug fit between the facets and spinous processes. Anatomic hooks are inserted into the first interspace 3–4 cm on either side of the sleeves. The shortest hook that will fit around the lamina is selected. The proximal hook is inserted under the lamina at the medial edge of the facet. Distal hooks are placed into narrow laminotomies that extend from the interspace to the laminar ridge formed by the distal insertion of the ligamentum flavum (17,21) (Fig. 19.8).

Reduction is accomplished with rod-sleeve instrumentation. A Harrington distractor should not be used, since it will lengthen the spine without fully correcting kyphosis and could tent the cord over the gibbus. To correct the deformity, first pass one rod through the upper hook and position the sleeve near the middle of the rod. Grossly reduce the spine by pushing "down" on the distal end of the rod while pulling "up" on the distal hook until the end of the rod can be engaged into the hook with a spreader (Fig. 19.9).

To facilitate reduction, a long rod and sleeve can be used on the opposite side of the spine as a reduction level (19). Resistant kyphosis can often be reduced in stages. Begin with straight rods, and sequentially replace them

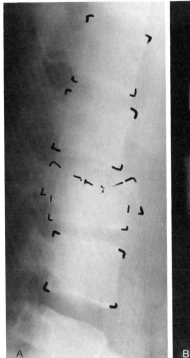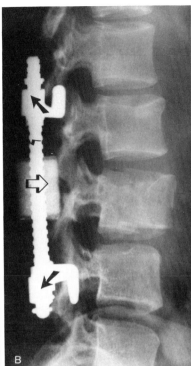

Figure 19.9. Rod-Sleeve Method. *A,* Lateral radiograph of L3 burst fracture with moderate fragment retropulsion. *B,* Complete reduction and fixation was accomplished with the Rod-Sleeve Method. Universal rods provide the distraction needed to restore vertebral height. Sleeves provide the 3-point loading needed to restore normal lumbar lordosis and substantial indirect reduction of the retropulsed fragment. Note that instrumentation and fusion extend across only three interspaces (L1-L4).

with progressively larger sleeves (19,26). When both rods are engaged with the proper size sleeve, complete the reduction by advancing the sleeves with a spreader until they are centered over the superior facet of the fractured vertebrae. Sleeves of sufficient size should produce a slight bow in the rods. Apply incremental distraction over at least 20 minutes. Confirm reduction with a lateral x-ray and consider intraoperative myelography or ultrasound for incomplete paraplegics. Finally, secure hook position with C-washers and perform a lateral fusion with fresh iliac bone (17,21).

Bridging Sleeve Technique

If a wide laminectomy has been performed or if the preoperative CT scan shows an unstable arch, the Bridging Sleeve technique is recommended. An unstable posterior arch is characterized by major pedicle comminution, widely displaced pedicles that are discontinuous with major body fragments, or by depressed laminar fractures (17). If the posterior arch is "unstable," use two pairs of sleeves centered over the facets of the first intact posterior arch above and below the fractured vertebrae (Fig. 19.10).

To assemble the Bridging Sleeve construct, hooks are inserted 3 cm proximal and distal to the edge of the sleeve pairs. Reduction is performed in the same manner as the Standard Sleeve technique. The resulting 4-point loading construct is longer, but achieves the same anatomic alignment and stability as a Standard Sleeve construct (19).

After surgery, patients with both the Standard and Bridging Sleeve techniques are typically protected in a polypropylene total contact orthosis for 6 months (19). When bracing is not possible, surgeons can supplement fixation with a pair of sublaminar wires proximal and distal to the sleeves and/or supplement proximal fixation with a bilaminar Anatomic hook claw (16,24,43).

Results

Excellent clinical results in late alignment and few complications are consistently reported for the Rod-Sleeve Method. Investigators have found it effective for the treatment of thoracic and lumbar burst fractures, fracture-dislocations, and dislocations (14,32,37,38–40). The largest spinal injury series published to date used the Rod-Sleeve Method for 135 thoracolumbar fractures. Surgery was performed early, averaging 19 hours from

Figure 19.10. Bridging Sleeve Construct. *A* and *B*, Reduction and fixation of L1 burst fracture with displaced pedicles following laminectomy to remove fractured lamina displaced into the canal. Sleeves are centered over the first intact facets above and below the injury. The resulting 4-point loading corrects kyphosis and vertebral height with very stable fixation. Proper sleeve selection causes slight bowing of the rods (*dotted straight line*) for continued dynamic loading in lordosis. (Case courtesy of Dr. Alan Levine, Baltimore, MD.)

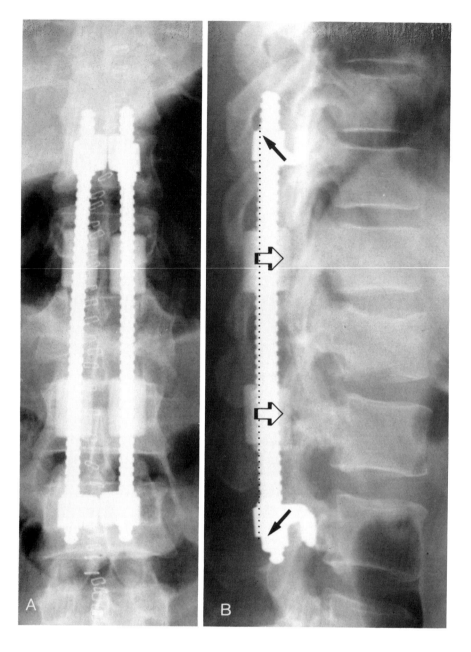

injury. The Rod-Sleeve Method successfully corrected all kyphosis and provided sufficient *in*direct decompression of the canal in 96% of the incomplete paraplegics. There were few complications, and no patient sustained neurologic worsening. At 2-year follow-up, average kyphosis was only 1.3,° substantially better than reported with alternative techniques (19).

Hanley and Starr recently reported a prospective series of 22 thoracolumbar junction fractures treated with the Rod-Sleeve Method. This series was also free of major complications. It reported correction of kyphosis to 3° and restoration of canal areas to 86% of normal via indirect decompression (33).

A series of 44 unstable burst fractures treated with early rod-sleeve reduction and 7-year average follow-up was recently presented. Anterior grafting was not performed in any of the cases, yet there was average reconstitution of 91% of the crushed vertebral body area. Average kyphosis across the fractured vertebra and disc space was limited to only 3° after 5–10-year follow-up (25).

Use of the Rod-Sleeve Method has grown rapidly in North America. Surgeons have found it to be the easiest available method for treating most thoracolumbar injuries with a remarkably low rate of serious complications and excellent long-term results (31,33,37,38). Accordingly, use of the Rod-Sleeve Method now approximates 2,000 cases per year in North America. Considering the widespread success and excellent late alignment using this method, there is little reason to accept the increased difficulty and risk of pedicle screw fixation for spinal injuries about the thoracolumbar junction.

DISTRACTION/LORDOSIS (D-L) CONSTRUCT

The D-L construct typically attaches to three consecutive lumbar vertebrae with spinal screws. Fixed-angle distraction screws are used proximally to maintian lordosis during distraction. Low hook linkages connect the proximal and distal screws to Universal Rods. Midposition connectors are extended to apply lordosis (17,22) (Fig. 19.11). The D-L construct is used successfully in the treatment of low-lumbar burst fractures (41), instability with stenosis, and degenerative lumbar spondylolisthesis (13,34).

Low Lumbar Fractures

For L4 or L5 burst fractures, screws are attached to the vertebrae on either side of the fractured body. Screws are also placed in the pedicles of the fractured vertebrae, since the stout L4 or L5 pedicles almost always remain intact. Midposition connectors are extended to restore lordosis, and the proximal hooks are ratcheted to restore height. The connectors are then further extended to translate the fractured vertebral body, together with any residual retropulsed fragments, anteriorly away from the cauda equina (Fig. 19.12). The D-L construct can be combined with a laminectomy to remove fracture fragments or enlarge stenotic foramina when needed (14,17).

Results of the first 16 low lumbar fractures treated with the D-L construct were presented in 1988. The D-L restored good alignment without the need to instrument adjacent normal lumbar vertebrae. It also provided sufficiently stable fixation to permit early patient ambulation. At 1-year follow-up, 89% vertebral height was maintained, and lordosis at the fracture level was restored to 6.° Fusion occurred in 94% of the cases. Complications were limited to one hook dislodgement and one radiculopathy, a considerable improvement over previous experience with hook fixation across the lumbosacral junction (41).

The Spinal Fixation Study Group series now includes 118 cases using the D-L construct to reconstruct low lumbar burst fractures. Results remain similar to the initial prospective study cited above, but with a lower rate of complications and a primary union rate of 90%.

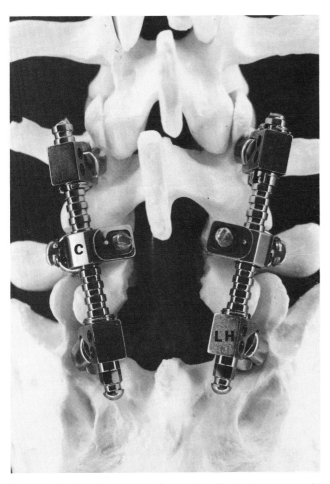

Figure 19.11. Distraction/Lordosis (D-L) Construct. AP model photograph showing D-L construct following L5 laminectomy. Screws are placed in L4, L5, and S1. Universal rods are attached to the screws with low hook linkages (LH) oriented in distraction at L4 and S1. Adjustable connectors (C) are extended to restore lordosis.

Degenerative Spondylolisthesis

For instability with borderline stenosis from bulging discs or narrowed foramina, the D-L construct will restore normal lordosis, flatten bulging discs, and enlarge foramina to reduce the amount of direct decompression required. For degenerative listhesis between L3-L4, or L4-L5, distraction restores normal height to flatten bulging discs and enlarge foramina, while lengthening the midposition connectors causes the lower two vertebrae (i.e., L5 and sacrum) to rotate into flexion underneath the slipped proximal vertebrae (L4). This reduces the listhesis and counteracts translation instability. The resulting indirect decompression lessens the amount of intracanal surgery needed to decompress the cauda equina (Fig. 19.13).

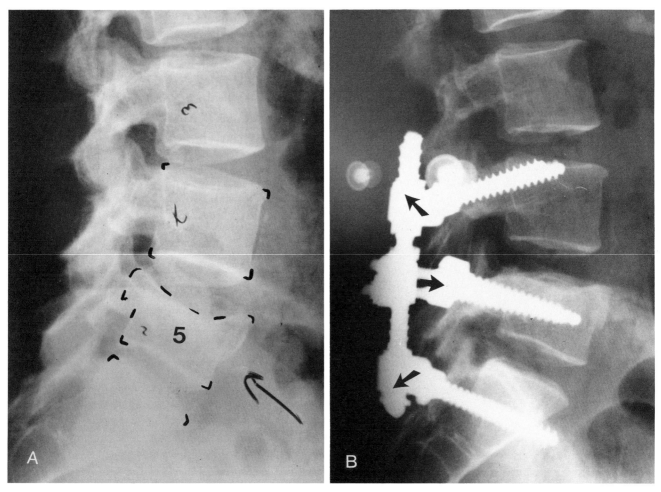

Figure 19.12. L5 Burst Fracture Treated with D-L Construct. *A,* L5 burst fracture with considerable fragment retropulsion. *B,* The D-L Construct provided L4-S1 distraction combined with anterior translation via the intact pedicles of fractured L5. This yielded considerable reduction of the retropulsed fragments and restoration of normal lumbosacral height and lordosis. (Case courtesy of Dr. Alan Levine, Baltimore, MD.)

The D-L construct has been used for the treatment of 347 cases with degenerative spondylolisthesis. It has consistently yielded successful reduction of listhesis, relative indirect decompression and a primary union rate of 85%.

KYPHOREDUCTION CONSTRUCT

The Kyphoreduction construct is used in the treatment of posttraumatic kyphosis and less frequently to treat Scheuermann's and congenital kyphosis. It is combined with a unilateral distraction rod and transverse loading in the correction of kyphoscoliosis.

Biomechanics

The Kyphoreduction construct evolved from the author's experience correcting posttraumatic kyphosis several weeks after injury with the sequential rod-sleeve technique described earlier. Early experience with the Kyphoreduction construct and stress-relaxation approach to the surgical correction of chronic spine deformity was first reported in 1987 (26). The Kyphoreduction construct makes use of viscoelastic stress-relaxation to greatly increase the amount of correction possible without the need for anterior release of vertebrectomy. Stress-relaxation is facilitated by the very gradual application of an extension moment over several hours. This is followed by compression to shorten the posterior column and promote axial loading.

Technique

Prior to surgery, flexion-extension films or tomograms are performed to detect the presence of either an anterior bony bridge or significant retropulsed bone responsible

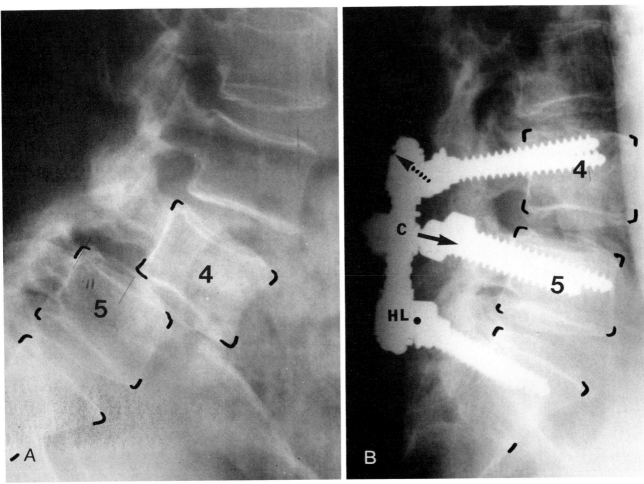

Figure 19.13. Treatment of Degenerative Spondylolisthesis with the D-L Construct. *A*, Severe L4-L5 degenerative spondylolisthesis with L5 radiculopathy. *B*, Correction of listhesis and L5 root impingement using the D-L Construct. After dis- traction to restore L4-L5 disc height, adjustable connectors (*C*) are extended to rotate L5 and the sacrum anteriorly about the S1 hook linkage (HL) into normal alignment under L4. (Case courtesy of Dr. Al Rhyne, Charlotte, NC.)

for neurologic deficit. If either is found, a preliminary anterior resection is performed. Otherwise, only posterior instrumented reduction is necessary (24).

At surgery, patients are placed over transverse rolls. If the posterior column is fused, an osteotomy is performed, along with partial facetectomies. Proximal attachment is achieved with bilaminar hook claws and distal fixation with one or two pairs of pedicle screws. To construct the bilaminar claws, hooks are placed over the most proximal lamina to be instrumented. Universal rods are contoured into normal sagittal alignment and then passed cephalad through the hooks and affixed with washers. A second pair of hooks is ratcheted underneath the adjacent distal lamina to complete the proximal claws. Sleeves of the appropriate size are passed over the rods and centered over the apical facets. Pedicle connectors are assembled between the rods and distal pedicle screws. Connectors

are shortened over a 1–3 hour period, depending on the rigidity of the deformity. After 3-point loading, sequential compression is applied with the ratcheted Universal rods to shorten the posterior column and facilitate subsequent axial loading (16,24) (Fig. 19.14).

Results

The Kyphoreduction construct has become one of the most gratifying new procedures. A prospective study of 15 cases of posttraumatic kyphosis reduced and stabilized with the Kyphoreduction construct was recently reported. The average patient was 44 years old and presented 4 years after spinal injury. Three patients had anterior bony bridges or retropulsed bone that required preliminary anterior surgery. The 12 remaining cases required no surgery anterior to their spinal cords. Rather,

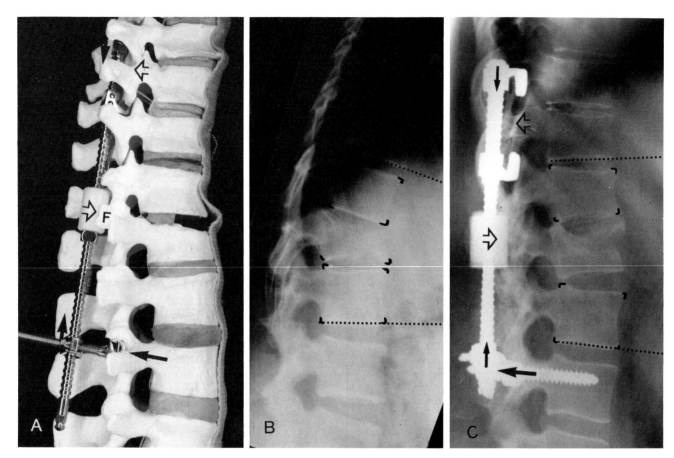

Figure 19.14. Kyphoreduction Construct. *A,* Model showing partial reduction of post-traumatic L1 deformity. Proximal fixation is obtained with bilaminar claws using low Anatomic hooks about the lamina of T9 and T10. Distal fixation is achieved with L3 screws. Medium sleeves provide the fulcrum at the level of injury. Adjustable connectors between the distal rods and L3 screws are gradually shortened to correct kyphosis and then ratcheted up the rod to shorten the posterior column and apply compression across the facets and fusion mass. *B,* Preoperative radiograph 2 months following L1 fracture with fixed kyphotic deformity. *C,* Postoperative radiograph demonstrating full correction of deformity using stress relaxation alone without the need for anterior surgery. The slight bow in the rods provides dynamic lordosis to maintain reduction until union. (Case courtesy of Dr. Thomas Bauman, Salt Lake City, UT.)

kyphosis was reduced using the principle of intraoperative stress-relaxation via the Kyphoreduction construct. Thirty-two degrees of average preoperative kyphosis at the fracture level was corrected to 2°. After 2-year average follow-up, union was documented by quantitative motion studies. Late kyphosis averaged only 5°, representing an 84% improvement of their preoperative kyphosis. Complications were confined to one transient impotence following anterior surgery and one asymptomatic single linkage dislodgement. There was no case of neurologic worsening (29).

Through 1990, the Kyphoreduction construct has been used in 49 posttraumatic cases by members of the Spinal Fixation Study Group. Clinical results using the Kyphoreduction construct for posttraumatic deformities have been excellent and free of major complications. Av-

erage correction of deformity exceeds 80% and successful fusion has occurred in 96% of cases after an operation. On late follow-up, there is minimal loss of correction. Hence, anterior grafting does not appear necessary when anatomic alignment is restored.

Spondylo Construct

For many years, in-situ posterolateral fusion plus/minus root decompression has been the standard surgical treatment for spondylolisthesis. Although some surgeons consider the results satisfactory, many others encounter open problems. For example, a higher rate of fusion *nonunion* occurs with spondylolisthesis than other spinal disorders, averaging about 35% (1). *Slip progression* after attempted fusion occurs in 33% of cases (1). *Neurologic deficit,* especially cauda equina syndrome, is reported in 6% of cases when in situ fusion is attempted for grade 3 or 4 spondylolisthesis (45). Even if fusion is successful, patients with high-grade spondylolisthesis are left with abnormal spine mechanics, a foreshortened trunk, and cosmetic deformity.

Indications

The reduction and fixation of spondylolisthesis offers a number of potential advantages. *Effective fixation*: (*a*) stops progression of the deformity; (*b*) lessens postoperative pain; (*c*) permits full root decompression without fear of further slippage. *Full reduction and fixation* also: (*d*) decompresses sacral roots; (*e*) promotes union; (*f*) limits fusion length; (*g*) restores normal spine mechanics and body posture; and (*h*) can improve the patient's appearance and self-image.

Hence, if the surgeon is well trained in current instrumentation methods, reduction/fixation is worthy of consideration for adolescents or adults in need of surgery for spondylolisthesis. Reduction is probably the procedure of choice for patients with:

1. Cauda equina syndrome;
2. Progressive slips surpassing 40%;
3. Nonunion or slip progression after in situ fusion;
4. Major deformity causing decompensation or emotional distress; or
5. Recurrent pain or deficit plus two or more risk factors for in situ fusion failure.
   Risk factors include:
   a. Slip angle of more than 25°;
   b. Trapezoidal L5 vertebral body;
   c. Rounded sacral endplate;
   d. Hyperlordosis (L2-S1) exceeding 50°;
   e. Excess lumbosacral mobility;
   f. Over 40% slip in an adolescent female;
   g. L5 radiculopathy requiring decompression; or
   h. Signs of sacral root stretch.

Biomechanics

The concept of gradual instrumented reduction for spondylolisthesis was developed by the author during the mid-1980s (10). The goal was to achieve *full* correction of the spondylolisthesis deformity with *less* surgery and morbidity than former methods. Four principles were combined to accomplish this goal: (1) sacral fixation at two points to provide a sufficient moment arm to restore and maintain lumbosacral lordosis; (2) the simultaneous application of distraction, posterior translation of the lumbar spine, and sacral flexion (lordosis) to reverse the spondylo deformity; (3) use of viscoelastic

stress-relaxation to gradually lengthen contracted anterior structures and eliminate the need for anterior release of discectomy; and (4) full correction of sagittal alignment to promote union of posterolateral grafts and eliminate the need for anterior fusion.

Surgical Technique

Grade 1–4 spondylolisthesis is reduced in a single-stage posterior operation. After L5 laminectomy, the fibrocartilage and osteophytes overlying the L5 roots are removed to fully decompress the roots and expose the L5 pedicles. Bicortical screws are inserted into L5 and across the ala at S1 and S2. Fixation to L4 is required only for grade 4 slips and those grade 3 slips with substantial lumbosacral kyphosis or scoliosis (Fig. 19.15).

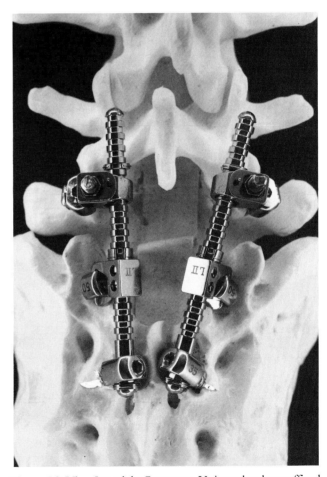

Figure 19.15. Spondylo Construct. Universal rods are affixed to the sacrum with standard screws at S1 and straight-hole screws at S2. Rod orientation is set with hook linkages between the rod and screw at S1. Ring connectors between the rods and L5 vertebral body are ratcheted up the rods to restore height, shortened to translate the lumbar spine posteriorly and flex the sacrum.

Reduction is accomplished by the gradual application of corrective forces with instrumentation (Fig. 19.16). There is no need to cross the canal or disturb the disc. Height is gradually restored by distracting between L5 and the sacrum using finely ratcheted Universal rods. Posterior translation of the lumbar spine and flexion of the sacrum is accomplished by gradually shortening connectors between the L5 screws and the spinal rods. Distraction and translational forces are replenished every 5–10 minutes. Generally, 30–45 minutes of reduction time is required for each grade of deformity. When radiographs document full reduction, all distraction is released to permit axial loading across the anterior column. The instrumentation is then locked in position and lateral fusion performed. Wake-up tests and SEP peroneal nerve monitoring is employed for reduction of grade 4 spondylolisthesis.

When advanced spondylolisthesis progresses to spondyloptosis, the lumbar spine rotates into flexion and drops within the pelvis to greatly shorten the course of the L4 and L5 roots. Special surgical techniques are required to safely accomplish reduction of spondyloptosis without excessive L4 and L5 root stretch. Most patients with spondyloptosis are successfully reduced by staged gradual instrumented reductions 1 week apart. Severe spondyloptosis deformities may also require sacral dome osteotomy to shorten the spine (18). After reduction/fixation for either spondylolisthesis or spondyloptosis, lateral iliac fusion is performed, and the patient is ambulated with brace protection.

Results

A prospective study of 25 consecutive patients with L5-S1 spondylolisthesis has been reported by the author (15). Eighteen patients had grade 2-4 spondylolisthesis, and seven had spondyloptosis. Patients ranged from 12 to 59, with an average age of 25. Slip correction averaged 91% at an average 2-year follow-up. The 33° preoperative slip angle was reduced to a mean of 4° kyphosis (90% correction). In addition, 35-mm average trunk height (L1-S1) was restored with a 43-mm average trunk height increase for patients with spondyloptosis. Patients ambulated at discharge in a total contact orthosis with thigh extension. Complications for patients with spondylolisthesis were remarkably few. Only one patient with borderline spondyloptosis developed unilateral dorsiflexion weakness. There were no dislodgements, one donor site infection, one temporary dural leak, and one patient required repair of a nonunion.

To date, 318 cases of L5-S1 spondylolisthesis have been documented by members of the Spinal Fixation Study Group (3,16). One-hundred and sixty-four of these

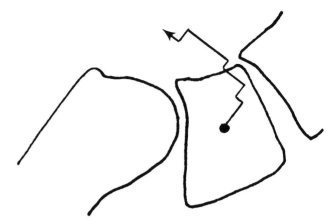

Figure 19.16. Spondylo Reduction. Reduction of spondylolisthesis requires initial distraction to dislodge L5 from the sacral dome, followed by sequential posterior translation and distraction to rotate the lumbar spine around the apex of the dome and finally, gentle compression to restore lumbosacral lordosis and to promote axial loading.

cases with over 1-year follow-up have been analyzed with overall results similar to the author's complications included 3% transient radiculopathy, 1% neurologic deficit, 1% infection, and 2% midsacral screw pullout. Solid fusion was documented in 87%. Hence, results to date suggest that gradual instrumented reduction is an effective and relatively safe new alternative for the treatment of spondylolisthesis (Fig. 19.17).

On the other hand, the gradual instrumented reduction of spondyloptosis is far more challenging and associated with more frequent complications. We have learned that complications vary according to the severity and duration of the deformity, the amount of prior surgery, and the age of the patient. Average expectations are for a 15% incidence of radiculopathy, usually unilateral weakness of ankle dorsiflexion. We have not seen any case of cauda equina syndrome of plantarflexion weakness. Failure of midsacral fixation and nonunion often complicated our early spondyloptosis reductions, but have become infrequent with advances in surgical technique. Despite our favorable early experience, instrumented reduction for spondyloptosis remains an investigational procedure.

SCOLIOSIS CONSTRUCTS

The six devices that comprise the Edwards Modular System can be combined in various ways to treat a wide array of scoliosis deformities ranging from idiopathic thoracic to degenerative lumbar scoliosis with lateral listhesis. The Scoliosis constructs are characterized by versatility of fixation and three-dimensional adjustability. Scoliosis constructs provide segmental compression, distraction, lateral loading, and/or active derotation.

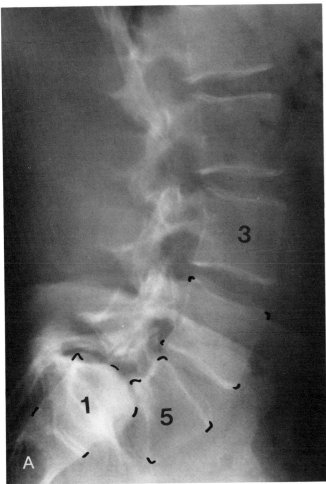

Figure 19.17. Correction of High-Grade Spondylolisthesis. *A,* Grade IV spondylolisthesis in a 25-year-old male. Note the middle of L5 is opposite the middle of the S1 body. *B,* The Spondylo Construct provided gradual distraction, posterior translation of the lumbar spine, and sacral flexion to restore normal trunk height, spine alignment and lumbosacral lordosis. There was no need for anterior surgery or discectomy. There was no postoperative root deficit or other complications. Successful union was documented after 12 months. (Case courtesy of Dr. Mark Rosenthal, Baltimore, MD.)

Technique

For most thoracic scoliotic patterns, concave distraction is applied with ratcheted Universal rods attached by Anatomic hooks proximally and pedicle or sacral screws distally. Short segment compression across the convex apex is provided by the Universal rods attached with hooks in the thoracic spine or screws in the lumbar spine. Active derotation is accomplished by shortening connectors between the concave apex and contoured distraction rod. Additional correction of scoliosis is often obtained with transverse loading between the spinal rods (16,43).

Kyphoscoliosis is treated with a Kyphoreduction construct on convexity and distraction rod with apical connectors on the concavity. After partial correction, the rods are gradually approximated with adjustable crosslinks.

One of the most frequent scoliosis patterns treated with Edwards modular instrumentation is degenerative lumbar scoliosis with lateral listhesis. These are typically elderly patients with a fixed lumbosacral obliquity, lateral listhesis causing radicular pain and a relatively flexible lumbar scoliosis above. Our surgical goal is relief of low back pain and radiculopathy with the minimum amount of surgery and length of instrumentation. This is accomplished by erecting rods from the sacrum proximally to the listhetic vertebra. The proximal lumbar scoliosis is rarely symptomatic and is not instrumented if lumbosacral reconstruction combined with proximal lumbar flexibility can restore coronal compensation. After any necessary partial facetectomies or root decompressions, concave lumbosacral distraction is combined with convex compression to correct the lumbosacral obliquity and re-

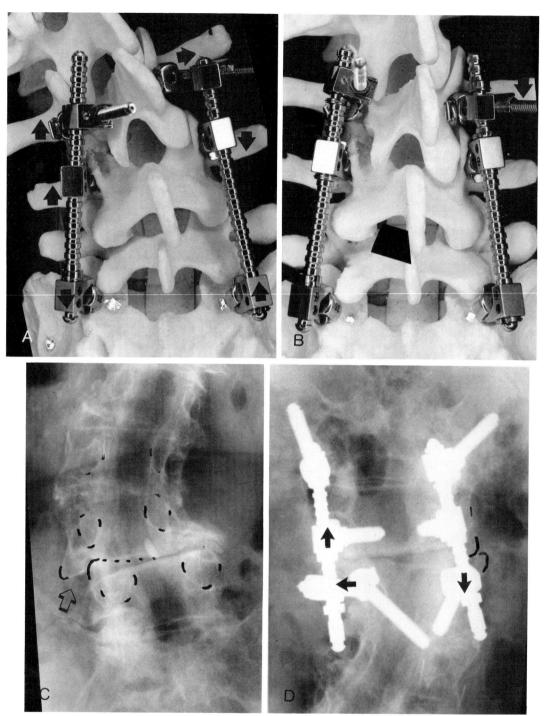

Figure 19.18. Lateral Listhesis Construct. *A*, Model demonstrates lumbosacral obliquity with lateral listhesis of L3 on L4. The lateral listhesis construct attaches to L3, L4, and S1 with spinal screws. The L4-S1 hook linkages on the left side are oriented to provide distraction, while those on the right are oriented to provide compression. The S1 screws are directed medially to position the rods as far laterally as possible for maximum rotational moments to reduce lumbosacral obliquity. In order to correct the L3-L4 lateral listhesis, the L3 connectors are first distracted to dislodge the vertebrae and then shortened to translate the proximal spine to the right. *B*, After left L4-S1 distraction and right compression to correct L4-S1 obliquity and lateral translation of L3, the right L3 connector is compressed to further reduce the lumbosacral scoliosis. Washers are applied to maintain final hook and connector positions. *C*, Preoperative radiograph of a 68-year-old female status-postdecompressive laminectomy with degenerative lumbosacral scoliosis and severe L4-L5 lateral listhesis with radiculopathy. *D*, Postoperative radiograph taken 6 months after surgery demonstrates considerable correction of the listhesis using the lateral listhesis construct. Anterior release was not required. Full fusion occurred, and both back pain and radiculopathy resolved.

322

store a level base for the listhetic vertebra. Pedicle screws and connectors are then used to reduce the proximal lateral listhesis. The reduction sequence generally involves: (*a*) concave distraction; (*b*) lateral translation of slipped vertebrae; (*c*) compression across convexities; and (*d*) lateral loading between the rods. The principles of sequential reduction and stress-relaxation are used in the correction of scoliosis, as with kyphosis and spondylolisthesis (Fig. 19.18).

Results

Scoliosis constructs represent out most rapidly evolving procedures; hence, meaningful long-term results are not available. However, early results suggest that careful planning combined with the gradual application of corrective forces to directly oppose all elements of the scoliosis deformity will yield greater correction of deformity with less surgery than other techniques.

REFERENCES

1. Amundson G, Edwards CC, Garfin SR: Spondylolisthesis. In Rothman RH, Simeone FA, eds. The spine (3rd ed). Philadelphia: WB Saunders, 1991 (in press).
2. Armstrong GWD, Connock SHG: A transverse loading system applied to a modified Harrington instrumentation. Clin Orthop 1975;108:70–75.
3. Bradford DS, Boachie-Adjei O: Reduction of spondylolisthesis. In: Evarts CM, ed. Surgery of the musculoskeletal system (2nd ed). New York: Churchill-Livingstone 1990;2129–2142.
4. Connock SHG, Armstrong GWD: A transverse loading system applied to a modified Harrington instrumentation. J Bone Joint Surg 1971;53A:194 (Abstract).
5. Cotrel Y: Techniques nouvelles dans le traitement de la scoliose idiopathique. Internat Orthop 1978;1:247.
6. Edwards CC: The spinal rod-sleeve method: Its rational and use in thoracic and lumbar injuries. Orthop Trans 1982;6:11–12.
7. Edwards CC: The sacral fixation device: Design and preliminary results. Proc Scoliosis Res Soc 1984;135.
8. Edwards CC: The sacral fixation device: A new alternative for lumbosacral fixation. Warsaw: Zimmer, 1985.
9. Edwards CC: A new method for direct sacral fixation: Rationale and clinical results. Orthop Trans 1986;10:541–542.
10. Edwards CC: Reduction of spondylolisthesis: Biomechanics and fixation. Orthop Trans 1986;10:543–544.
11. Edwards CC: Spine stabilization: Analysis of surgical options. In: Lane J, ed. Fracture healing. New York: Churchill-Livingstone 1987;215–256.
12. Edwards CC: Spinal screw fixation of the lumbar spine: Early results treating the first 50 cases. Orthop Trans 1987;11:99.
13. Edwards CC: Early results correcting spondylolisthesis. Orthop Trans 1989;13:72.
14. Edwards CC: Thoracolumbar trauma: Posterior reduction and fixation with the Modular Spinal System. Semin Spine Surg 1990;2:8–18.
15. Edwards CC: Prospective evaluation of a new method for complete reduction of L5-S1 spondylolisthesis using corrective forces alone. Orthop Trans 1990;14:549.
16. Edwards CC: Spinal reconstruction using a modular system: Surgical manual III. Baltimore: Spinal Research Foundation, 1990.
17. Edwards CC: Reconstruction of acute lumbar injury. Op Tech Orthop 1991;1:106–122.
18. Edwards CC: Reduction of spondylolisthesis. In: Dewald R, Bridwell K, eds. Spinal disorders. Philadelphia: JB Lippincott, 1991 (in press).
19. Edwards CC, Levine AM: Early rod-sleeve stabilization of the injured thoracic and lumbar spine. Orthop Clin NA 1986;17:121–146.
20. Edwards CC, Levine AM: Fractures of the lumbar spine. In: Evarts CM, ed. Surgery of the musculoskeletal system (2nd ed). New York: Churchill-Livingstone, 1990;2237–2275.
21. Edwards CC, Levine AM, Murphy J, et al: New techniques in spine stabilization. Warsaw: Zimmer, 1982.
22. Edwards CC, Levine AM, Weigel MC: A modular system for 3-dimensional correction of lumbosacral deformities. Orthop Trans 1987;11:19.
23. Edwards CC, Levine AM, York JJ, et al: A new spinal hook: Rationale and clinical trials. Proc: Scoliosis Res Soc 1984;134.
24. Edwards CC, Rhyne A: Late treatment of post-traumatic kyphosis. Semin Spine Surg 1990;2:63–69.
25. Edwards CC, Rhyne AL, Weigel MC, et al: 5–10 year results treating burst fractures with rod-sleeve instrumentation and fusion. Orthop Trans 1991:15 (in press).
26. Edwards CC, Rosenthal MS: A new method for correcting late post-traumatic kyphosis. Orthop Trans 1988;12:257.
27. Edwards CC, Weigel MC: A prospective study of 51 low lumbar nonunions. Orthop Trans 1988;12:608.
28. Edwards CC, Weigel MC: Treatment of 56 lumbosacral non-unions with compression instrumentation. Presented at AAOS, 1989.
29. Edwards CC, Weigel MC: Early results correcting chronic post-traumatic kyphosis with a new Kyphoreduction construct and stress-relaxation. Orthop Trans 1991;15 (in press).
30. Edwards CC, York JJ, Levine AM, et al: Determinants of spinal hook dislodgement. Orthop Trans 1986;10:8.
31. Garfin SR: Thoracolumbar spine trauma. In: Orthopaedic knowledge update. Park Ridge: AAOS, 1990;425–440.
32. Garfin SR, Mowery CA, Guerra J, et al: Confirmation of the posterolateral technique to decompress and fuse thoracolumbar spine burst fractures. Spine 1985;10:218–223.
33. Hanley EN, Starr JK: Junctional burst fractures. Orthop Trans 1991;15 (in press).
34. Herkowitz HN, El-Kommos H: Instrumentation of the lumbar spine for degenerative disorders. Op Tech Orthop 1991;1:91–96.
35. Johnston CE, Ashman RB, Baird AM, et al: Effect of spinal construct stiffness on early fusion mass incorporation. Spine 1990;15:908–912.
36. Johnston CE, Ashman RB, Corin JD: Mechanical effects of cross-linking rods in Cotrel-Dubousset instrumentation. Orthop Trans 1987;11:96–97.
37. King AG: Burst compression fractures of the thoracolumbar spine. Orthopaedics 1987;10:1711–1719.
38. Kurz LT, Herkowitz HN, Samberg LC: Management of major thoracic and thoracolumbar spinal injuries. Spine: State of the Art Review 1989;3:243–268.
39. Levine AM, Bosse M, Edwards CC: Bilateral facet dislocations in the thoracolumbar spine. Spine 1988;13:630–640.
40. Levine AM, Friedman C, Edwards CC: The use of a short rod-sleeve construct for fixation of thoracolumbar spine trauma. Orthop Trans 1990;14:264.

41. Levine AM, Garfin S, McCutcheon M, et al: The operative treatment of L4 and L5 burst fractures. Orthop Trans 1989;13:753.

42. McCutcheon ME, Cohen M: Early clinical results for painful nonunions of the lumbar spine treated with Edwards Modular Spine Fixation. Orthop Trans 1991;15 (in press).

43. Murphy MJ: Thoracolumbar spine reconstruction. In: Orthopaedic knowledge update. Park Ridge: AAOS, 1990;441–453.

44. Panjabi MM, Abumi K, Duranceau J, et al: Biomechanical evaluation of spinal fixation devices: Stability provided by eight internal fixation devices. Spine 1988;13:1135–1140.

45. Schoenecker PL, Cole HO, Herring JA, et al: Cauda equina syndrome of the in-situ arthrodesis for severe spondylolisthesis at the lumbosacral junction. J Bone Joint Surg 1990;72A:369–377.

46. Zindrick MR, Wiltse LL, Widell EH, et al: A biomechanical study of intrapeduncular screw fixation in the lumbosacral spine. Clin Orthop 1986;203:99–111.

TWENTY

Isola Spinal Implant System: Principles, Design, and Applications

Marc A. Asher, Walter E. Strippgen, Charles F. Heinig, and William L. Carson

INTRODUCTION

The Isola effort was born out of frustration with existing means of surgical treatment of patients with deformed and/or mechanically insufficient (unstable) spines. Our effort formally began in January 1985, and our original intent was to perfect sacral fixation (3). Because our first implant component resembled a butterfly, we named it *Isola*, a butterfly species.

Our work began with implant design and in vivo animal studies (approved by the Animal Care Committee). This was followed by a limited custom clinical trial (approved by the Human Subjects Committee) (June 1985–July 1986) in 15 patients, 4 with sacral butterfly implants. There were no neurologic or infection complications in the group. One patient, a 48-year-old female, died of metastatic carcinoma of the cervix 14 months postoperatively. She and her husband believed the spinal stabilization provided acceptable pain relief. Radiographically, she had sacral implant loosening. An autopsy was not obtained. A second patient, a 16-year, 5-month-old male with severe psychomotor retardation, died 36 hours after his second stage scoliosis surgery due to a central venous pressure line penetration of the right atrium and cardiac tamponade (48). The autopsy revealed a slight loosening of the sacral implant. Thus, we became very skeptical of sacral fixation as the sole foundation for long spine implant constructs, and we directed our pelvic fixation efforts toward improving iliac fixation. We initially developed a combined iliosacral and iliac fixation construct (Fig. 20.1). Subsequently, we focused our efforts on further improving the Luque-Galveston type fixation, as described by Allen and Ferguson (1), a fixation that continues to gain support (12,15,46,53). A third patient, a 12-year, 4-month-old male with severe psychomotor retardation, died approximately 18 months postopera-

tively of unrelated problems. His spine reconstruction was quite satisfactory 15 months after surgery when he was last examined.

Three patients required revision. The sacral implant in one broke 8 months postoperatively. An 11-year, 5-month-old male with nonfamilial dysautonomia lost considerable scoliosis correction that had been markedly improved with a fully segmented single spinal rod implantation. A 71-year-old female with degenerative scoliosis developed thoracolumbar junction pseudarthrosis and had breakage of the flat-threaded, ¼″ spinal rods. These three patients have had successful revision surgery including realignment, restabilization, and pseudarthrosis repair.

All 12 living patients have eventually had satisfactory outcomes with stable, balanced spines. Based on the results of this work, we made several important observations, including the following:

1. The sacrum alone is unreliable for long fixation;
2. Two longitudinal members are necessary for construct stability;
3. A bolt connection is more stable than a screw connection;
4. The split rod connection has yet to fail;
5. A dual (bypass) connection is essential;
6. The Morris-type connection is cumbersome;
7. Threaded rods are fatigue-prone;
8. Transverse connection of longitudinal members improves stability (4);
9. Strong smooth rod clamping is possible (4);
10. Motion segment malalignment and/or destabilization adjacent to a stable spine segment should be avoided (8,22).

Our original goal of perfecting sacral fixation was altered, as it became apparent that there were many other

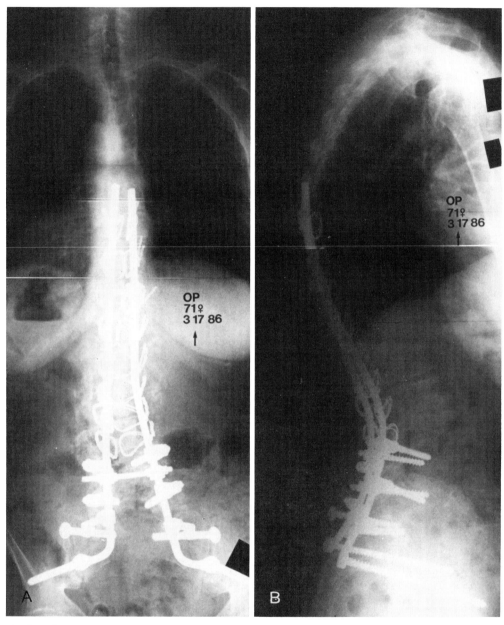

Figure 20.1. *A,* Standing PA. *B,* lateral radiographs of a 71-year-old female with extensive degenerative disc disease il-lustrating an early custom Isola implant utilizing an iliac screw and iliosacral screw pelvic foundation.

dorsal spinal instrumentation problems. The principal problems related to internal and external profile, sim-plicity, stability, strength, versatility, and revisability. With this background, development of a comprehensive dorsal, thoracolumbosacroiliac implant system, applica-ble in the full range of ages, deformities, and instabilities, became our objective (7).

The Isola spinal implant system is based on the prin-ciples and designs conceived by Paul R. Harrington, M.D. (33,34). These include precise description of the

spinal deformity *with special emphasis on spinal balance;* lamina, transverse process, iliosacral, and pedicle anchors; segmental fixation; anatomically compatible dimensions; proper instrumentation sequence; and data banking. Many serious students of spinal disease and deformity have enlarged on these beginnings, and we acknowledge our debt to them (1,2,20,21,27,28,31,37,41-44,47,52, 57,60).

The Isola system is completely compatible with and should be considered an extension of the variable screw placement system (VSP), developed by Arthur D. Steffee, M.D. (54). VSP and Isola provide the spinal surgeon with a complete implant armamentarium for the surgical management of deformity and instability of the thoracolumbosacroiliac spine.

The goals of the Isola spinal implant system are as follows:

1. Relief of constrictive, translational, and/or angular deformity as needed;
2. Access to the full range of anchor sites possible and to as many or as few of these sites as needed;
3. Provision of stability and strength to the point that the need for external support is minimized;
4. Application of a full range of supplemental techniques to improve deformity correction (35) and provide stability; and
5. Preservation of as many motion segments in as near anatomic position as possible (40).

PRINCIPLES

Spinal instrumentation involves much more than just metal implants. Patient selection is probably the most important single variable. Patient preparation, operative segment selection, unoperated segment preservation, and surgical technique are also key elements of the Isola spine system.

Preoperative planning involves not only the establishment of an accurate diagnosis(es) but also the determination of its relationship to the patient's symptoms. The possibilities of spinal cord and nerve abnormality, tumor, osteopenia, and altered pain behavior must always be considered. The effects of malnutrition, smoking habit, previous surgery, age, obesity, activity level, patient expectation, and possible metal allergy on the outcome of any proposed implant surgery should also be evaluated. Appropriate studies, referrals, and treatments help deter-

Table 20.1.
Spinal Deformity and Mechanical Insufficiency Classification

Deformity
  Constriction (e.g., degenerative, trauma, tumor)
  Translation (e.g., spondylolisthesis)
  Angulation (e.g., scoliosis, hyperkyphosis)
Mechanical Insufficiency
  Primary
    Acute (e.g., trauma)
    Chronic (e.g., degenerative, tumor)
  Secondary
    Resection (e.g., facetectomy)
    Overload (e.g., malalignment, stress concentration)

Table 20.2.
Possible Surgical Needs of Patients with Spinal Deformity and/or Instability

Decompression
  Direct
  Indirect
Realignment
  Corrective mechanical forces
  Destabilization
    Discectomy
    Osteotomy
Stabilization
  Location
    Anterior
    Posterior
  Method
    Implant
    Arthrodesis

mine if implant surgery is necessary and increase the likelihood of its success if it is required (13).

Regardless of the disease, deformity and/or instability (mechanical insufficiency) are the spine's physical manifestations that require treatment. These deformities and instabilities are subdivided in Table 20.1.

The three surgical issues that must be addressed, though not necessarily in every patient, are decompression, realignment, and stabilization (Table 20.2).

An underlying principle of the Isola system in the treatment of deformities and instabilities is their analysis in *three dimensions for 6° of freedom of motion* (56) (Fig. 20.2).

Translational and angular position and deformity may be determined on the basis of a global or local cartesian coordinate axis system. With the global (gravity-based) axis system, the origin is placed at the center of the superior end plate of S1, the vertical Z axis a gravity line, and the Y axis parallel to a line connecting the anterior superior iliac spines. Recumbent x-rays, of course, preclude the use of a global (gravity-based) axis system.

With the local axis system, the origin is at the center of the vertebral body, the vertical z axis passes through the endplate centers, and the y axis is parallel to a line joining the base of the pedicles.

Angular position and deformity signs are determined by the right-hand convention, in which counterclockwise is positive when the origin is viewed along the $X(x)$, $Y(y)$, or $Z(z)$ axis from positive to negative.

Clinically, translational and angular position and deformity observations are made in the coronal and sagittal planes. Thus, true three-dimensional analysis of spine deformity is currently not being practiced. However, a working three-dimensional 6° of freedom of motion anal-

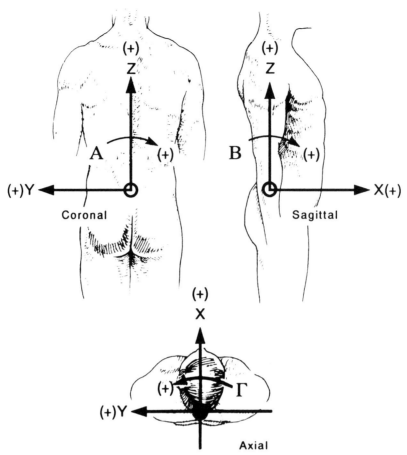

Figure 20.2. The three anatomic planes and six motion segment possibilities with a right-hand orthogonal (90° angle) coordinate axis system. Shown is a global axis system for the conventional anatomical planes of the human body with the origin at the center of the superior endplate of S1 and the gravity line as the Z axis. The planes are coronal (YZ), sagittal (XZ), and axial (transverse) (XY). Positive directions for translation and angulation are indicated by arrows. (Partially redrawn from ISO 2631-1978 Guide to Evaluation of Human Exposure to Whole Body Vibration, 1978).

ysis can be done with conventional radiographs, which should be obtained on 91-cm (36″) cassettes at a 183-cm (72″) tube-film distance to minimize magnification.

Of the 6° of freedom of motion, only axial plane angulation cannot be determined directly from the described biplanar radiographs. However, axial plane angular position and deformity, in degrees, have been shown to correlate with the percent translation of the convex pedicle between the sides of the vertebral body, as viewed in the coronal plane (9,49,50).

It is widely recognized that scoliosis is a three-dimensional deformity (23,25,30,51,55). However, it is generally described on the basis of curve patterns that consider only the coronal plane (39). An attempt to classify deformities on the basis of coronal and sagittal plane observations without even considering the axial plane leads to an unmanageable classification of at least 14 curve patterns (5).

The common translational and angular positions and deformities utilized to describe spinal deformity are shown in Figures 20.3A–D.

A major principle underlying the use of the Isola system for the treatment of spinal deformity is that *coronal plane angular deformities (scoliosis) do not occur in synchrony with the normal sagittal plane curves, and their apices and radii are different.* Maximal thoracic dorsal displacement normally occurs in the sagittal plane at T5-T6 and maximal lumbar anterior displacement at L4. The radii of kyphoses and lordoses angulation are not constant, being shorter near the cephalad and caudad ends, respectively, and longer as the thoracolumbar junction inflection point is reached (10) (Fig. 20.4). Although thoracic scoliosis most commonly apexes at T8-T9, and lumbar scoliosis at L2, the apex may occur at any level from L2-L4, and, in addition, the radius of curvature is nearly constant. Coronal and sagittal plane deformities do not necessarily

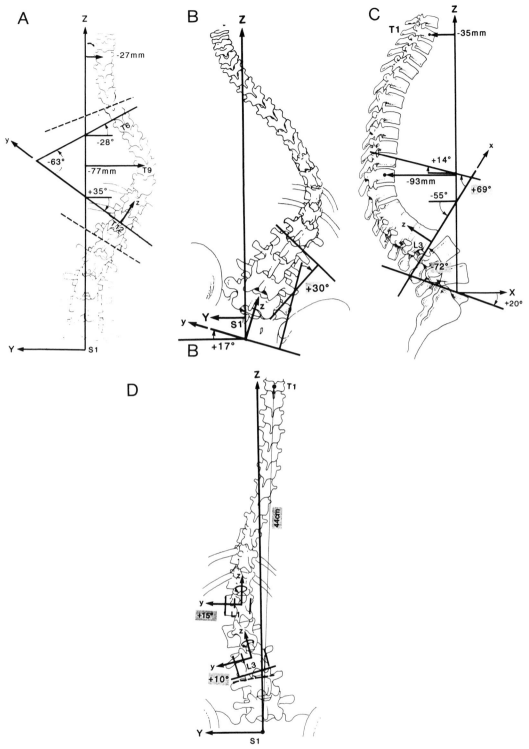

Figure 20.3. *A*, Drawing of a standing 36″ (91-cm) coronal plane radiograph (viewed PA) of a 14-year-old female with idiopathic scoliosis, thoracic curve pattern, illustrating the commonly determined global (YZ) and local (yz) translational and angular positions. In these and subsequent drawings, numbers with plain background are measured with respect to the global XYZ coordinate axes and numbers with shaded background measured with respect to the local xyz coordinate axes. *B*, Drawings of a sitting 36″ (91-cm) coronal plane radiograph (viewed PA) of an 18-year-old male with neuromuscular scoliosis, illustrating the pelvic angular position (+17°) determined from the global coordinate system and the lumbosacral (Cobb) angle (+30°) determined from the local (in this case pelvic) coordinate system (yz). *C*, Drawing of a standing 36″ (91-cm) sagittal plane radiograph (viewed RL) of a 12-year-old female with congenital kyphoscoliosis, illustrating the common global (XZ) and local (xz) displacement and angular positions determined. *D*, Drawing of a standing 36″ (91-cm) coronal plane radiograph (viewed PA) of a 15-year-old female with idiopathic scoliosis, thoracolumbar curve pattern, showing axial length (44 cm) and axial plane apical angular position (+15°), as well as lower end vertebra angular position (+10°) (Perdriolle method). This illustrates that the axial plane global angular position of the lower end vertebra (L3) may not be 0°.

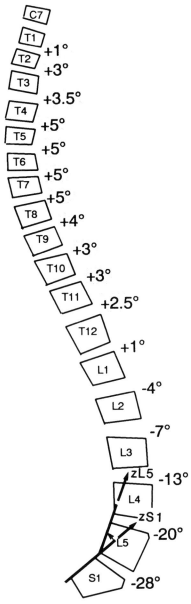

Figure 20.4. Normal segmental angular sagittal plane position. Maximum sagittal plane displacement occurs dorsally at T5-T6 and ventrally at L4 (Adapted with permission from the segmental sagittal angulation data of Bernhardt and Bridwell, Spine 14:717–721, 1989).

(26). Clinical observations suggest that the same is often true for the axial plane. This helps explain the diversity of scoliosis deformities seen, underscores the need to avoid pattern thinking, reinforces the need for three-dimensional analysis of spinal deformity, and emphasizes the importance of identifying and selecting those degrees of freedom of motion to which corrective forces and moments are necessary to correct the deformity satisfactorily.

The biomechanical function of the spine must also be appreciated in the analysis and treatment of spinal deformities and instabilities. In the sagittal plane, the spine can be considered as three load-bearing columns (24). Seventy-five percent or more of the spine's compressive load is transferred through the anterior and middle columns (38). It is necessary to identify mechanical incompetence of these columns and to make allowance in the treatment plan for their restoration. In the posterior column linkages, the facets are particularly important in providing sagittal plane stability in the thoracic spine and axial plane stability in the lumbar spine. The greatest rotational stability for the lumbar spine, however, appears to be provided by intervertebral discs (32) and is the principal reason why axial plane angular deformity ("rotation") is so difficult to correct. This should be remembered when either restoring stability or establishing instability to correct deformity.

The spine's deep dorsal musculature is broad, and the extensor force developed is large. Preservation of its mass and innervation, which is provided by the dorsal rami, is important. The dorsal rami are located just lateral to the axilla formed by the transverse process and the pars interarticularis, and an attempt to protect them seems appropriate, even though it is not always achievable.

OPERATIVE PLAN

Operative

Since these surgeries often involve extensive reconstruction, patient positioning, anesthesia, monitoring, radiographic imaging, and postoperative care require attention to detail. It is essential for the patient and family to understand that serious complications, though uncommon, including death, paralysis, infection, pseudarthrosis, implant loosening or breakage, and chronic residual pain, can occur.

The surgical principles are preservation and, where necessary, restoration of: (*a*) neural canal/foramen patency; (*b*) overall coronal and sagittal plane spinal balance; (*c*) three-dimensional segmental translational and angular alignment of the immobile, as well as the mobile, motion segments; (*d*) provision for short- and long-term stabil-

end at the same level. For instance, it is well recognized that some thoracic coronal plane curves are associated with thoracolumbar junction kyphosis. For these reasons, we do not believe that direct transfer of coronal plane deformity to the sagittal plane is realistic.

Although there is some disagreement on the following points (23), we have found that the magnitude of coronal and sagittal plane deformities does not always correlate

ity; and (*e*) preservation of as many motion segments as possible. The techniques include direct (dorsal, midline, subarticular, foraminal, extraforaminal, and ventral) and indirect (reduction and ligamentotaxis) decompression; realignment by application of corrective mechanical forces, aided by destabilization (osteotomy [dorsal, ventral, and dorsal and ventral], resection, or discectomy); and restabilization (in the short term by spinal implants and in the long term by arthrodesis [intra- and extraarticular]). All are accepted techniques that continue to be refined.

Postoperative

Postoperative care is the same as for any other patient who had undergone major surgery. An intensive care unit is almost always needed for at least 24 hours. Ambulation is usually begun 3–5 days postoperatively. An orthosis or cast may be needed; however, use of either depends upon many factors, including length and levels of instrumentation, ventral column competence for load sharing, bone quality, patient reliability, and surgeon preference.

Of course, every effort should be made to avoid complications. However, inevitably complications may occur, and when they do, early recognition, careful patient communication, and appropriate treatments are usually effective.

Rehabilitation needs vary considerably, depending upon the patient's age, disease process, and needed surgery. Important considerations in the recovery process include appropriate rest and nutrition, progressive aerobic conditioning through walking, smoking abstinence, and trunk muscle strengthening.

DESIGN

The implant component design objectives are user friendliness, minimal internal and external profile, simplicity through inventory control, versatility through angular and translational variability, and VSP compatibility. The implant dimensions are standardized to permit maximum flexibility and versatility in use. The mechanical objectives are the provision of stability, strength, and durability adequate to hold restored spinal alignment during the healing of spine arthrodesis. The dimensions to which all round and hex components can be related are 3.2 mm (1/8"), 4.76 mm (3/16"), 6.35 mm (1/4"), 7 mm (9/32"), 8 mm (5/16") and 9.5 mm (3/8").

The implant categories are anchors (screws, posts, hooks, and wires); longitudinal members (rods, plates, eye rods, and plate-rod combinations); longitudinal member to anchor connectors (continuous, bolt, knot, and closed and split connectors); longitudinal member to longitudinal member connectors (transverse, dual [bypass], and tandem [end-to-end]); and accessories (washers, nuts, and set screws).

Anchors

Pedicle Screws. The screws used with the Isola system are the same as the VSP screws (Fig. 20.5*A*). The machine-threaded portions allow sagittal plane translational variability through the use of washers. Sagittal plane angular variability can be allowed for during placement because of the larger sagittal than coronal plane diameter of the pedicle. Over the past 5 years, a number of steps, including an integral nut and tapered minor diameter thread, have been taken to improve the fatigue life of the VSP screws (29,45).

Iliac: Screws. These screws are designed for placement between the iliac cortical tables. They provide versatility for the pelvic fixation anchor site by providing for subsequent connection with a longitudinal member (Fig. 20.5*B*).

There are two sizes, 6.25-mm diameter with a 60-mm length and 7.0 diameter with an 80-mm length. The 9.5-mm hex junction and 4.76-mm, 10-32 machine-threaded connector portion of the screw are the same as the VSP screw, except that the machine-threaded 10-32 portion is shorter so that the 3.2-mm (1/8-inch) hex drive portion protrudes just above the eye rod or slotted connector and nuts.

Posts, Iliac. This anchor is the same as a Luque-Galveston post, which is the portion of a continuous rod that is contoured for placement between the cortical tables of the ilium (Fig. 20.5*C*). It is the lowest profile means of anchoring a construct to the ilium.

Hooks. The hooks have been designed with special emphasis on profile and inventory control.

Drop-Entry (Closed Body) Hooks. Different height hook openings (notches) provide low profile in the sagittal plane. A shortened hook body provides low profile along the z or vertical axis. A shortened hook blade provides low profile in the spinal canal (Fig. 20.6*A*). Clinical placement of the hook, while already passed on to the longitudinal rod member, is facilitated by the drop-entry design (Fig. 20.6*B*). The underlying principle is that when the hook is loose on the rod, the blade of the hook can rotate up to a 15° angle to the rod in the sagittal plane. This is possible because of the dorsal oval enlargement of the rod receptacle hole on the hook opening end of the hook body. As the hook set screw is tightened to the rod, there are two results: (1) the sagittal plane angle

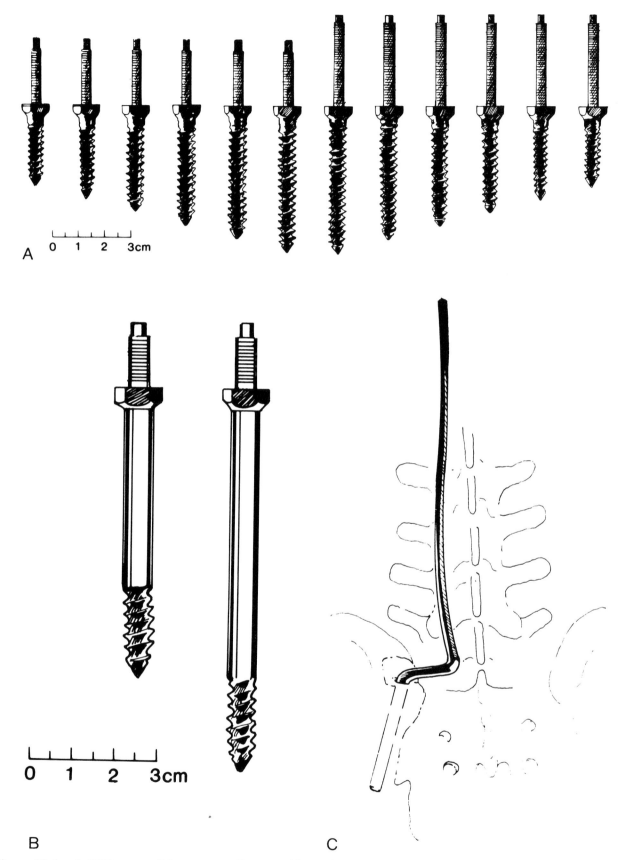

Figure 20.5. *A*, VSP screws, 7.0-mm outer diameter with size ranges of 25–50 mm in 5-mm increments; and 23- or 33-mm machine-threaded lengths for connection. A narrower size range of 6.25- and 5.5-mm screws are available. *B*, Iliac screws. *C*, Iliac (Luque-Galveston) posts.

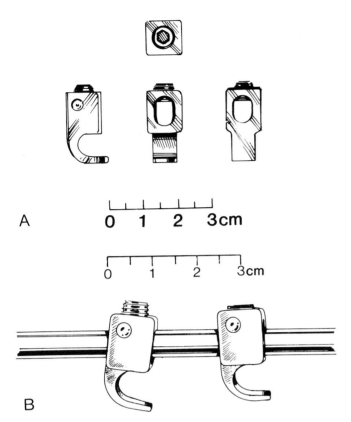

Figure 20.6. *A*, Four views of hook showing low profile. *B*, Drop-entry concept.

of the hook blade becomes nearly parallel with the rod (there is a built-in 5° angulation of the blade related to the body that also helps the seating on the rounded underside of the lamina or transverse process fixation site); and (2) the hook blade tightens against the bone fixation site. Secure connection of the hook to a straight or curved smooth rod is provided by the V-groove (Figs. 20.7*A* and *B*) hollow-ground (Figs. 20.7*C* and *D*) (VHG) design in which the rod is driven into the V-groove by a 6.35-mm (¼″) set screw. The recommended set screw torque is 6.8 Nm (60″/lb). This is readily achieved with the 3.2-cm (⅛″) Allen wrench, the endpoint being the feeling that the shoulder of the Allen wrench is about to give way. The drop entry feature makes it possible to place hooks while on the rod, by doing some local bone sculpting, and the VHG feature makes it possible to achieve a secure attachment to smooth rods.

The drop-entry hook is available in four sizes for both the 6.35-mm (¼″) and the 4.76-mm (³⁄₁₆″) rods (Fig. 20.8). The nominal hook throat heights for the 6.35-mm hooks are 6.5, 8.0, 9.5, and 11 mm. For the 4.76-mm hooks, they are 5.0, 6.5, 8.0, and 9.5 mm. These opening

dimensions were selected because of extensive experience with the Harrington 1253 and 1254 hooks having a 9.5-mm throat opening and the Harrington-Moe pediatric hook with a 6.5-mm throat opening. In addition, numerous lamina measurements were studied to determine proper hook opening heights (11). The successful usage of a custom 1253 body, 1254 blade Harrington hook since 1979 was also very helpful in determining hook design.

The hooks may be placed over or under the lamina or transverse processes. Because of the shortened body length, intrasegmental transverse process-lamina claws can be formed that are strong and stable (14). When placing over the lamina, it is important to use hooks with the smallest throat height that still allow the spinal rod to pass just over the lamina. In this manner, overpenetration of the hook toe into the spinal canal is avoided.

Top-Entry (Open-Body) Hooks. Because of our emphasis on profile and inventory control, the Isola spinal implant system was designed to be viable without top entry hooks, relying instead on the drop-entry concept for the hooks as well as top entry allowed by wires and VSP screws. Clinical application in over 300 patients in the last 2 years has supported this concept. However, in response to requests, a top-entry hook with a VHG connection has been developed incorporating design ideas contributed by Robert W. Gaines, Jr., M.D. (Fig. 20.9). The sliding cap closes the hook, but final stability is not achieved until the set screw is tightened. This provides a strong stable connection in all 6° of freedom of motion.

One major advantage of hooks over screws is their relative insensitivity to osteoporosis (18).

Wires. Sublaminar wires are strong anchors (19) for providing sequential posterolateral displacement at the apex of a scoliotic deformity and for reducing or preventing positive angular displacement (forward flexion) in the sagittal plane. They also provide excellent variable position connections that allow sequential deformity reduction and accommodate residual deformity. Both the potential risks (59) and the safety (61) of their use have been well documented. The base of spinous process wires provides a safe means of delivering a modest lateral and dorsal displacement force at the apex of a flexible scoliotic deformity (27). Because wires resist vertical axis translation poorly, placement at construct ends is not usually recommended.

Wires provided are 16-gauge, either single-strand with beaded ends or double-preformed for sublaminar passage and double-18-gauge with button (Fig. 20.10).

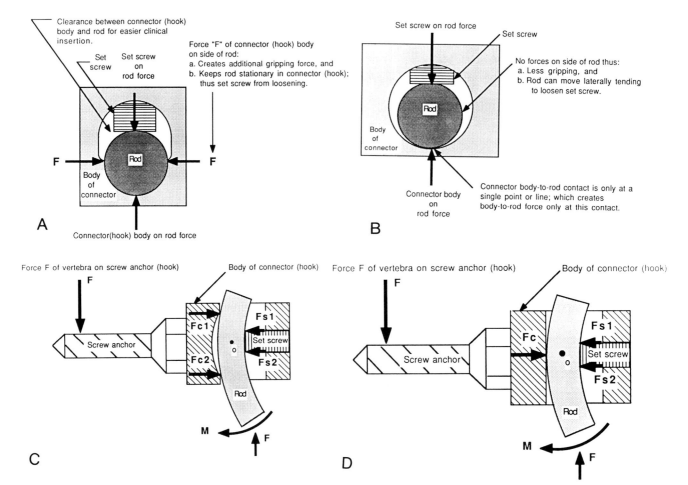

Figure 20.7. *A,* Isola V-groove connection design. *B,* Conventional hole with set screw connection design. *C,* Isola hollow-ground connection design on curved rod showing: (*a*) double body-to-rod contact creating better fit to curved rod; and (*b*) double body-to-rod forces Fc1 and Fc2 creating superior mechanical strength and durability. *D,* Conventional hole with set screw connection on curved rod showing: (*a*) single body-to-body contact; and (*b*) single body-to-rod force Fc.

Longitudinal Members

The longitudinal members are smooth rods, eye rods, and plate-rod combinations. In addition, VSP plates can be integrated into the implant construct.

Rods. Rods are smooth because of their superior bending and fatigue strength (29). They also provide infinite position adjustability of connectors along (axial translation) and about (transverse angulation) the rods.

The rods are provided in two diameters, 4.76 mm (³⁄₁₆″) and 6.35 mm (¼″) (Fig. 20.11*A*). There is one standard length, 46 mm (18″). Additionally an extra-long 61-cm (24″) rod is available. Either rod is cut to the appropriate length at the time of surgery, thus minimizing rod inventory. The remaining portions are often use-ful for later procedures, such as fractures, where shorter rods are required.

Eye Rods. The eyelet, or hole, at one end of a rod provides a low-profile connection to the iliac screws or to an end pedicle screw (Fig. 20.11*B*).

Eye rods are available in two dimensions, 4.76 mm (³⁄₁₆″) and 6.35 mm (¼″), and a 46-cm (18″) length. Because the rods are cut to required length during surgery, inventory is reduced.

Plate-Rod Combinations (PRC). The PRCs allow use of screws, hooks, and/or wires on the same continuous longitudinal member (Figs. 20.12*A* and *B*).

There are PRCs in both the 6.35-mm (¼″) and

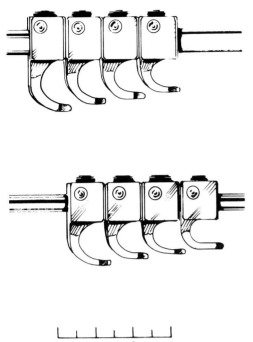

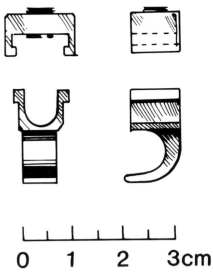

Figure 20.9. Top-entry (open-body) hook.

Figure 20.8. Drop-entry hooks for 6.35- and 4.76-mm rods.

4.76-mm (³⁄₁₆″) rod diameter. The plate portion is standard-size VSP (16-mm wide) for those PRCs with 6.35-mm (¼″) rod portions. For those PRCs with 4.76-mm (³⁄₁₆″) diameter rod size, the plate portion is the reduced width (12.7 mm). The plate portion sizes are single, double-half, one and one-half, and two slots. The length of the rod portion on each is 20.3 cm (8″). A 30.5-cm (12″ inch) rod is available by special order.

Longitudinal Member to Anchor Connectors

Continuous. This is the simplest and lowest profile connection, consisting of a bend(s) in the rod so that one of the bent sites enters an anchor site (Fig. 20.5C). It requires no special implant components. It is easily made with the Isola variable radius benders.

Bolt. In this standard VSP plate to VSP screw connection, the plate is securely sandwiched and fastened between two nuts. The bolt connection is unlike a screw connection, which relies on bony contact with the longitudinal

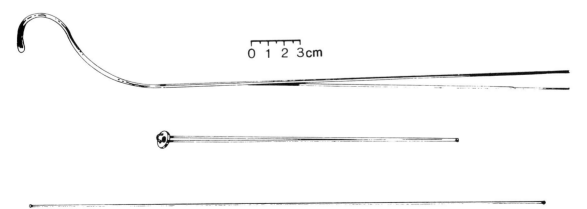

Figure 20.10. Wires: double-preformed, double with button, and single-strand beaded.

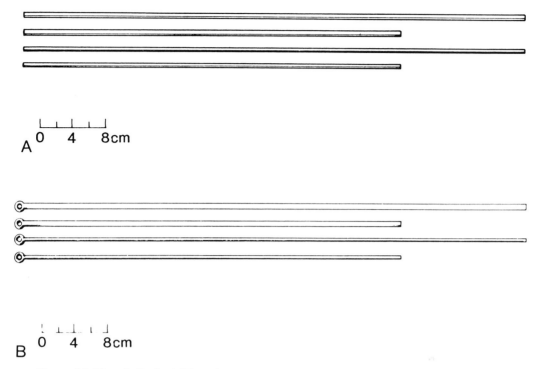

Figure 20.11. *A*, Rods, 6.35- and 4.76-mm diameters, 46- and 61-cm lengths. *B*, Eye rods.

member for stability and is subject to the claw hammer screw pullout effect (17).

Knot. The anchor wire is connected to the longitudinal member with a twist knot, eliminating the need for an added component. The knot most resistant to untwisting is a double twist (19).

Closed and Split Connectors. These connectors are designed to provide a stable, strong, and durable screw-to-connector-to-rod union. To provide secure fixation to the rod, the V-groove hollow ground (VHG) design is used in all connectors and hooks (Figs. 20.7*A*–*D*). The VHG strength results from the combined effects of wedging the rod between the sides of the connector body (V-groove) and attaining contact between connector and either straight or bent rods only near the outer edges of the connection (hollow-ground). This mechanism results in early realization of gripping strength during set-screw (closed or top-entry connector) or hex-nut (split connector) tightening. Each set screw and nut should be checked at least once before closure. The endpoint for tightness is the feeling that the shoulder of the wrench (Allen) or of the nut is about to round off.

Closed connectors are slipped over the end of the rod before placing the rod. These connectors are stronger than split connectors and should be used whenever possible, particularly at ends of constructs where the greatest load is transferred from the spinal column to the longitudinal members of implant constructs. Split connectors have the advantage that they can be added any time by placing them over the rod after it is in position.

Closed Connectors. These have a closed VHG connector body for attachment to rods and a slotted hole for connection to the machine-threaded portions of a pedicle or iliac screw. Closed connectors are designed for versatility by reducing the three-dimensional morphologic constraints on implant component connection, while allowing and controlling complex multiplanar displacements and angulations among implant components as corrective forces are applied. There are four styles of closed, slotted connectors for each size rod: straight, angled, extended straight, and extended angled (Figs. 20.13*A*–*D*).

The slotted connectors have a 16-mm long plate portion; the extended version is 24 mm. The slotted and extended slotted connectors have the plate portion extending straight laterally from the VHG body. The angled and extended angled versions have the VHG body placed at a 20° angle from the plate portion to avoid possible interference with the sacrum. The slot in the plate provides coronal plane position versatility by allowing at-

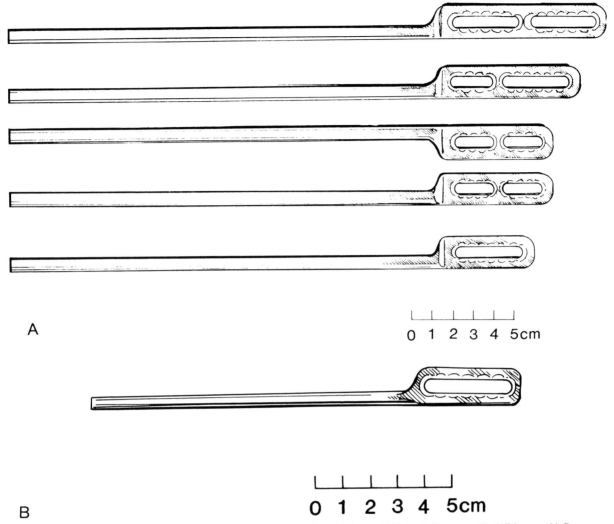

0 1 2 3 4 5cm

A

0 1 2 3 4 5cm

B

Figure 20.12. *A*, Plate-rod combination (PRC) with 6.35-mm (¼″) rod diameter. *B*, 4.76-mm (³⁄₁₆″) rod diameter.

tachment of the rod to the screws at variable distances from the rod in the coronal plane. The rod is secured to the connector with a 6.35-mm (¼″) set screw. The pedicle or iliac screw is secured to the slotted portion of the connector with an 8-mm (⁵⁄₁₆″) hex nut placed on the 4.76-mm, 10-32 machine thread of the screw.

Sagittal plane angular versatility is made possible by the oval configuration of the pedicle with the large diameter located in the sagittal plane. Sagittal plane AP position versatility dorsal to the pedicle entry site is provided by washers placed on the 4.76-mm, 10-32 machine thread of the screw between the connector and the integral nut of the screw.

Infinitely adjustable axial plane angular and longitudinal position versatility is provided by the ability to lo-

cate the VHG connector anywhere along or around the smooth rod.

Split Connectors. These consist of two matching halves (jaws) (Fig. 20.14). Each jaw is the same as the unthreaded jaw on the transverse and dual (bypass) connectors. The split connector allows the closest lateral attachment of the screw anchor relative to the rod longitudinal member. The force necessary to squeeze the jaws together is provided by an 8-mm (⁵⁄₁₆″) hex nut. The recommended torque is 7.3 Nm (65″/lb), a force easily achieved with the cannulated locking wrench. This hex nut is also used in the transverse connector. Rod gripping strength is achieved by the VHG-designed jaws and posteriorly placed heels about which the jaws pivot (Figs.

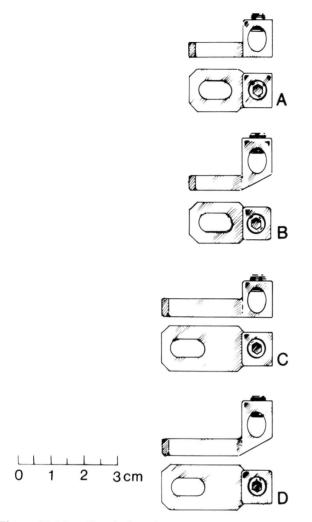

Figure 20.13. Closed, slotted connectors (6.35 mm shown; 4.76 mm also available). *A*, Straight. *B*, Angled. *C*, Extended straight. *D*, Extended angled.

ruption of circular continuity around the rod inherent in any split connections. Thus, split connectors are not recommended for carrying flexion-extension loads when load sharing does not exist. Their use at the ends of constructs should be limited to those situations in which adjacent vertebral segments that are stable anteriorly can be secured to form an end foundation.

There is one style of split connector provided in the sizes for the 6.35-mm and 4.76-mm rod.

Longitudinal Member to Longitudinal Member Connectors

Transverse connection to paired longitudinal members of a spinal implant construct increases stability and avoids unstable linkage configurations and the associated collapse of the construct until sufficient load sharing with the instrumented segment of the spinal column occurs. Transfixation may also be used to control excessive forces and moments internal to the construct that otherwise might cause premature failure of the implant itself or of the bone implant interface (16).

Extending a longitudinal member by either side-to-side or end splicing with dual (bypass) or tandem (end-to-end) connection may be desirable as a step in an instrumentation sequence (e.g., deformities in different planes at different levels) or in revision surgery.

Transverse Connectors. Two sizes of transverse connectors are available; one for 4.76-mm and one for 6.35-mm

20.15*A* and *B*). After 9 months' implantation in the unfused canine spine, a clinically insignficant loosening of 17% has been observed (22).

The axial (Figs. 20.16*A* and *B*) and torsional (Figs. 20.17*A* and *B*) gripping strengths of closed and split VHG connectors have been studied and compared with other connections. It is important to realize that split connectors are not as strong as closed connectors and must be used with discretion. For example, the comparative axial loosening strengths for the 6.35-mm (¼″) versions are 1600 newtons for the closed connector and 640 newtons for the split connector. The comparative torsional loosening strengths for the same versions are 4.8 Nm for the closed connector and 1.9 Nm for the split connector. These differences are the result of the inter-

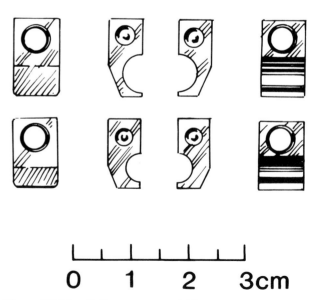

Figure 20.14. Split connectors, 6.35 mm (*top*) and 4.76 mm (*bottom*).

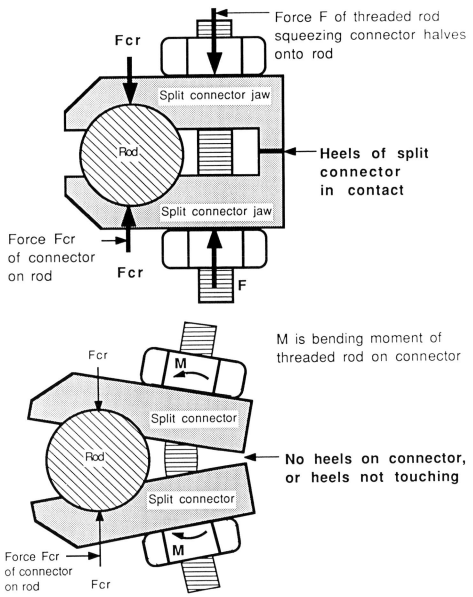

Figure 20.15. *Top,* Heels on jaws of split-type connectors in contact give greater rod gripping strength. *Bottom,* Split type of connectors with NO heels (or heels not in contact) create less rod gripping and are more prone to fatigue failure.

diameter longitudinal members (Fig. 20.18). There are two clamping jaws with unthreaded cross-member holes and one jaw each with right- and left-hand threaded cross-member holes. The cross member, a 4.76-mm diameter, turnbuckle-style left- and right-hand threaded, 10-cm long rod, is the same for both sizes so that, if necessary, a 4.76-mm connector can be placed on one side and a 6.35-mm connector on the other.

The unthreaded jaws are held together against the threaded jaws with 8.0-mm (⁵⁄₁₆″) hex nuts, one right-hand and the other left-hand threaded (36). These nuts have displayed no tendency toward loosening after 9 months' implantation in the unfused canine spine (22).

Dual (Bypass) Connectors. A dual connector assembly (Fig. 20.19) is made by combining one-half (either left or right) of a transverse connector with a dual connector jaw. The assembly consists of one-half of a transverse connector cross-member, the appropriate-size transverse connector threaded dual connector jaw (for either 4.76-

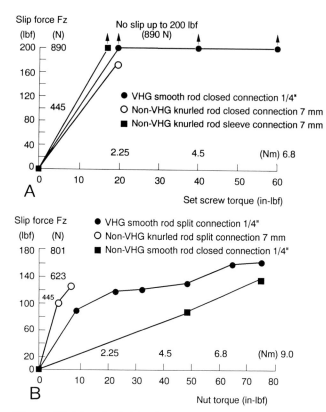

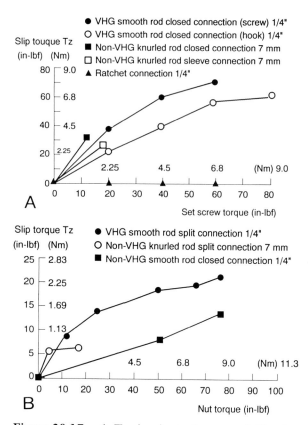

Figure 20.16. *A,* Axial gripping strength Fz of connection types expressed as a function of set screw torque. *B,* Axial gripping strength Fz of connection types expressed as a function of nut torque.

Figure 20.17. *A,* Torsional gripping strength Tz of connection types expressed as a function of set screw torque. *B,* Torsional gripping strength Tz of connection types expressed as a function of nut torque.

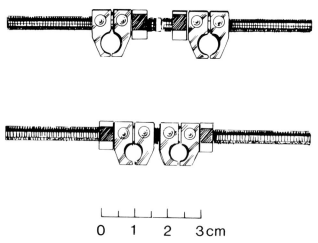

Figure 20.18. Transverse connector assemblies for 6.35- and 4.76-mm rods. Nut position, inside or outside, is determined by the length of span between longitudinal members. Nuts are placed inside when possible.

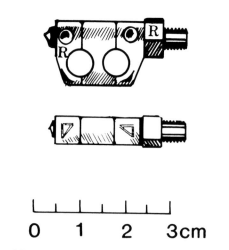

Figure 20.19. Dual (bypass) 6.35-mm (¼″) connector.

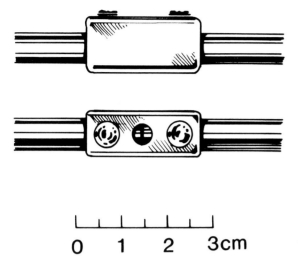

Figure 20.20. Tandem 6.35-mm (¼″) (end-to-end) connector.

or 6.35-mm rods), a matching unthreaded jaw, and an 8.0-mm (⁵⁄₁₆″) hex nut of the appropriate right- or left-hand thread. Three dual connector jaws are available, making it possible to connect any combination of 6.35- and 4.76-mm rods. The VHG design feature is included in this connector.

Dual connectors add tremendous versatility to the system by making it possible to attach rods that have been secured to separate foundations and brought together in a reduction maneuver. They also permit splicing of rods to plates and across fractured rods. It is necessary for two dual connectors to complete each connection.

Tandem Connectors (End-to-End). A tandem connector allows rods to be connected end-to-end. It is available to connect 4.76- or 6.36-mm rods (Fig. 20.20) or a combination of the two. The VHG connector design feature is included in this connector.

Accessories, VSP

Washers. Two 11-mm diameter washers of either 3- or 5-mm height (Fig. 20.21) provide sagittal plane positioning variability of a connector or longitudinal member on a screw anchor. The washers also increase strength of the connection between the screws and longitudinal slots of plates and PRCs. Washers elevate the connector or longitudinal member dorsally to avoid interference with bony structures, such as facet joints, and allow for more room for bone graft underneath the connector or longitudinal member.

Although not commonly used, the washers or 8.0-mm (⁵⁄₁₆″) nuts (right- and left-hand) may also be used to enlarge the diameter and thus strengthen the transverse rod of wide transverse rod connections.

A 12.7-mm diameter washer with a 15° angle provides sagittal plane angular position adjustability between screws and plate-type components that use acorn nuts in nests to form the connection.

Set Screws and Nuts. All VHG connections are secured with a 6.35-mm (¼″) set screw that accommodates a 3.2-mm (⅛″) hex end screw driver.

The right-hand threaded 8.0-mm (⁵⁄₁₆″) nut is supplied as a separate component for attachment of closed and split connectors to screw anchors. It is the same nut used on transverse and dual connectors (right-hand thread portion). Left-hand thread nuts may also be obtained individually as needed.

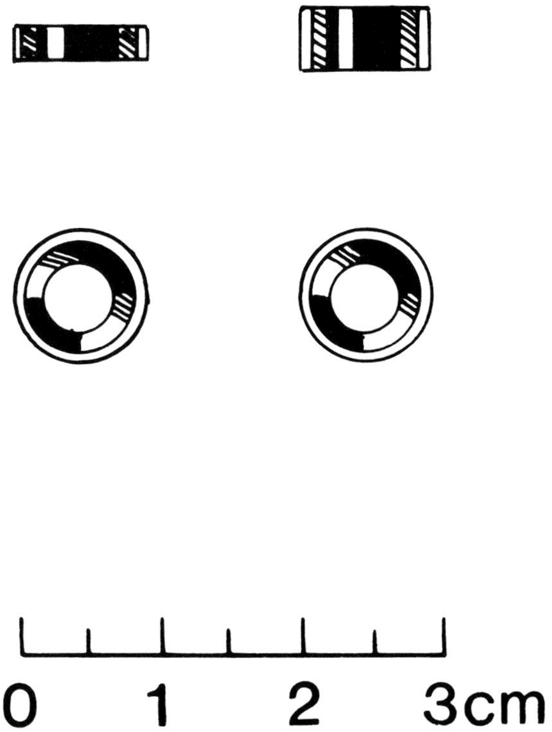

Figure 20.21. Washers, 11-mm outer diameter, 3- and 5-mm heights.

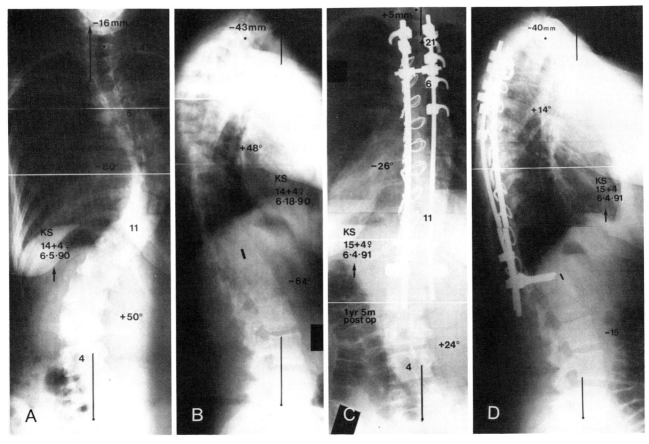

Figure 20.22. *A–D,* A 14-year, 4-month-old female whose standing preoperative radiographs, PA (*A*) and lateral (*B*), show a right thoracic major curve that is marginally flexible ([80–60] ÷ 80 × 100 = 25%). T12 is a neutral vertebra and L1-L2 the stable disc. Sagittal plane alignment of the thoracolumbar junction is normal, and the kyphosis apex at T8 is only slightly lower than normal. Standing 1-year, 5-month postoperative radiographs, PA (*C*) and lateral (*D*), are shown. The procedure included right thoracoplasties and left rib osteotomies. Although her correction and balance are satisfactory, it is apparent that her instrumentation could have been stopped at T12.

APPLICATIONS

There are a number of instruments that are unique to the Isola spine system. These include cannulated locking wrenches, a table-top rod cutter, and variable radius benders.

Techniques

The visual-tactile-anatomic approach to pedicle screw and iliac screw post or screw placement is emphasized (54). Drill placement is not utilized. Some method of intraoperative biplanar radiographic exposure should be available.

An adjacent sublaminar wire may be used to approximate a rod and drop-entry hook to the spine. It is essential to select a hook with the minimum throat height necessary to seat under the lamina while allowing the rod to pass directly over the top of the lamina. Furthermore, it is important not to place a hook in a canal that is compromised in size. When preparing transverse process-lamina claws, enough lamina must be preserved to complete the claw. Recent experiments utilizing osteoporotic human thoracic vertebra have shown that a transverse process—lamina claw is as strong and stable as a transverse process—pedicle hook claw. Sublaminar wires, either single or doubled, are as strong as the two claws but are less stable, especially the single wire (14).

Longitudinal member length is determined by measuring the distance along the path of the curved spine from the facet joint above to the facet joint below the end segments of the spine to be instrumented. A single suture stabilized by three hemostats works well for following the path of the curved spine, which is held as straight as possible by external three-point pressure. The suture is removed and straightened for rod marking. To this distance .5-1 cm may need to be added, depending upon the flexibility of the spine. Using this technique, in situ cutting of the longitudinal members is rarely necessary. Because rods are relatively inexpensive, it is better to resize and shape a new rod than to persist very long with a rod that is not best sized or shaped.

Longitudinal member contouring is based on two principles: 1. preservation or restoration of sagittal plane alignment; and 2. removal of coronal plane deformity. It is essential to remember that the apex and location of abnormal coronal plane curves (scoliosis) and sagittal plane deformities (hyperkyphosis, hypokyphosis, hyperlordosis, and hypolordosis), as well as the normal sagittal plane position, are usually different from the apex of the normal sagittal plane curves. Also consider that the curve radius of a pathological curve is usually more or less constant for that curve, whereas the radius of the normal sagittal plane curve is constantly changing. A major principle in the application of the Isola spine system in the treatment of spinal deformity is to contour the longitu-

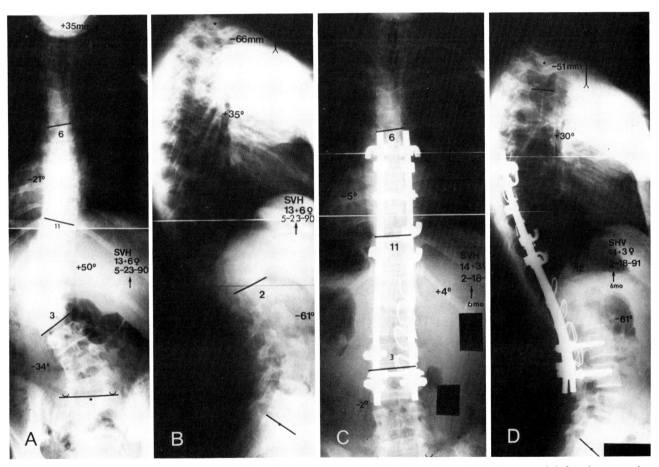

Figure 20.23. *A–D,* A 13-year, 6-month-old female whose standing preoperative radiographs, PA (*A*) and lateral (*B*), show a left thoracolumbar major, right thoracic minor curve pattern with a fully lumbarized S1 vertebra and imbalance to the right of 35 mm. She does not have thoracolumbar junction kyphosis. Standing radiographs taken 6 months postoperatively, PA (*C*) and lateral (*D*), show good deformity correction and balance restoration with instrumentation from one vertebra below the upper end vertebra of the thoracic curve and one vertebra below the lower end vertebra. Because of the fully lumbarized S1 vertebra, she still has three normal motion segments below her instrumentation.

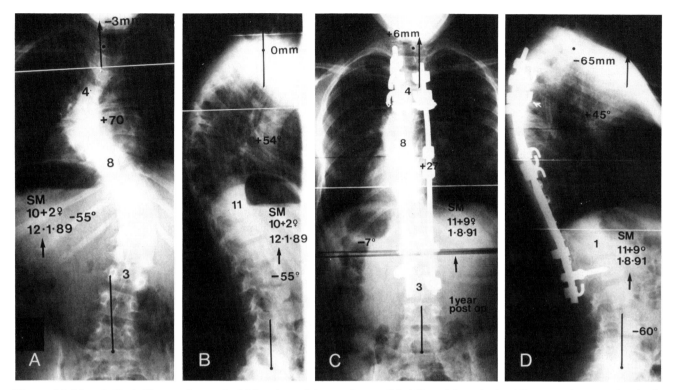

Figure 20.24. *A–D,* A 10-year, 8-month-old female, weighing 22.3 kg, with progressive kyphoscoliosis secondary to neurofibromatosis. Standing preoperative radiographs, PA (*A*) and lateral (*B*), show that size and etiology of the deformities necessitates treatment of all three: left major scoliosis, thoracic hyperkyphosis, and right compensatory thoracolumbar scoliosis. Standing radiographs taken 1 year postoperatively are shown, PA (*C*) and lateral (*D*). The procedure consisted of a same-day sequential 5th rib resection thoracotomy, anterior discectomy and fusion as well as strut grafting of the apex of the curve, followed by dorsal instrumentation and fusion. Because of the patient's small size, 4.76-mm (³⁄₁₆″) components were utilized.

dinal member as would be desired for normal sagittal plane angular position. *The Isola spine technique specifically does not attempt to directly displace coronal plane deformity into sagittal plane alignment, as the two very seldom coincide. The Isola principle is to realign the spine onto a longitudinal member shaped for the expected normal sagittal plane alignment.* Every effort is made to remove most, if not all, of the coronal plane deformity. Thus, continuous or staged anterior, concurrent transdiscal (L2-L5), or transpedicular destabilization may be necessary. The variable position connections allowed by the slotted connectors and wires and the limited elastic deformity possible for the longitudinal members make it possible to accommodate some residual coronal plane deformity. When necessary, some coronal plane deformity can be bent into the longitudinal members. A videotape detailing use of the variable radius benders is available (6).

Clinical Applications

Some examples of the use of the implants and techniques are shown as follows: Adolescent idiopathic scoliosis, right thoracic curve pattern (Fig. 20.22*A–D*); adolescent idiopathic scoliosis, left thoracolumbar major and right thoracic minor curve pattern (Fig. 20.23*A–D*); neurofibromatosis kyphoscoliosis with large compensatory scoliosis (Fig. 20.24*A–D*); neuropathic hyperkyphosis (Fig. 20.25*A–D*); L2 burst fracture (Fig. 20.26*A–F*); degenerative disc disease and mild scoliosis (Fig. 20.27*A–D*); degenerative disc disease, spinal stenosis, and postlaminectomy two-level spondylolisthesis (Figs. 20.28*A–D*); and L4-5 and L5-S1 disc disease and sagittal plane instability following prior instrumentation and fusion to L4 for idiopathic scoliosis (Figs. 20.29*A–D*).

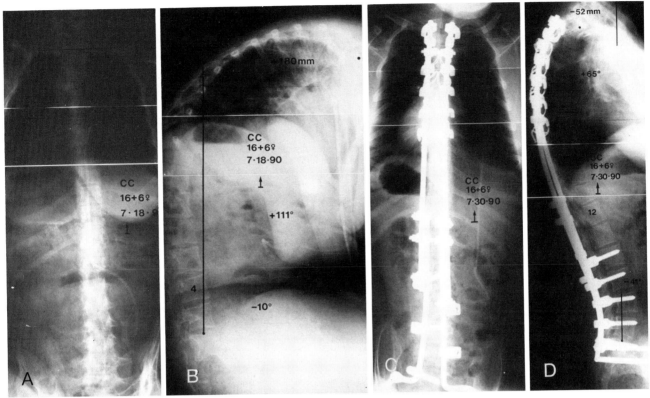

Figure 20.25. *A–D,* A 16-year, 6-month-old female non-ambulatory patient with psychomotor retardation and progressive neuropathic hyperkyphosis, sitting preoperative radiographs, PA (*A*) and lateral (*B*). The hyperkyphosis is completely flexible, and there is no coronal plane deformity. Sitting postoperative radiographs, PA (*C*) and lateral (*D*), show good correction of patient's deformities with establishment of stable and strong foundations at both ends of the instrumentation to the point that no external immobilization was necessary, as confirmed by follow-up 1 year later with no loss of correction.

Problems

Implant problems have been few. Because there was some iliac screw breakage at the thread-collar shaft junction, we shortened the thread length and tapered the root of the thread in order to improve biomechanical characteristics. Transverse connector breakage adjacent to the inside nut or connector jaw in long breakage adjacent to the inside nut or connector jaw in long constructs, including the pelvis, has occurred on a few occasions. This can be avoided or minimized by limiting the expanse of transverse connector rod exposed by contouring the longitudinal member rods so as to limit the length of transverse connection necessary and by placing the nuts or, if space permits, stacking them adjacent to the medial mobile jaws. The only major implant problem to date has been screw breakage at the end of constructs in which anterior load sharing was either not provided for or was inadequate. A screw specifically designed for this purpose is currently being developed. Until it is available, use of constructs spanning three or four motion segments is to be considered when treating marked anterior column instability, such as burst fractures, as this greatly decreases the load experienced by individual screws (58). It is important to recheck each set screw and nut for tightness, the endpoint being the feeling that the shoulder of the wrench (Allen) or of the hex nut is about to round off.

CONCLUSION

The Isola implant system is a comprehensive thoracolumbosacroiliac dorsal implant system applicable in all

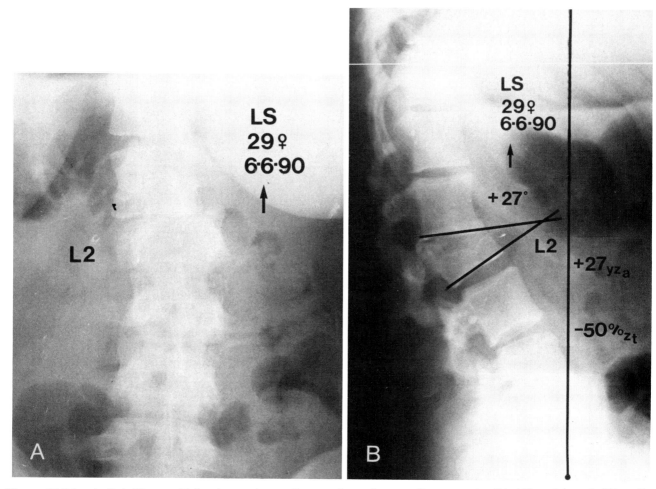

Figure 20.26. *A–F,* A 29-year-old female was thrown from her car at the time of a motor vehicle accident and sustained a left diaphragmatic rupture as well as a lumbar spine fracture. She had no radicular findings or symptoms. Because of her other injuries, treatment of her spine fracture was delayed, and she remained neurologically normal. Standing radiographs taken 25 days after injury, PA (*A*) and lateral (*B*), show an L2 burst fracture. Intraoperative PA (*C*) and lateral (*D*) radiographs were taken after ligamentotactic reduction and during preparation for transpedicular grafting. Standing radiographs, PA (*E*) and lateral (*F*), taken 1 year postoperatively, show maintenance of body height and fusion forming across the L1-L2 disc space anteriorly.

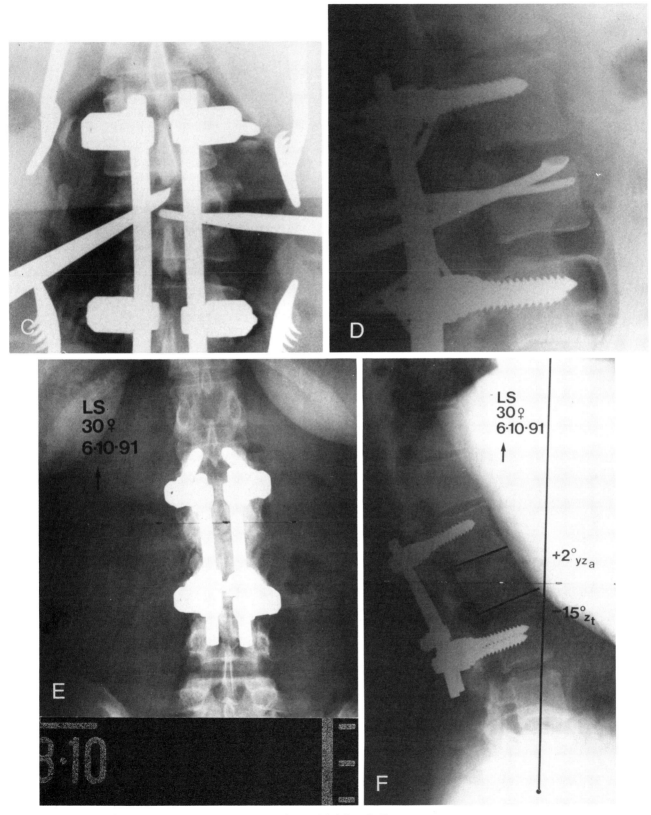

Figure 20.26. *C–F.*

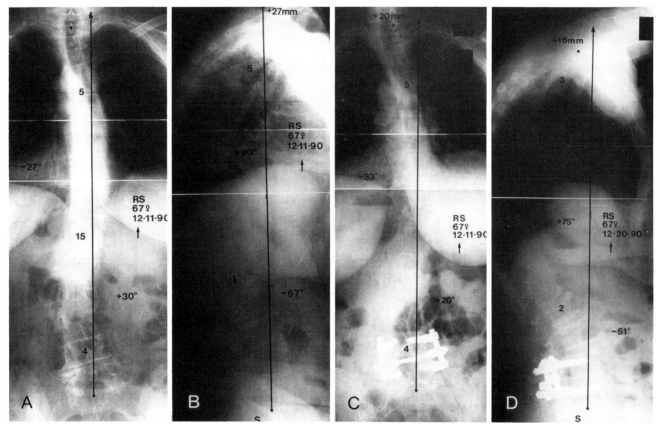

Figure 20.27.   *A–D.*

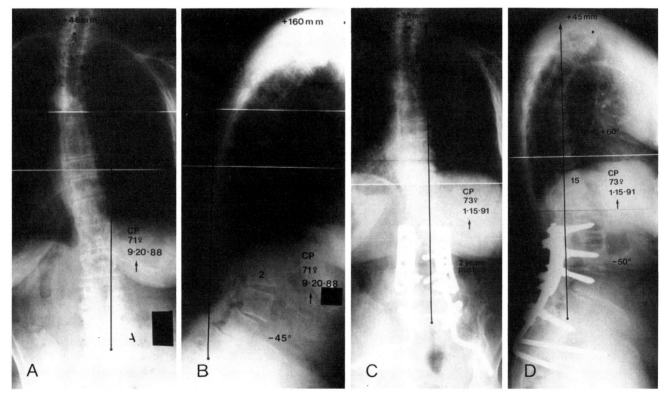

Figure 20.28.   *A–D.*

Figure 20.27. *A–D,* A 67-year-old female with low back pain, neurogenic claudication due to L4-L5 stenosis, and mild degenerative scoliosis whose preoperative standing PA (*A*) and lateral (*B*) radiographs are shown. Because of the focal nature of her problem at L4-L5, limited surgery was undertaken in spite of her more global degenerative disease process. Standing postoperative PA (*C*) and lateral (*D*) radiographs show the placement of one motion segment fixation. The procedure included decompression and left hemiposterior lumbar interbody fusion utilizing a block each of sterilely procured and sterilely processed bicortical allograft and bicortical autograft. The procedure relieved most of her symptoms.

Figure 20.28. *A–D,* A 71-year-old female with central stenosis had undergone decompressive laminectomy several years earlier. She had subsequently developed two-level spondylolisthesis, marked sagittal plane imbalance, and minimal coronal plane imbalance, as shown on her standing preoperative PA (*A*) and lateral (*B*) radiographs. Her sagittal plane position could be realigned in the recumbent supine position. Operative procedure consisted of preparing a lower foundation and reducing an upper foundation to it. Her standing PA (*C*) and lateral (*D*) radiographs 2 years postoperatively are shown.

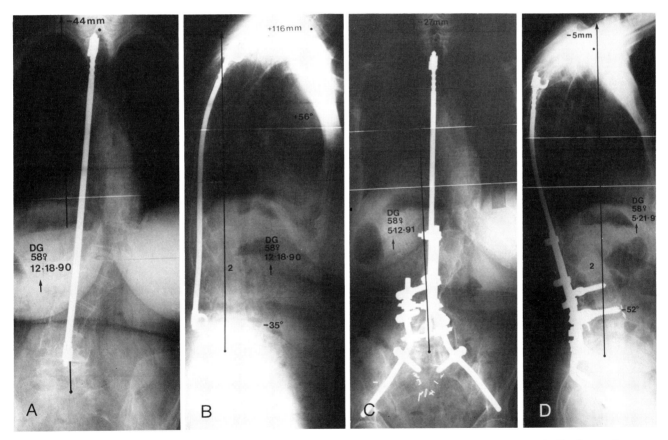

Figure 20.29. *A–D,* A 58-year-old female had had Harrington instrumentation and fusion 14 years previously and had recently developed back pain, moderate sagittal plane imbalance, and minimal coronal plane imbalance, as shown on her standing preoperative PA (*A*) and lateral (*B*) radiographs. Normal sagittal plane alignment could be restored passively. For this reason, dorsal instrumentation and fusion was performed first. Because of the patient's osteoporosis, fixation to the upper portion of her spine would have been very difficult without utilizing her existing stable Harrington rod, as shown on her standing postoperative PA (*C*) and lateral (*D*) radiographs. Prior to these radiographs, a second-stage transperitoneal anterior L4-L5 and L5-S1 discectomy with bi- and tricortical allo- and autografting had been performed.

ages to all deformities and instabilities of the human spine. It is designed to minimize internal and external profile, maintain simplicity and versatility, and be compatible with the VSP. Its successful use depends on a thorough understanding of both the three-dimensional 6° of freedom of motion characteristics of the spinal deformity and/or instability being treated and the biomechanics of the implant system components and the clinical constructs developed with them.

Acknowledgments. The authors wish to acknowledge Arthur D. Steffee, M.D.; Samuel Chewning, M.D.; Terry Stahurski, M.S.; Tom Flatley, M.D.; Mark Brown, M.D., Ph.D.; and Jan Brunks; Janice Orrick, R.N.; and Barbara Funk.

REFERENCES

1. Allen BL, Ferguson RL: The Galveston technique for L rod instrumentation of the scoliotic spine. Spine 1982;7:276–284.
2. Armstrong GWD, Connock SHG: A transverse loading system applied to a modified Harrington instrumentation. Clin Orthop 1975;108:70–75.
3. Asher MA, Strippgen WE: Anthropometric studies of the human sacrum relating to dorsal transsacral implant designs. Clin Orthop 1986;203:48–62.
4. Asher M, Carson WL, Heinig C, et al: A modular spinal rod linkage system to provide rotational stability. Spine 1988;13:272–277.
5. Asher M, DeSmet A, Cook L, et al: Classification of adolescent idiopathic scoliosis curve patterns: A three-dimensional analysis. Orthop Trans 1989;12:260.
6. Asher MA, Strippgen WE, Heinig CF, et al: Spinal rod and plate bending technique. AAOS 1991:VT-210015; NASS 1990:V0-33.
7. Asher MA, Strippgen WE, Heinig CF, et al: Isola spine implant system: Principles and practice. Cleveland: AcroMed, 1991, ISBN 0-932845-45-2.
8. Asher MA, Lark D: Eggshell procedure in the dog: A means of technique development. Orthop Trans 1991;15:245.
9. Barsanti CM, deBari A, Covino BM: The torsion meter: A critical review. J Pediatr Orthop 1990;10:527–531.
10. Bernhardt M, Bridwell KH: Segmental analysis of the sagittal plane alignment of the normal thoracic and lumbar spines and thoracolumbar junction. Spine 1989;14:717–721.
11. Berry JL, Stahurski TM, Asher MA: A morphometric description of human thoracic and lumbar vertebral lamina. Trans Orthop Res Soc 1991;16:638.
12. Boachie-Adjei O, Dendrinos GK, Ogilvie JW, et al: Management of adult spinal deformity with combined anterior-posterior arthrodesis and Luque-Galveston instrumentation. J Spinal Disorder 1991;4:131–141.
13. Brown M: Clinical perspectives of intervertebral discs. In: New perspectives on low back pain. Frymoyer JW, Gordon SL, eds. Chicago: Am Acad Orthop Surgeons Press, 1989;133–146.
14. Butler T, Asher M, Jayaraman G, et al: The strength and stability of some dorsal thoracic anchor and anchor sites in osteoporotic spines. Trans North American Spine Society Annual Meeting, July 31–August 3, 1991, Keystone, Colorado (poster exhibit), Trans Scoliosis Research Society Annual Meeting, September 24–27, 1991, Minneapolis, Minnesota (Poster Exhibit), and Trans Combined Meeting of the Orthopaedic Research Societies of U.S.A., Japan and Canada, October 21–23, 1991, Banff, Alberta, Canada (poster exhibit).
15. Camp JF, Candle R, Ashman RD, et al: Immediate complications of Cotrel-Dubousset instrumentation to the sacropelvis: A clinical and biomechanical study. Spine 1990;15:932–941.
16. Carson WL, Duffield RC, Arendt M, et al: Internal forces and moments in transpedicular spine instrumentation—the effect of pedicle screw angle and transfixation—the 4R-4bar linkage concept. Spine 1990;15:893–901.
17. Carson WL, Redman RS, Richards K: Bending stiffness and strength of VSP, Isola, CD, TSRH and Luque longitudinal member to bone screw connection subconstructs. Trans Scoliosis Research Society Annual Meeting, Minneapolis, Minnesota, September 24–27, 1991.
18. Coe JD, Herzing MA, Warden KE, et al: Load to failure strengths of spinal implants in osteoporotic spines—A comparison study of pedicle screws, laminar hooks, and spinous process wires. Trans Orthop Res Soc 35th Annual Meeting, 1989:71.
19. Crawford RJ, Sell PJ, Ali MS, et al: Segmental spinal instrumentation: a study of the mechanical properties of materials used for sublaminar fixation. Spine 1989;14:632–635.
20. Cotrel Y, Dubousset J: New segmental posterior instrumentation of the spine. Orthop Trans 1985;9:118.
21. Cotrel Y: New instrumentation for surgery of the spine. London: Freund, 1986.
22. Dalenberg D, Asher M, Jayaraman G, et al: The effect of a stiff spinal implant and its loosening on bone mineral content in canines. Trans North American Spine Society Annual Meeting, July 31–August 3, 1991, Keystone, Colorado.
23. Deacon P, Dickson RA: Vertebral shape in the median sagittal plane in idiopathic thoracic scoliosis. A study of true lateral radiographs in 150 patients. Orthopaedics 1987;10:893–895.
24. Denis F: The three column spine and its significance in the classification of acute thoracolumbar spine injuries. Spine 1983;8:817–831.
25. DeSmet AA, Tarlton MA, Berridge AS, et al: The top view of analysis of scoliosis progression. Radiology 1983;147:369–372.
26. DeSmet AA, Asher MA, Cook LT, et al: Three dimensional analysis of right thoracic idiopathic scoliosis. Spine 1984;9:377–381.
27. Drummond D, Guadagni J, Keene JS, et al: Interspinous process segmental spinal instrumentation. J Pediatr Orthop 1984;4:397–404.
28. Dwyer AF, Newton NC, Sherwood AA: An anterior approach to scoliosis. A preliminary report. Clin Orthop 1969;62:192–202.
29. Geiger JM, Udovic NA, Berry JL: Bending and fatigue of spine plates and rods and fatigue of pedicle screws. Scientific exhibit AAOS 56th Annual Meeting, Las Vegas, NV, February 1989.
30. Graf H, Dubousset J: Tridimensional study of scoliotic spines: Application to infantile scoliosis. Orthop Trans 1981;5:23–24.
31. Hack HP, Zielke K, Harms J: Spinal instrumentation and monitoring. In: Bradford DS, ed. The pediatric spine. New York: Thieme, 1985;491–517.
32. Haher TR, Felmy W, Baruch H, et al: The contribution of the three columns of the spine to rotational stability: A biomechanical model. Spine 1989;14:663–669.
33. Harrington PR: Treatment of scoliosis: correction and internal fixation by spine instrumentation. J Bone Joint Surg 1962;44A:591–610.
34. Harrington PR, Tullos HS: Reduction of severe spondylolisthesis in children. South Med J 1969;62:1–7.
35. Heinig CF: Eggshell procedure in segmental spinal instrumentation. In: Luque E, ed. Segmental spinal instrumentation. Thorofare, New Jersey: Slack, 1984;221–234.

36. Isola transverse rod connectors: Principles and techniques. Cleveland: AcroMed, 1989.

37. Jacobs RR, Schlaepfer F, Mathys R Jr, et al: A locking hook spinal rod system for stabilization of fracture-dislocations and correction of deformities of the dorsolumbar spine. A biomechanical evaluation. Clin Orthop 1984;189:168–177.

38. King AI: A review of biomechanical models. J Biomech Eng 1984;106:97–104.

39. King HA, Moe JH, Bradford DS, et al: The selection of fusion levels in thoracic idiopathic scoliosis. J Bone Joint Surg 1983; 65A:1302–1313.

40. Lee CK: Accelerated degeneration of the segment adjacent to a lumbar fusion. Spine 1988;13:375–377.

41. Luque ER, Cardoso A: Treatment of scoliosis without arthrodesis or external support. A preliminary report. Orthop Trans 1977;1:37–38.

42. Luque ER, Cardoso A: Segmental correction of scoliosis with rigid internal fixation. A preliminary report. Orthop Trans 1977;1:136–137.

43. Luque ER: Segmental spinal instrumentation for correction of scoliosis. Clin Orthop 1982;163:192–198.

44. Luque ER: Segmental spinal instrumentation. Thorofare, New Jersey: Slack, 1984.

45. Marcinek SA, Njus GO: Technical paper #30A-789, University of Akron, 1989.

46. McCord DH, Cunningham BW, Shono YU, et al: Biomechanical analysis of lumbosacral fixation. Trans North American Spine Society Annual Meeting, July 31–August 3, 1991, Keystone, Colorado.

47. Moe JH, Winter RB, Bradford DS, et al: Scoliosis and other spinal deformities. Philadelphia: WB Saunders, 1978:499–503.

48. Montesano PX, Asher MA, Schlehr FJ: Fatal cardiac tamponade resulting from a central venous catheter: a case for open-chest cardiac resuscitation. J Spinal Disorders 1989;2:52–55.

49. Nash C, Moe J: A study of the vertebral rotation. J Bone Joint Surg 1969;51:223–228.

50. Perdriolle R: La Scoliose. Maloine SA, ed. Paris, 1979;79–82.

51. Raso VJ, Gillespie R, McNeice GM: Determination of the maximum plane of deformity in idiopathic scoliosis. Orthop Trans 1980;4:23.

52. Roy-Camille R, Saillant G, Mazel C: Internal fixation of the lumbar spine with pedicle screw plating. Clin Orthop 1986;203:7–17.

53. Saer EH, Winter RB: Long scoliosis fusion to the sacrum in adults with nonparalytic scoliosis: an improved method. Spine 1990;15:650–653.

54. Steffee AD, Biscup RS, Sitkowski DJ: Segmental spine plates with pedicle screw fixation. A new internal fixation device for disorders of the lumbar and thoracolumbar spine. Clin Orthop 1986; 203:45–53.

55. Stokes IAF, Bigalow LC, Moreland MS: Three dimensional spinal curvature in idiopathic scoliosis. J Orthop Res 1987;5:102–113.

56. Stokes IAF: Three dimensional study group, ad hoc committee of SRS working document, 1991.

57. Uhtoff HK, Armstrong G: Symposium, New horizons in spinal surgery. Clin Orthop 1988;227:2–142.

58. Voth B, Duffield RC, Carson WL: Finite element analysis of internal forces and moments in bilevel and trilevel spine instrumentation: The effects of pedicle angle, transfixation, vertebra offset and variations in vertebra size. Master's degree thesis University of Missouri–Columbia, August 1991.

59. Wilber RG, Thompson GH, Shaffer JW, et al: Postoperative neurological deficits in segmental spinal instrumentation. A study using spinal cord monitoring. J Bone Joint Surg 1984;66A:1178–1187.

60. Wiltse LL: Symposium, Internal fixation of the lumbar spine. Clin Orthop 1986;203:2–231.

61. Winter RB, Anderson MB: Spinal arthrodesis for spinal deformity using posterior instrumentation and sublaminar wiring. A preliminary report of 100 consecutive cases. Int Orthop 1985;9:239–245.

TWENTY-ONE

Zielke Instrumentation of the Spine

James W. Ogilvie

INTRODUCTION

Correcting coronal plane deformities of the spine can be done with several modes of force application. The earliest attempts were with external bracing. References to a brace-like device applied by the armorer of the French surgeon Ambrose Paré date to the 15th century (20). This involves direct lateral pressure or transverse force at the apex of the curve to correct the deformity. It remains a fundamental principle behind current orthotic treatment philosophy of scoliosis.

Bending moments on the upper and lower limbs of a scoliotic curve are the basis for such devices as the turn-buckle or hinged cast. This method of external fixation is cumbersome and has been replaced by operative and internal fixation.

Early attempts at correction and internal fixation of scoliosis used the concept of distraction. Harrington distraction rods utilize this method of correction (9,12). Earlier, Adam Gruca utilized compression springs and turnbuckle jacks surgically placed in the spine to effect correction (10). This is a highly efficient means of correcting curves greater than 55°. However, as the curve diminishes in magnitude with progressive distraction, more force is needed for incremental correction. In other words, the efficiency of the distraction force expressed as degrees of correction per unit of force diminishes rapidly (29).

Compressive force applied to the convex side of a scoliotic curve has also been used for correction of the coronal plane deformity and also to reduce kyphosis or produce lordosis.

Although Von Lackum had performed anterior surgery for scoliosis in 1933, it was Dwyer, in 1969, who proposed the combination of anterior discectomy and the application of a compressive device across the convexity of the vertebral bodies (5,6,28). This is a powerful corrective force, and when combined with the appropriate placement of interbody bone grafts, an excellent scoliosis correction can be obtained (1,14,17). The Dwyer device is not rigid internal fixation. The staples in the vertebral body are connected with a flexible cable, and once fixed to the cable through a crimping process, they are not adjustable (22,23,25). Postoperative bracing is needed until interbody arthrodesis has occurred.

ZIELKE DESIGN

In 1976, Zielke introduced a modification of the Dwyer procedure that has offered the ability to correct not only the coronal plane deformity but the rotational deformity of scoliosis (30,31). The vertebral body screws are connected by a threaded rod, providing infinite adjustment to the compression force. In addition, the application technique allows more controllable production of lordosis. The generic designation of ventral derotation spondylodesis (VDS) is applied to the Zielke procedure.

The advantages of VDS are an excellent fusion rate, good overall correction of the scoliosis, and most importantly, fewer levels required to fuse. This allows more mobile motion segments to remain distal to the fusion mass. Considerable evidence exists to support the concept that the presence of two or less mobile motion segments distal to a lumbar fusion predisposes to an unacceptably high incidence of degenerative disc disease (3). Using the conventional criteria of determination for fusion limits in posterior distraction instrumentation, many lumbar or thoracolumbar curves that formerly would require fusion down to L4 can be ended at L3 or above (Fig. 21.1).

VDS SURGICAL TECHNIQUE

Hodgson has described the anterior surgical approach to the entire spine for the treatment of tuberculosis (13). The reader is referred to his classic article for a more detailed account.

With the patient in the right lateral decubitus position for a left lumbar curve, the operating table is flexed to

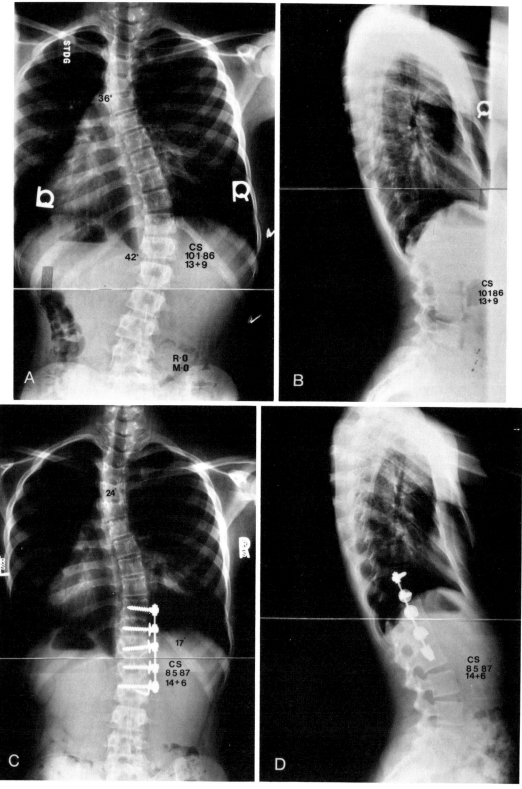

Figure 21.1. *A,* This 13-year, 9-month-old premenarchal female with thoracolumbar idiopathic scoliosis was treated unsuccessfully with an orthosis. An anterior-posterior radiograph demonstrates a scoliosis of 42°. *B,* The lateral radiograph shows no kyphosis above the area of the lumbar spine to be instru- mented with VDS. *C,* At 9 months following VDS, the patient's curve has been corrected to 17° and in the lateral projection. *D,* There is an acceptable sagittal contour. Patient wore a brace for 6 months after surgery.

enhance subsequent exposure. When exposing the lumbar spine in preparation for VDS, care must be exercised in the exposure to avoid injury to the vessels and internal organs. The aorta, as opposed to the vena cava, is a substantial structure that is both resistant to casual injury and capable of being repaired, should one inadvertently transgress it. This is convenient when dealing with idiopathic lumbar curves that are usually to the left. Most idiopathic thoracolumbar curves are to the right and require added care in dealing with the great vessels.

The bed of the tenth rib is ideal for approaching the diaphragm. If the eleventh rib is used, the bed of the rib is also the lateral insertion of the diaphragm, and dissection is more difficult. Following blunt dissection of the retroperitoneal plane, the peritoneum and its contents are reflected anteriorly and medially to expose the lumbar spine. After obtaining a radiograph to confirm the levels of dissection, ligation of the segmental vertebral vessels is then done over the extent of the fusion levels. The surgeon then proceeds with meticulous removal of the intervertebral disc and placement of the bone graft in the disc space. Zielke screws are placed in the midbody of each vertebra to be fused. The derotation and lordosing bridge is attached to the threaded rod that is anchored to each screw. Compression is applied in the corrected position, thus locking the spine in the lordotic and derotated position. Placement of the intervertebral bone graft should be anterior to the line of compression to help create or maintain lordosis. Excess rod is trimmed, and the wound is closed anatomically. A chest tube is necessary, usually for 48–72 hours, for evacuation of the hemothorax. When the patient's ileus has cleared, and he/she is able to stand, an underarm thoracolumbosacral orthosis (TLSO) is fitted. This is worn until interbody fusion has occurred, generally 6 months.

INDICATIONS FOR VDS

Indications for VDS are a lumbar or thoracolumbar scoliosis that is not rigid due to degenerative changes in the facets, resulting in ankylosis. If posterior surgical correction of a lumbar or thoracolumbar scoliosis is contraindicated because of mitigating local skin conditions, previous infection, or loss of posterior elements such that posterior instrumentation and fusion are technically impossible, i.e., myelomeningocele, VDS may be the best option. However, if posterior instrumentation is to be used in a second-stage posterior surgery, even a semirigid anterior construct such as Zielke VDS may limit the correction. As a result of implementing the Luque technique of segmental fixation, the author has discontinued the use of Zielke VDS in two-stage myelomeningocele spine surgery. When a rigid deformity exists, anterior discec-

tomy and bone graft without instrumentation followed by second-stage Luque-Galveston fixation has provided excellent results.

As a precondition to VDS, there must not be a significant (>30°) compensatory thoracic curve that is rigid. If the lower curve is corrected with VDS and the upper curve is rigid, trunk decompensation may result. Usually, a thoracic curve greater than 35–40° or with a significant rib cage deformity precludes the use of VDS in the lumbar spine. Despite careful anterior placement of the intervertebral bone graft, VDS usually produces some degree of kyphosis (18,19). Its use is therefore contraindicated in a lumbar curve where kyphosis preexists.

Moe and colleagues reported an 84% correction of idiopathic scoliosis deformities with the Zielke device, while Kaneda and colleagues achieved an 82% improvement (15,16,18). Moe noted a 40% correction in the unoperated compensatory thoracic curve.

COMPLICATIONS

Despite the generally good results in those patients where VDS is an appropriate alternative, some disadvantages exist (19). The anterior thoracolumbar surgical approach introduces a new set of possible complications sometimes unfamiliar to orthopaedists. Due to the high profile of the instrumentation, it should not be placed under the iliac vessels and is therefore not applicable to the L5 and S1 vertebral bodies. Chylothorax, injury to the ureter, spleen or great vessels, retroperitoneal fibrosis, and incisional hernia can result (2,3,7,8,24). The long anterior lateral incision may be cosmetically unacceptable, especially in young women. In today's demanding and sophisticated patient population, there is frequently resistance to wearing a TLSO for 6 months.

Recently, there have been long term follow-up studies that also point to previously unappreciated problems with VDS. Trammell and associates have reported a 31% failure of fixation and a 12% pseudarthrosis rate in a group of 26 adults treated with the Zielke procedure (27). They identified rigid curves greater than 60° and patients older than 50 years as high-risk groups for complications. Puno and coworkers reported an average 54% loss of correction in the operated curves in 33 of 34 patients when followed for more than 2 years (21). Ten of 34 patients had loss of correction in the unoperated thoracic curve also. Hammerberg and associates reported a 20% pseudarthrosis rate in 25 patients undergoing VDS for single lumbar or thoracolumbar curve when followed for 30–60 months (11). When compared with the levels that would have been selected for Harrington distraction instrumentation, they were able to preserve one additional motion segment in the lumbar spine in 23 of 25 patients. Clearly, the

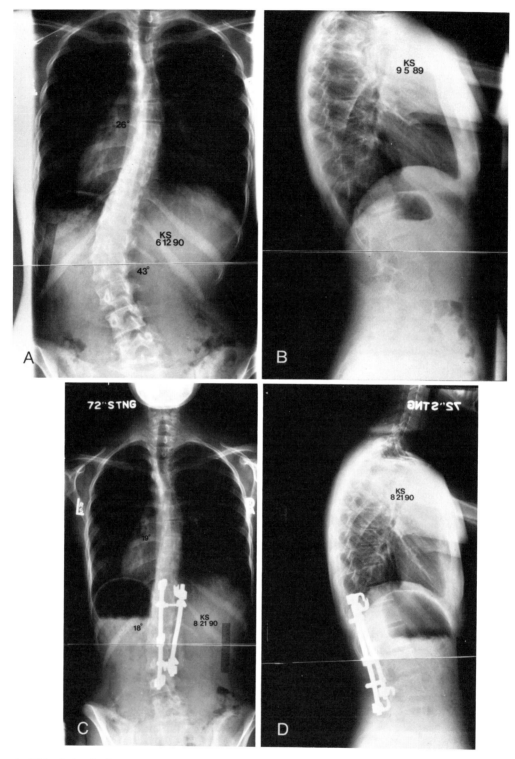

Figure 21.2. *A,* This skeletally immature female with tho-racolumbar idiopathic scoliosis had curve progression to 43° in spite of orthotic treatment. *B,* The lateral radiograph did not demonstrate an abnormal sagittal alignment. *C,* Two months after Cotrel-Dubousset instrumentation, the scoliosis measured 18°. The patient wore no brace following surgery. *D,* The sagittal contour is satisfactory.

Dwyer or Zielke apparatus can be effective in the preservation of motion segments distal to a lumbar fusion. The price to be paid includes significant constraints and complications.

COTREL-DUBOUSSET INSTRUMENTATION

In 1985, a new posterior spinal instrumentation was introduced by Cotrel and Dubousset (4). It is reported to correct spinal deformity through a system of multiple posterior element hooks attached to knurled 7-mm rods and applied through a derotation maneuver. This corrected not only the coronal and sagittal plane deformity, but also applied a derotational force to the spine to improve the torsional deformity. Although the exact mechanism of correction with Cotrel-Dubousset (C-D) instrumentation remains controversial (26), its use has become very popular. Originally designed for application to right thoracic curves, C-D has been implemented in other curve pattern surgeries.

Lumbar and thoracolumbar scoliosis deformities that were previously prime candidates for VDS, can now be treated with C-D instrumentation (Fig. 21.2). The rigidity of the construct allows brace-free convalescence. For routine lumbar and thoracolumbar idiopathic scoliosis surgery, the author's first choice of instrumentation is now the C-D instead of Zielke VDS. The important goal of preserving at least three mobile motion segments distal to the fusion can be achieved with a more cosmetically acceptable posterior midline scar and without the use of a postoperative orthosis. More control over lumbar lordosis is possible with C-D than VDS. Thus, if some degree of kyphosis is present, C-D is not contraindicated.

The advantages of C-D and other currently available variable hook-rod spinal instrumentation constructs compared with Zielke VDS in the treatment of idiopathic lumbar and thoracolumbar scoliosis are: (*a*) no postoperative bracing; (*b*) the ability to spare motion segments distal to the fusion mass comparable to that achieved with Zielke VDS; (*c*) avoidance of the anterior surgical approach with its less cosmetic incision; (*d*) the option of extending instrumentation to the thoracic compensatory curve if indicated; and (*e*) better control of lumbar hypolordosis or kyphosis. This compelling list of differences has relegated the Dwyer apparatus and Zielke VDS to a place of historical interest in the development of spinal instrumentation.

SUMMARY

Zielke ventral derotation spondylodesis (VDS) is a powerful method of correcting selected lumbar and thoracolumbar curves. The curve must not have a kyphotic component, since this procedure tends to reduce lordosis and may result in an unacceptable sagittal plane contour. If a rigid compensatory thoracic curve coexists, correction of the lumbar curve will produce trunk decompensation and an unacceptable shift of the trunk. With this device, it is usually possible to save additional mobile motion segments distal to the lumbar fusion, thus decreasing the likelihood of subsequent lumbar degenerative disc disease.

From 1969 to the mid-1980s, the Dwyer apparatus and, later, the Zielke device were unique in their ability to correct lumbar scoliosis and maintain distal motion segments. With the evolution of rigid posterior derotation instrumentation with the Cotrel-Dubousset or other variable hook rod constructs such as the Texas Scottish Rite Hospital system, the advantages of VDS can now be achieved with greater ease, reliability, and safety without the disadvantages of anterior surgery.

The Dwyer and Zielke anterior devices deserve a prominent place in the history of spinal instrumentation for scoliosis, but their clinical application is no longer indicated for routine lumbar and thoracolumbar curves.

In salvage surgery for lumbar scoliosis, VDS still has a limited role if instrumented correction is indicated and posterior surgery is not possible.

REFERENCES

1. Bauer R, Mostegl A, Eichenauer M: An analysis of the results of Dwyer and Zielke instrumentation in the treatment of scoliosis. Arch Orthop Trauma Surg 1986;105:302–309.
2. Chan FL, Chow SP: Retroperitoneal fibrosis after spinal fusion. Clin Radiol 1983;34:331–335.
3. Cochran T, Irstam L, Nachemson A: Long term anatomic and functional changes in patients with adolescent idiopathic scoliosis treated by Harrington rod fusion. Spine 1983;8(6):576–584.
4. Cotrel Y, Dubousset J: New segmental posterior instrumentation of the spine. Orthop Trans 1985;9:118.
5. Dwyer AF: Experience in anterior correction of scoliosis. Clin Orthop 1973;93:191.
6. Dwyer AF, Newton NC, Sherwood AA: An anterior approach to scoliosis. Clin Orthop 1969;62:192.
7. Eisenstein S, O'Brien JP: Chylothorax: A complication of Dwyer's anterior instrumentation. Br J Surg 1977;64(5):339–341.
8. Flynn JC, Price CT: Sexual complications of anterior fusion of the lumbar spine. Spine 1984;9:489–492.
9. Gaines RW, Leatherman KD: Benefits of the Harrington compression system in lumbar and thoracolumbar idiopathic scoliosis in adolescents and adults. Spine 1981;6:483.
10. Gruca A: The pathogenesis and treatment of idiopathic scoliosis. A preliminary report. J Bone Joint Surg 1958;40A:570–584.
11. Hammerberg KW, Rodts ME, DeWald RL: Zielke instrumentation. Orthopaedics 1988;11:1365.
12. Harrington PR: Treatment of scoliosis. Correction and internal fixation by spine instrumentation. J Bone Joint Surg 1962;44A:591–610.
13. Hodgson AR, Stock FE: Anterior spinal fusion. Br J Surg 1957;44:266.
14. Hsu LC, Zucherman J, Tang SC, et al.: Dwyer instrumentation

in the treatment of adolescent idiopathic scoliosis. J Bone Joint Surg 1982;64B:536–541.

15. Kaneda K, Fujiya N, Satch S: Results with Zielke instrumentation for idiopathic thoracolumbar and lumbar scoliosis. Clin Orthop 1986;205:195–203.

16. Kaneda K, Satch S, Fujiya N: Analysis of results with Zielke instrumentation for thoracolumbar and lumbar curvatures. Nippon Seikeigeka Gakkai Zasshi 1985;59:841–851.

17. Michel CR, Onimus M, Kohler R: The Dwyer operation in the surgical treatment of scoliosis. Rev Chir Orthop 1977;63:237–255.

18. Moe JH, Purcell GA, Bradford DS: Zielke instrumentation (VDS) for the correction of spinal curvature. Analysis of results in 66 patients. Clin Orthop 1983;180:133–153.

19. Ogiela DM, Chan DP: Ventral derotation spondylodesis: A review of 22 cases. Spine 1986;11:18–22.

20. Paré A: Opera Ambrosii Parei. Paris: Apud Jacobum, Du-Puys, 1582.

21. Puno RM, Johnson JR, Ostermann PA, et al: Analysis of the primary and compensatory curvatures following Zielke instrumentation for idiopathic scoliosis. Orthop Trans 1989;13:507.

22. Schafer MF: Dwyer instrumentation of the spine. Orthop Clin North Am 1978;9:115–122.

23. Schafer MF, Page D, Shen G: Mechanical evaluation of the Dwyer screw-cable attachment. Spine 1979;4:398–400.

24. Silber I, McMaster W: Retroperitoneal fibrosis with hydronephrosis as a complication of the Dwyer procedure. J Pediatr Surg 1977;12:255–257.

25. Stephen JP, Wilding K, Cass CA: The place of Dwyer anterior instrumentation in scoliosis. Med J Aust 1977;12:206–208.

26. Thompson JP, Transfeldt EE, Bradford DS, et al: Decompression after Cotrel-Dubousset instrumentation of idiopathic scoliosis. Spine 1990;15:927–931.

27. Trammell TR, Benedict F, Reed D: Anterior spine fusion using Zielke instrumentation for adult thoracolumbar and lumbar scoliosis. Orthop Trans 1989;13:506.

28. Von Lackum HL, Smith AF: Removal of vertebral bodies in the treatment of scoliosis. Surg Gynecol Obstet 1933;57:250.

29. White AA, Panjabi MM: Clinical biomechanics of the spine. Philadelphia: JB Lippincott, 1978;105.

30. Zielke K: Ventral derotation spondylolisthesis. Results of treatment of cases or idiopathic lumbar scoliosis. Author's translation. Z Orthop 1982;120:320–329.

31. Zielke K, Stunkat R, Beaujean F: Ventrale derotationsspondylodesis. Author's translation. Arch Orthop Unfallchir 1976;85:257–277.

TWENTY-TWO

Anterior Kostuik-Harrington Distraction Systems

John P. Kostuik

INTRODUCTION

History records the first surgical procedure for a spinal cord injury was performed by Paul of Aegina (625–690 AD).

Since that time, the treatment of injuries of the spine with or without neurologic deficit and, in particular, those involving the thoracic and lumbar spine, has moved from bed rest to postural reduction, to laminectomy with or without posterior fusion. The fusion, when done, has sometimes been in conjunction with varying forms of internal fixation used posteriorly such as wires, plates, and springs.

Because of the high failure rate of posterior fixation devices such as wires and plates, the conservative postural reduction approach of Sir Ludwig Guttman, Frankel, and Bedbrook (2,16,18,19) for fractures of the spine column was adopted in many spinal centers throughout the world. However, the results of reduction by this method were not universally obtained (32,38,42).

The report of Harrington (23) in 1962 and that of Dickson-Harrington-Erwin (10) in 1978, led to considerable efforts in an attempt to achieve stabilization of fracture-dislocations of the thoracic and lumbar spine. Improved fixation, using the Harrington distraction rods to provide three-point fixation, results in a more anatomic reduction of the vertebral column, particularly the anterior column. This has obviated the need of laminectomy which frequently increases the neurologic deficit and may result in an increasing kyphosis (32,36,50).

Until recently, in most centers in North America, Harrington instrumentation has become the preferred mode of stabilization for injuries of the thoracic and lumbar spine. This form of fixation has enhanced the speed with which rehabilitation of spinal injury patients may commence.

Although accepted by many as a panacea, Harrington instrumentation has not proven to be so, particularly with regard to burst injuries of the thoracic and lumbar spine. Initial reports on the use of Harrington distraction rods using three-point fixation failed to differentiate between different fracture patterns (5,10,51). It was suggested that applying a distractive force would result in a realignment of bony fragments and disimpact the neural canal. The fragments achieved correction through attachment to the posterior and/or anterior longitudinal ligament.

Numerous reports have subsequently appeared to demonstrate lack of universal correction, especially in burst injuries of the spine (3,6,9,24–28,35,39,41,48,49). The author has also experienced similar cases in which late neurologic deficit improved after secondary anterior cord decompression and fusion. Henceforth, it has become the author's policy to perform anterior surgery together with anterior fixation for some burst injuries of the spine. Royle (43) and Ito in 1934 were the first to describe anterior spinal cord decompression. The technique, however, remained unpopular until Hodgson and Stock (22) in 1956 reported on anterior decompression for tuberculous lesions of the spine that had resulted in paraplegia.

Subsequently, there has been an increasing number of reports of anterior decompression for related problems such as tuberculosis, pyogenic osteomyelitis, rigid kyphotic deformities, and more recently, tumor, both primary and metastatic, and burst fractures. Most of these procedures have included anterior debridement, resection, and fusion without the use of internal fixation.

Wenger (33) in 1953 was first to describe the use of an anterior distractive device, which ultimately failed. Use of anterior spinal devices still remains unpopular largely because of their lack of ready availability and fear of complications.

In 1969, Dwyer (12) illustrated the use of an anterior corrective device in the treatment of certain spinal deformities, namely scoliosis in the thoracolumbar spine. Hall (20) in 1977 reported on the use of modified Dwyer instrumentation and anterior stabilization of the spine.

Dunn (11) reported on the use of an anterior distractive stabilizing device for the treatment of burst injuries. In the author's experience, this device is bulky and leaves little room for an anterior interbody graft.

Anterior distractive devices or fixation devices generally fall into the following categories: external plates, external rods, and interbody distractors. External devices include the Kostuik-Harrington (27,28), Dunn (11), Slot (46), and Zielke (53), the A-O plate, Armstrong (C.A.S.P.) plate, and the I-Beam plate of Yuan (52). Interbody devices include Rezaian (40) device or temporary devices such as the Pinto distractor.

Plates provide fixation only, whereas most distractive devices are corrective as well. Reports on anterior interbody fusion in the lumbar spine indicate varying rates of union from 18–100%. In most series, the nonunion has been 10–20%. Accordingly, many surgeons are reluctant to perform anterior surgery in the lumbar spine. In the author's experience, the incidence of nonunion has been 5% with the use of Kostuik-Harrington (27,28) devices for kyphotic deformities, as in burst injuries, or for long fusions in Scheuermann's kyphosis corrected anteriorly with anterior distraction. The incidence of nonunion using double Zielke instrumentation anteriorly, where posterior surgery was not believed to be reasonable or feasible, was 12% in salvage surgery for degenerative lumbar disc disease (in this author's hands).

Morscher (37), and Malcolm and Bradford (32) have reported on the use of interbody grafts. With regard to posttraumatic kyphosis, Malcolm and Bradford (32) have reported on the use of interbody grafts and found a 50% incidence of nonunion and loss of correction with the use of interbody grafts alone without fixation or without second-stage posterior surgery. Morscher (37) stated that interbody grafts were unable to withstand the loads without fixation. White (48) has stated that iliac crest interbody grafts cannot withstand the loads in the erect position, although they may in the recumbent position. Fibular cortical strut grafts may withstand these loads; however, revascularization is slow—over 6 months. While testing in a cyclical and dynamic fashion in the laboratory, using calf spines, the author has noted that a single anterior fixation rod device used alone does not provide good control over rotation and lateral bending. As a result, when rod systems are to be used, supplementary fixation with a second rod as a neutralization rod is recommended, preferably coupling the two rods. Laboratory testing indicates that these devices, although not as rigid as segmental wiring or posterior Harrington instrumentation, do provide sufficient stability to allow for early rehabilitation and ambulation generally with the use of an external orthosis rather than a body cast. The use of anterior fixation devices precludes the necessity of posterior fusion or instrumentation in the majority of cases, assuming that the posterior elements are intact. The use of anterior devices shortens hospitalization, the necessity of a second procedure, and possible morbidity. However, if the posterior elements are absent, comminuted, or if more than one vertebral body has been resected, a second-stage posterior stabilization and fusion in addition to the anterior fixation are necessary.

Biomechanics of Kyphotic Deformities

Definition

In angulation >40,° the thoracic spine in the sagittal plane is considered to be abnormal. In the cervical and lumbar spine, 5° or more of fixed posterior angulation is defined as a kyphotic deformity.

Anatomic Considerations

The spinal column is essentially divided into two, consisting of the anterior elements and the posterior elements. Anything anterior to the posterior longitudinal ligament is considered an anterior element.

From a viewpoint of burst fractures of the spine and CT scanning, the three-column concept is used. The anterior column consists of the anterior longitudinal ligament and the anterior two-thirds of the body. The middle column consists of the posterior third and cortex of the body, with the centering longitudinally. The posterior column consists of the remaining posterior structures. Muscles that apply loads to the spine can temporarily alter the spatial arrangement of the vertebrae. The resting positions of the spine are dictated by the osseous and ligamentous components. Physiologic thoracic kyphosis is determined primarily by osseous structures, and the lordotic curves of the cervical and lumbar spine are determined more by ligamentous structure.

The posterior elements are under tension, and the anterior elements are under compression. Kyphosis may occur when either of these two components is disrupted. Posteriorly, the laminae and yellow ligaments are major structures resisting tension. Osteoporotic fractures are the most common cause for loss of anterior support.

Nonphysiologic loads, both in magnitude and direction, may also result in a kyphotic deformity (Fig. 22.1). An increase in the moment arm, that is, the amount of angulation present, also plays an important role in the production of kyphosis. The more angulation there is, the greater chance for additional angulation under a given load.

As a result of an increasing angulation, one develops an increase in the moment arm, which results in an in-

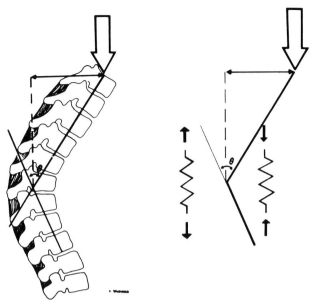

Figure 22.1. Biomechanics of kyphosis—on the left, there is a kyphotic deformity showing a cobb angle of 58°. Vertically directed physiological forces shown by the large arrow work at a moment arm at length. On the right, the deformity is depicted schematically, showing that the posterior elements resist tensile loading. The anterior elements resist compressive loading. Factors contributing to kyphosis include: (*a*) increase in physiologic load (*white arrow*); (*b*) increase in moment arm; (*c*) weakening of posterior elements; (*d*) weakening of anterior elements.

crease in eccentric loading, and may result in increasing wedging and subsequent increase in angulation. These angular deformities play a role in the adult and in the child. Wedging accentuates angulation and effectively increases the moment arm, which in turn increases eccentric loading, causing a vicious cycle.

Biomechanical Considerations Involved with Treatment

The treatment of severe kyphosis involves one or more steps including, if necessary, adequate decompression of the spinal cord and the application of forces to correct deformity. The corrective forces consist of axial traction and sagittal plane bending moments (transverse loading). Correction moment is better axially than transversely if the cobb angle is greater than 53°. These correctional forces reverse the role of the anterior and posterior structures. The biomechanical concepts of creep and relaxation play a role in the treatment of spinal deformities. Creep plays a particular role where axial correction is used in the reclining position. Relaxation of tissues plays a role in axial correction with the patient erect. This is due to the viscolastic properties of bone and ligaments.

Pathomechanics of Fusion (Grafts)

Posterior fusions in a kyphotic deformity are generally under tension. They are usually thin and susceptible to stress fractures and, indeed, may bend.

A posterior fusion is usually considered more stable the greater its length. Despite this, pseudarthrosis rates and failure to maintain correction are as high as 40% in the treatment of Scheuermann's disease in adults (27,28). Conversely, anterior fusions are under compression and are, therefore, ideal.

If one considers a kyphotic deformity as a bent column and the middle of the column the neutral axis, the more one moves away from this netural axis toward the concavity, the more the moment arms are reduced, and the more effective the support. Ideally, bone grafts for fusion kyphosis should be placed as far as feasible from the neutral axis on the compressive side and should include all vertebrae that are in the deformity.

Instrumentation

The Kostuik-Harrington instrumentation provides adequate rigidity and stability, provided it is used in a rectangular or parallelogram fashion (Figs. 22.2 and 22.3).

The assets of the system are its versatility, ease of application, and adaptability. The system allows for ease of correction and deformity and early ambulation. Instrumentation is simple. A standard Harrington distraction instrumentation is all that is required, together with a crimper for the screw heads where heavy compression rods are used in conjunction with distraction. Crimping the collar-ended heads over the heavy compression rod is faster and as effective as using nuts. Equipment consists of a collar-ended screw and a distraction (rachet) screw. The heads of either screw are compatible with the standard round end of the Harrington rods. The screw heads are attached to cancellous threads, which come in three lengths. Ideally, the maximum length is used and the excess cut after measuring the depth with a depth gauge and adding 2-3 mm. This assures penetration of the contralateral cortex of the vertebral body.

Indications

The anterior Kostuik-Harrington system is used for all forms of kyphotic deformities, both acute and chronic for the following indications: (*a*) burst injuries of the spine; (*b*) posttraumatic kyphosis; (*c*) Scheuermann's disease; (*d*) rigid round back; (*e*) postlaminectomy kyphosis and instability; (*f*) iatrogenic lumbar kyphosis (flat back syndrome); (*g*) kyphosis secondary to tumor; and (*h*) kyphosis secondary to osteoporosis with fracture.

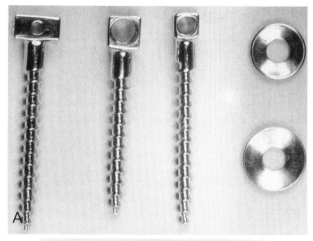

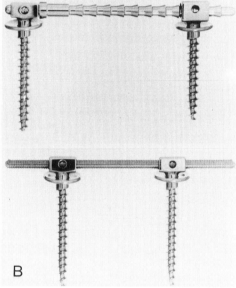

Figure 22.2. *A,* Kostuik screws, distraction screw (rachet end), and collar-ended screw (for compression rods and end of distraction rod). *B,* Kostuik-Harrington system. Round-ended Harrington rod distraction screw (rachet end), coillar-ended screw, washers, and heavy compression Harrington rod on the right.

Clinical Studies

Between January 1981 and April 1988, the author (27,28) used the Kostuik-Harrington system in the following situations: acute burst injuries (100), posttraumatic kyphosis (45), Scheuermann's disease (37), rigid round back (4), acute rigid kyphosis (4), postlaminectomy kyphosis (45), iatrogenic lumbar kyphosis (flat back syndrome) (70), kyphosis secondary to tumor (10), and kyphosis secondary to osteoporosis with fracture (4), for a total of 319 cases. The screws were used posteriorly for pedicle fixation for a variety of reasons (pseudarthrosis,

multiple-level degenerative disease, and tumor) in 50 cases.

COMPLICATIONS RELATED TO INSTRUMENTATION AND FUSION

To date, the instrumentation has been used in 319 cases anteriorly and 50 cases of pedicle fixation posteriorly. There have been mimimal complications.

Screw breakage totaled 35. The majority, 24, were performed with the older, thin-shank untapered screw. Twenty-three of these occurred with burst fractures and four in Scheuermann's kyphosis, three in posttraumatic kyphosis, and four in pedicles. There was no loss of correction despite the fractured screws, except for four cases.

Two distraction rods fractured at the junction of the rachet-rod area, a well-recognized point of stress concentration. There were no abnormal sequelae with these rod fractures. In addition, two heavy compression rods fractured.

Vertebral body fracture occurred in eight cases. All occurred intraoperatively in osteoporotic bone. Three occurred in the same person. All cases were salvaged by the insertion of methylmethacrylate bone cement and the application of screws within the fractured body. The use of bone cement in osteoporotic vertebral bodies is recommended and appears to provide excellent holding power. The body is drilled with a standard drill and measured for depth. The drill hole is then enlarged with the aid of a curette, and packed with cement. The screw is then inserted over a washer and can be turned after the cement hardens.

There have been no vascular injuries or neurologic injuries.

SURGICAL APPROACHES

For anterior decompression, the author prefers to use the left side since the aorta tends to protect the left common venous iliac system. Damage to arterial vascular structures is more difficult and frequently results in greater blood loss. The only indication for an anterior approach in trauma is for burst injuries, late posttraumatic kyphosis, or concomitant vascular injury.

For injuries to L5 and occasionally to L4, posterior decompression can be done by removing the posterior elements, preferably "en bloc" and by pushing the bony fragments anteriorly and removing any displaced disc fragments or by employing distraction and lordosis by means of an internal fixator. Generally, in fractures proximal to L5, an anterior approach is preferred by the author. A left flank approach is satisfactory for lesions of L3-L5. The iliolumbar and segmental vessels must be

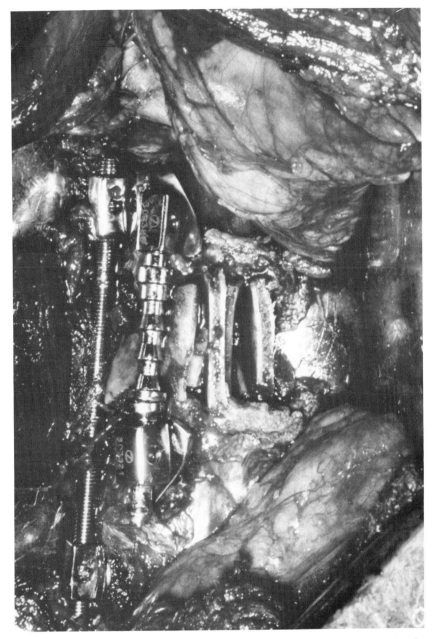

Figure 22.3. Intraoperative photograph of the Kostuik-Harrington system in place.

ligated, and the psoas should be resected off at the lateral aspect of the vertebral bodies. For L2 and L3, the 12th rib is used in a retroperitoneal approach. For exposure of T11-L1, a thoracoabdominal approach should be used.

For approaches more proximal in the thoracic spine, generally, an incision is made two ribs above the desired vertebral level, e.g., a fracture of T9 is approached through the bed of the 7th rib. If the ribs are horizontal, one can go one rib proximal to the affected vertebral body.

Technical Points

Some important surgical guidelines with regard to Kostuik-Harrington follow.

1. Use an awl to start the screw holes.
2. Ideally, place the screws for distraction at midbody (slightly anterior in fractures and slightly posterior in other kyphoses).
3. Pierce the far cortex.

4. Use staples where possible (screw length should be measured with a depth gauge, and add 2–4 mm).
5. Ideally, placement of the distraction screw(s) should allow ease of rod insertion.
6. During distraction, apply manual pressure posteriorly to help correct the kyphotic deformity and lessen forces on the screws.
7. In Scheuermann's disease, place both rods first and distract both concurrently.
8. In burst fractures, distract to a predetermined length (normal body plus two disc heights as measured from the lateral x-ray of patient). Place the bone graft, preferably iliac crest bicortical or tricortical grafts, slightly longer than the gap. Rib graft can be added. Add a second heavy Harrington compression rod, and crimp the screw heads lightly. Nuts may be used instead of crimping the screw heads.
9. Cut any excess rod length.

Ligation of the segmental vessels two levels proximal and distal to the affected site at any level allows for satisfactory mobilization of the major vascular structures and prevents their abutment against any foreign materials. Care must be taken to avoid the abutment of any screw heads or prominent metal components against the aorta or the common iliac artery.

SPECIFIC INDICATIONS FOR KOSTUIK-HARRINGTON INSTRUMENTATION

Acute Fractures

Current indications for anterior fixation of spinal fractures with or without decompression of the neural elements are:

1. Acute burst injuries with neurologic injury, involving the anterior and middle column with retropulsion of bone fragments into the canal.
2. Late burst injuries that are 7 days or more postinjury with or without neurologic injury.
3. Burst injuries without neurologic injury that show greater than 50% retropulsion of material into the spinal canal by CT scan. The level of injury is also considered when assessing the degree of canal compromise.

The region of the cauda equina will tolerate much greater bone intrusion into the canal than the more proximal cord level. As much as 85% canal occlusion has been noted in the area of the cauda equina without neurologic sequelae, while as little as 20% have resulted in severe paraparesis in the area of the cord.

There are no available data on the long term sequelae, especially spinal stenosis, of significant canal bone intrusion, although Bohlman (3) and Malcolm (32) have reported on the late development of spinal stenosis following such injuries.

Burst injuries with no neurologic injury and less than 7 days old are stabilized posteriorly using the AO internal fixator. A postoperative CT scan is done in all cases where posterior instrumentation is used and where there is significant (greater than 20%) canal occlusion by bone fragments.

Technique

A lateral decubitus left-sided approach is preferred. The incision is usually two levels above the fracture (i.e., 10th rib for fracture at T12). The anterior one-fourth of the body is left, and the dura is fully decompressed (Fig. 22.4A and B). The Kostuik screws are inserted, and distraction is then done (Fig. 22.4C). C-clamps are applied to the rachet end of the distraction rod after distraction is completed. The bone graft is then inserted. A rib strut is added if available. A heavy compression rod is inserted into the collar-ended Kostuik screws, which are angled forward from the near posterior part of the body to the contraanterolateral cortex of the body (Fig. 22.4D). Slight compression is applied, and the screw heads are lightly crimped. Recently, crosslinkage has been added to create a more stable quaralateral frame. A case using this procedure is illustrated in Figure 22.5.

Postoperative immobilization has usually been with a plastic molded orthosis or a body cast in noncompliant patients. Ambulation was dependent on the degree of neurologic damage. Early transfers and walking were permitted.

Posterior distractive devices that include built-in lordosis, i.e., AO internal fixator, may decrease the need for anterior surgery for acute burst injuries. A randomized prospective study by Esses, Kostuik and Botsford (13) comparing the use of the AO internal fixator with Kostuik-Harrington instrumentation showed no statistical differences for correction of kyphotic angulation, instrumentation, failure fusion rate, or neurologic recovery. The Kostuik-Harrington was significantly better at achieving canal clearance by virtue of the anterior decompression.

RESULTS

By April, 1988, a total of 100 cases were dealt with by the anterior technique just described (26). There were four nonunions, including three cases early in the series where, in retrospect, second-stage posterior fusion and instrumentation should have been added because of severe posterior column comminutions.

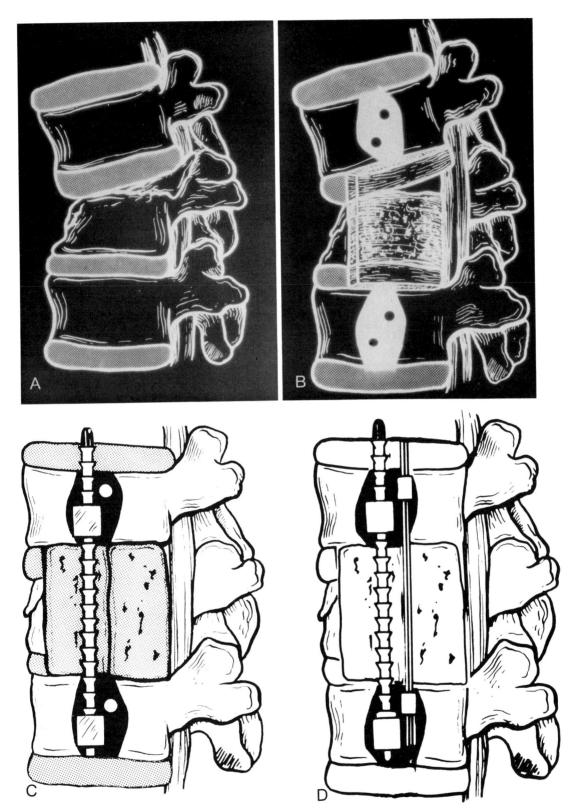

Figure 22.4. *A,* Burst fracture. *B,* Dura decompressed anterior ¼ of body is left as graft. *C,* Anterior lateral rod is inserted to reduce kyphosis bone graft (iliac crest) is added. *D,* Second heavy Harrington compression rod is added to increase stability. Slight compression is applied. Collar-ended screw heads are crimped.

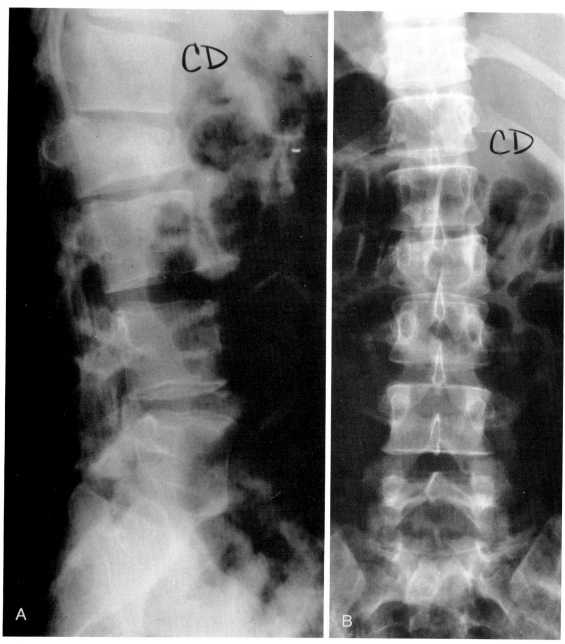

Figure 22.5. A 20-year-old male fell 12 meters, sustaining a L2 burst injury. His neurologic status improved from Frankel B to Frankel D at 2 years follow-up. *A,* Lateral views of a burst fracture; neurological assessment Frankel Grade B. *B,* Preoperative anterior posterior view. Note widening of pedicles of L2. *C,* CT scan demonstrates significant canal occlusion. *D,* Postoperative lateral demonstrates fusion at 2 years with good correction of deformity after anterior decompression, grafting, and stabilization. *E,* Postoperative anteroposterior radiograph.

There were 23 screw fractures, with the majority occurring in the earlier model of untapered screws. One rod fractured. The average neurologic improvement was 1.6 Frankel grades in the partial paraplegics with a range of 2.0–1.0. Greater improvement was seen when the case was done earlier after injury. There were no early or late neurologic or vascular problems.

If there is severe posterior element comminution or severe posterior instability, delayed second-stage posterior instrumentation and fusion are recommended.

Neurologically, complete paraplegia occurred at T11, T12, L1, and L2. No root recovery occurred despite early decompression (less than 24 hours). Four patients with Frankel grade B were treated within 6 hours of injury.

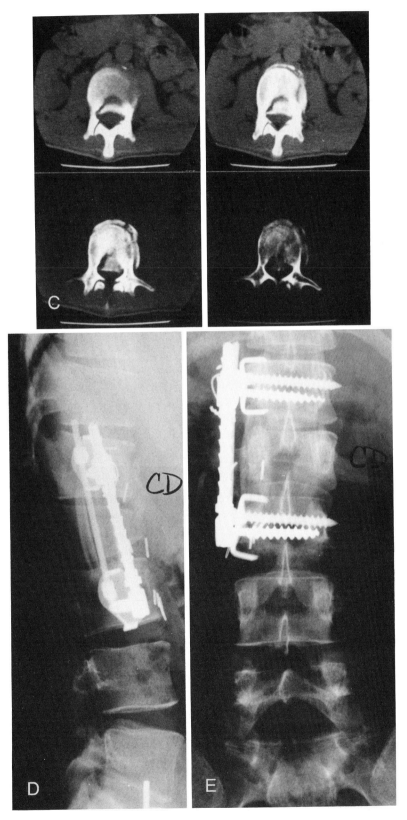

Figure 22.5. *C–E.*

The level of injury was T12, L1, L2, and L3. All improved to Frankel grade D with return of bowel and bladder function.

No correlation as to degree of canal intrusion was possible, except that compromise was greater than 50%. Thirty-one patients had decompression between 6–48 hours, and an average improvement of Frankel 1.6 grades was noted. This is the overall neurologic recovery in all 53 partial paraplegic patients.

When decompression was done between 48–72 hours in 22 patients, the average recovery was 1.0 grades in partial paraplegics. The trend suggests that the earlier the decompression, the greater the neurologic recovery. However, the numbers are far too small to be significant, and there are other variables such as age, level of injury, and degree of injury.

Thirty-six of the 57 cases with neurologic involvement presented with loss of bowel and bladder function. Four of these were complete paraplegics and remained so. Of the remaining 32 cases, 10 required continued intermittent catheterization. These were all lesions in the area of the conus medullaris (L1). The rest had satisfactory to normal bladder control.

As far as pain relief was concerned, four patients complained postoperatively of severe incisional flank pain and dysthesia (postthoracotomy syndrome). Two were relieved by extradural rhizotomies, one by phenol intercostal blocks, and one refused further treatment.

Six patients complained of significant late low back pain in the lumbosacral area. In four, this was disabling and prevented work. All six underwent discography. Two were found to have reproducible symptoms at the L4-L5 discs and four at the L5-S1 discs on discography. All discs showed early radiographic changes of degeneration.

All patients were 22 years of age or less without prior history of low back pain. Two patients have undergone L5-S1 fusions; one with complete relief of pain. The other patient continues to complain of pain; however, third-party litigation is still pending.

The etiology of the pain and disc degeneration is felt to originate with the spinal injury. Burst injuries are essentially axially loading injuries with a secondary anterior flexion moment component. Distal soft tissue (disc) injuries are felt to be possible, similar to multiple-level bone injuries that may occur with such a mechanism of injury.

COMPLICATIONS

Osteomyelitis occurred in one patient, necessitating removal of the anterior fixation devices once union occurred. A partial sequestrectomy of the grafted area was necessary. The fixation devices were not loose at the time of removal. Wound healing occurred by secondary intention.

Superficial wound or donor site infections occurred in six cases, and were treated by local wound care. Pulmonary embolism occurred in one case. This was prior to the current use of routine anticoagulation. Atelectasis occurred in seven cases; two required ventilation for 48 hours. Routine urinary antisepsis did not prevent urinary tract infection in most paraplegics, requiring more specific antibiotic treatment.

No major pressure sores developed during the acute care period, which lasted from 10–30 days (average 24 days), until admission to a convalescent or paraplegic rehabilitation center. There were no early or late neurologic or vascular injuries.

Of the 13 cases where screw breakage occurred, two developed a nonunion, as described earlier. Two cases were also associated with rod breakage. No broken screws have been removed.

POSTTRAUMATIC KYPHOSIS

The indications for surgery included pain and deformity, which were present in all 45 patients. Neurologic lesions occurred in 22 patients, including 10 with residual paraparesis from the original injury and 12 who developed slow and progressive signs and symptoms of spinal stenosis.

Preoperative assessment included CT scanning, metrizamide myelography, discography, done above and below the fracture (four levels) and facet blocks (if no previous posterior fusion). Discograms and facet blocks are done to be sure all painful levels are incorporated in the subsequent surgery.

The technique for acute burst fracture is used. If CT scanning shows little or no canal intrusion, the dura does not need to be decompressed. Previous posterior fusions do not need an osteotomy (Fig. 22.6).

RESULTS

Screw breakage occurred in three of 45 patients. Pain relief was good to excellent in 37 of the 45 cases. Neurologic improvement can be seen 20 years after the initial fracture.

Of the 10 paraparetics, four improved more than one grade on the Frankel scale after decompression. All 12 spinal stenosis cases improved after anterior decompression.

SCHEUERMANN'S KYPHOSIS (27,28)

Studies of the surgical treatment of Scheuermann's kyphosis by posterior instrumentation indicate a progressive

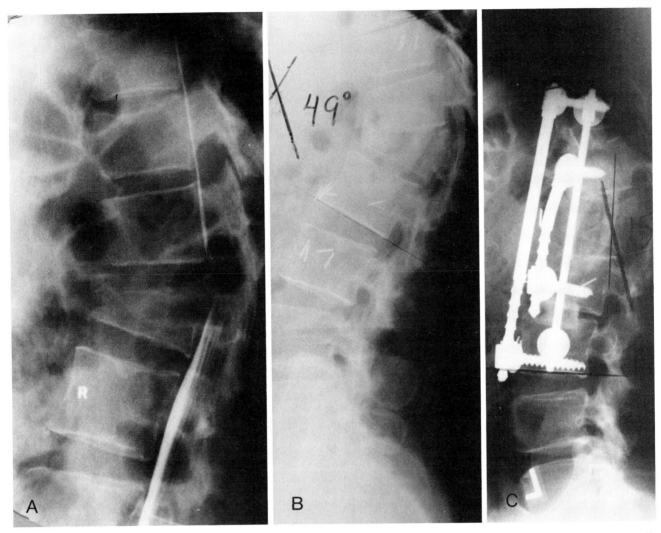

Figure 22.6. *A*, A 34-year-old female with acute burst fracture with neurologic deficit. *B*, Postoperative at 2 years shows loss of correction with graft collapse and a recurrence of her neurologic deficit. *C*, Reduction of kyphosis by Kostuik-Harrington system.

loss at long-term follow-ups. Loss of correction is due to fusion on the tensile side of the spine, high pseudarthrosis rates (up to 40%), and late stress fractures secondary to repetitive cyclic loading on the tensile side of the spine.

Anterior interbody fusion alone does not provide an adequate correction of the deformity. Anterior instrumentation and interbody fusion were thus developed. The goal is to stabilize and correct the kyphotic deformity by a mechanically sound procedure with minimal postoperative immobilization and minimal complications. Biomechanically, this system provides axial distraction and reduces bending moments, placing the fusion mass under compression far from the neutral axis.

Surgical Technique

For thoracic deformities, a thoracotomy via the 5th or 6th rib is performed. The scapula is mobilized. If there is an associated right thoracic scoliosis, a left-sided approach is preferred. The segmental vessels are clipped, and the spine is exposed from T2-T12 (or where appropriate). All discs and endplates back to the posterior annulus are removed. Ratchet and collar-ended screws are inserted. The screws must pierce both cortices of the body and are placed as far posteriorly as possible. The rods are inserted and may be contoured. Distraction of both rods is carried out concurrent with application of manual pressure posteriorly. C-clamps are used to secure the rods.

Bicortical iliac crest grafts are inserted under compression (Fig. 22.7). The grafts should be slightly larger than the interspace. Supplementary rib is also used. In osteoporotic bodies, cement may be used to hold the screws in place.

Surgical Indications

Surgical indications in the skeletally mature are pain (apical or low back), deformity (75° or greater), spinal cord compression (rare), and progression of kyphosis. In the skeletally immature, surgical indications include failure of bracing techniques and deformity (65° or greater) which is rigid.

Early Results

The preliminary early results (27,28) of anterior interbody fusion and modified Kostuik-Harrington anterior instrumentation from 1982–1987 included 36 patients with an average age of 27.5 years (range 21–62). The preoperative curve was 75.5°. Postoperatively, the curve was reduced to 56° with instrumentation. After follow-up, the average curve was 60° (Fig. 22.8). Six patients had progression of their curves within their fusions. One patient underwent subsequent surgery, and one patient had a pseudarthrosis. The complications were minimal, with four screw fractures.

Postoperatively patients were immobilized in a plastic orthosis for 6 months. The average hospital stay was 12 days.

Acute Angular Kyphosis

Moe, Winter, and Bradford (34) have clearly outlined indications and treatment protocol for the treatment of acute angular kyphosis of either a congenital, developmental, or infectious nature. General principles in the treatment of acute angular kyphosis consist of decompression of the neural canal, traction for correction of de-

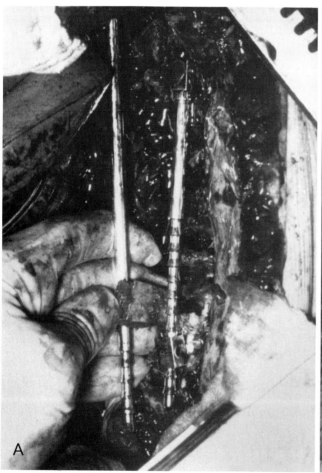
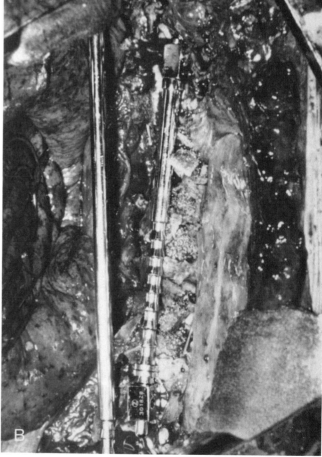

Figure 22.7.   *A*, Scheuermann's kyphosis. The spine has been exposed from T2-L2. The Kostuik-Harrington rods have been inserted to correct the deformity. A bicortical graft is inserted at each disc space together with small bone chips. *B*, Grafting completed.

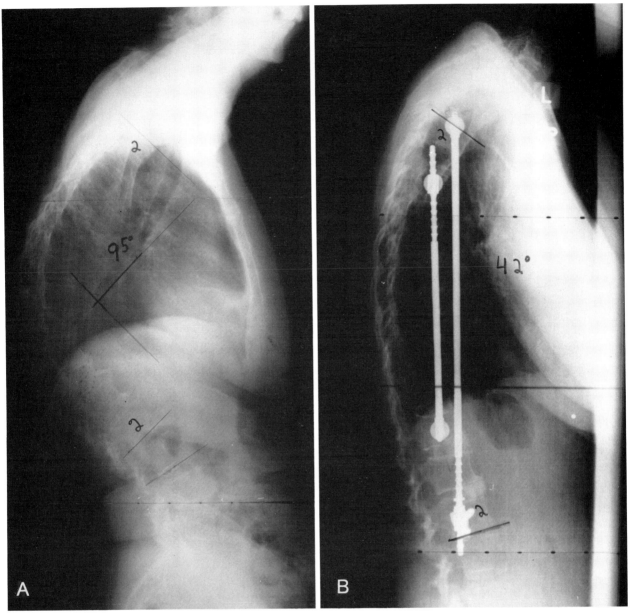

Figure 22.8. *A*, A 49-year-old female with deformity of 95° from T2-L2, with associated pain. *B*, Postoperative lateral radiograph demonstrates the deformity reduced to 42°. Pain was relieved.

formity, if indicated, strut grafting anteriorly, and supplementary posterior fusion with instrumentation.

The use of anterior instrumentation has decreased the need for posterior instrumentation and fusion in the treatment of this problem (Fig. 22.9). The principles of decompression and strut grafting, plus or minus traction where indicated, remain the same.

We prefer to use iliac crest strut grafts rather than fibular grafts. The iliac crest grafts were supplemented with rib grafts.

Fibular grafts take up to 2 years to revascularize and are quite weak, particularly at their ends at 6 months following implantation. Iliac crest grafts revascularize quickly. Bicortical grafts are generally used in all treatment of all forms of kyphosis, but tricortical grafts may be used in the presence of osteoporosis.

IATROGENIC LOSS OF LUMBAR LORDOSIS

Posterior instrumentation (Harrington) to L5 and S1 may result in excessive loss of lordosis. Pseudarthrosis rates for fusion to the sacrum in adults with Harrington rods are as high as 50% and may lead to loss of lordosis.

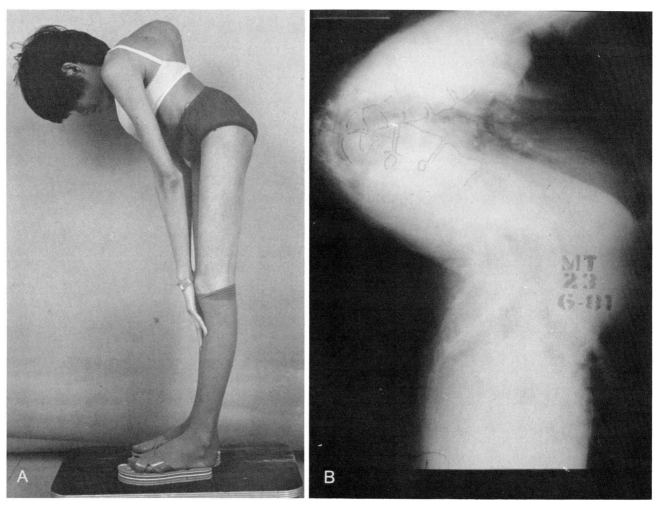

Figure 22.9. *A*, Severe angular kyphosis with spastic paraparesis in a 23-year-old female due to congenital deformity. *B*, The deformity is about 160°. *C*, Intraoperative photograph. This procedure was preceded by a posterior release and multiple posterior osteotomies. Note decompression posterior to the rib struts. The aorta lies anterior to the rod. *D* and *E*, Postoperative lateral and AP views. Curve has been reduced to 105°.

Pseudarthrosis rates (29,30) in adolescents with fusions to L5 or S1 are 12% with Harrington rods and may lead to loss of lordosis. Loss of lordosis (flat back) occurred in 50% of posterior fusions to the sacrum in adults and was significant in half of these (29,30). Children with flat backs develop problems in adulthood, as they no longer can compensate for the loss of lordosis after age 35. Frequently, the development of degenerative changes below a previous fusion ending at L3-L4, or L5, as shown by Cochran and Nachemson (8), may lead to loss of anterior disc height, loss of lordosis, and a flat back.

The prevention of iatrogenic lumbar kyphosis or flat back syndrome can be achieved with attention to strict detail if fusion to the sacrum is necessary. The use of prebent Harrington rods together with sacroiliac hooks or midline hooks is not considered ideal, since distraction is still necessary.

Segmental wiring with Luque (29) contoured rods into lordosis has helped and has decreased the pseudarthrosis rates to 20% over Harrington instrumentation, where fusion to the sacrum is necessary. However, the incidence of pseudarthrosis is still, we think, somewhat high.

In mobile curves with preservation of lordosis, anterior Zielke (53) instrumentation followed by a second-stage posterior pedicle fixation from L3 to the sacrum will assure correction, fusion, and preservation of lordosis. In rigid curves, especially kyphoscoliotics, the procedures of choice are multiple-level anterior discotomies filling the disc spaces with morselized bone graft followed by a second-stage posterior Cotrel-Dubousset instrumentation and fusion in order to derotate the spine and restore lordosis. Those are performed 7–10 days after the first stage (29).

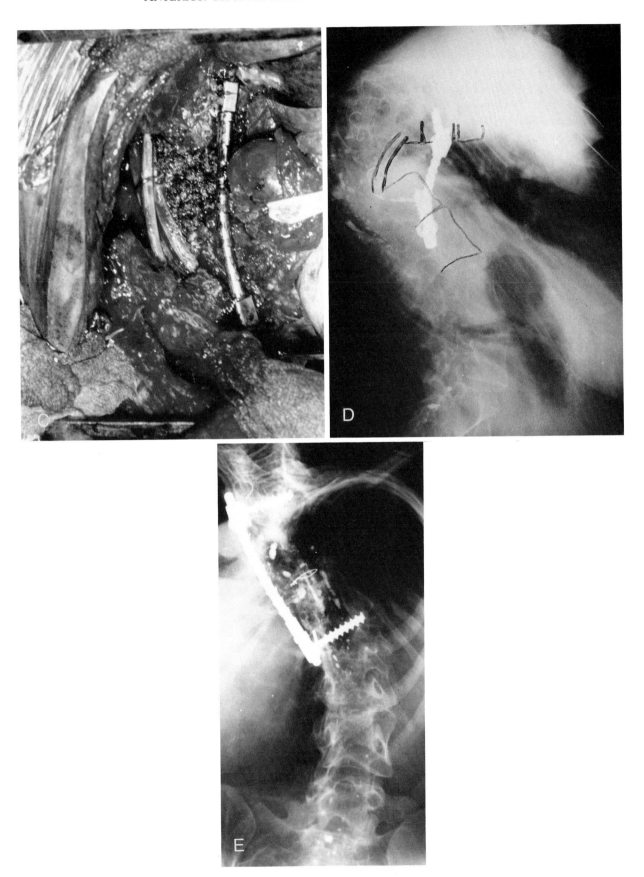

Figure 22.9. *C–E.*

Materials

This study is a restrospective review of 56 scoliotic patients (4 females, 52 males). The average age was 40, with a range of 15–60. Of the 56 patients, 45 were idiopathic. The number of previous operative procedures was 27. Previous posterior instrumentation extended to L4 (4), L5 (5), and S1 (47).

Surgical Technique

A combined single-stage posterior and anterior approach is used incorporating two incisions, flank and posterior. Incisions are joined if a quadrilateral wedge removal is required. An anterior osteotomy in the presence of a previous fusion is done. Alternatively, the disc and endplates at the selected level are removed (usually L3-L4 or

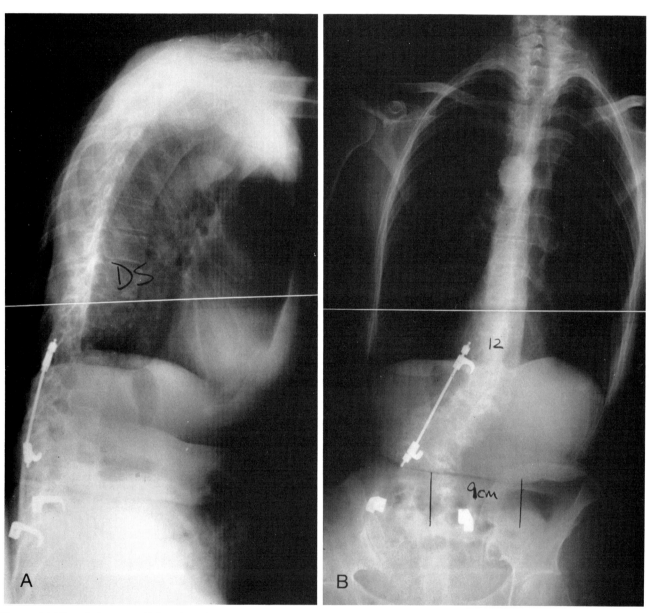

Figure 22.10. A 41-year-old female with iatrogenic flat back. *A,* Precorrection painful lumbar kyphosis (8° of lordosis) due to lumbar distraction—distraction rod has been removed. *B,* Note imbalance of AP plane of 9 cm. *C,* Osteotomy closed posteriorly with Dwyer cables simultaneously as anterior wedge opens with anterior distraction device. AO plate added to control rotation. *D* and *E,* Postosteotomy. *Note:* Restoration of lordosis with complete relief of pain. Lordosis measures 37°. Balance has been restored in AP plane.

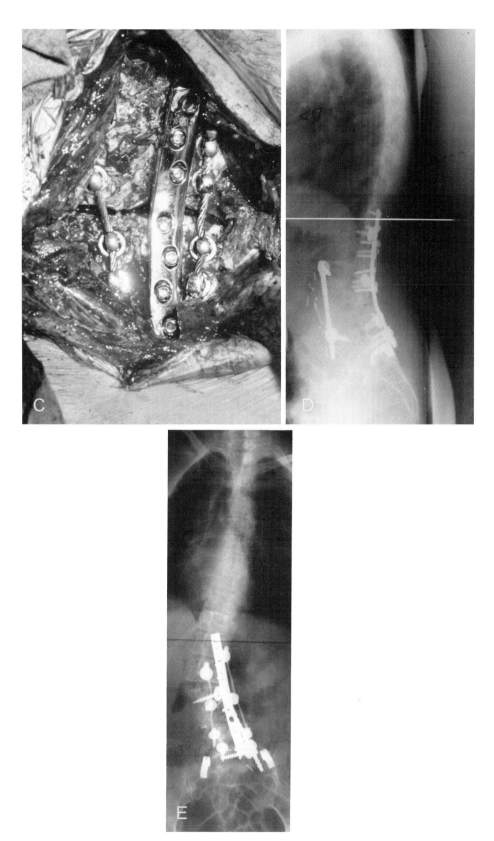

Figure 22.10. *C–E.*

at the same level as a preexisting pseudarthrosis). The anterior instrumentation is inserted (Fig. 22.10). The posterior osteotomy is done (1–1.5 cm of bone is removed). Posterior instrumentation is used consisting of Dwyer screws and cables placed in the fusion mass lateral to the dura. The anterior osteotomy is opened with the anterior Kostuik-Harrington system simultaneously as the posterior osteotomy is closed with the Dwyer instrumentation. A bone graft (iliac crest) is applied anteriorly in the open wedge. A contoured neutralization plate is applied centrally and posteriorly for rotational control, together with a posterior bone graft.

Results

The average preoperative lordosis was 21.5°, and at minimum of 2 years follow-up following osteotomy, the average lordosis was 49°, ranging from 5–78°, which was similar to the lordosis prior to initial posterior Harrington instrumentation.

Bone union occurred in all cases. Pain relief was obtained in 48 of 56 patients. Three patients lost partial correction due to partial anterior graft collapse.

Major complications included one death and three intraoperative major left common iliac vein tears. All three had had previous anterior surgery. There were two neurologic complications, one with persistent loss of bowel and bladder function.

Discussion

This chapter describes the uses for anterior fixation in the treatment of acute and chronic kyphosis of the thoracic and lumbar spine.

The anterior Harrington system, as described by the author (27,28), has been in clinical use for 12 years for a variety of reasons including the correction of acute kyphosis in burst injuries, late posttraumatic kyphosis, Scheuermann's kyphosis, acute angular kyphosis, and anterior fixation for posterior pseudarthrosis in 319 cases (27,28) up to April, 1988.

There have been 26 screw fractures: 13 in acute fractures; three in late posttraumatic kyphosis; three used anteriorly for correction of Scheuermann's kyphosis; one for a congenital kyphosis; and three used posteriorly for pedicle fixation in degenerative disease; and one in a case of previous posterior decompression for tumor over three levels.

There have been four broken rods, two in acute burst injuries. A total of 1,400 screws and 700 rods have been used to date.

In the treatment of acute burst injuries or late posttraumatic kyphosis, the devices serve to readily correct the kyphosis and provide stability, allowing for early rehabilitation and ambulation. The ease of application allows for its variable use in many areas of the spine. The uppermost level of vertebral body insertion has been T2 and the lowest level, L5. Although the screws are available in three lengths, they can be readily shortened by cutting the tips. The use of washers or staples prevent toggling of the screw within the cancellous vertebral body. In cases of severe osteopenia, methylmethacrylate bone cement can be used to enhance screw fixation.

Using these anterior fixation devices precludes the necessity of any posterior fusion or instrumentation, except where significant posterior element comminution or laminectomy is present. Use of this system shortens hospitalization, and allows for early rehabilitation and ambulation with the use of an external orthosis rather than a body cast.

References

1. Batchelor JS: Anterior interbody spinal fusion. Guy's Hosp Rep 1963;112:61.
2. Bedbrook GM: Spinal injuries with tetraplegia and paraplegia. J Bone Joint Surg 1979;61b:267.
3. Bohlman HH, Freehafer A, Dejak J: The results of treatment of acute injuries of the upper thoracic spine with paralysis. J Bone Joint Surg 1985;67A:360.
4. Bohlman HH, Eismont FS: Surgical techniques of anterior decompression and fusion for spinal cord injuries. Clin Orthop 1981;154:57.
5. Bradford DS, Akbarnia BA, Winter RD, et al: Surgical stabilization of fracture and fracture dislocation of the thoracic spine. Spine 1977;2:185.
6. Breig A: The therapeutic possibilities of surgical bioengineering in incomplete spinal cord lesions. Paraplegia 1972;9:173.
7. Chou D, Armstrong G, O'Neal J, et al: The contoured anterior spinal plate. (C.A.S.P.) Presented Scoliosis Research Society, Amsterdam, Holland, September 1989.
8. Cochran T, Irstam L, Nachemson A: Longterm anatomic and functional changes in patients and adolescent idiopathic scoliosis treated by Harrington rod fusion. Spine 1983;8:576–584.
9. Dewald RL, Fister JS, Savino AM: The management of unstable burst fractures of the thoracolumbar spine. Presentation Scoliosis Research Society, Denver, Colorado. September 1982.
10. Dickson JH, Harrington PR, Erwin WD: Results of reduction and stabilization of the severely fractured thoracic and lumbar spine. J Bone Joint Surg 1978;60A:799.
11. Dunn H: Personal communication.
12. Dwyer AF: Experience of anterior correction of scoliosis. Clin Orthop 1973;93:191.
13. Esses SI, Kostuik JP, Botsford D: A prospective randomized comparison of the use of the AO internal fixator and Kostuik-Harrington instrumentation for the treatment of burst fractures. Presented NASS, Quebec City, July 1989.
14. Flynn JC, Hoque MA: Anterior fusion of the lumbar spine. J Bone Joint Surg 1979;61A:1143.
15. Freeebody B, Bendal R, Taylor RD: Anterior transperitoneal lumbar fusion. J Bone Joint Surg 1971;53B:617.
16. Frankel HL, Hancock DO, Hyslop G, et al: The value of postural reduction in the initial management of closed injuries of the spine with paraplegia and tetraplegia. Part 1, Paraplegia 1969;7:179.

17. Goldner JL, McCollum DE, Urbaniak JR: Anterior disc excision and interbody spine fusion for chronic low back pain. In: Orthop Clin North Am 1971;2:543–568.

18. Guttmann L: Initial treatment of traumatic paraplegia. Proceedings of the Royal Society of Medicine 1954;47:1103.

19. Guttmann L: Spinal deformities in traumatic paraplegics and tetraplegics following surgical procedure. Paraplegia 1969;7:38.

20. Hall JE, Micheli LJ: The use of modified dwyer instrumentation in anterior stabilization of the spine. Presentation at Scoliosis Research Society, Hong Kong, October 1977, Montreal, September 1981.

21. Harmon PH: Anterior extra peritoneal disc excision and vertebral body fusion. Clin Orthop 1960;18:169.

22. Hodgson AR, Stock FE: Anterior spinal fusion. A preliminary communication on radical treatment of Pott's Disease and Pott's Paraplegia. Br J Surg 1956;44:266–275.

23. Harrington PR: Treatment of scoliosis. J Bone Joint Surg 1962;44A:591.

24. Kaneda K, Abume K, Fujiya M: Burst fractures of the thoracolumbar and lumbar spine with neurological involvement. Anterior decompression and fusion with instrumentation. Presentation, Scoliosis Research Society, Denver, Colorado, September 1982.

25. Kostuik JP: Anterior spinal cord decompression for lesions of the thoracic and lumbar spine. Techniques, new methods of internal fixation, results. Spine 1983;8:512–531.

26. Kostuik JP: Anterior fixation for burst fractures of the thoracic and lumbar spine with or without neurological involvement. Spine 1988;13:286–293.

27. Kostuik JP: Anterior Kostuik-Harrington distraction systems for the treatment of kyphotic deformities. The Iowa Orthopedic Journal 1988;8:68–77.

28. Kostuik JP: Anterior Kostuik-Harrington distraction systems for the treatment of kyphotic deformities. Spine 1990;15:169–180.

29. Kostuik JP: Treatment of scoliosis in the adult thoracolumbar spine with special reference to fusion to the sacrum. The Orthopaedics clinics of North America 1988;2:371–381.

30. Kostuik JP, Richardson W, Maurais G, et al: Combined single stage anterior and posterior osteotomy for correction of iatrogenic lumbar kyphosis. Spine 1988;13:257–266.

31. Kostuik JP, Matsuzaki H: Anterior stabilization, instrumentation, and decompression for post-traumatic kyphosis. Spine 1989;14:379–386.

32. Malcolm BW, Bradford DS, Winter RB, et al: Post-traumatic kyphosis. J Bone Joint Surg 1981;63A:891.

33. Milgram J: Hospital for joint diseases. New York, NY. Personal communication.

34. Moe JH, Winter RB, Bradford DS, et al: Scoliosis and other spinal deformities. Philadelphia, W.B. Saunders, 1978.

35. Moon MS: Anterior interbody fusion in fractures and fracture disclocations of the spine. Int Orthop 1981;5:143.

36. Morgan TH, Wharton GW, Austin GN: The results of laminectomy in patients with incomplete spinal cord injuries. Paraplegia 1971;9:14.

37. Morscher E: Personal communication.

38. Nicholl EA: Fractures of the dorso-lumbar spine. J Bone Joint Surg 1949;31B:376.

39. Paul RL, Michael RH, Dunn JE, et al: Anterior transthoracic surgical decompression of acute spinal cord injuries. J Neurosurgery 1975;43:299.

40. Rezaian SM, Dombrowski ET, Ghista DN: Spinal fixator for the management of spinal injury (the mechanical rationale). Engin. Med. 1983;12:95.

41. Riska EB: Antero-lateral decompression as a treatment of paraplegia following a vertebral fracture in the thoracolumbar spine. Int Orthop 1977;1:22.

42. Roberts JB, Curtis PH Jr: Stability of the thoracic and lumbar spine in traumatic paraplegia following fracture or fracture dislocation. J Bone Joint Surg 1970;52A:1115.

43. Royle ND: The operative removal of an accessory vertebra. Austral Med J 1928;1:467.

44. Sacks S: Anterior interbody fusion of the lumbar spine. J Bone Joint Surg 1965;47B:211.

45. Sacks S: Anterior interbody fusion of the lumbar spine. Indications and results in two hundred cases. Clin Orthop 1966;44:163.

46. Slot GH: A new distraction system for the correction of kyphosis using the anterior approach. Presentation, Scoliosis Research Society, Montreal, Quebec, September 1981.

47. Stauffer RN, Coventry MB: Anterior interbody lumbar spine fusion. Analysis of Mayo Clinic series. J Bone Joint Surg 1972;54A:756.

48. White AA III, Punjabi M, Thomas CL: The clinical biomechanics of kyphotic deformities. Clin Orthop 1977;128:8–17.

49. Whitesides TE, Shah SGA: The management of unstable fractures of the thoracolumbar spine. Spine 1976;1:99.

50. Whitesides TE: Traumatic kyphosis of the thoracolumbar spine. Clin Orthop 1977;128:78.

51. Yosipovitch Z, Robin GC, Makin M: Open reduction of unstable thoracolumbar spinal injuries and fixation with Harrington rods. J Bone Joint Surg 1977;59A:1003.

52. Yuan H: Personal communication.

53. Zielke K: Ventral derotation spondylodese: behandlungsergebnisse bein idiopathischen lumbarskoliosen. Orthop 1982;120:320–329.

TWENTY-THREE

The Contoured Anterior Spinal Plate

Gordon W. D. Armstrong and Donald Chow

INTRODUCTION

The need for a specialized spinal plate was perceived somewhat fortuitously when in 1980, a 38-year-old patient was sent to us for treatment, with a particularly difficult problem of instability of the spine secondary to an L1-L2 fracture that had occurred 12 years previously. He had developed a ball and socket type of joint at this level (Fig. 23.1) that had been aggravated by previous extensive laminectomy so that his level of anaesthesia was at T7. He was totally paraplegic and was unable to sit for more than a few minutes because of a collapsing kyphosis.

A two-stage procedure was undertaken. The first entailed posterior Harrington compression rods of large diameter with fusion from T6-L4. The second stage was an anterior bone grafting using fibular and cancellous bone at the L1-L2 level, which was supplemented with an AO femoral plate applied to the lateral side of the spine to give additional stability (Fig. 23.2). This produced a satisfactory fusion, and the patient has been able to carry on an active and productive life with no complications after a 10-year period.

It was apparent to us in carrying out this anterior plating that the AO femoral plate was less than ideal for vertebral body fixation, as the screw holes allowed only one or two screws to be placed in each vertebra. It was also felt to be too narrow for the spine, particularly in the lumbar area. This stimulated us to develop a specialized plate for the spine. We ultimately succeeded, with the help of the Biomedical Engineering group at the National Research Council of Canada under the direction of Dr. Robin Black.

The plate, which is attached to the lateral aspect of the spine and spans from two to five vertebrae, is noteworthy for its ease of application and its inherent strength. It is presently used from T10–L5 levels.

A search of the literature disclosed that a previous clamp had been devised by Humphries (10) in Cleveland in 1961. This had been placed anteriorly on the spine directly under the vessels, and was therefore regarded as being potentially hazardous. The Dunn device (8) was noted to be somewhat bulky, and vascular complications subsequently led to its withdrawal from use.

Ryan (12), in Australia, devised a bolted plate with a single attachment to each vertebral body. Our concern was that the single bolt in the vertebral body provided less resistance to rotation than could be obtained with multiple points of fixation.

In considering the surgical requirements of a specialized plate, we desired to have an implant with a low cross-sectional profile that approximated the curve of the vertebral body. We particularly wanted a device that was simple in design and easy to apply using cancellous screws. Another requirement was to have an option for more than two fixation points to each vertebral body.

The mechanical requirements included:

1. Strong mechanical fixation with a control of motion in 6 degrees of freedom for each motion unit.
2. Restoration of axial loading in continuity in the three columns of the spine (2).
3. Its ability to maintain stress levels below the materials endurance limit.
4. The ability of the construct strength to exceed that of the associated anatomic structures.

INITIAL PLATE DESIGN

The first plate used clinically (Fig. 23.3) had built-in compression capabilities similar to the dynamic compression plate. We discontinued this because it was felt that compression could be obtained by other means in the presence of cancellous bone. This implant was applied at the L4-L5 level to repair a pseudarthrosis in a 250-lb female patient, with a very satisfactory result. We noted at operation, however, that the lower end of the rectangular plate was in contact with the overlying iliac vessels

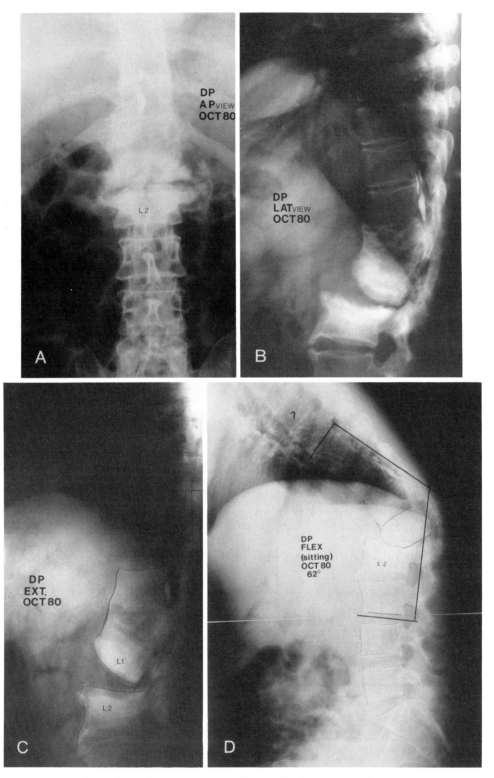

Figure 23.1.   Preoperative views of unstable spine due to old L1-L2 injury. *A,* AP. *B,* Lateral. *C,* Extension. *D,* Sitting.

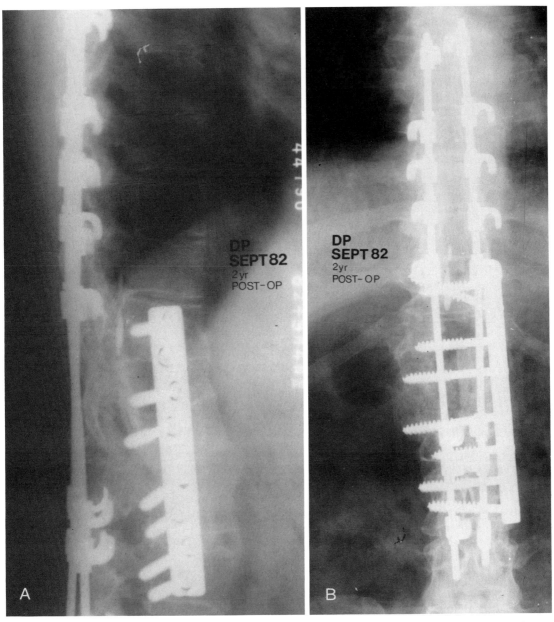

Figure 23.2. *A* and *B*, Postoperative views showing use of AO femoral plate and Harrington compression rods.

that crossed it. As a result, we designed a plate with a tapered end specifically to be used at the L5 level to avoid this problem (Fig. 23.4).

We also found that the original plate was too wide (3 cm), and it was subsequently narrowed to 2.5 cm. The present plate spans 2–5 vertebral bodies, and varies in length from 6–16 cm (Fig. 23.5). It is 0.5 cm in thickness, and except for the plate designed for the L5 level, is rectangular in shape and contoured to fit the vertebral body (Fig. 23.6). The surface is smooth, and the corners are rounded.

Fixation to the spine is by fully threaded 6.5-mm cancellous screws, which are obtained in 2.5-mm increments in length, as exact measurements should be carried out to avoid prominence of the screw tips.

Experience with the Dwyer instrumentation convinced us that it was necessary for the screw to grip the opposite cortex of the vertebral body for extra holding power. We adhered to this principle for the contoured plate. The design of the plate provides five screw holes overlying each vertebral body for a maximum choice of placement (Fig. 23.7). We suggest that a minimum of three can-

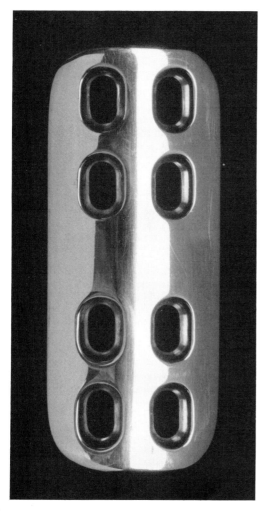

Figure 23.3. First design of a contoured anterior plate.

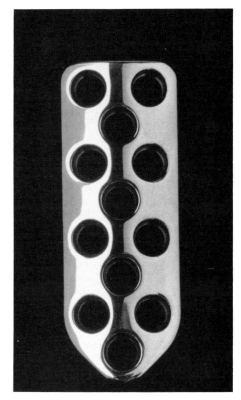

Figure 23.4. Tapered plate for use at L5 level.

cellous screws in a triangular pattern be used for each vertebra.

For better screw fixation, 1–2 cc of liquid cement (polymethylmethacrylate) is injected into each screw hole in patients where the bone is osteoporotic, especially in tumor patients. Also, if the screw head is underlying a blood vessel, it is wise to use the same technique. Testing of the plate using eccentric loading to determine the contribution of multiple screws showed that two screws provided a strength of 2.5 Nm, three screws, 3.7 Nm and five screws, 18.9 Nm (3). Our conclusion was that the more screws that could be inserted into the vertebral body, the greater the strength of the construct as the screws share in the load-bearing force. We have not seen fragmentation of the vertebrae occur following insertion of the maximum number of screws.

DRILL GUIDE

A special drill guide (Fig. 23.8) has been designed that has a contoured portion which is slipped around to the opposite side of the vertebral body. The sliding sleeve, which fits exactly into the screw hole in the plate, is pushed into the hole using a "syringe grip" (Fig. 23.9). The wing nut is then tightened to secure the guide in place prior to drilling. A special depth gauge passed through the drill guide measures exact screw length.

The necessity of a drill guide has been questioned by some surgeons experienced in anterior spinal instrumentation. However, we advise that it should be used, mainly as a safety precaution, because multiple screws increase the risk of penetration of the spinal canal. The guide should also minimize the risk of vascular injury by the drill. It avoids angulation of the screw, e.g., disc penetration, and it should also prevent penetration of the surgeon's glove by the drill point.

INDICATIONS

The indications for the device include:

1. Reconstruction after tumor resection of vertebral bodies;
2. Stabilization following anterior decompression of vertebral fractures;
3. Pseudarthrosis repair;
4. Fusion for severe degenerative disc disease; and
5. Inadequate posterior instrumentation.

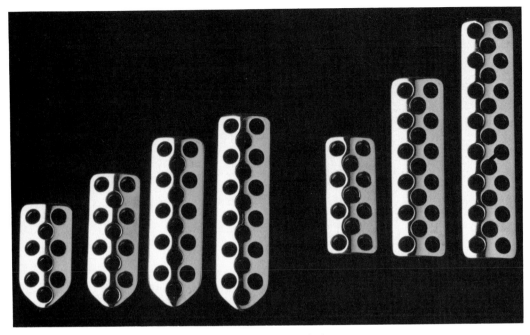

Figure 23.5. Series of plates.

Tumors of the Vertebral Body

Up to 70% of metastases from breast tumors to the spine lodge in the vertebral bodies (11), and anterior compression frequently causes neurological damage. This is best treated by anterior decompression and replacement either by an allograft, fibular autograft, or a cement construct.

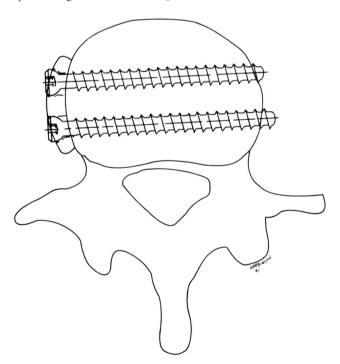

Figure 23.6. Cross-section of vertebral body to show contour of plate and fully threaded cancellous screws.

These implants are then stabilized by a plate that attaches to the adjacent vertebral bodies, and should also attach to the grafts or cement, giving a solid construct.

With the creation of a longer plate that extends from L1-L5, it is possible to resect two or three vertebral bodies. Preoperative MRI scanning is important to delineate the extent of the vertebral involvement.

Fractures

In a recent review of 1,019 fractures of the thoracic and lumbar spine by Gertzbein, presented to the Scoliosis Research Society (9), 62% were bursting injuries. These are a common cause of neurological deficit and many require anterior decompression and stabilization. We have used mainly fibular grafts supplemented by the bone removed from the vertebral body and disc spaces. In our experience, the addition of the contoured plate prevents tilting of the graft, and allows early mobilization of the patient.

Using Denis' (7) classification of bursting injuries, large fragments involving the whole of the posterior aspect of the vertebral body are seen in double endplate fractures (type A) and burst rotation injury (type D). Dural tearing has been seen anteriorly due to the sharp edge of the fragment in burst rotation injuries. In types B and C, in addition to the central fragment in the canal, the remaining portion of the vertebral body is split into halves, producing an unstable bed for a graft. In our center, we have decompressed the whole of the vertebral body in all the different types of bursting injuries requiring anterior procedures.

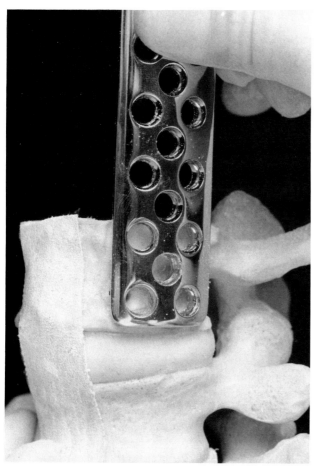

Figure 23.7. Plate provides option of five screws for each vertebral body.

One major advantage of the contoured anterior spinal plate in spinal injuries is in the management of combined type of injuries seen in burst fractures with posterior disruption. Prior to the availability of the plate, we used two separate approaches to manage this fracture. The first was anterior, to decompress the vertebral fragments from the dura and insert a bone graft. The second was a posterior incision in the midline, to expose the spine and insert Harrington compression rods over multiple levels

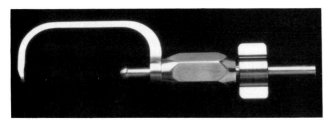

Figure 23.8. Drill guide showing contour, drill sleeve, and wing nut.

to repair the posterior instability. We now can significantly diminish the operating time by using only the anterior approach with decompression, grafting, and plate fixation.

Pseudarthrosis Repair

Failed posterior grafting, particularly at L4-L5 level is another indication for anterior fusion and plating.

Severe Degenerative Disc Disease

Multiple failed posterior procedures, e.g., laminectomies, leading to instability may respond to anterior fusion and plating through an area not previously disturbed surgically.

Combined Anterior and Posterior Approach

We have used the contoured anterior spinal plate to supplement posterior fixation in pseudarthrosis in scoliosis at the thoracolumbar junction.

SURGICAL TECHNIQUES

Standard anterior approaches are used. In general, we prefer to use a right-sided approach for the thoracic spine, unless the lesion is predominantly left-sided. This exposure of the vertebral bodies is made easier, since the position of the aorta is predominantly to the left side, and the venous system is quite small. In the lumbar area, the left side is preferred, as the aorta is less easily damaged than the vena cava, which is more friable.

To approach the lower lumbar spine (L4-L5, and upper sacrum), it is advisable to locate and double-ligate the ascending lumbar vein. This procedure is described in detail by Crock (6), and it allows retraction of the iliac vessels.

As in the Dwyer procedure, it is not possible to spare the sympathetic chain. The patient must be warned preoperatively about the difference in temperature and color in the lower extremities following surgery.

Following ligation of the segmental vessels in the midlateral portion of the vertebral bodies, the periosteum is incised vertically in patients, except for those undergoing tumor resection, and is elevated forward to the opposite side of the vertebral bodies and discs, normally over three levels. Since the segmental vessels lie exterior to the periosteum, they are protected from injury by it.

In burst fractures such as type B, the damaged disc is incised and explored. The central portion is impacted into the vertebral body. The posterior one-half of the vertebral body is removed piecemeal, and the rotated fragment can

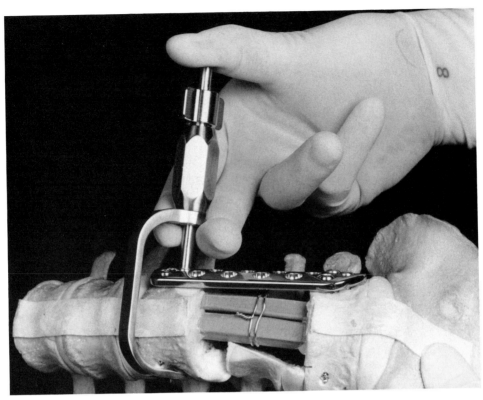

Figure 23.9. Use of drill using "syringe grip."

be seen tilted into the canal. The superior endplate may be turned 90°. The edge of this fragment is sought and is carefully rotated out of the canal with a small bone hook or curved curette. Often, a very large fragment can be extracted in one piece.

The canal is explored following removal of the posterior half of the vertebral body to make certain no residual fragments of bone are present, and that there is no pressure on the dura. The two intervertebral discs are then completely excised, and the endplates cleaned by curettage. Bone grafts, either fibular graft or bone bank strut, can be used. These are cut exactly to fit the defect between the two endplates. The distance between the two endplates can be opened up by bending the operating table to extend the spine; or, a special distraction-compression tool can be used. The grafts are then driven into place, and the table is flattened out, compressing the graft. The grafts should be checked to make certain they are vertically situated in the AP and lateral planes.

Cancellous bone removed from the vertebral body is then packed into the disc spaces and around the graft, with the dura being protected. The appropriate plate to bridge three vertebrae is then positioned on the lateral side of the spine, making certain that it is sufficiently far

from the vertebral foraminae. Two temporary 20-mm cortical screws are inserted at either end of the plate as positioning screws. The position of the plate is then checked, and, if necessary, radiographs are taken. The special drill guide and depth gauge are then used, and a minimum of three 6.5-mm fully threaded cancellous screws are placed in the two end vertebrae.

TECHNIQUE FOR CORPECTOMY FOR TUMOR

Following ligation of segmental vessels over a minimum of three vertebral levels, the great vessels are retracted. The periosteum in this instance is not elevated. The involved vertebrae are identified, and the discs adjacent to them are divided at the endplate of the normal vertebra above and below so that both discs are removed with the diseased vertebral body. The psoas muscle, having been retracted to allow visualization of the pedicle and the intervertebral foraminae above and below, allows adequate delineation of the pedicular edges. The pedicle is then cut vertically with a Kerrison rongeur to gain visual access to the underlying dura and anterior wall of the spinal canal. A thin retractor is then used to gently retract the dura, and when the plane has been established, a wide

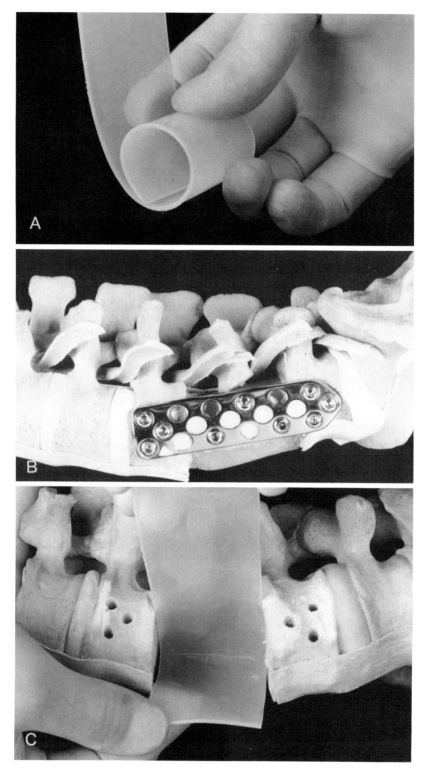

Figure 23.10. *A,* Polyethylene strip for use in molding cement constructs. *B,* Width of strip is cut to fit vertebrectomy site. *C,* Model of spine with methylmethacrylate construct and plate.

osteotome can be driven through the vertebral body at least two-thirds of the way across. A second wide osteotome is driven at right angle to meet it. In this way, a large segment of vertebral body can be removed in one piece. The remainder of the vertebral body is removed and the exciting nerve roots are visualized on the opposite side. The segmental vessel must be ligated on this side as well.

The endplates of the normal vertebrae above and below are curetted to remove all the cartilage, and several holes about 5-mm deep are made with a curette or drill to allow better fixation of the polymethylmethacrylate.

A sheet of thin polyethylene is then cut to fit exactly into the space between the two endplates in width, and should be about 20 cms in length (Fig. 23.10). It is then laid over the dura. The methylmethacrylate, having been shaped into a tube, is then inserted between the endplates and further shaped by the polyethylene material, whose ends are overlapped to form a tubular cover. As the cement is beginning to cure, the tube is gently compressed to force some of the cement into the endplates under pressure. When the cement is cured, the polyethylene is slipped out, leaving an adequate space in front of the dura, which must be inspected to make sure that there is no abnormal pressure on it. The contoured plate is then positioned with two short screws, and drill holes are made.

In our experience, the maximum number of screws should be inserted in tumor problems, and in addition, the screws are cemented in place (Fig. 23.11). At least two screws are then inserted through the plate into the cement construct for a distance of 2.5 cm. Cortical screws can be used for this purpose. This provides strong fixation and additional support to the whole construct.

In other problems such as pseudarthrosis repair, it is necessary to remove the bony prominence with a rongeur or osteotome at the level of the endplates in the adjacent vertebrae. Otherwise, the plate may rock over this prominence. Bone grafting of the disc space bridged by the plate is done prior to plate attachment.

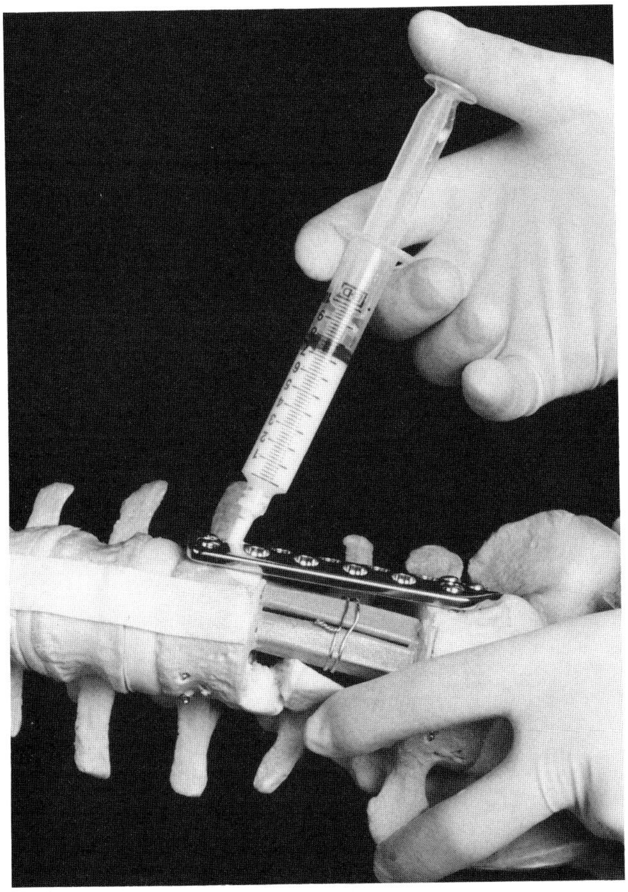

Figure 23.11. Low-viscosity cement is injected into screw holes, and the screw is reinserted.

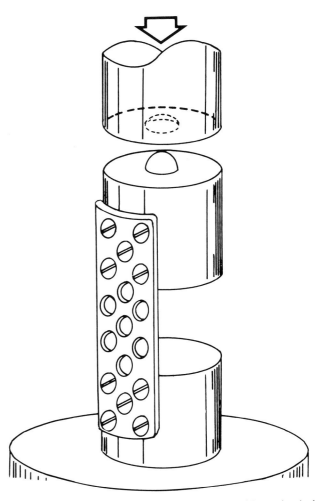

Figure 23.12. Eccentric loading model used in biomechanical testing.

Table 23.1.
Mechanical Characteristics of Spinal Plate[a]

3-point bending	
Rigidity	33 Nm/m^2
Strength[b]	23 Nm
Mean flexural rigidity	19 Nm^2
Eccentric loading of the unsupported plate[c]	
Bending yield strength	20 Nm (at 80 kg axial load)
Ultimate bending strength	30 Nm (at 123 kg axial load)

[a]From Black RC, Eng P, Gardner VO, et al. A contoured anterior spinal fixation plate. Clin Orthop 1988;227:135–142.
[b]Strength as defined by The American Society for Testing and Materials (ASTM) F382, 13:01, Philadelphia, ASTM, 1983.
[c]Simulates in vivo loading through a 24.5-mm offset of axial load.

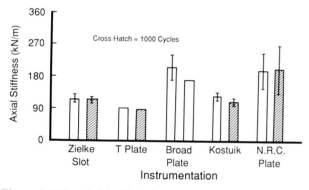

Figure 23.13. Axial stiffness comparison. NB: The contoured anterior spinal plate was initially designated the N.R.C. Plate (Reprinted with permission from Bone LB, Johnston CE II, Ashman RB, et al: Mechanical comparison of anterior spinal instrumentation in a burst fracture model. J Orthop Trauma 1988;2:195–201.)

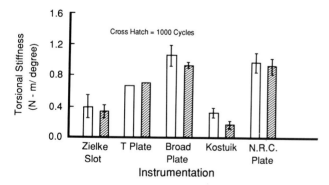

Figure 23.14. Torsional stiffness. NB: The contoured anterior spinal plate was initially designated the N.R.C. Plate (Reprinted with permission from Bone LB, Johnston CE II, Ashman RB, et al: Mechanical comparison of anterior spinal instrumentation in a burst fracture model. J Orthop Trauma 1988;2:195–201.)

BIOMECHANICAL CONSIDERATIONS

In the early development of the contoured anterior spinal plate system at the National Research Council of Canada, the mechanical characteristics of the spinal plate were determined using guidelines defined by the American Society for Testing and Materials (ASTM). The measurements included bending stiffness, bending yield point, torsional stiffness, torsional yield, axial stiffness under eccentric loading, and yield strength under eccentric loading. The eccentric loading conditions (Fig. 23.12) represented the worst case scenario, in which the plate bridged the vertebral space without any reconstruction strut to share axial loading forces. The results of this mechanical testing were initially published by Black et al. (3), and are outlined in Table 23.1.

Mechanical comparison of various types of anterior instrumentation in a burst fracture model were carried out by Bone et al. (4). Their testing of the Contoured Anterior Spinal Plate was compared with the Zielke slot rods, the Harrington-Kostuik constructs, the ASIF T plate, and the ASIF broad dynamic compression bone plate. The burst fracture model was created by performing a corpectomy of the L1 vertebrae with fresh human cadaveric spines, leaving the posterior elements intact. Each spine was then instrumented from T12-L2 with the various fixation systems. Initial axial and torsional testing was carried out and then repeated after applying 1000 cycles of a combined axial and torsional load. Their results (Figs. 23.13 and 23.14) revealed that axial stiffness and torsional stiffness of the contoured anterior spinal plate (CASP) were similar to the ASIF broad plate in that they were superior to the three other anterior instrumentation systems. The CASP system also had the least tensile stress,

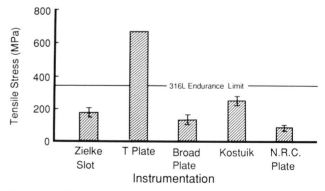

Figure 23.15. Tensile stress in relation to endurance limit of 316 L stainless steel. NB: The contoured anterior spinal plate was initially designated the N.R.C. Plate (Reprinted with permission from Bone LB, Johnston CE II, Ashman RB, et al: Mechanical comparison of anterior spinal instrumentation in a burst fracture model. J Orthop Trauma 1988;2:195–201.)

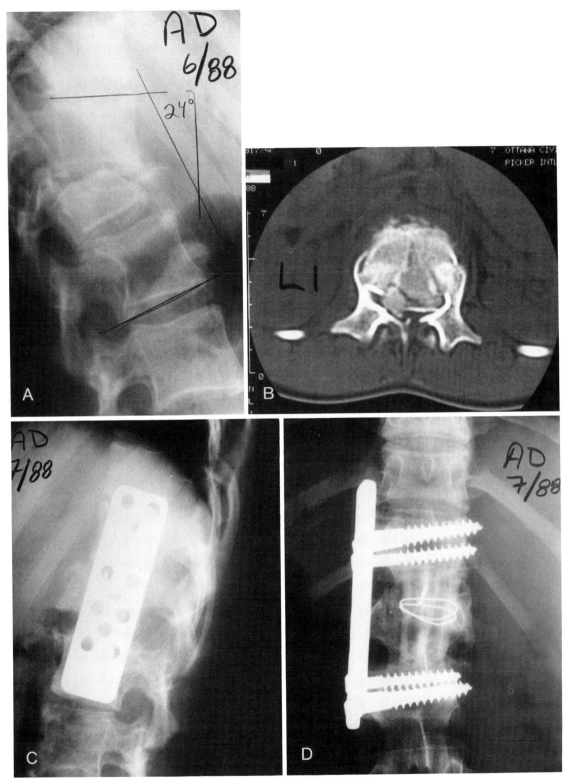

Figure 23.16. Burst fracture patient with partial paraplegia. *A,* Lateral view showing kyphotic deformity. *B,* CT scan with severe canal compromise. *C,* Lateral view following decompression. *D,* AP view showing fibular strut in place.

which was well below the endurance level for 316 L stainless steel (Fig. 23.15). Endurance limit is that stress below which fatigue failure is not predicted (13). It was noted that the thinner T plate exhibited a very high stress, and it was felt by the investigators that a thicker cross-sectional version of that plate might be required for surgical application.

Further tests at the National Research Council of Canada were carried out in which a polymethylmethacrylate strut was inserted in the area of the vertebrectomy. These tests revealed that loads of up to 2000 kg could be sustained through the construct without failure. The Council agreed that this would represent a load well beyond any expected physiological loading. These constructs are similar to those that are used in the spinal reconstruction of tumor patients.

CLINICAL TRIALS

Unfortunately, there is no readily available animal model that can test in-vivo cyclic loading generated by the upright human spine. The analysis of clinical trials is therefore of utmost importance. In 1990, a review of the first 25 patients instrumented with the contoured anterior spinal plate with a minimum 2-year follow-up was carried out (5). There were 15 male and 10 female patients. The age range was from 17–82, with an average age of 48.7 at the time of surgery. The indications included: acute burst fractures in six patients; remote burst fractures in four patients; six patients with severe degenerative disc disease; five patients with pseudarthrosis following failed posterior fusion; and four patients with spinal tumor, requiring anterior decompression. In the four tumor patients, a polymethylmethacrylate strut was used for the spinal reconstruction after vertebrectomy. In all the remaining 21 patients, the plate was used for spinal stabilization following a fusion procedure. Tricortical iliac crest bone was used for single-level disc fusions. Fibular strut grafting was used in the remaining fusion patients in which a partial vertebrectomy was carried out for an anterior decompression.

Except for the four tumor patients, the goal of the stabilization utilizing the plate was a fusion. If the fusion was not evident by plain radiographs, AP tomograms were taken. At the 2-year follow-up, all but two of the 21 patients undergoing a fusion procedure had achieved a solid fusion (Fig. 23.16). One of the remote fracture patients was noted to have some continued right midback pain. This was one of the first patients using the system, and only two screws per vertebra were used. As well, the screws did not completely traverse the vertebral body to obtain purchase on the contralateral cortex. Although no

definite pseudarthrosis could be seen at the junction of the fibular struts and adjacent vertebral bodies on the tomograms, there was definite breakage of the upper two screws (Fig. 23.17). The area was reexplored, and a solid fusion was found beneath the plate. The plate and the accessible screw portions were removed with a substantial but unexplained decrease in his pain.

The only pseudarthrosis in the first 21 procedures for fusion stabilization was in a 50-year-old woman referred to our spinal unit with an L4-L5 pseudarthrosis, and a history of seven previous posterior spinal procedures. Initially, she did very well for over a year. However, she noted the return of her pain, and on radiographic examination, development of an anterior pseudarthrosis along with breakage of two of her six screws were noted. At this time, she underwent a revision of her anterior pseudarthrosis with removal of the hardware and fibular

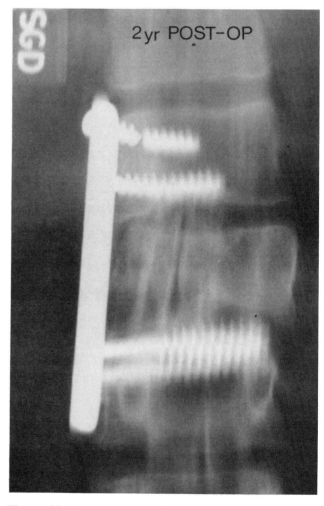

Figure 23.17. Tomogram of the first patient in our series showing breakage of upper two screws.

strut grafting, as it appeared that the previous tricortical iliac crest graft had collapsed. Investigations for infection were negative. She appears to have finally fused at this level at the time of her 1-year follow-up for this revision (Fig. 23.18).

Our initial results with the use of the plate system in tumors were disappointing, as two of the four patients had instrumentation failure secondary to recurrence of their metastatic disease in adjacent vertebrae. One patient had adenocarcinoma of the lung, while the other patient had renal cell carcinoma. Both patients required further surgery to stabilize their spine posteriorly. At our spine unit, we have since carried out plate instrumentation in 10 other patients with spinal tumors, requiring anterior decompression and stabilization. Although the follow-up

ranges between 5–26 months, we are fortunate that all 10 patients have maintained good stabilization.

COMPLICATIONS

The possible untoward side effects can be categorized into those associated with the anterior spinal approach used for the decompression-fusion procedure, and those specifically related to the plate instrumentation system. Complications associated with anterior spinal surgery are well outlined by Bauman and Garfin (1) as well as Watkins (14–15). The unavoidable consequences of the anterior approach such as peri-incisional anesthesia as well as interference of the ipsilateral sympathetic chain, should always be explained to the patient preoperatively.

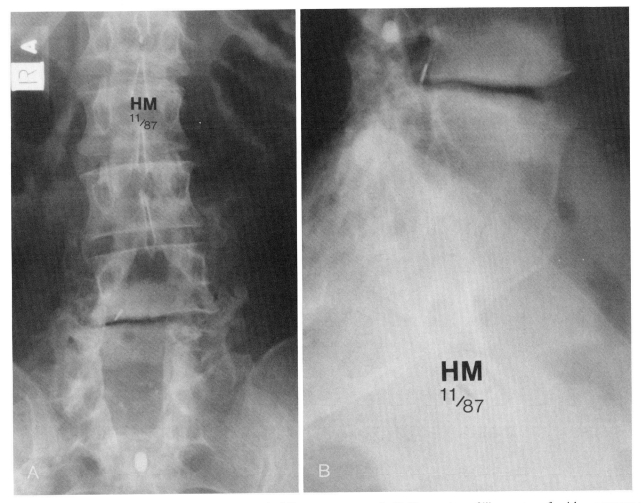

Figure 23.18. Patient with recurrent pseudarthrosis following multiple past operations. *A*, AP view. *B*, Lateral view. *C*, Initial contoured anterior spinal instrumentation after iliac crest strut graft. *D*, Resorption of iliac crest graft with recurrence of pseudarthrosis. *E*, Fusion using fibular strut graft.

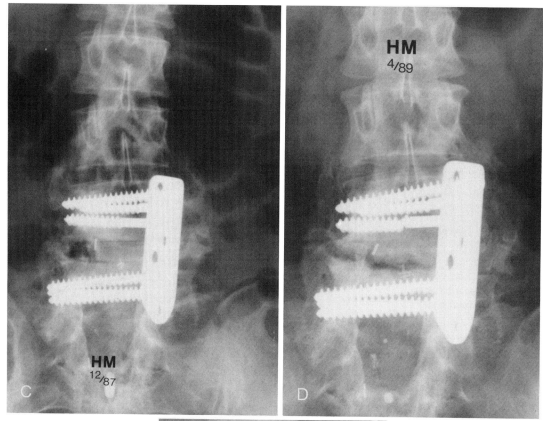

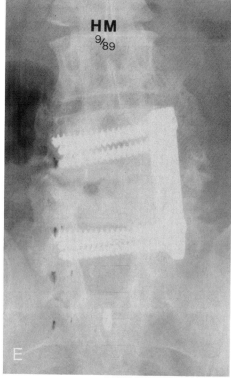

Figure 23.18. *C–E.*

The complication of instrumentation failure and loss of stabilization can occur in tumor patients due to further progression of their disease, as well as in patients who develop a pseudarthrosis. If symptomatic, this may require further surgery for restabilization. To date, 60 patients have been instrumented at our center with this plate system, and only three have required further surgery due to loss of stabilization (two tumor patients and one pseudarthrosis patient). All three patients were within our first 25 consecutive patient series. Also, to date we have not yet had a deep wound infection, although there have been two superficial wound infections that have responded to antibiotics. Screw breakage has been seen in four patients. So far, three have gone on to fusion, including the one patient who was reexplored. The other case was the pseudarthrosis patient who required further bone grafting anteriorly.

Screw backout has been noted in eight patients; however, backout greater than 5 mm has been seen only in two patients, one of whom was a metastatic renal cell carcinoma patient whose stabilization had completely failed. The other was an anterior interbody fusion patient who was extremely agitated during the first 2 postoperative weeks, but who went on to have an uneventful fusion with no further progression of screw backout over the next year (Fig. 23.19).

DISCUSSION

The fusion and stabilization results of the contoured anterior spinal plate system appear promising in fracture and degenerative disc disease patients. From reviewing the first 25 consecutive patients, the major problems appeared to be in the tumor patients. In the past 2 years, patient selection may have been modified somewhat with the recent availability of MRI scanning to our unit. The use of the MRI scan may show small deposits of metastatic tumor in adjacent vertebral bodies, which may necessitate extension of the stabilization. As well, the use of postoperative radiotherapy treatments may be required. After reviewing the first fracture patient who developed broken screws despite an adequate fusion, we have used three screws per vertebral body instead of two, which we recommend highly. In addition, with the use of the special drill guide now available, screw purchase of the contralateral vertebral cortex may decrease the incidence of screw breakage. The problem of screw backout and screw purchase in osteoporotic bone, especially in older tumor patients, has been addressed with augmentation of screw fixation with polymethylmethacrylate in the screw holes. Using fully threaded cancellous screws may also decrease screw backout, as there is no longer

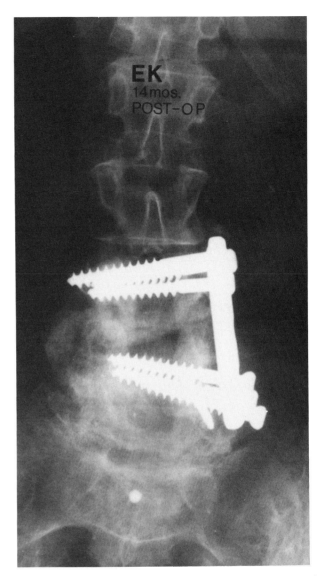

Figure 23.19. Backout of screws unchanged since second postoperative week.

any signficant smooth shank between the head and the 6.5-mm diameter threads.

Research is now underway to develop a screw that may improve the resistance to stress fracturing. This will be done by changing the pitch of the thread as well as by increasing the inner core diameter of the screw thread slightly. Preliminary data in our screw pullout tests have shown that the pullout strength does not change significantly, provided the outer diameter of the screw thread does not change.

The original contoured anterior spinal plate system was designed for the T10-L5 vertebral levels. Since then, a new series of anterior spinal plates has been designed for the thoracic spine up to the T3 level. This series of plates

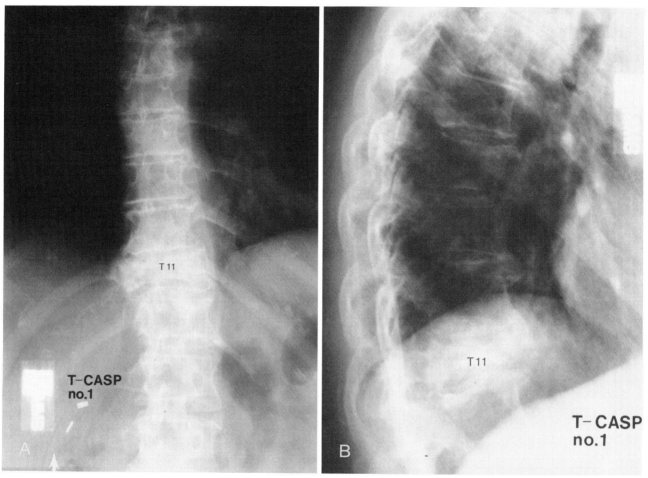

Figure 23.20. Woman with metastatic carcinoma. *A,* AP view. *B,* Lateral view. *C,* MRI scan showing tumor at T11 and L1. *D,* AP view showing instrumentation T8-L2. *E,* Lateral postoperative view.

involves contouring to fit the lateral aspect of the vertebral body. At the same time, a second contour in the sagittal plane has been created to fit the thoracic kyphosis. Our initial biomechanical testing reveals that this plate will far exceed the demands of physiological loading. Prototype plates have been used in five patients so far with good results (Fig. 23.20).

In summary, the contoured anterior spinal plate system is a promising new technique to complement anterior spinal surgery of fractures, tumors, and certain problems of severe degenerative disc disease including pseudarthrosis. The benefits include the relative ease of instrumentation and relative safety due to its low profile and lateral positioning. Accordingly, the authors find it preferable to previously available anterior spinal stabilization techniques.

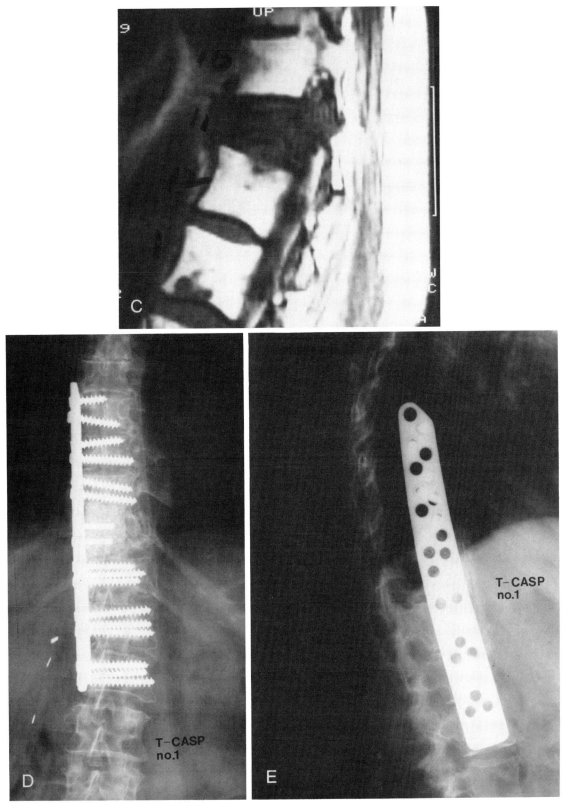

Figure 23.20. *C–E.*

REFERENCES

1. Bauman T, Garfin SR: Complications associated with anterior grafting. In: Garfin SR, ed. Complications of spine surgery. Baltimore: Williams & Wilkins, 1989;248–277.

2. Black RC, Eng P, Gardner VO, et al: A contoured anterior spinal fixation plate. Clin Orthop 1988;227:135–142.

3. Black R, St. George M, 1989; unpublished data.

4. Bone LB, Johnston CE II, Ashman RB, et al: Mechanical comparison of anterior spinal instrumentation in a burst fracture model. J Orthop Trauma 1988;2:195–201.

5. Chow D, Armstrong GWD, Feibel R, et al: The contoured anterior spinal plate: design rationale and results of the first 25 cases [abstract]. Scol Res Soc Meeting, Honolulu 1990;138.

6. Crock HV: Practice of spinal surgery. Berlin: Springer-Verlag, 1983;71–74.

7. Denis F: The three column spine and its significance in the classification of acute thoracolumbar spine injuries. Spine 1983;9:817.

8. Dunn HK: Anterior spine stabilization and decompression for thoracolumbar injuries. Orthop Clin North Am 1986;17:113.

9. Gertzbein S: 1990, personal communication.

10. Humphries AW, Hawk WA, Berndt AL: Anterior interbody fusion of lumbar vertebrae: a surgical technique. Surg Clin North Am 1961;41:1685.

11. Miller F, Whitehall R: Cancer of the breast metastatic to the skeleton. Clin Orthop 1984;184:121.

12. Ryan MD, Taylor TKF, Sherwood AA: Bolt-plate fixation for anterior spinal fusion. Clin Orthop 1986;203:196.

13. Shigley JE, Mitchell LD: Mechanical engineering design. New York: McGraw-Hill, 1983;270.

14. Watkins RG: Anterior lumbar interbody fusion-surgical complications. In: Garfin SR, ed. Complications of spine surgery. Baltimore: Williams & Wilkins, 1989;278–301.

15. Watkins RG: Cervical, thoracic, and lumbar complications-anterior approach. In: Garfin SR, ed. Complications of spine surgery. Baltimore: Williams & Wilkins, 1989;211–247.

TWENTY-FOUR

The Syracuse Anterior I-Plate

James C. Bayley, Hansen A. Yuan, and Bruce E. Fredrickson

INTRODUCTION

The Syracuse Anterior I-plate is a neutralization plate designed for anterior stabilization of the thoracolumbar spine. This chapter examines the history of anterior thoracolumbar spine surgery, describes the indications, approaches, and biomechanical data concerning the application of the I-plate, and evaluates the results of its use. Ultimately, it is hoped that the reader will become acquainted with the application of this device in the anterior treatment of the unstable spine due to tumor, infection, or following trauma.

HISTORICAL PERSPECTIVES

Anterior Surgery of the Thoracolumbar Spine

Historically, the spine was approached posteriorly. Laminectomy was performed for the removal of intraspinal tumors and drainage of infection as early as the 1800s. Independently, in 1911, Hibbs (32) and Albee (1) described laminectomy, decompression, and posterior arthrodesis for tuberculosis of the spine (Pott's disease). The classic paper of Mixter and Barr (54) detailing disc herniation as a common cause of sciatica, greatly expanded the popularity of posterior laminectomy for the treatment of spinal disorders.

The anterior approach to the thoracolumbar spine was pioneered by von Lackum and Smith (60) in 1933 for release of scoliosis. However, perhaps because of the unfamiliarity with this approach on the part of orthopaedic surgeons (9), or fear of catastrophic complications (55), the anterior route was not widely used until popularized by Hodgson and Stock in 1960 (34). They described in detail the anterior anatomic approach to the thoracolumbar spine and reported excellent results in the debridement and drainage of tuberculous abscesses of the spine. These findings were in marked contrast to other studies using posterior drainage procedures and/or medical treatment alone (48,52) for treatment of Pott's disease. Similarly, Harmon (28) advocated anterior fusion for severe spondylolisthesis at approximately the same time.

During this period, Smith and Robinson (58) were promoting the anterior approach to the cervical spine for treatment of spondylosis, herniated discs, and fractures. Success with this approach in numerous series (6,58) and extension of the principle of anterior treatment for anterior pathologic lesions (the Willie Sutton principle), popularized the anterior approach to the thoracolumbar spine. The simultaneous development of effective methods for internal fixation anteriorly in the spine expanded the use of this approach. Eventually, successful treatment of degenerated discs (the painful disc syndrome) through anterior interbody fusion increased the number of anterior procedures performed, so that the anterior approach to the lumbar spine is now the fourth most widely performed procedure in the lumbar spine (62). Thus, anterior surgery has become a versatile procedure to be used for many lesions in the thoracolumbar spine, including but not limited to infection (34), tumors (29), spondylolisthesis (7), degenerated discs (21), postlaminectomy instability (23), and most recently, fractures with neural compression (42).

Historical Development of Anterior Internal Fixation Devices for the Thoracolumbar Spine

Although first described by Lange in 1910 (43), the application of metal fixation devices to the spine came many years after routine use in the appendicular skeleton, such as in extremity fractures and joint replacements. The first series of anterior devices applied to the spine was by Humphries et al. (36) in 1959. They described a double clamp system for anterior fusion of L4 to the sacrum. Interestingly, the two senior authors were vascular, not orthopaedic surgeons. This report also predated the publication of Harrington's work (31), which is credited with popularizing posterior internal fixation for correction of scoliosis.

The plate-hook system of Humphries was never widely used due to the increasing popularity of the posterior approach to the spine for degenerative conditions. Dwyer in 1964 developed an anterior cable system applied to the convex side of thoracolumbar scoliotic curves. He published preliminary results in 1969 (16), indicating excellent early results in curve correction and successful arthrodesis. A more detailed report (17) described the approach and technique of device application, confirming the good initial results. However, other authors (27) found that the compression cable system caused excessive flattening of the lumbar lordosis, leading to a high rate of nonunion if the Dwyer system was not reinforced by posterior fixation. This prompted Zielke (65) to invent a rigid cable system that allowed better restoration of the lumbar lordosis and correction of scoliosis. Simultaneously, Werlinich (61) described a staple for anterior single level fusions in degenerative conditions.

Unfortunately, several significant complications were reported with the use of the Dwyer and Zielke systems. These included retrograde ejaculation in males (22), ureteral obstruction (37), injury to the spleen (33), and vena caval or aortic injury (18). Fear of these rare but catastrophic complications has limited the application of these bulky devices in the thoracolumbar spine.

In the area of fixation devices for traumatic injuries, the primary approach has been long posterior fixation, pioneered by Dickson and Harrington in 1977 (13). Although reduction of displaced spinal fractures and successful fusion was excellent with this apparatus (20), concerns were raised about the length of fusion (five to seven levels, including three to five normal levels) required for adequate mechanical leverage to produce and maintain fracture reduction (24).

Additionally, it was apparent that in burst injuries, the most common fracture, neural compression is from the anterior direction. Anterior debridement of fracture fragments therefore would potentially be a more effective means to decompress the spinal canal (41). These factors prompted a reevaluation of the anterior approach to thoracolumbar fractures. However, decompression via the anterior route significantly destabilizes the anterior and middle vertebral columns. In the cervical spine, stability can be restored by interference fit of bone graft alone following decompression (5). Unfortunately, due to higher compression and increased lateral bending loads in the lumbar spine compared with the cervical spine, bone grafts unsupported by internal fixation are significantly less stable there (45). Clearly, improved internal

fixation devices were required to make anterior decompression successful.

For this reason, Dunn (15) in 1984 introduced a device for anterior distraction and fusion in the thoracolumbar spine, specifically for treatment of fractures. His system consists of two rods linked by bridges fixed to the vertebral bodies on either side of the fracture by staples and bone screws. Because the rods are threaded, distraction and compression, as required, can be applied to the spine. This allows restoration of spinal alignment following anterior decompression of fracture fragments as well as compression of the cortical bone graft spanning the decompressed vertebrae. Most importantly, the device is stable enough to eliminate the need for supplementary posterior instrumentation. Dunn's initial series reported only three pseudarthroses in the first 48 patients, with no loss of alignment or recurrent neural compression. Although initial results were promising, the prominence of this instrumentation and its proximity to major vessels led, in inexperienced hands, to several cases of vessel perforation (8). The device is currently not available in the United States.

A similar implant has been developed in Canada. The Kostuik-Harrington device (41) combines a Harrington distraction rod in front and a compression rod further back on the body clamped to the vertebrae by specially modified bone screws. Attachment of these screws to the intact vertebrae adjacent to the fractured level by special staples prevents toggling of the screws. Kostuik's early results (40) were excellent: general improvement in partial spinal cord injuries with anterior decompression, no cases of nonunion, few device-related problems, and no early or late vascular complications. The device has not gained any widespread popularity in the United States.

A third dynamic device has recently been introduced by Kaneda (39) who encountered a high failure rate with the Zielke apparatus in lumbar spine fractures. The Kaneda device is similar to the Dunn device in that it consists of two threaded rods for compression or distraction, attached to the intact vertebrae by two bone screws apiece through a staple that fits over the vertebral endplates. A crosslinking clamp recently introduced provides significantly improved rigidity. In the largest series reported (39), there was significant neurologic improvement in all partial spinal cord injuries and no loss of fixation. This device is currently under clinical investigation in the United States.

The main advantage of these three devices is that they allow direct dynamic distraction of the vertebrae followed by direct compression of implanted bone graft after decompression of the neural elements. All are extremely rigid once inserted. The major disadvantage is that the bone screws and connecting rods are prominent, which may increase the danger of early or late injury to the great vessels, especially if the device is inadvertently placed anteriorly on the vertebral body instead of directly laterally, as intended (15). Additionally, the rigidity of the device may promote stress shielding in interposed vertebrae and bone graft (50).

In contrast to these bulky devices that allow direct compression of the bone graft, two plate systems have been developed for anterior application to the thoracolumbar spine. In 1988, Black and Armstrong (4) introduced a multiholed low-profile plate for lateral placement on the lumbar vertebral bodies. The plate is available in the United States in three lengths for use following decompression of tumors and burst fractures, disc degeneration, and pseudarthroses.

Yuan et al. (64), in 1988, introduced the Syracuse I-plate for anterior stabilization of the thoracolumbar spine following decompression of tumors and burst fracture fragments. The remainder of this chapter will be devoted to a description of the I-plate, biomechanical data comparing the I-plate with several other devices, a review of the indications for its use, and a summary of the published clinical results to date.

THE SYRACUSE I-PLATE

The lack of a firm fixation device for anterior stabilization led to the development of a modified plate in 1985 by Yuan, Mann, et al., called the Syracuse I-plate. Initial experimental data showed that a standard AO/ASIF DC or neutralization plate was not sufficient to resist rotational or translational forces because of the narrowness of the plate and the parallel nature of the vertebral screws applied through the plate. An AO/ASIF DC plate was therefore modified into an I configuration (Fig. 24.1) by broadening the upper and lower ends, removing the intervening holes, and curving the plate to wrap around the vertebral bodies. Two of the four remaining holes in the I-plate were configured in dynamic compression mode to allow compression across the bone graft as the screws were tightened. The screws used in the initial plate were standard 6.5-mm cancellous bone screws.

Further in-vitro biomechanical testing showed that with cyclic loading, the cancellous screws were prone to toggle in the plate, which led to premature screw breakage and pullout. This occurred because of the flexibility of screw orientation in the dynamic compression holes. If any graft resorption or settling developed, the screws loosened and protruded out of the plate. With in vivo application, this area of increased motion would eventually disappear after graft incorporation. It was predicted, however, that failure of fixation could occur before primary bone healing. Therefore, the concept of using dynamic compression through the plate was abandoned.

To minimize screw toggling, a revised I-plate was devised (Fig. 24.2). The holes were reconfigured to a neutralization mode. However, when longer screws were inserted, the distal tips frequently collided, making insertion of the second screw in each vertebra difficult.

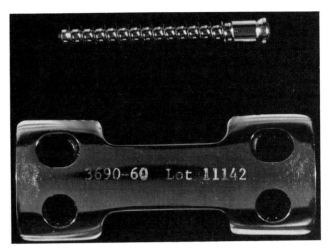

Figure 24.1. The original I-plate. The two posterior holes (*top*) are configured in dynamic compression mode.

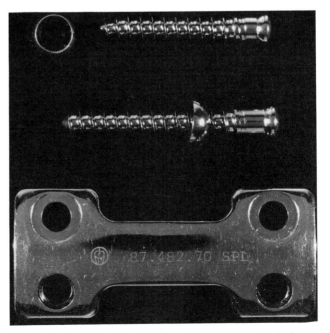

Figure 24.2. The revised I-plate. The two posterior holes are indented to allow countersinking of the grommet.

Therefore, a grommet was added to give additional height to the posterior screw and offset screw lengths, allowing the second screw to glide by the first. Additionally, this grommet provided improved stability to the posterior screw, limiting toggle. Unfortunately, the grommet was found to be somewhat prominent, defeating the purpose of the plate. Thus, the screws were again redesigned to fit better into the plate, reducing toggle but maintaining the low-profile nature of the I-plate. This is the version presently in use.

The current I-plate (Fig. 24.3) functions as a neutralization plate after compression has been applied across the bone graft. The plate is 3-mm thick and angled so that 60° of curvature separates the two holes. The plate is applied with two screws inserted into each intact vertebral body above and below the involved vertebra.

The plate comes in lengths of 70 mm, 80 mm, and 90 mm. The plate that allows placement of the screws in the middle of the intact vertebral bodies should be selected. The screws are modified AO/ASIF 6.5-mm cancellous screws (Fig. 24.4). They consist of a standard hexagonal head and a 4-mm long nonthreaded 6.5-mm shank. This nonthreaded shank engages the plate, minimizing toggle. The screws are available in 5-mm increments from 40–80 mm. When fully seated (Fig. 24.5), the screws lie flush with the surface of the plate. Thus, the vascular structures are at negligible risk, unless the screws disengage or otherwise back out.

BIOMECHANICAL DATA

To determine whether in-vivo use might succeed, the relative and absolute strength of the I-plate was determined in a series of in vitro experiments. The rigidity of four anterior fixation systems, including the original I-plate, the current I-plate, the Kostuik-Harrington system, and the Kaneda device was studied in a burst fracture model (46). These four implants were attached to T12 and L2 in human cadaver spines after resection of the posterior two-thirds of the vertebral body of L1, simulating an unstable burst fracture. Using a block of wood to simulate an interposed bone graft, the specimens were loaded in an Instron testing apparatus to 400 N and a bending moment of 10–14 Nm. Resultant angular motion was measured.

Decompression and block insertion alone resulted in reduced stiffness in all directions. Thus, as expected, this caused a more unstable construct, as seen in the in vivo unstable burst fracture. All four anterior systems tested improved the stiffness of the fracture construct, except the Kostuik-Harrington device, which was significantly less stable in flexion. It was postulated that the anterior distraction rod of this system holds the vertebra away from the bone graft so that displacement occurs in forward flexion. In turn, this leads to increased motion, and thus less stability, between the vertebral endplate and the graft.

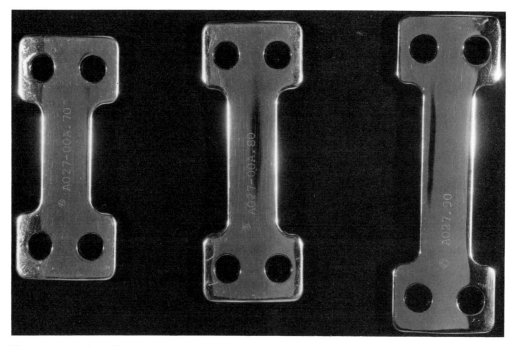

Figure 24.3. The current I-plate. Three lengths (70 mm, 80 mm, 90 mm) are available. The plate chosen should fit so that the screws are in the midportion of the vertebrae adjacent to the resected vertebral body.

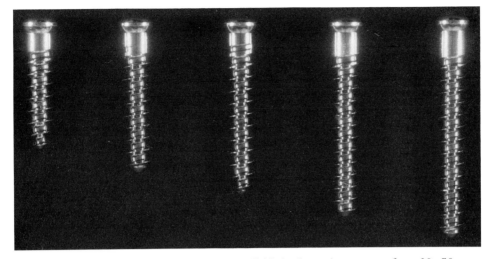

Figure 24.4. Available screws. These are available in 5-mm increments, from 30–50 mm.

Among the four anterior devices tested, the current I-plate was the most stable in flexion and extension, but was less stable than the Kaneda device in lateral bending. All four devices were more stable in resisting torsional loads than the block alone, but slightly less stable when compared with the intact spine.

This study also showed that all constructs were more stable than the intact spine in extension if the anterior longitudinal ligament is preserved. It was postulated that, in extension, this ligament resists tensile forces. Thus, as is noted below, the anterior longitudinal ligament should be preserved by placing the I-plate laterally on the vertebral body and leaving the anterior soft tissues intact.

In a second experiment (47), the current I-plate was compared with a posterior system, the AO/ASIF fixateur interne. A burst fracture was created in human cadaver spines by weight drop. By cross-over studies, the fixateur interne and the I-plate were compared for stiffness in flexion, extension, lateral bending, and rotation in either direction. When the posterior ligamentous structures, i.e., the supra- and interspinous ligaments, facets and facet capsules, and ligamentum flavum were preserved, both systems provided increased stability in flexion, extension and lateral bending compared with the intact spine. In axial rotation, the I-plate was as stable as the intact spine, but the fixateur interne without crosslinking was less stable. However, when the posterior ligamentous structures were damaged, as may occur in a flexion/distraction type of injury, the I-plate was significantly less stable in all directions than the intact spine. In this situation, the fixateur interne was as stable as the intact spine in all directions, except lateral rotation. Recent unpublished experiments have shown that crosslinking the rods of the fixateur interne by wire may significantly improve its stability in lateral bending.

In conclusion, the current I-plate is as stable as the other anterior fixation devices tested. It is also as stable as the short-segment internal fixator when posterior structures are intact, but is quite unstable, compared with a normal intact spine when any significant posterior disruption has occurred. The degree of posterior disruption can usually be ascertained prior to surgery by knowledge of the mechanism of injury and by critical evaluation of the radiographs. Thus, choice of an anterior system vs. a

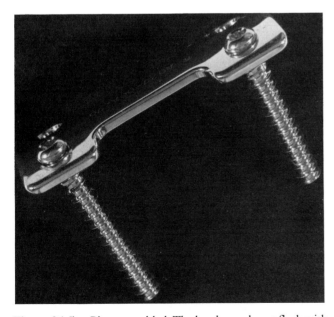

Figure 24.5. Plate assembled. The heads are almost flush with the plate, providing a very low-profile implant.

posterior system can be made ahead of time, and will depend on the presence of posterior ligamentous disruption.

INDICATIONS FOR USE OF THE I-PLATE

Fractures of the spine occur most commonly at the thoracolumbar junction (13), and frequently involve flexion-compression injuries. Prior to the routine use of myelography and CT scanning, these fractures were listed as simple compression fractures. The reason for neurologic injury in these injuries was not well understood. Holdsworth in 1970 (35) described the concept of the burst fracture, recognizing the role of retropulsed fragments of bone in causing spinal cord or cauda equina injury. Later, the three-column spine model was popularized by Denis (10). He argued that a middle column, consisting of the posterior vertebral cortex and posterior longitudinal ligament, determined ultimate spinal stability. Damage to this middle column by fracture or tumor led to an unstable spine, potentially requiring surgical stabilization.

Treatment of unstable thoracolumbar injuries in the early part of this century consisted of prolonged bed rest. Later, Guttmann (25) popularized postural reduction on a specialized frame to reduce and maintain these fractures. This treatment, however, required 3 months of bed rest in hyperextension with all attendant complications. Although internal fixation of the thoracolumbar spine was first described by Lange in 1910 (43), it was not until Harrington's report of his distraction rods (31) that a reliable implant was found to achieve distraction. Initially, the Harrington system was used to treat scoliosis. Dickson, Harrington, and Erwin (13) reported success with Harrington distraction rods in the treatment of unstable spine fractures. This became the standard method of treatment of fractures throughout the 1980s. McAfee, Yuan, and Lasda (51) found that posterior decompression through laminectomy and fragment impaction resulted in improved neural recovery when combined with Harrington distraction rods, if surgery is performed early.

Posterior distraction alone, because it relies on indirect reduction, was found to frequently result in inadequate reduction, especially if surgery is delayed or in the presence of extensive comminution (5). Additionally, with posterior distraction and instrumentation, the spine is under tension, not compression. This may potentially lead to a weaker fusion mass, a higher nonunion rate, and implant failure (5). Recently, studies have shown late collapse following distraction instrumentation due to hardware failure or after removal of implants (24).

Thus, it is potentially more advantageous to decom-

press and fuse the spine anteriorly in cases of anterior impingement of neural structures due to fracture or tumor. Early series of anterior fusions based on this concept used bone graft without internal fixation for posttraumatic instability, and reported a high incidence of nonunions and late collapse (21,44). Most failures were due to graft fracture or loss of position. Similarly, the use of polymethylmethacrylate not reinforced by metal fixation resulted in a high rate of failure (49). Thus, it was clear that, in cases of extensive bone loss or resection, supplementation with internal fixation was required. Dewald (11) advocated a second stage posterior fusion using Harrington rod instrumentation following anterior debridement and grafting. This provides more stability with a lower rate of late collapse, but subjects the patient to a second major surgery; posterior distraction may also occasionally dislodge the previously placed anterior strut graft.

In the recent past, standard treatment for spinal fractures with, or at risk for, significant displacement has been posterior fixation with Harrington or Luque rods (11,13,44,51). This usually entailed fusing two or three motion segments above and below the fracture, permanently immobilizing five or six motion segments. While such immobilization is not a problem in the relatively stiff thoracic spine, such an extensive fusion can lead to late complications in the lower thoracic and lumbar spine (53). The once-popular technique of rodding long but fusing short has been shown to have a deleterious effect on immobilized joints (38) and has fallen into disfavor. Problems encountered with long fusions in the lumbar spine have included: loss of lumbar lordosis or flatback (2), premature disc and facet degeneration (53), neurologic injury (26), and chronic backache. Thus, methods of short fusion have been sought.

One recent approach to short fusion has been posterior transpedicular fixation with immobilization of only two motion segments. Initial pedicle fixation systems included the Roy-Camille plate (57), and the VSP system of Steffee (59). Because these are plate systems, their ability to reduce displaced fractures of the spine is limited (45). Recently, pedicle fixation systems with the ability to distract through threaded connecting rods have been developed. These include the Fixateur Interne (12) and the Olerud device (56). However, these posterior systems rely on indirect reduction of anterior fractures to relieve spinal cord compression. Potentially, this may not be successful, especially if the posterior longitudinal ligament and/or posterior annulus are disrupted (63). Prolonged delay between fracture and surgery may prevent indirect reduction by a posterior system (19). In this situation, anterior decompression is indicated.

With the anterior approach, the spinal cord is under direct vision, ensuring adequate decompression. Associated nerve root injuries can be evaluated and/or decompressed. In cases of multiple trauma, retroperitoneal and intraperitoneal injuries can be repaired through the same incision. Thus, direct anterior decompression and fusion of unstable burst fractures have several advantages over indirect posterior reduction and fusion, as long as stability can be adequately restored (41,42).

A second important area where spinal cord compression occurs anteriorly is in metastatic and primary malignancies. Neoplasms of the vertebral column occur most commonly in the vertebral body (3). Vertebral destruction leads to progressive kyphosis and spinal cord compromise, due to epidural spread of tumor or by retropulsed bone fragments from the pathologically involved vertebra. Debridement of vertebral bodies replaced by tumor may provide palliation and may prevent further neurologic deterioration (3). It must be done anteriorly, as posterior reduction will have no effect on the anterior tumor mass. However, because radiation is frequently used to control spread of any residual tumor, bone graft incorporation into adjacent uninvolved bone is frequently inadequate, resulting in late collapse. Thus, debridement of tumor and bone grafting must be supplemented with internal fixation. Methylmethacrylate was initially used alone (30), but has been shown to have a high failure rate when followed long term (49).

Two indications currently exist for using the Syracuse I-plate in lesions from T11-L5. One is for stabilization of the vertebral column following resection of single-level bony neoplasms, whether primary or metastatic. The anterior approach provides immediate stabilization, allows early irradiation to control residual tumor, and eliminates the necessity of a second posterior operation for stabilization.

The second indication for use of the I-plate is in unstable burst fractures with or without neurologic injuries. This is especially true if a delay between injury and surgery has occurred. In cases of complete spinal cord injury where stability is an issue, a posterior approach, whether by hook and rod or by pedicle fixation, may be appropriate. In patients with partial neurologic deficits due to anterior spinal cord compression or in intact patients with significant cord compromise, anterior debridement and grafting supplemented with the I-plate and cortical bone graft is indicated. If the posterior ligamentous structures are damaged, such as in a flexion-distraction injury or dislocation (both three-column injuries), the I-plate can be used, but must be combined with adequate external support or secondary posterior internal fixation.

SURGICAL APPROACHES AND I-PLATE APPLICATION

A thoracolumbar retroperitoneal approach is used for the lower thoracic and upper lumbar vertebrae. For placement at L2 or below, a lateral retroperitoneal approach is done. The lumbosacral angle is too acute for placement of the current plate design, preventing its use below L5. The spine is usually approached from the patient's left side, since any incidental vascular lacerations are more easily repaired if they occur to the aorta rather than to the thin-walled vena cava. Also, a right-handed surgeon usually finds it easier to place the posterior screws from the left side. However, either a left or right approach can be used at the discretion of the surgeon. Spinal cord monitoring equipment, if available, should be used to document spinal cord decompression and warn of any neurologic injuries during surgery. The approaches described will be from the left.

Thoracoabdominal Approach

The patient should be positioned so that the affected vertebra is over the bend in the table to enhance exposure and provide lateral distraction on the side of I-plate fixation. A double-lumen endotracheal tube is helpful to allow deflation of the left lung. The patient is placed in the right lateral decubitus position resting slightly backwards on a kidney rest or sandbag. The entire left side is prepped and draped from axilla to hip including the iliac crest. Autologous or allograft fibula can be used if necessary. An incision is made over the 10th rib from the posterior axiallary line extending anteriorly and inferiorly to the lateral margin of the rectus sheath. Using electrocautery, the subcutaneous tissue is incised down to the rib through the periosteum. Anteriorly, the external and internal oblique muscles along with the transversus abdominis are incised or split in line with the fibers, if possible. The cartilaginous tip of the 10th rib, called the keystone, is incised sharply and the rib exposed extrapleurally by use of Doyon rib elevators. The rib is osteotomized as far posteriorly as possible, at least as far as the costotransverse junction. The rib is used to provide extra bone graft, or it can be used for a vascularized graft. The thoracic cavity is entered through the rib bed, and the anterior attachment of the diaphragm to the tip of the 10th rib identified. By gentle finger dissection, the retroperitoneum is entered through the incised keystone, and by blunt dissection, the plane between the diaphragm and the retroperitoneum is developed as far posteriorly as possible. The diaphragm is then incised at least 1 cm from its peripheral attachment and the central portion tagged with heavy suture for later reattachment. It is important to leave a peripheral rim of diaphragm for this closure; the rim, however, is denervated by this maneuver, so it should not be overly generous. The retroperitoneum is stripped from the undersurface of the diaphragm back to the crura. Anteriorly, the peritoneum is detached by blunt dissection from the anterior abdominal wall as far forward as the rectus sheath. The crura of the diaphragm are then taken down and tagged, leaving a small peripheral portion for reattachment. This exposes the vertebral bodies from T10-L2.

The vertebra to be removed is identified. If this is not obvious, an x-ray may be taken with a marker over the suspected body. The lung is deflated and packed off, using a soft retractor. A rib spreader is used to widen the space between the 9th and 11th rib. The peritoneum is gently retracted anteriorly.

The discs are readily identifiable by their glistening bulge and are safe to approach. The segmental vessels lie on the middle of the vertebral bodies, away from the discs. The vessels are gently elevated from the periosteum using right angle clamps and ligated with sutures or clips.

Two ligatures are tied on the proximal end nearest the aorta. Ligation must be done at least 1 cm from the vertebral foramen to avoid interfering with the anastomotic network of blood supply to the cord. The critical artery of Adamkiewicz supplies the spinal cord anywhere from T4-L1 (30). Most authors state that three adjacent segmental vessels on the same side can be ligated without arterial compromise; no series report any serious neurologic sequelae as long as this precaution is taken. Ligation of the segmental vessels allows the aorta and vena cava to be mobilized, falling away from the vertebral column. The vertebrae are then stripped subperiosteally back to the neural foramen and pedicles, and forward to the anterior longitudinal ligament. The pathologic vertebra is debrided using osteotomes, rongeurs, or a high-speed burr. To ensure complete decompression of the spinal cord, the dural sac must be visualized from the near to the far pedicle. The authors find it easier to start at the far pedicle so that the dural sac does not bulge into the field as debridement is carried across the posterior cortex of the body. Following complete debridement, the I-plate is affixed.

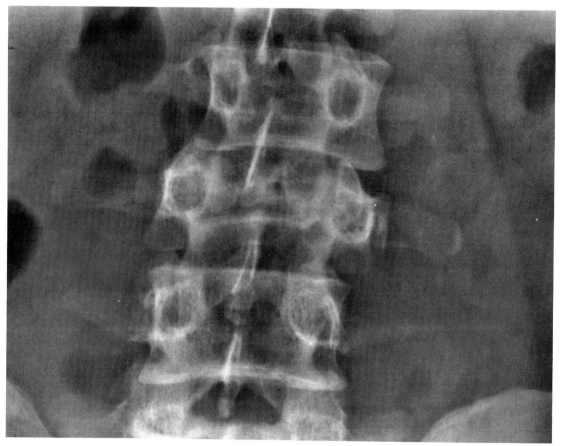

Figure 24.6. AP x-ray of a typical burst fracture of L3, illustrating compression, widened pedicles, and lateral translocation.

Closure is begun by inserting a #24 chest tube through a separate stab incision. The crura of the diaphragm are repaired using nonabsorbable suture, and a running suture is used to close the diaphragm. This may be supplemented with multiple interrupted sutures for added strength. Prior to closure, the lung is checked for air leaks by filling the thoracic cavity with saline and watching for bubbles. The ribs are approximated and sutured together with heavy suture and the muscle layers closed separately.

Postoperatively, the patient is fitted in a body cast or plastic TLSO. He/she is then allowed progressive ambulation. The chest tube is removed when no air leak is evident and drainage is minimal.

Retroperitoneal Approach

For exposure of L1-L5, an extraperitoneal approach through the 12th rib is used. The patient is anesthetized and positioned as in a thoracoabdominal approach. The 12th rib is palpated and the skin incised over this, extending anteriorly and inferiorly to the lateral border of the rectus sheath. For exposure of the lower lumbar vertebrae, the incision is extended distally toward the pubis; laterally to the rectus sheath. Using electrocautery, the subcutaneous tissue is incised down to the external oblique muscle, which can usually be split by blunt dissection in line with its fibers. The internal oblique and transversus abdominis are cut with electrocautery, being careful not to enter the peritoneum deep to the transversus abdominis muscle. The retroperitoneal space is then entered using blunt dissection and the peritoneum gradually mobilized forward and retracted. The periosteum of the 12th rib is incised and the rib removed as far back as the costo-transverse junction. Once again, the cartilaginous tip of the 12th rib is used as a keystone for locating the junction of the peritoneum and retroperitoneum. By blunt dissection, the interval between the retroperitoneum and the diaphragm is opened, and the peritoneal contents retracted anteriorly. If any tears are made in the peritoneum, they should be closed with running absorbable suture when identified. For surgery at L2 and below, the diaphragm does not have to be incised.

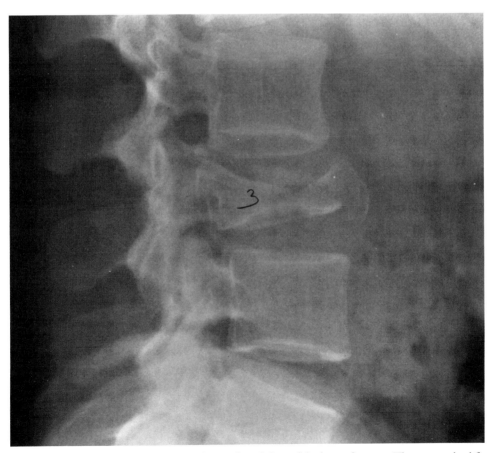

Figure 24.7.   Lateral x-ray of L3, illustrating compression and wedging of the burst fracture. The retropulsed fragment is difficult to see due to the overlying pedicle.

The psoas muscle is then identified but not entered. The disc spaces are the best landmarks and can be identified as the protruding white bulges. At the anterior border of the psoas muscle, the segmental vessels are located at the waist of the vertebral bodies; they are ligated using right angle clamps as in a thoracoabdominal approach. This frees up the vascular structures, which are retracted anteriorly. The vertebrae are then stripped subperiosteally as far posteriorly as the vertebral foramen and forward to the anterior longitudinal ligament. This also mobilizes the psoas muscle posteriorly, as well as the sympathetic chain, which normally lies in the muscle or on its anterior aspect. After debridement of the vertebra is performed, and the I-plate affixed, the wound is closed in separate layers over a drain. Because the thoracic cavity is not entered in this approach, no chest tube is required. Postoperative care is the same as for a thoracoabdominal approach.

Placement of the I-plate

Prior to or following adequate debridement of the affected vertebral body, the discs and cartilaginous endplates on either side must be removed. The authors prefer a sharp osteotome or Cobb elevator, which avoids damage to the cortex of the adjacent vertebrae. This exposes the subchondral bone of the two intact vertebrae on either side. The bend in the table or the elevated kidney rest is elevated by the anesthesiologist. This opens up the space between the intact vertebral bodies. A large spreader clamp is placed between the vertebrae and distracted in order to restore height to the spinal column.

Once the alignment of the vertebral column has been restored, the distance between the midportions of the vertebral bodies is measured and the appropriate plate length chosen. Through a separate incision, a full-thickness piece of iliac crest is harvested and cut so that it will just fit in the space between the spread vertebrae. The authors prefer to use two tricortical pieces with the ends abutting the vertebral endplates because of the theoretical advantage of increased graft incorporation and avoidance of allograft-related disease transmission. Alternatively, a piece of autologous or allograft fibula, tibia, or femur can be used.

The grafts are then placed into position and secured by pounding in both ends symmetrically until wedged in the center of the bodies tightly. The ends of the graft should contact the subchondral bone directly. A trough is not cut into cancellous bone, as this may lead to the graft later settling further into cancellous bone.

The bend in the table is then straightened, putting the graft under compression. The I-plate is placed as poster-

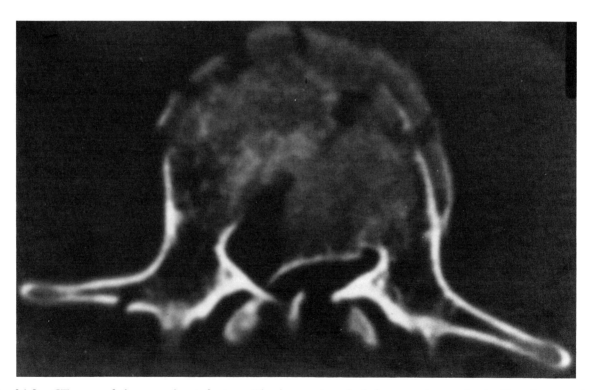

Figure 24.8. CT scan of the same burst fracture. The large retropulsed fragment is noted, significantly narrowing the spinal canal.

olaterally as possible on the vertebrae, and the posterior holes drilled with a 3.2-mm drill bit. The holes are not tapped. The depth is measured to the opposite cortex using the depth gauge, and the appropriate-length 6.5-mm screws tightened in the two posterior holes. The screws should just penetrate the opposite cortex. Care must be taken to direct the screws transversely, as any posterior aiming of the screws risks their entrance into the spinal canal. Both anterior screw holes are then drilled, measured, and the screws placed. These should be directed in a slightly posterior direction for best purchase. The I-plate is designed so that the screws are separated by 60°. If the screws are placed slightly convergent, this provides good translational and rotational stiffness. Because the graft is compressed prior to plate application, the I-plate should be considered as a neutralization plate, not a compression plate.

An illustrative case for the use of the I-plate is shown in Figures 24.6–24.10. AP (Fig. 24.6) and lateral (Fig. 24.7) x-rays demonstrate a typical burst fracture of L3 with approximately 40% posterior and 65% anterior compression. There is a small degree of lateral translocation on the AP x-ray. The CT scan (Fig. 24.8) demonstrates a large fragment of bone displaced into the vertebral canal, with at least 80% canal compromise. The right transverse process is fractured, as well as the lamina.

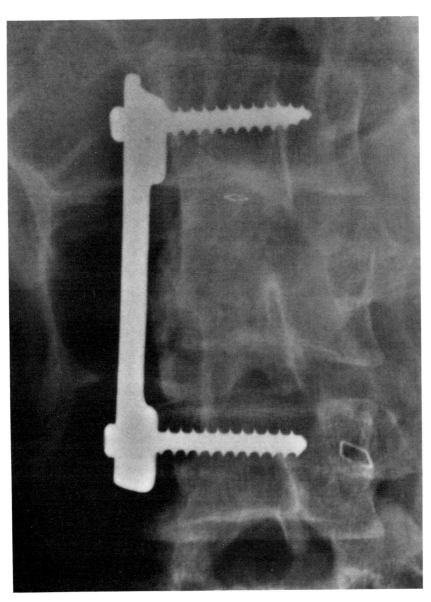

Figure 24.9. AP x-ray of the burst fracture after decompression, bone graft insertion, and I-plate application. The plate is positioned directly laterally, and the screws are in the midportion of the vertebral bodies.

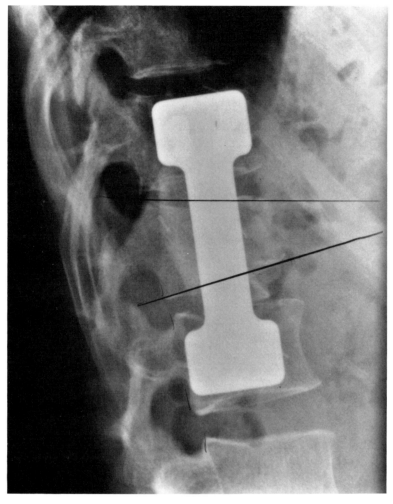

Figure 24.10.   Lateral x-ray of the burst fracture after I-plate application. The intact vertebral bodies, L2 and L4, are parallel. Height and alignment have been restored.

Following decompression of the burst fracture, distraction by spreader clamp and insertion of two pieces of autologous tricortical iliac crest graft, the I-plate was applied. AP (Fig. 24.9) and lateral (Fig. 24.10) x-rays demonstrate restoration of vertebral body height and alignment. The plate is shown directly laterally on the vertebral column, and the screws are in the midportion of the adjacent intact vertebral bodies away from the disc spaces and endplates. Although the fractured vertebra appears still somewhat wedged, the endplates of the adjacent vertebrae are noted to be parallel, indicating full restoration of alignment.

RESULTS OF I-PLATE INSERTION

The first series of patients in whom the I-plate was used was reported in 1988 (64). Sixteen patients underwent successful anterior debridement and fusion with bone graft and the I-plate. Of these 16, 10 had acute burst fractures, two had old unreduced burst fractures with kyphosis of more than 20°, and four had primary or metastatic tumors. The ages ranged from 14–72 years, with a mean of 30 years. All fractures occurred from T12–L3, and eight of 10 patients with acute fractures had partial neurologic deficits. Of these, seven improved neurologically with anterior decompression and I-plate insertion. Degree of spinal canal compromise was improved significantly in six of seven in whom postoperative CT scanning was done. Among the four patients with neoplasms, all had good pain relief; however, one developed increased kyphosis of 20° and scoliosis of 17° due to osteoporotic settling of the graft.

Complications in this initial series were few. One case of screw breakage occurred in an asymptomatic patient.

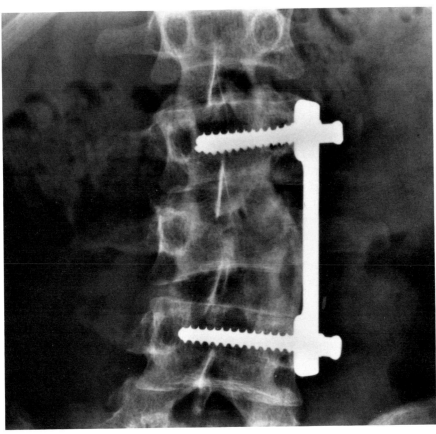

Figure 24.11. AP x-ray of failed I-plate application. Due to bone graft collapse and posterior comminution, the opposite cortex and graft have collapsed. The screws toggle, loosen, and protrude out of the plate.

One patient of the 16 suffered displacement of the bone graft, despite implantation of the I-plate. He was placed on prolonged bed rest, and his fracture eventually healed without further neurologic complication.

Since the publication of the original series, many more patients have undergone anterior decompression and fusion with the I-plate. With more experience, surgeons are recognizing the limitations of this device. As predicted by the in-vitro biomechanical data (45), any degree of posterior ligamentous disruption will negate the stability provided by the anterior I-plate. Figure 24.11 illustrates the long-term follow-up of a patient who suffered a flexion-distraction injury of L2. He underwent anterior retroperitoneal decompression of the burst fragments and insertion of an I-plate. Despite excellent initial correction, his spine eventually became unstable in lateral bending. An x-ray at 6 weeks postoperatively (Fig. 24.11) revealed displacement of the screws due to toggling of the plate. Hardware removal was required due to the danger of vascular injury by the loose screws. Ideally, in this case, the extent of posterior disruption should have been rec-

ognized. The anterior decompression and fusion was appropriate to relieve his canal compromise, but the I-plate should have been protected by subsequent posterior fusion and internal fixation.

Follow-up in patients with osteoporosis has revealed that graft resorption or subsidence occurs at an increased rate in these patients. This may lead to loosening of the I-plate and subsequent screw migration.

DISCUSSION

To summarize, the I-plate is an excellent device for anterior stabilization of the lower thoracis and lumbar spine following decompression of burst fractures or neoplasms. Biomechanically, it is as stable as the other anterior devices currently available, and has a lower profile than the Kaneda or Dunn devices. It must be combined with a strong bone graft intercalated between intact vertebrae on either side of the damaged vertebra. The presence of posterior disruption or significant osteoporosis is a contraindication to the use of the I-plate alone, or to any currently available anterior instrumentation. In these cases, it should be protected by subsequent posterior internal fixation.

Recently, the Morscher plate has been developed for anterior fixation of the cervical spine. This plate incorporates titanium inserts placed into the vertebral body which expand when screws are placed for fixation. This expansion substantially increases the pullout strength of the plates, and significantly lessens the chance of the screw backing out.

Because these two problems have occurred occasionally with the I-plate in the thoracolumbar spine, a second modification of the I-plate is currently under development. The new plate will incorporate the Morscher screw design to eliminate backing out and screw toggling.

Clearly, continued development of the I-plate will bring improvements. It is hoped that as further refinements are made, the indications for the use of the Syracuse I-plate will be expanded.

REFERENCES

1. Albee FH: Transplantation of a portion of the tibia into the spine for Pott's disease. A preliminary report. JAMA 1911;57:885–889.
2. Balderston R, Winter R, Moe J: Fusion to the sacrum for non-paralytic scoliosis in the adult. Orthop Trans 1984;8:170.
3. Berrettoni BA, Carter JR: Mechanisms of cancer metastasis to bone. J Bone Joint Surg 1986;68A:308–312.
4. Black RC, Gardner VO, Armstrong GWD, et al: A contoured anterior spinal fixation plate. Clin Orthop Rel Res 1988;227:135–142.
5. Bohlman HH, Eismont FJ: Surgical techniques of anterior decompression and fusion for spinal cord injuries. Clin Orthop Rel Res 1981;154:57–67.
6. Bohlman HH, Freeajfel A, Dejak J: Spinal cord injuries and late anterior decompression of spinal cord injuries. J Bone Joint Surg 1975;57A:1025–1031.
7. Bradford DS, Gotfried Y: Staged salvage reconstruction of grade IV and V spondylolisthesis. J Bone Joint Surg 1987;69A:191–201.
8. Brown LP, Bidwell KH, Holt RJ, et al: Aortic erosions and lacerations associated with the Dunn anterior spinal instrumentation. Presented at the Scoliosis Research Society, 1985.
9. Capener N: Spondylolisthesis. Brit J Surg 1932;19:374–382.
10. Denis F: The three column spine and its significance in the classification of acute thoracolumbar spine injuries. Spine 1983;8:817–831.
11. Dewald RL: Burst fractures of the thoracic and lumbar spine. Clin Orthop Rel Res 1984;189:150–161.
12. Dick W: The "fixateur interne" as a versatile implant for spine surgery. Spine 1987;12:882–900.
13. Dickson JH, Harrington PR, Erwin WD: Results of reduction and stabilization in the severely fractured thoracic and lumbar spine. J Bone Joint Surg 1978;60A:799–806.
14. Dommisse GF: The blood supply of the spinal cord: A critical vascular zone in spinal surgery. J Bone Joint Surg 1974;56B:225–235.
15. Dunn HK: Anterior stabilization of thoracolumbar injuries. Clin Orthop Rel Res 1984;189:116–124.
16. Dwyer AF, Newton NC, Sherwood AA: An anterior approach to scoliosis. Clin Orthop Rel Res 1969;62:192–202.
17. Dwyer AF, Schafer MF: Anterior approach to scoliosis: Results of treatment in fifty-one cases. J Bone Joint Surg 1974;56B:218–224.
18. Dwyer AP: A fatal complication of paravertebral infection and traumatic aneurysm following Dwyer instrumentation. J Bone Joint Surg 1979;61B:239.
19. Esses SI: The AO spinal internal fixator. Spine 1989;14:373–378.
20. Flesch JR, Leider LL, Erickson DL, et al: Harrington instrumentation and spine fusion for unstable fractures and fracture-dislocations of the thoracic and lumbar spine. J Bone Joint Surg 1977;59A:143–153.
21. Flynn JC, Hoque MA: Anterior fusion of the lumbar spine: End-result study with long-term follow-up. J Bone Joint Surg 1979;61A:1143–1150.
22. Flynn JC, Price CT: Sexual complications of anterior fusion of the lumbar spine. Spine 1984;9:489–492.
23. Freebody D, Bendall R, Taylor RD: Anterior transperitoneal lumbar fusion. J Bone Joint Surg 1971;53B:617–627.
24. Gertzbein SD, MacMichael D, Tile M: Harrington instrumentation as a method of fixation in fractures of the spine: A critical analysis of deficiencies. J Bone Joint Surg 1982;64B:526–529.
25. Guttmann L: Initial treatment of traumatic paraplegia. Proc Royal Soc Med 1954;47:1103–1121.
26. Hales DD, Dawson EG, Delamarter R: Late neurologic complications of Harrington rod instrumentation. J Bone Joint Surg 1989;71A:1053–1057.
27. Hall JE: Current concepts review: Dwyer instrumentation in anterior fusion of the spine. J Bone Joint Surg 1981;63A:1188–1190.
28. Harmon PH: Anterior extraperitoneal lumbar disk excision and vertebral body fusion. Clin Orthop Rel Res 1960;18:169–176.
29. Harrington KD: Anterior cord decompression and spinal stabilization for patients with metastatic lesions of the spine. J Neurosurg 1984;61:107–117.
30. Harrington KD: The use of methyl-methacrylate for vertebral body replacement and anterior stabilization of pathological fracture-dislocations of the spine due to metastatic malignant disease. J Bone Joint Surg 1981;63A:36–46.
31. Harrington PR: Treatment of scoliosis. J Bone Joint Surg 1962;44A:591–602.
32. Hibbs RA: An operation for progress in spinal deformities. A preliminary report of three cases from the service of the Orthopaedic Hospital. NY Med J 1911;93:1013–1016.
33. Hodge WA, Dewald RL: Splenic injury complicating the anterior thoraco-abdominal surgical approach for scoliosis. J Bone Joint Surg 1983;65A:396–397.
34. Hodgson AR, Stock FE: Anterior spine fusion for the treatment of tuberculosis of the spine. J Bone Joint Surg 1960;42A:295–310.
35. Holdsworth F: Fractures, dislocations and fracture-dislocations of the spine. J Bone Joint Surg 1970;52A:1534–1551.
36. Humphries AW, Hawk WA, Berndt KL: Anterior fusion of the lumbar spine using an internal fixation device. J Bone Joint Surg 1959;41A:371–376.
37. Johnson RM, McGuire EJ: Urogenital complications of anterior approaches to the lumbar spine. Clin Orthop Rel Res 1981;154:114–118.
38. Kahanovitz N, Bullough P, Jacobs PR: The effect of internal fixation without arthrodesis on human facet joint cartilage. Clin Orthop Rel Res 1984;189:204–208.

39. Kaneda K, Abumi K, Fujiya M: Burst fractures with neurologic deficits of the thoracolumbar spine: Results of anterior decompression and stabilization with anterior instrumentation. Spine 1984;9:788–795.

40. Kostuik JP: Anterior fixation for burst fractures of the thoracic and lumbar spine with or without neurological involvement. Spine 1988;13:286–293.

41. Kostuik JP: Anterior fixation for fractures of thoracic and lumbar spines with or without neurologic involvement. Clin Orthop Rel Res 1984;189:116–124.

42. Kostuik JP: Anterior spinal cord decompression for lesions of the thoracic and lumbar spine: Techniques, new methods of internal fixation and results. Spine 1983;8:512–531.

43. Lange F: Support for the spondylotic spine by means of buried steel bars, attached to the vertebrae. Am J Orthop Surg 1910;8:344–355.

44. Malcolm BW, Bradford DS, Winter RB, et al: Post-traumatic kyphosis: A review of forty-eight surgically treated patients. J Bone Joint Surg 1981;63A:891–899.

45. Mann KA, Found EM, Yuan HA, et al: Biomechanical evaluation of the effectiveness of anterior spinal fixation systems. Orthop Trans 1987;11:378.

46. Mann KA, Yuan HA, Found EM, et al: A biomechanical study of the stability of thoracolumbar anterior decompression surgery and anterior spinal fixation. Spine (in press).

47. Mann KA, McGowan DP, Fredrickson BE, et al: A biomechanical investigation of short segment spinal fixation for burst fractures with varying degrees of posterior disruption. Spine 1990;15:470–478.

48. Martin NS: Pott's paraplegia: A report in 120 cases. J Bone Joint Surg 1971;53B:596–608.

49. McAfee PC, Bohlman HH, Ducker T, et al: Failure of stabilization of the spine with methlymethacrylate. J Bone Joint Surg 1986;68A:1145–1157.

50. McAfee PC, Farey ID, Shirado O, et al: A quantitative histologic study of stress shielding with transpedicular instrumentation: A canine model. Orthop Trans 1990;14:37–38.

51. McAfee PC, Yuan HA, Lasda N: The unstable burst fracture. Spine 1982;7:365–373.

52. Medical Resource Council Working Party on Tuberculosis of the Spine: Five year assessments of controlled trials of ambulatory treatment, debridement and anterior spinal fusion in the management of tuberculosis of the spine: Studies in Bulawayo (Rhodesia) and in Hong Kong. J Bone Joint Surg 1978;60B:163–177.

53. Michel CR, Lalain JJ: Late results of Harrington's operation: Long-term evaluation of the lumbar spine below the fused segments. Spine 1985;10:414–420.

54. Mixter WJ, Barr JS: Rupture of the intervertebral disc with involvement of the spinal canal. NEJM 1934;211:210–215.

55. Newman PH: Editorial: Lumbo-sacral arthrodesis. J Bone Joint Surg 1965;47B:209–210.

56. Olerud S, Karlstrom G, Sjostrom L: Transpedicular fixation of thoracolumbar vertebral fractures. Clin Orthop Rel Res 1988;227:44–51.

57. Roy-Camille R, Saillant G, Mazel C: Internal fixation of the lumbar spine with pedicle screw plating. Clin Orthop Rel Res 1986;203:7–17.

58. Smith GW, Robinson RA: The treatment of certain cervical spine disorders by the anterior removal of the intervertebral disc and interbody fusion. J Bone Joint Surg 1958;40A:607–613.

59. Steffee AD, Biscup RS, Sitakowski DJ: Segmental spine plates with pedicle fixation: A new internal fixation device for disorders of the lumbar and thoracolumbar spine. Clin Orthop Rel Res 1986;203:45–53.

60. von Lackum HL, Smith AF: Removal of vertebral bodies in the treatment of scoliosis. Surg Gynecol Obstet 1933;57:250–256.

61. Werlinich M: Anterior interbody fusion and stabilization with metal fixation. International Surg 1974;59:269–273.

62. White AA: Editorial comment on anterior interbody fusion. In: Lumbar spine surgery. St. Louis: CV Mosby 1990;432.

63. Yuan HA, Donovan D, Edwards W, et al: Contribution of the posterior annular attachments in the reduction of vertebral burst fractures. Presented at Orthopaedic Trauma Assoc. Sixth Annual Meeting, Toronto, CA, 1990;43.

64. Yuan HA, Mann KA, Found EM, et al: Early clinical experience with the Syracuse I-plate: an anterior spinal fixation device. Spine 1988;13:278–285.

65. Zielke K: Derotation and fusion: anterior spinal instrumentation. Presented at the Twelfth Annual Meeting of the Scoliosis Research Society, Hong Kong, 1977.

Kaneda Anterior Spinal Instrumentation for the Thoracic and Lumbar Spine

Kiyoshi Kaneda

INTRODUCTION

Anterior spinal instrumentation for the thoracic and lumbar spine was first applied by Dwyer and colleagues in 1964 for the correction of scoliosis, using a cable and screw system (7,8). The Dwyer system provided limited stability through the compressive effect of one vertebral body against another. The flexible cable resists only the tension force, and the elastic connection of the implants may lead to cable or screw failure, with the development of subsequent pseudarthrosis. Furthermore, kyphosis may result following this type of fixation (5). Zielke and Pellin (30), and Zielke and colleagues (31), modified the Dwyer system by substituting a compression rod with nuts for the cable, and introduced the derotator to correct rotation and kyphosis. The results with Zielke instrumentation in the treatment of thoracolumbar scoliosis were reported by Moe and colleagues (25), Kaneda and coworkers (17), and Puno and colleagues (27).

The Zielke instrumentation system was designed for correction and stabilization of scoliosis. The Zielke system, with its small threaded rod, was not designed originally to withstand the compression force in the anterior vertebral column following subtotal or total corpectomy, or correction of kyphosis.

Hall and Micheli (13) reported a modification of the Dwyer system using a solid rod instead of a cable. Kostuik (21) has reported extensively on the anterior spinal fixation system using a Dwyer-Hall vertebral plate and Harrington distraction rod (anterior Kostuik-Harrington system) in the treatment of spinal fractures. Slot (29) reported a distraction rod instrumentation using the Zielke system for anterior correction of kyphosis. The Dunn device was developed for the treatment of burst fractures (6), but the use of the Dunn device (Type III) was complicated by aortic rupture due to erosion by the device (15). Dunn's work has contributed greatly to the development of anterior spinal devices.

I started the use of my own anterior device (Kaneda device) for reconstruction of the spine following anterior decompression of thoracolumbar burst fractures with neurologic deficit (16,17). This anterior spinal instrumentation system has been developed and improved through extensive clinical experience. Biomechanical testing of the Kaneda device shows favorable results in the literature (9,12,22). Using a corpectomy model of a calf spine, Gurr et al. (12) evaluated the Kaneda device, among others. They found that the Kaneda device, which extends fixation only one vertebral level cephalad and one level caudad to the site of corpectomy, compares favorably with both the Cotrel-Dubousset instrumentation and Steffee transpedicular screw systems, which required incorporation of two additional motion segments. Also, the great stability with the Kaneda device may preclude additional posterior procedures. Furthermore, the Kaneda device does not result in a significant reduction in stability before a solid fusion is achieved, and is not associated with any long-term adverse sequelae related to its proximity to the abdominal viscera.

COMPOSITION OF THE KANEDA ANTERIOR SPINAL DEVICE

The Kaneda anterior spinal device (Fig. 25.1) consists of the vertebral plate, vertebral screw, paravertebral rod, nut, and transverse fixators. The vertebral plate has tetra-spikes, which are fixed into the lateral vertebral body. The vertebral screw is tapered and self-tapping with a neck diameter of 6.0 mm. The diameter of the paravertebral rod is 5.5 mm. The nuts are fixed into the screw head holes on the rod from both sides. The top and bottom vertebral bodies are fixed with an ordinary plate

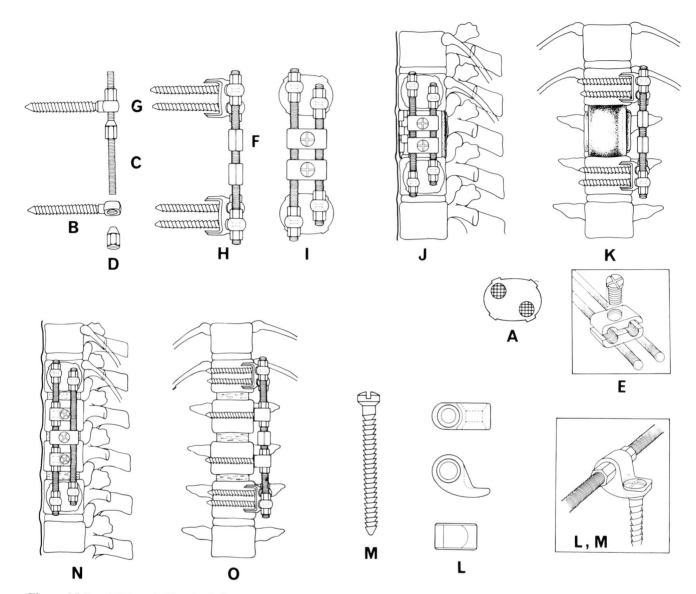

Figure 25.1. CKD. *A*, Vertebral plate. *B*, Vertebral screw. *C*, Paravertebral rod. *D*, Nut. *E* and *F*, Transverse fixators. *G*, Relationship between the screwhead hole and nuts. *H* and *I*, Final construction of the implants. *J* and *K*, Application of the Kaneda device to the 12th thoracic vertebral body and the 2nd lumbar vertebral body. *L* and *M*, One-hole vertebral plate and screw for multisegmental fixation. *N* and *O*, Multisegmental fixation.

and screws, and the vertebral bodies between the top and the bottom are fixed with the one-hole vertebral plate and screw. The anterior and posterior paravertebral rods are coupled with the transverse fixators. The rod of the multisegmental fixation system is flexible (the rod diameter is 4.0 mm). If the deformity is easily correctable, the rigid paravertebral rod will be applicable.

The Kaneda device can withstand both compressive and distractive forces. Either compressive or distractive forces can be applied by turning the nuts on the rods.

Biomechanically, the transverse fixators are very important for elimination of rotatory and flexion-extension instability.

INDICATIONS FOR THE KANEDA DEVICE IN THE THORACOLUMBAR SPINE

Anterior procedures in the thoracolumbar spine are generally done for spinal canal decompression and for stabilization. Specific indications may include deficient bone anteriorly to trauma, tumor, infection, degenerative disease, congenital causes, or deformity. Kyphosis following laminectomy or posttraumatic kyphosis should also be approached anteriorly. The Kaneda device has been utilized for all of the above indications, and the use of this device for injuries, degenerative diseases, deformity, and tumor will be discussed in this chapter.

Indications for the Kaneda Device in Thoracolumbar Spinal Injuries

The recent classification of thoracolumbar spinal injuries has been based on the mechanism of injury to the middle column. Denis (1,2), and McAfee and coworkers (24) discussed the importance of the middle column in determining the stability of an injured spine. The authors' classification of thoracolumbar spinal injuries is as follows:

1. Wedge compression fractures (anterior, lateral);
2. Burst fractures (Type A–E, according to Denis' classification);
3. Flexion-distraction injuries (chance fracture, seatbelt type: one- or two-level lesions);
4. Combined type of burst fracture and flexion-distraction injury;
5. Fracture-dislocations (flexion-rotation, flexion-distraction, and shear); and
6. Isolated fractures of the posterior element.

Combined type of burst fracture and flexion-distraction injury in this classification has not been reported yet. The mechanism of this injury appears to be a combination of axial load followed by flexion-distraction force, disrupting both the middle and posterior columns. In the author's series, this type of injury usually results from being thrown out of a car or from falling from a significant height. In the treatment of this type of injury, posterior instrumentation procedures utilizing a compressive force may result in worsening of neurologic status by increasing the retropulsion of bony fragments in the spinal canal. Anterior decompression and stabilization are the initial treatments of choice, but in some cases, posterior stabilization with instrumentation may have to be added for additional stability.

Fracture-dislocations (translational injury with vertebral body comminution (24) and the combined burst and flexion-distraction injury are unstable injuries due to the loss of the posterior and the middle column. All acute fracture-dislocations should be managed posteriorly by utilizing segmental or transpedicular instrumentations.

Flexion-distraction injuries are associated with a disruption of the posterior column; therefore, posterior compression stabilization should be performed. Neurologic deficits following thoracolumbar spinal injuries (except for fracture dislocations) are usually due to anterior spinal canal impingement by retropulsed bone or disc fragments. Anterior spinal canal decompression is therefore indicated in these cases. This approach allows decompression and correction of deformity under direct vision. Since kyphosis may be a contributory factor to neurologic compromise this deformity should be corrected surgically.

Burst fractures of L-3 or above can be treated effectively by anterior decompression and stabilization with the Kaneda device as a single-stage operation. This device affords enough stability to enable early ambulation with the maintenance of anatomic alignment and progression to a solid fusion (18).

Burst fractures at L4 or L5 with a neurologic deficit can be managed successfully by posterior decompression and stabilization. Recently, reduction of the retropulsed bony fragments into the spinal canal by application of distraction force has been attempted with various transpedicular screw systems (3,4). Gertzbein and colleagues (11) reported on spinal canal clearance in burst fractures using the Synthes (AO) internal fixator. They concluded that ligamentotaxis is most efficient when carried out in the first 4 days. The best improvement in clearance was apparent in cases with an initial canal compromise of 34–66%; however, the extent of improvement, even in this group, is not dramatic, with an average of 31% encroachment still remaining and, in some cases, as high as 50%. Therefore, they recommended that when canal clearance is essential, anterior decompression is the treatment of choice.

All fresh fracture-dislocations should be treated by posterior reduction and stabilization with instrumentation. However, old fracture-dislocations having an incomplete neurologic deficit with or without progressive kyphosis are best treated by anterior spinal canal decompression, correction of kyphosis, and stabilization. Rarely, some patients with a residual kyphosis following anterior decompression and fusion will require a posterior fusion and instrumentation. Also, chronic wedge compression fractures or flexion-distraction injuries with severe kyphosis but without neurologic deficit cannot be handled adequately by a posterior procedure alone. They require anterior correction and stabilization. Posterior approach alone in this type of posttraumatic kyphosis will be inadequate in the correction of kyphosis, and relapse may also occur due to anterior instability. If neurologic deficit is associated with this type of posttraumatic kyphosis, anterior reconstruction with the Kaneda device will be indicated following anterior decompression and correction of kyphosis.

Lately, compression of the spinal cord or the cauda

equina due to osteoporotic vertebral collapse with kyphosis has been reported by many authors (14,19,20,23). We have treated 28 patients with this problem by anterior decompression and stabilization with correction of kyphosis. The tricortical iliac crest was too weak and thin to be used as an anterior strut graft between the vertebral bodies above and below the resection; therefore, a bioactive ceramic vertebral spacer (A.W. glass ceramic: artificial ceramic vertebral body) and the Kaneda device for reconstruction were used. The iliac crest or fibula was poor in maintaining the correction of kyphosis because the bone graft tends to collapse into the osteoporotic vertebral body. The artificial ceramic vertebral body with wide cross-sectional area has maintained correction of kyphosis while attaining a bonding at the ceramic-bone interface.

Thoracolumbar Degenerative Diseases with Neurologic Deficit

Degenerative disc disease or spondylosis may be associated with the spinal cord compromise at the thoracolumbar spine. The causes of the spinal cord compression are disc herniation, posterior vertebral osteophyte, or ossification of the posterior longitudinal ligament. Posterior decompression of the spinal cord through the spinal canal is not safe in this area. The most suitable procedure is a direct anterior decompression, correction of any spinal malalignment, bone graft fusion, and stabilization with the Kaneda device.

Thoracolumbar and Lumbar Scoliosis or Kyphosis

The Kaneda anterior multisegmental device may be used for thoracolumbar scoliosis or thoracolumbar kyphoscoliosis (idiopathic, posttraumatic, congenital, neurogenic, or other causes). Postoperative maintenance of correction has been satisfactory in 12 cases for over 2 years. We have previously demonstrated satisfactory properties of the Kaneda multisegmental anterior device (the flexible rod diameter is 4.0 mm; two-rod system) biomechanically) (26). Both Dwyer and Zielke instrumentations can correct scoliosis in the AP plane, but iatrogenic kyphosis may result. In our small series treating thoracolumbar scoliosis with the Kaneda multisegmental systems, kyphosis in the fusion area has not been observed. This appears to be secondary to biomechanical stability in all planes. A larger series with longer follow-up will be needed before further conclusions are made.

Spinal Tumors (Primary or Metastatic)

Of the primary malignant tumors, multiple myeloma, Ewing's sarcoma, malignant lymphoma, chondrosarcoma, chordoma, and osteosarcoma have been encountered. The first three are treated effectively by radiation or chemotherapy, or both. Osteosarcoma is quite uncommon. In a patient with osteosarcoma, cure is usually not a realistic goal, and treatment should also consist of radiation and systemic chemotherapy. Salvage surgery may consist of decompression or posterior stabilization. Chordoma in the thoracolumbar spine is rare. If a resectable primary malignant tumor is associated with bony destruction and neurologic damage, anterior reconstruction with the Kaneda device and bone grafting is indicated following en bloc resection or total spondylectomy.

Metastatic tumors to the spine are relatively easy to diagnose, but proper management may be challenging. Problems associated with metastatic tumors in the spine are pain, instability, or neurologic compromise. At present, treatment of metastatic tumors to the spine is palliative. Therefore, it is usually directed at reducing pain, enhancing structural stability, and improving or at least maintaining neurologic function (10).

When surgical intervention is required to restore stability or protect against anticipated loss, it must be carefully planned to reestablish the structural deficit. Acute compromise of the spinal cord or cauda equina function by tumor may necessitate surgical decompression, which may itself further impair stability. The posterior surgical approaches are technically easier for reconstruction of the metastatic tumor of the spine and may offer better immediate stability than the anterior approaches. But the main lesion of the metastatic spine tumor is usually located anteriorly in the vertebral body. Laminectomy only for decompression may bring about temporary improvement of neural function, but it will result in increase of instability and kyphosis with deterioration of neurologic status. Patients with metastatic spinal tumor can be benefited by aggressive anterior decompression and stabilization procedures, when appropriate (10).

Indications for anterior decompression to spinal metastasis with neurologic deficit should depend on the nature of the tumor, the neurologic status, the three-dimensional anatomy of the metastatic vertebra, and the patient's general status. We have performed anterior decompression and reconstruction with a ceramic vertebral body and the Kaneda device for metastatic tumors. All patients were treated preoperatively with chemotherapy and radiation, which minimized tumor size and bleeding during surgery. All the patients who received anterior reconstructive surgery with a ceramic vertebral body and the Kaneda device showed improvement in their quality of life due to decreased pain, restoration of spinal stability, and improvement or maintenance of neural function.

SURGICAL TECHNIQUES

The patient is placed in the right lateral decubitus position approaching the left portion of the spine below T9 or T10 and in the left lateral decubitus position above T9 or T10 (Fig. 25.2A). Maintenance of a secure position is essential during the procedure, using a firm strapping or positioners. Peripheral nerves should be protected, and the iliac crest or the fibula must be available for bone graft harvesting.

The anterior approach utilized depends on the level of the vertebral lesion (Fig. 25.2B and C). The thoracolumbar junction (T12, L1) is usually approached by the extrapleural (or transpleural) and retroperitoneal route. The thoracic vertebral bodies above T9 or T10 are usually exposed by thoracotomy, and the lumbar spine by the retroperitoneal approach. Application of the Kaneda device should be on the lateral aspect of the vertebral bodies (on the right side above T9 or T10 due to the thoracic aorta, and on the left side below T9 or T10). Placing the Kaneda vertebral plate anterolaterally increases the risk of canal penetration by the screw; therefore, the plates should be fixed on the lateral aspect of the vertebral bodies. The segmental vessels in the area of dissection are ligated and cut. The iliopsoas muscle is bluntly dissected

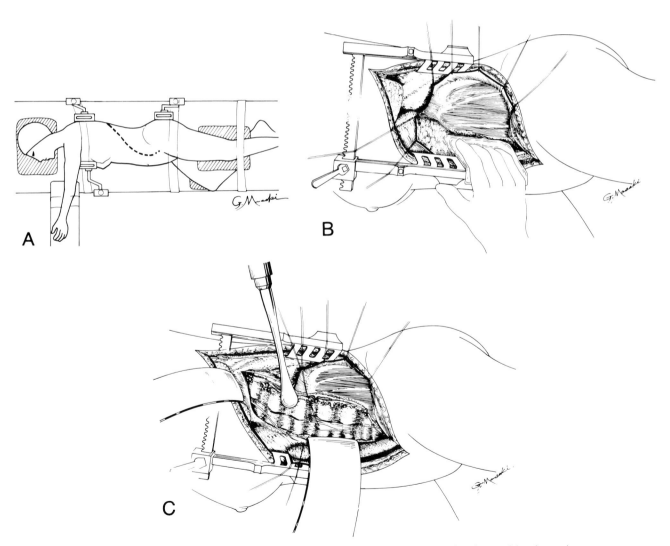

Figure 25.2. *A,* Patient's positioning. *B* and *C,* Exposure of the thoracolumbar and lumbar spine.

off the spinal segments to be instrumented. The lateral aspect of the vertebral bodies must be well exposed for proper application of the Kaneda device implants.

The lateral aspect of the spinal column opposite the area of the exposure should be gently exposed with a finger or a long-handle nerve root retractor, and a thick sponge should be packed to protect the great vessels. The great vessels and the psoas muscle are gently retracted to fully expose the vertebral bodies. Next, the discs above and below the lesion are meticulously excised. Hemostasis is assured throughout by cautery, bone wax, and gelfoam (Fig. 25.3A).

The vertebral body with lesion is then excised in the area, as shown on the inset. At first, the vertebra is excised with a chisel or an osteotome (Fig. 25.3B). Anterior spinal canal decompression is performed using instruments such as gouges, curettes, rongeurs, or air-powered instruments. The spinal canal is approached through the neural foramen. The retropulsed bone or pathological lesion should be completely removed to decompress the dural sac. During this procedure, posterior longitudinal ligament is usually left intact, unless there is a specific indication to remove it. Removal of the posterior longitudinal ligament may result in significant bleeding from the epidural vein (Fig. 25.3C).

Once the decompression is complete, appropriate-sized

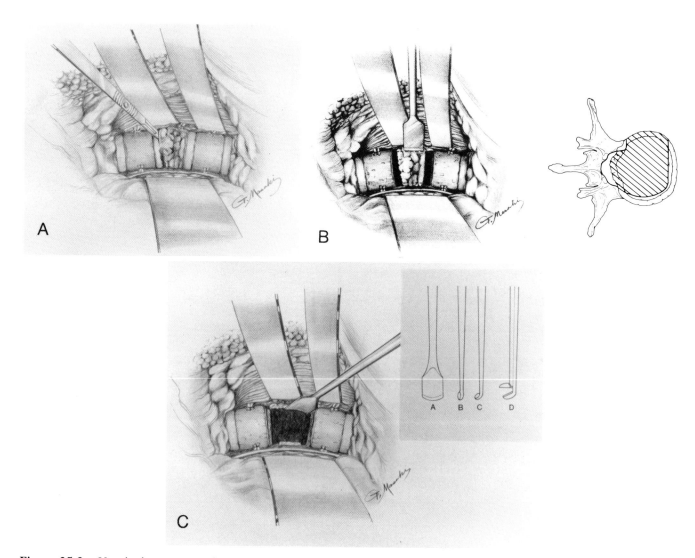

Figure 25.3.   Vertebral exposure and vertebrectomy for anterior decompression. *A,* Excision of the discs above and below the injury. *B,* Excision of the vertebral body with lesion. The inlet shows the area of vertebrectomy. *C,* Anterior decompression using several kinds of instruments (gouge, *A,* curette, *B* and *C,* and curette punch-pituitary rongeur, *D*).

vertebral plates are tapped into place, holding the plate with the plate holder. The plate must be positioned so that a trapezoidal configuration of the Kaneda construct is created. This means that the anterior rod of the Kaneda device should be longer than the posterior rod (Fig. 25.4A).

The posterior screw is directed 10–15° anteriorly away from the spinal canal. The anterior screw must be directed transversely to the frontal plane across the vertebral body, thereby triangulating the fixation. The screw must be driven home so that the base of the screw head contacts firmly the vertebral plate (Fig. 25.4B).

The transverse diameter of the vertebral body is measured in order to choose the most appropriate screw length, using the vertebral gauge. Direct palpation on the contralateral side must be performed to ensure penetration of the screw tip and so that the penetrated screw tip does not protrude beyond the vertebral body more than 2 or 3 mm, and to guarantee that its path is straight across the vertebral body. Great care must be taken during palpation to avoid injury to the contralateral segmental vessels or the great vessels (Fig. 25.4C).

Once the screws are in place and the length is proper, correction of the kyphotic deformity is achieved by the use of the spreader between the anterior-most screwhead holes. If the kyphotic deformity cannot be corrected because of tension in the contractured anterior longitudinal ligament in old posttraumatic kyphosis, the ligament should be divided at the disc level using an angled curette-rongeur, which is safer than other instruments. The defect following vertebrectomy is then measured with the intervertebral scale, and an appropriate-length tricortical iliac crest is obtained to fill the defect (Fig. 25.4D).

If distraction force is applied between the two screwhead holes above and below with the spreader (Fig. 25.4D) in a fresh burst fracture associated with a flexion-distraction injury, the posterior column will be widened. To avoid this complication, the posterior rod should be applied first, before the spreader is applied to the anterior screw holes. The rod attached to the posterior screwhead holes will work as a fulcrum when correcting kyphosis, thereby avoiding an increase in the posterior horizontal split (flexion-distraction injury), and will, in fact, usually approximate the deficit (Fig. 25.4E).

Bone grafting should be done in a meticulous manner. Bone grafts consisting of the tricortical iliac crest, the rib strut taken during exposure, and the bone chips from the resected vertebral body are inserted (Fig. 25.4F). The iliac crest should be strong, wide, and long enough to share load with the implants. If the fibular strut graft is used with an iliac crest, the strut will be much stronger. The tricortical iliac crest and the rib struts are tapped into place. Bone chips are packed into the defect between the

anterior bony wall and the iliac crest with a bone impactor. Gelfoam is used over the posterior longitudinal ligament or the dura (Fig. 25.4G).

Appropriate-length paraspinal rods that span the screw holes above and below are chosen. Before insertion into the holes of the screwheads, the inner nuts are placed in proper orientation on the rods (Fig. 25.4H). Once the distal-end nuts are added, a compression force is applied to the strut graft by tightening the nuts on the proximal and distal end of each paraspinal rod. The importance of this maneuver cannot be overemphasized. The Kaneda device relies directly on the load transmission through the strut graft with healthy, strong tricortical iliac crest graft for secure fixation and for long-term healing. If firm compression on the graft for secure fixation and for long-term healing is not provided during instrumentation, the construct will fail.

The transverse fixators (the rod coupler) are applied to the paravertebral rods, creating a rectangular configuration. The deeper side of the transverse fixator is introduced with the holder. The inlet shows the holder and a piece of the transverse fixator (Fig. 25.4I).

Once two sets of the transverse fixators are applied firmly, the nuts must be tightened firmly to secure the rod-screwhead junctions. Overcompression may create an iatrogenic scoliosis; consequently, after tightening the nuts and the transverse fixators properly, AP x-rays should be obtained. Any lateral curvature may be corrected by adjusting the nuts. Once the instrumentation has been completed, the appropriate closing procedures should be performed step by step.

Postoperatively, the patient may ambulate with a polypropylene thoracolumbosacral orthosis (TLSO) 3–4 days after surgery. Usually, a brace will be worn for 20–24 weeks.

Surgical Techniques with the Kaneda Multisegmental Fixation Device for Thoracolumbar Spondylosis

At the lower thoracic, thoracolumbar, and upper lumbar spine (T10-T11 to L1-L2 disc levels), disc herniation or spondylosis with neurologic deficit is not rare. Neural decompression in these areas is not safe if done posteriorly; hence, we perform anterior decompression and stabilization.

In most patients with thoracolumbar spondylosis, there is a kyphotic deformity with instability over several intervertebral disc levels. Anterior reconstruction with the Kaneda multisegmental fixation device has brought about correction of kyphosis and stabilization following anterior decompression. Anterior decompression in this type of pathology is achieved by discectomy and/or resection

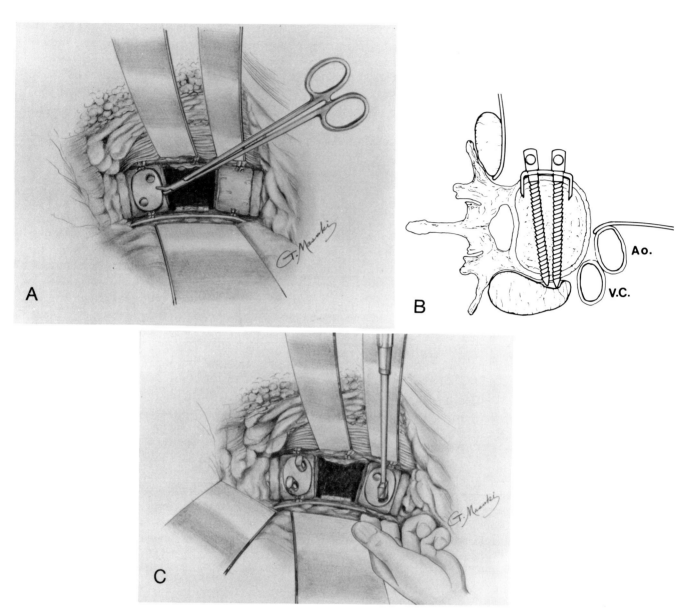

Figure 25.4. *A,* Application of the vertebral plate. *B,* Direction of the screw insertion. *C,* Checking for penetration of the screw chip on the contralateral vertebral cortex. *D,* Correction of kyphosis and insertion of an iliac crest as a strut. *E,* Correction of kyphosis in patients with combined burst fracture and flex- ion-distraction injury. *F,* Transverse section of bone grafting (*X,* iliac crest, *Y,* rib, *Z,* bone chip from the resected vertebral body). *G,* Bone grafting. *H,* Application of the paraspinal rods. *I,* Application of the transverse fixators and tightening of the nuts.

of the posterior vertebral osteophytes. Therefore, stabi- lization is attained by interbody fusion at multiple disc spaces instead of anterior strut grafting following verte- brectomy. Following decompression, the ordinary ver- tebral plates are fixed to the most cephalad and caudal vertebral bodies. Next, the 5.5-mm rod with a one-hole plate(s) and nut(s) is inserted into the screwhead holes on the top and bottom vertebrae. The nuts are attached on the rod at both ends. Tightening the nuts in the cor-

rected position is conducted after bone grafting of the intervertebral spaces with iliac bone and/or rib. Three-dimensional correction of the spinal column align- ment is then performed. Following application of the posterior rod, the anterior rod application is performed by the same procedures. Correction of kyphosis is per- formed by bone grafting into the intervertebral spaces and by turning the nuts after fixation of the one-hole plate to every intermediate vertebral body. Every level is

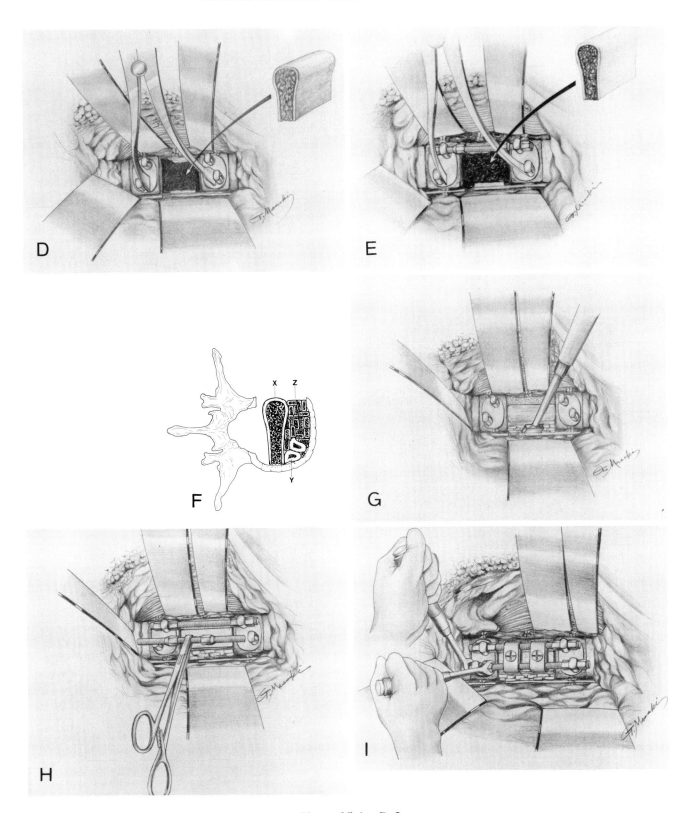

Figure 25.4. *D–I.*

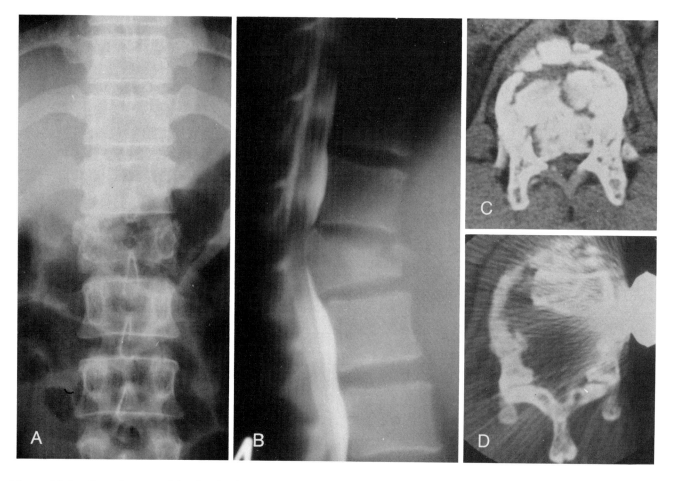

Figure 25.5. Burst fracture of the first lumbar vertebra with neurologic deficit in a 26-year-old man. *A,* Preoperative AP view. *B,* Myelography. *C,* Preoperative CT scan. *D,* Postoperative CT scan. *E* and *F,* Postoperative scans 4 years later. The meylography and preoperative CT showed the spinal canal com- promise with retropulsed massive bony fragments. *D,* Shows complete removal of the spinal canal fragments by anterior de- compression. *E* and *F* show complete reconstruction with solid fusion and good alignment.

secured to the rod with two screws. It is possible to correct both kyphosis and scoliosis, but adequate bone grafting of the resected disc spaces cannot be overem- phasized.

Kaneda Device for Thoracolumbar or Lumbar Scoliosis

After resecting the discs in the fusion area, the ordinary vertebral plates are fixed on the top and bottom vertebral bodies. If the scoliotic curve is rigid, the flexible rod (measuring 4 mm in diameter) is used with the one-hole plates and nuts on the intermediate levels. The curve is relatively flexible, the semirigid rod (5.5-mm diameter) is used. After inserting the rod into the screwhead holes on the most cephalad and caudal vertebral bodies, a compression force is applied to correct scoliosis. After packing bone chips (usually sectioned rib) into the disc spaces, a screw is inserted into each intermediate vertebral body, and the nuts are tightened on the rod, while ap- plying force at the scoliotic/kyphotic apex for correction of deformity. Zielke derotator instrumentation can be used, as described in the Zielke technique manual. In the author's experience, pushing the hump with the assistant's palm is very helpful. An AP x-ray is taken before closure to check the lateral curvature as overcorrection may occur in a flexible curve.

Postoperatively, a thoracolumbosacral orthosis is uti- lized for 20–24 weeks. The external orthosis may perhaps be omitted when considering the results of the biome- chanical tests, but postoperative bracing is still recom- mended in clinical practice.

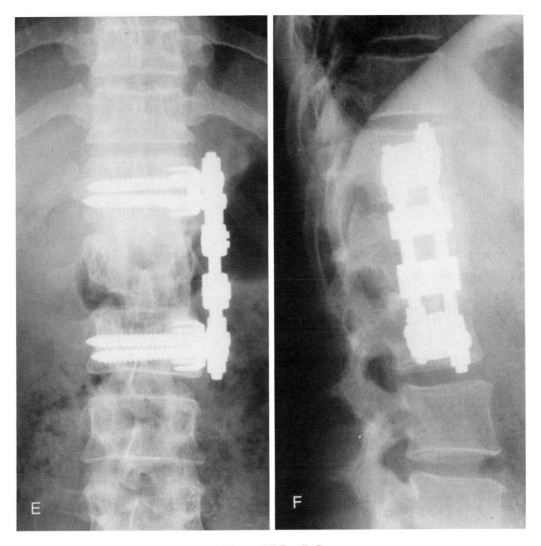

Figure 25.5. *E–F.*

RESULTS WITH THE KANEDA DEVICE

Thoracolumbar Burst Fractures with Neurologic Deficit

The main indication for the Kaneda device in the treatment of spinal injuries is thoracolumbar burst fractures with or without neurologic deficit. The author described the results in his series of the first 100 consecutive patients who had sustained a thoracolumbar burst fracture with neurologic deficit. All of them were treated by anterior decompression and reconstruction with the Kaneda device between 1980–1985. These results were reported at the Annual Meeting of the American Academy of Orthopaedic Surgeons, Anaheim, CA, 1991. The materials were as follows: During 1980–1985, 100 consecutive patients (72 males, 28 females) who sustained thoraco-

lumbar burst fracture with neurologic deficit were treated by the surgical procedures described. Ages at surgery ranged from 13–69 years, with an average of 41 years and 4 months. Time from injury to surgery was within 2 weeks in 20 patients, 2 weeks-1 month in 24, and over 1 month in 56. The onset of neurologic deficit was immediate after injury in 86 patients, and delayed from 1 month–16 years with an average of 4 months in 14. The levels of fractures included 14 T12, 51 L1, 21 L2, 7 L3, 4 L4, 1 T12-L1, 1 L1-L2, and 1 L3-L4. Classification by Denis (1) was Type A (24%), Type B (59%), Type C (5%), Type D (8%), and Type E (4%). All of the patients were followed-up except for one who died from bleeding due to rupture of an esophageal varice at 2 years and 7 months after surgery. The length of follow-up was 42–98 months, with an average of 4 years and 5 months

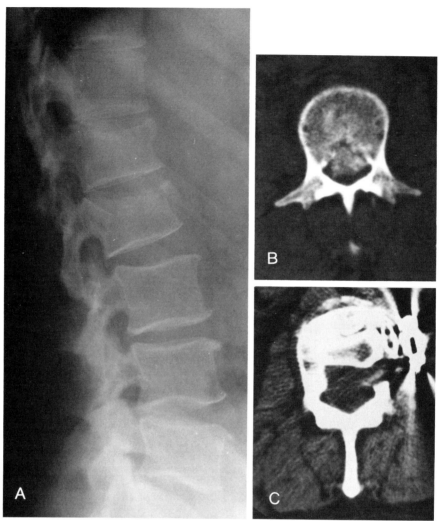

Figure 25.6. Burst fracture of the first lumbar vertebra with neurologic deficit and compression fracture of the 12th thoracic vertebra in a 54-year-old man; *A*, Preoperative CT scan. *B* and *C*, Pre- and postoperative CT scan. *D* and *E*, At follow-up, postoperative scans 2 years and 7 months later. Anterior spinal canal decompression and multilevel fusion (interbody fusion at T12-L1 and iliac crest strut graft at L1-L3) with the Kaneda device resulted in satisfactory neurologic recovery and stable fusion with good alignment.

after surgery. The preoperative Frankel grade in 90 patients (excluding 10 who had lesion of the pure conus medullaris) were: A, 2; B, 5; C, 4; and D, 79. These improved to: A, 2; B, 0; C, 1; D, 8; and E, 79. Postoperatively, no patients showed neurologic deterioration. Sixty patients (spinal cord injury in 42 and cauda equina injury in 18) had a bladder dysfunction preoperatively. Their recovery at follow-up was complete (no difficulty in urination) in 48, incomplete (occasional incontinence, but no need for self-catheterization) in 5, and no recovery (self-catheterization) in 7.

Radiologic evaluations of bony union were assessed by the functional x-rays (flexion-extension lateral) and oc-casionally by tomograms. In the first 54 consecutive patients, the transverse fixators (Figure 25.1*E*, *F*) were not used, and in the second 46 consecutive patients, the transverse fixators were applied. The solid fusion rate was 88.9% (48 of 54) in the former group and 95.7% in the latter. This difference was statistically significant (p < 0.01). Their relationship between the fracture levels and the pseudarthrosis rate was as follows: 0:14 at T12; 0:51 at L1; 2:21 at L2 (9.5%), 3:7 at L3 (42.9%), and 3:4 at L4 (75%). Each of the eight patients with pseud-arthrosis was treated successfully by posterior fusion with instrumentation in the same area as the anterior fusion. Kyphosis was present in 92 patients at the time of ad-

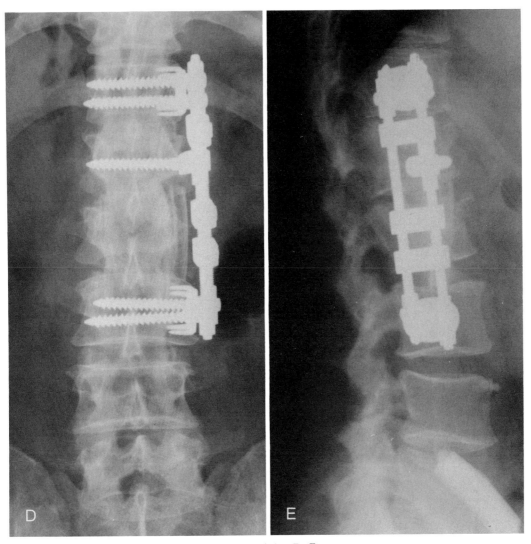

Figure 25.6. *D–E.*

mission. In the early surgery group, within 1 month after injury (48 patients), the average kyphosis was 18.5° (12–24°) preoperatively, 6.6° at discharge (0–11°), and 7.3° (0–12°) at follow-up. In the late surgery group (52 patients) over 1 month after injury, the average kyphosis was 21.9° (16–44°) preoperatively, 10.3° (0–18°) at discharge, and 12.1° (0–24°) at follow-up. Loss of correction in kyphosis was below 2°. Complications were not serious, except one with postoperative deep infection, who had severe urinary tract infection preoperatively. This patient developed pseudarthrosis, which was managed successfully by appropriate antibiotic therapy and posterior fusion with instrumentation. Hardware failures occurred in seven of eight patients with pseudarthrosis. Screw breakage accounted for six failures, while a rod and screw breakage occurred in one. No implant has been

removed, as all pseudarthroses have been successfully repaired by posterior fusion with instrumentation in the same area (solid fusion was obtained in all at follow-up). One death without any relation to surgery was noted at 2 years and 7 months after surgery after returning to work. There were no vascular or iatrogenic neurologic complications.

Case 1 (Fig. 25.5):

This 26-year-old man sustained a lesion of the conus medullaris and the cauda equina by burst fracture of the first lumbar vertebra. His neurologic status was Frankel C with bladder dysfunction. He was transferred to us 5 days after injury. The preoperative myelogram and CT scan demonstrated compression of the spinal cord with the massive retropulsed bony fragments. Anterior decompression by the extrapleural and retroperitoneal approach was conducted. The postoperative CT scan showed complete removal of the fragments in the spinal canal. Neurologic recovery was remarkable. At the final follow-up of 4 years, motor function in the lower extremities and the bladder-bowel function were almost normal. Spinal stability and alignment were well maintained.

Case 2 (Fig. 25.6):

This 56-year-old man fell down from a height and sustained an L1 compression fracture and an L2 burst fracture with a lesion of the cauda equina (Frankel D). Anterior decompression and

iliac crest strut graft at L1-L3 and interbody fusion at T12-L1 were conducted with the Kaneda device (multisegmental fixation system) 7 days after the injury. Spinal canal decompression was complete. Neurologic recovery was prompt and complete at the final follow-up, 3 years postoperatively. Spinal reconstruction was stable with a good alignment. One of the grafted ribs did not incorporate due to separation.

In treatment of thoracolumbar burst fractures with neurologic deficit, anterior decompression and reconstruction with the Kaneda device as a one-stage operation resulted in acceptable improvement and establishment of a stable corrected spine.

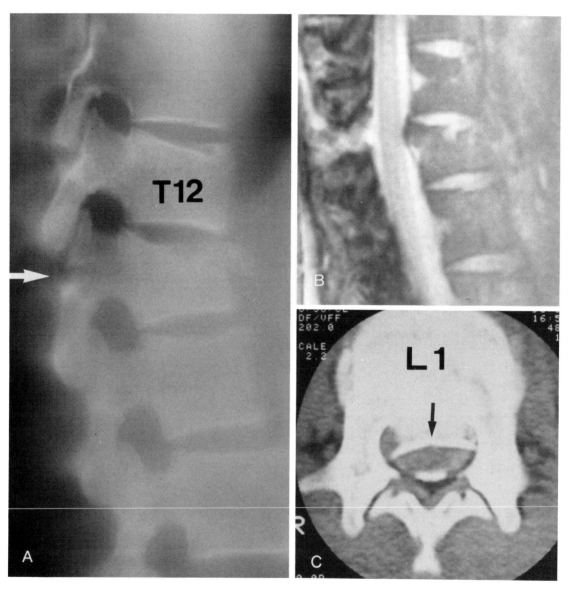

Figure 25.7. Combined type of burst fracture with flexion-distraction injury at the first lumbar vertebra with neurologic deficit in a 29-year-old woman. *A*, Preoperative tomogram. *B*, Preoperative MRI showed posterior horizontal splitting (flexion-distraction injury). *C*, Preoperative CT and MRI scans show a burst fracture with the retropulsed bony fragments in the spinal canal. *D* and *E*, Postoperative scans; 3 years later, stabilization and spinal alignment seem to be complete. Neurologic status became normal.

Posterior reinforcement was not necessary, except in patients with pseduarthrosis. Anterior decompression and stabilization with the Kaneda device are recommended for treatment of thoracolumbar burst fractures above L4 with or without neurologic deficit. The L5 burst fracture cannot be stabilized with the Kaneda device or any other anterior device because of the iliac vessels.

Combined Flexion-Distraction Injury and Burst Fracture

This specific injury, especially when complicated by a neurologic deficit, poses challenges at surgery. If posterior compression instrumentation is applied for reduction of the posterior horizontal injury (flexion-distraction injury at the posterior column), retropulsion of bone may increase due to the compression force. On the other hand, simple distraction force will worsen the posterior horizontal gap and increase the kyphotic deformity. If this type of spinal injury is combined with a neurologic deficit, anterior decompression and anterior spinal reconstruction should be considered. In a severe posterior injury associated with a dislocation or translation, anterior instrumentation alone may be inadequate to achieve enough stability; therefore, posterior reinforcement should be considered. In the author's series of 25 patients who sustained combined burst fracture and flex-

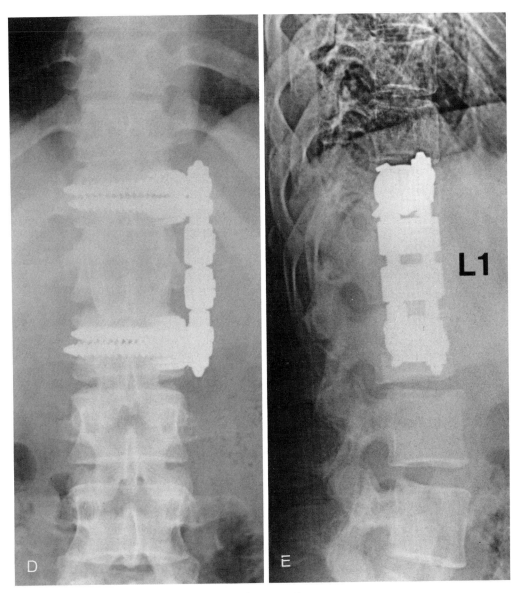

Figure 25.7. *D–E.*

ion-distraction injury with neurologic deficit, all patients were treated by anterior decompression and stabilization with the Kaneda device. Two patients showed increasing kyphosis postoperatively due to instability in the posterior column. Accordingly, posterior instrumentation with fusion was added. Twenty-three of 25 patients have obtained solid fusion with correction of kyphosis, and each one demonstrated improvement. As described in the section on surgical technique, application of the posterior rod before undertaking correction of kyphosis with spreader should be conducted. Then posterior rod will work as a fulcrum in correcting kyphosis.

Case 3 (Fig. 25.7):

This 29-year-old woman jumped from a second floor window. Immediately after the injury, she sustained lesion of the conus medullaris and the cauda equina. A preoperative lateral tomogram, CT and MRI scans revealed a flexion-distraction injury and burst fracture. The arrow on the laminogram shows the posterior horizontal splitting, and CT scan illustrates retropulsion of the posterior vertebral body into the spinal canal. Anterior decompression and stabilization with the Kaneda device resulted in stable reconstruction with correction of kyphosis.

VERTEBRAL COLLAPSE WITH NEUROLOGIC DEFICIT IN THE OSTEOPOROSIS SPINE

Between 1986 and 1989, 28 patients with osteoporosis had posttraumatic vertebral collapse (Kuemmell disease). All were followed for over 1 year after surgery. Posterior reinforcement with instrumentation and fusion was added in three patients because the bioactive ceramic vertebral spacer was collapsing into the vertebral body above or below. There was no clear zone between the ceramic spacer and the vertebral bodies in 16 of 28 patients including the presence of newly formed bone or autogenous grafted bone. Nine patients had a "clear zone" between the vertebral body and the ceramic, but they did not demonstrate abnormal motion or displacement of the ceramic vertebral spacer. Bonding between the ceramic surface and the vertebral bone is usually recognizable by x-ray 12–18 months after surgery. The Kaneda device provides the initial stabilization between the vertebral bodies and the ceramic surfaces. This is absolutely essential for obtaining the biologic bonding between the bioactive ceramic spacer and bone. At surgery, bone cement (methyl methacrylate acetate) was applied to the screw holes if fixation was inadequate due to osteoporosis.

From our preliminary survey, the combination of the Kaneda device and a bioactive ceramic vertebral spacer (artificial vertebral body) has provided a reliable construct following anterior decompression and correction of kyphosis in osteoporotic patients. Reconstructive surgery may be difficult in patients with osteoporotic vertebral collapse and neurologic deficit, if both the Kaneda device and the bioactive ceramic vertebral spacer are not available.

Case 4 (Fig. 25.8):

A 66-year-old female sustained a T12 vertebral compression fracture following mild trauma and was treated with a brace. Three months after the injury, she complained of leg weakness and urinary difficulty. Her thoracolumbar kyphosis increased gradually along with back pain. At admission, she had neurogenic bladder with paresis of both the legs and feet (Frankel D). Her preoperative films disclosed spinal cord compression by a T12 burst fracture with osteoporosis. She was treated with an anterior decompression and reconstruction with the Kaneda device. The iliac crest was too soft and thin to be used as a strut graft in the gap after removal of the crushed vertebral body; therefore, a bioactive A.W. glass ceramic vertebral spacer was utilized. Recent follow-up (3 years and 4 months) revealed that she was neurologically intact, and her reconstructed spine was stable, maintaining correction of her kyphosis (from preoperative 29° to 13°). The implanted bioactive ceramic spacer was surrounded firmly with the incorporated grafted autogenous bone (Fig. 25.8).

THORACOLUMBAR DEGENERATIVE DISEASES

During these 5 years, 18 patients with neurologic deficit due to thoracolumbar spondylosis were treated by anterior decompression and reconstruction with the Kaneda device. Anterior decompression, by discectomy and resection of the posterior vertebral osteophytes with or without vertebrectomy was performed. The Kaneda multisegmental fixation system was used in 10 of 18 patients, and all resulted in a solid bony fusion. Neurologic recovery depended upon the preoperative status, and there was no neurologic deterioration.

Case 5 (Fig. 25.9):

This 52-year-old female presented with neurogenic bladder, severe perineal pain, and difficulty in walking due to paraparesis. She had noticed her leg weakness for about 2 years before admission. The preoperative examinations on MRI, myelogram and myelogram/CT disclosed compression of the epiconus medullaris, the conus medullaris, and the cauda equina, by the vertebral osteophytes and a bulged disc at T11-T12, T12-L1 and L1-L2, respectively. These intervertebral disc spaces were slightly unstable. Anterior decompression and stabilization, as described, were performed. At follow-up, her neurologic findings were almost completely normal, and anterior fusion with the Kaneda device from T11-L2 was solid.

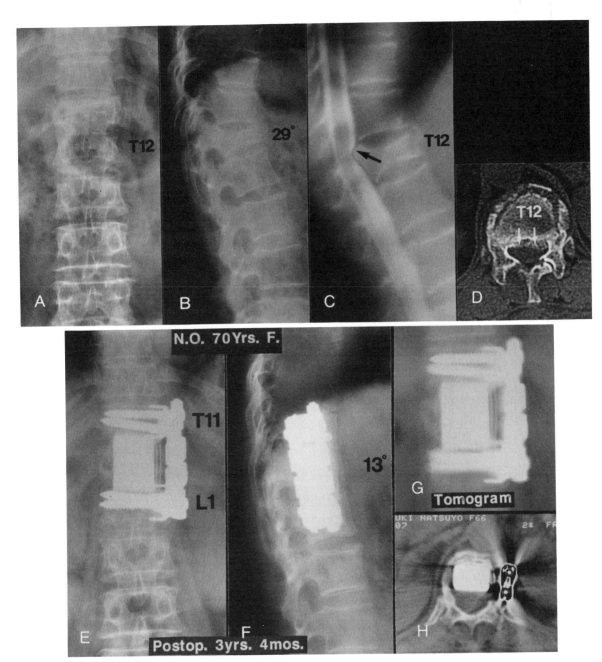

Figure 25.8. Vertebral collapse with neurologic deficit due to osteoporosis in a 66-year-old woman. *A* and *B*, Preoperative scans. *C* and *D*, Preoperative myelography and CT scan showed spinal cord compression at the 12th thoracic vertebra with the retropulsed bony mass. *E*, *F*, and *G*, Postoperative films showed solid fusion. *G*, Postoperative tomogram demonstrated firm bonding between vertebral body and the bioactive A. W.-glass ceramic artificial vertebral body. *H*, Postoperative CT scan showed no displacement or migration of the the ceramic to the spinal canal.

THORACOLUMBAR OR LUMBAR SCOLIOSIS

Indications for the Kaneda multisegmental fixation system in scoliosis are the same as for the Zielke system. Eleven patients with idiopathic scoliosis and one paralytic lumbar scoliosis were treated. The idiopathic cases were successfully treated by the Kaneda device alone. The paralytic case was stabilized by both front and back procedures. Correction rate averaged 92%. Resultant kyphosis in the fusion area was not seen as in cases treated with the Dwyer or Zielke system.

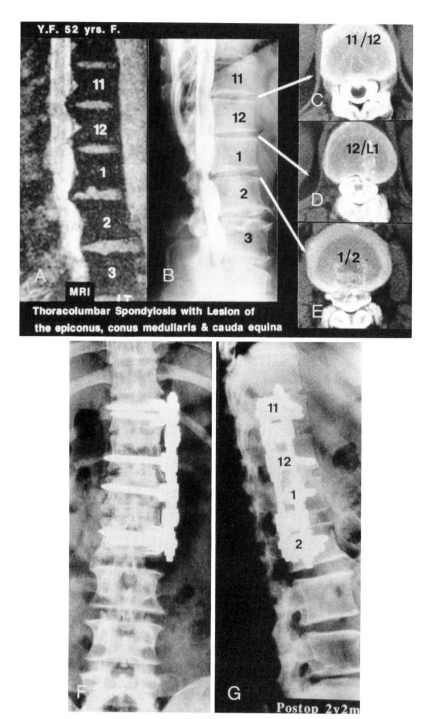

Figure 25.9. Thoracolumbar multiple spondylosis with neurologic deficit in a 52-year-old man. *A,* Preoperative MRI scan. *B,* Preoperative myelogram. *C–E,* Myelo-CT demonstrated compression of the epiconus, conus medullaris, and cauda equina. *F* and *G,* Postoperative pictures 2 years and 2 months at follow-up; multiple interbody fusion with the Kaneda device was solid with a good alignment.

Case 6 (Fig. 25.10):
This 15-year-old girl presented with idiopathic thoracolumbar scoliosis with a decompensated curve of 48° from T10-L2. Only the major curve was corrected and fused. Postoperatively, at 2 years follow-up, her spinal column remains nicely balanced in the coronal and sagittal planes, with solid fusion.

SPINAL TUMORS—METASTATIC SPINAL TUMORS—INDICATIONS FOR ANTERIOR DECOMPRESSION IN SPINAL METASTATIC TUMORS

The neurologic status must be considered carefully when considering an anterior decompression for patients with spinal metastasis. Twenty-one patients with a metastatic spinal tumor were treated by vertebral resection, replacement with the bioactive ceramic vertebral spacer, and fusion with the Kaneda device following radiation and chemotherapy. The initial stabilization was obtained successfully. In most patients, neurologic recovery followed. The surgical reconstruction appears to be effective in raising the quality of life by decreasing pain and in creating spinal stability.

At the latest follow-up, 11 of 21 patients died, with an average survival time of 11 months (3–29 months) after surgery. Ten of the 11 patients who died showed no tumor recurrence at the reconstructed portion of the spine. They died due to metastasis to other organs. Their

postoperative quality of life had been greatly improved by relief of pain and restoration of the activities of daily living. The other 10 patients are alive with a stable spine. Patients with breast cancer metastasis demonstrated the best postoperative course. Chemotherapy and/or radiation have been continued periodically in these patients.

Case 7 (Fig. 25.11):
A 48-year-old male suffered from severe back pain and paraparesis due to tumorous destruction of the L1 vertebra from a ureter cancer metastasis. The preoperative AP plain film and lateral myelogram showed destruction of the L1 body and compromise of the spinal canal. Even after radiation, paraparesis continued. Anterior decompression by partial vertebrectomy, replacement with the bioactive ceramic vertebral spacer, and fixation with the Kaneda device achieved improvement of neurologic function and almost complete pain relief. The postoperative films were taken 12 months after surgery.

COMPLICATIONS RELATED TO THE SPINAL INSTRUMENTATION

Complications related to the Kaneda device have not been seen, except for instrumentation failures in pseudarthrosis cases. The instrumentation failures include screw and rod breakage. All of these were associated with pseudarthrosis. There were no vascular complications, neurologic deterioration, or other organ system injuries. In the author's series with approximately 300 patients, no hard-

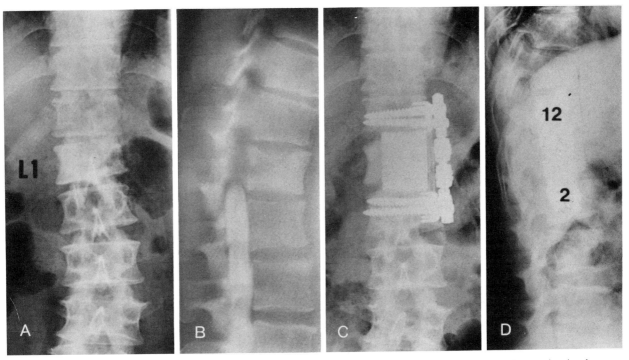

Figure 25.10. *A–D.* Idiopathic thoracolumbar scoliosis in a 15-year-old girl. *C–D.* Correction maintained.

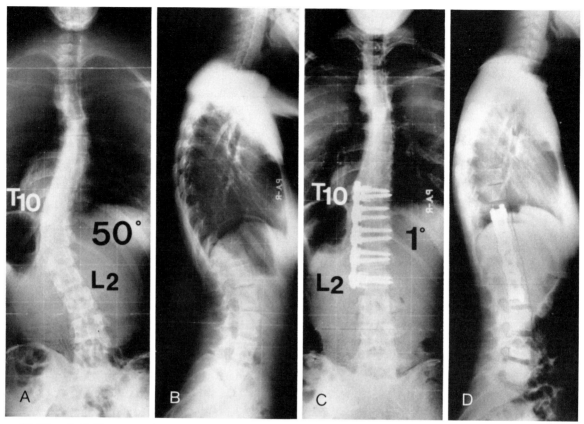

Figure 25.11. *A–D*. Tumorous destruction of the L1 vertebra from a ureter cancer metastasis. *C–D*. Correction maintained.

ware has ever been removed. Pseudarthrosis has been repaired successfully by posterior fusion with instrumentation in each case.

CONCLUSION

General indications for the use of the Kaneda device, composition of the Kaneda device, and surgical techniques, results, and complications have been described. The indications for the Kaneda device include thoracolumbar burst fractures with neurologic deficit, combined burst fracture and flexion-distraction injury with neurologic deficit, posttraumatic vertebral collapse with neurologic deficit in osteoporosis, thoracolumbar spondylosis with neurologic deficit, thoracolumbar scoliosis, and metastatic spinal tumors. Based on current results, the Kaneda device can be recommended for use in anterior spinal reconstruction following vertebrectomy, discectomy, or resection of the vertebral lesions for various disorders of the thoracolumbar spine. When using this device, one must use meticulous techniques of bone grafting as well as precise instrumentation.

REFERENCES

1. Denis F: The three column spine and its significance in the classification of acute thoracolumbar spinal injuries. Spine 1983; 8:817–831.
2. Denis F: Spinal instability as defined by the three-column spine concept in acute spinal trauma. Clin Orthop 1984;189:65–76.
3. Dick, Kluger P, Magerl F, et al: A new device for internal fixation of thoracolumbar and lumbar spine fracture: The fixateur interne. Paraplegia 1985;23:225–232.
4. Dick W: The fixateur interne as a versatile implant for spine surgery. Spine 1987;12:882–900.
5. Dunn HK: Spinal instrumentation. Part 1. Principles of posterior and anterior instrumentation. In: AAOS Instructional Course Lectures, vol. 32. St. Louis: CV Mosby, 1983;192–202.
6. Dunn HK: Anterior stabilization and decompression for thoracolumbar injuries. Orthop Clin North Am 1986;17:113–120.
7. Dwyer AF, Newton NC, Sherwood AA: An anterior approach to scoliosis—preliminary report. Clin Orthop 1969;62:192–202.
8. Dwyer AF: Experience of anterior correction of scoliosis. Clin Orthop 1973;93:191.
9. Fredrickson B, Yuan H: Internal fixation. In: Weinstein JN, Wiesel SW, eds. The lumbar spine. Philadelphia: WB Saunders, 1990; 941–956.
10. Friedlaender GE, Southwick WO: Tumor of the spine. In: Rothman RH, Simeone FA, eds. The spine. Philadelphia: WB Saunders, 1982;1022–1040.

11. Gertzbein SD, Crow P: Spinal canal clearance in burst fractures using the AO internal fixator. Presented at the Scoliosis Research Society. Amsterdam, 1989.

12. Gurr KR, McAfee PC, Shih CM: Biomechanical analysis of anterior and posterior instrumentation system after corpectomy: A calf spine model. J Bone Joint Surg 1988;70A:1182–1191.

13. Hall JE, Micheli LJ: The use of modified Dwyer instrumentation in anterior stabilization of the spine. Presented at the Scoliosis Research Society, Hong Kong, 1977, and Montreal 1981.

14. Hashimoto T, Kaneda K, Abumi K: Relationship between traumatic spinal canal stenosis and neurological deficits in thoracolumbar burst fractures. Spine 1988;13:1268–1272.

15. Jendrisak MD: Spontaneous abdominal aortic rupture from erosion by a lumbar spine fixation device. A case report. Surgery 1986;99:631.

16. Kaneda K, Abumi K, Fujiya K: Burst fractures with neurologic deficits of the thoraco-lumbar spine. Results of anterior decompression and stabilization with anterior instrumentation. Spine 1984; 9:788–795.

17. Kaneda K, Fujiya N, Satoh S: Results with Zielke instrumentation for idiopathic thoracolumbar and lumbar scoliosis. Clin Orthop 1986;205:195–203.

18. Kaneda K, Hashimoto T, Abumi K: Presented at the Annual Meeting of the Scoliosis Research Society, Amsterdam, 1989.

19. Kaplan PA, Orton DF, Asleson RJ: Osteoporosis with vertebral compression fractures, retropulsed fragments, and neurologic compromise. Radiology 1987;165:533.

20. Kempinsky WH, Morgan PP, Boniface WR: Osteoporotic kyphosis with paraplegia. Neurology 1985;8:181.

21. Kostuik: Anterior spinal cord compression for lesions of the thoracic and lumbar spine. Techniques, new methods of internal fixation results. Spine 1983;8:512.

22. Mann KA, Found EM, Yuan HA, et al: Biomechanical evaluation of the effectiveness of anterior spinal fixation systems. Orthop Trans 1987;11:378.

23. Maruo S, Takekawa K, Nakano K: Paraplegie infalge von Wirbel kompressionsfrakturen bei seniler Osteoporose. Z Orthop 1987;125:320.

24. McAfee PC, Bohlman HH, Yuan HA: Anterior decompression of traumatic thoracolumbar fractures with incomplete neurologic deficit using a retroperitoneal approach. J Bone Joint Surg 1985; 67A:89–104.

25. Moe JH, Winter RB, Bradford DS, et al: Scoliosis and other spinal deformities. Philadelphia: WB Saunders, 1978;521–526.

26. Nather A, Bose K: The results of decompression of cord or cauda equina compression from metastatic extradural tumors. Clin Orthop 1988;169:103.

27. Puno RM, Johnson JR, Osterman PAW, et al: Analysis of the primary and compensatory curvatures following Zielke instrumentation for idiopathic scoliosis; ventral derotation spondylodesis. Spine 1986;11A:8.

28. Shono Y, Kaneda K, Yamamoto I: Comparative biomechanical study of Zielke, Kaneda, and C.D. instrumentations using calf spine—scoliotic model. (Submitted to Spine 1991).

29. Slot GH: A new distraction system for the correction of kyphosis using the anterior approach. Presented at the Scoliosis Research Society, Montreal, 1981.

30. Zielke K, Pellin B: Neue Instrumente und Implantate zur Erganzung des Harrington Systems. Z Orthop Chir 1976;114:534.

31. Zielke K, Berthet: Ventrale derotationsspondylodese—Vorlanfiger bericht uber 58 falle. Beitr Orthop Traumatol 1978;25:85.

TWENTY-SIX

Principles, Indications, and Complications of Spinal Instrumentation: A Summary Chapter

Jerome M. Cotler, J. Michael Simpson, and Howard S. An

INTRODUCTION

With the explosion of new and advanced forms of spinal instrumentation, the proper techniques and details of spinal fusion should not be forgotten or dismissed. Since first introduced by Albee (2) and Hibbs (51) in 1911, arthrodesis has been one of the most important and frequently employed operations of the spine. Certainly, advances in instrumentation have improved our ability to deal with deformity, trauma, tumor, and degenerative conditions, but without successful bony arthrodesis, all instrumentation will ultimately fail. The incidence of pseudarthrosis is variable, depending on the type and degree of pathology, technique of fusion, instrumentation, immobilization, and host factors. Such failures account for significant patient morbidity.

There are four general reasons to perform an arthrodesis of the spine. These include: (*a*) prevention of progression of spinal deformity as in kyphosis, spondylolisthesis, and scoliosis; (*b*) maintenance of corrected deformity; (*c*) reestablishment of spinal stability of the spine following disruption of its structural integrity; and (*d*) diminished pain through elimination of motion between spinal segments.

A review of all known techniques and indications for spinal fusion is beyond the scope of this text. However, in brief, the biomechanical and technical principles of spinal arthrodesis will be discussed, along with broad indications and advantages of each instrumentation class.

PRINCIPLES AND BIOMECHANICS OF SPINAL FUSION

The results of attempted spinal fusion are dependent on several factors including the surgical preparation of the fusion site, influence of both systemic and local factors, ability of the graft material to stimulate a healing process, and the biomechanical features of graft positioning.

It is well known that only a few osteocytes survive transplantation. Therefore, it seems logical that optimization of the tissue bed is essential in providing a proper healing environment. Minimization of soft tissue trauma and proper decortication designed to provide a maximally exposed surface area of bone is ideal. Avascular or severely traumatized tissue should be removed from the graft bed, as it inhibits the necessary vascularization process. Decortication of a large surface area enhances the potential for vascular ingrowth, allows delivery of more osteoprogenitor cells, and, if successful, results in a mechanically superior large fusion mass. Attention to such surgical detail will optimize outcome.

There are several important considerations to make in choosing the type and source of graft material. The graft may be needed to provide structural stability or simply to induce or assist in the process of osteogenesis. It is generally believed that autogenous iliac crest remains the single best source of graft material combining osteogenic, osteoconductive, and osteoinductive properties (13). Iliac autograft generally results in higher rates of successful fusion and improved quality of the fusion mass. The ilium offers various contours to fit particular needs, while avoiding immunologic reactions, transmission of disease, availability, and storage problems associated with allograft. However, under certain conditions, the results with allograft have been reported to equal those of autograft, while avoiding donor site complications (18,85,91,96,116). Donor site complications reported include pain, hematoma, nerve injury, arterial injury, cosmetic deformity, infection, herniation, and fracture. Additionally, infection rates have not been shown to increase when using allograft material (104).

Several alternative graft materials are currently under

investigation including tricalcium phosphate, hydroxy-apatite, demineralized bone matrix, and bone morpho-genetic protein. Future use and efficacy of alternative materials remain unclear until further laboratory and clin-ical investigative studies are completed.

Certain basic biomechanical principles to graft posi-tioning must be understood. The basic biomechanical premise for graft positioning is that to prevent or mini-mize movement about any single axis of motion, the fusion mass should be placed at a maximum distance from the instantaneous axis of rotation. This concept is nicely demonstrated for sagittal plane motion in Figure 26.1, and is related to the principles of both leverage and area moment of inertia. This same biomechanical principle applies to both lateral bending and axial rotation. Lee and Langrana (65) recently published results of a bio-mechanical study evaluating various types of fusion in the lumbar spine. In 16 fresh cadavers, anterior, posterior, and bilateral lateral fusions were tested under compressive bending loads. All types of fusion increase both axial and bending stiffness, but unfortunately increase stress at ad-jacent unfused segments. Anterior fusions provided the stiffest construct, followed by bilateral lateral and pos-terior fusions, respectively. The bilateral lateral fusion placed the least stress on unfused segments. It was there-fore thought to be the best of the three constructs. Pos-terior fusion permitted moderate anterior motion and placed the highest amount of stress on adjacent motion segments.

Additional biomechanical considerations pertaining to specific graft constructs and instrumentation will be made during the course of the remaining text.

UPPER CERVICAL SPINE: ANTERIOR CONSTRUCTS

Anterior C1-C2 Screw Fixation

Barbour first introduced this technique as a method of internal fixation for odontoid fractures (5). It involved placement of screws bilaterally from the lateral mass of C1 to the body of C2, the angle of insertion determined by placing the drill bit on the anterior surface of the mastoid process to the tip of the C1 transverse process with the patient's head in a neutral position (Fig. 26.2). This technique offers rigid fixation and is possibly in-dicated in cases where the posterior arch of C1 is not available for arthrodesis, as in congenital absence or hypoplasia of the posterior ring or in postlaminectomy conditions. The disadvantage of the technique is related to the bilateral exposure required for screw placement, difficult anatomical approach, and unfamiliarity of the

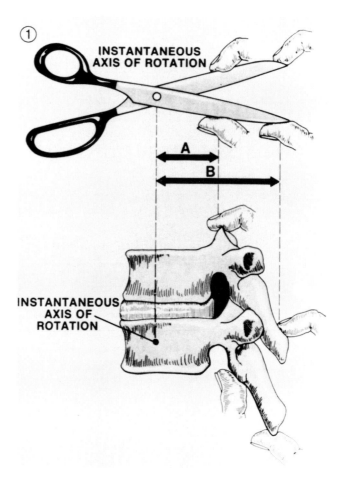

Figure 26.1. To prevent opening of the scissor blades by holding them together, it is distinctly easier to pinch the blades together at the tips (distance B) rather than at the midpoint of the blade (distance A). Because distance B is further away from the instantaneous axis of rotation, there is greater leverage. The same concepts apply to the vertebral functional spinal unit. Flexion, separation, or opening of the spinous processes is more easily prevented by placing the fingers at the tips of the spinous processes (distance B) rather than at the facet joints (distance A). Thus, a healed bone graft at distance B is more effective in presenting a flexion moment than one closer to the instanta-neous axis of rotation. (Reprinted with permission from White AA, Panjabi MM: Clinical biomechanics of the spine. Phila-delphia: JB Lippincott, 1990;533.)

surgeon with the approach and technique of the proce-dure.

Anterior Screw Fixation of the Dens

Bohler introduced a method of anterior screw fixation for fracture and nonunion of the odontoid (7). The tech-nique involves insertion of one, or two (preferred), screws across the fracture as the primary treatment for this par-

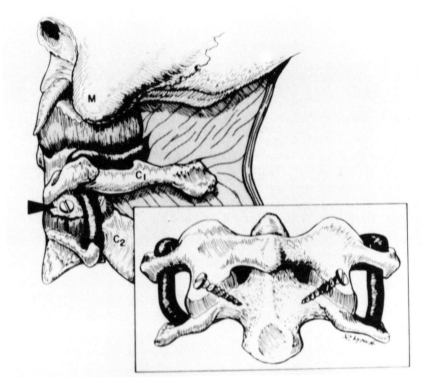

Figure 26.2. The Barbour technique of anterior C1-C2 screw fixation. Bilateral exposure is required through difficult anatomic regions with potential complications. C1-C2 articular cartilage is removed, and the space filled with autogenous cancellous bone. Screw fixation provides immediate stability and is especially useful in cases where the posterior arch of C1 is not available for arthrodesis. (Reprinted with permission from White AA, Panjabi MM: Clinical biomechanics of the spine. Philadelphia: JB Lippincott, 1990;543.)

ticular injury (Fig. 26.3). The obvious advantage of the technique is to provide rigid, biomechanically sound fixation without disruption of the C1-C2 articulation, thus preserving significant axial rotation. However, the author has failed to expand on the complications associated with this procedure. Possible neurologic and vascular complications may result from the procedure because of the proximity of these structures and unfamiliarity of the operating surgeon. Based on a recent multicenter study reviewing treatment of odontoid fractures, it appears that other methods of treatment are safer and more successful, and therefore preferable in the treatment of such injuries (17). However, this method may be preferable for displaced odontoid fractures associated with posterior C1 arch fracture.

UPPER CERVICAL SPINE: POSTERIOR CONSTRUCTS

Occipitocervical Fusion

Occipitocervical fusion may be required for a variety of conditions including occipitocervical instability, neuro-logic compromise, infection, tumor, or intractable pain referable to the occipitocervical articulation. The majority of patients requiring this procedure have involvement of this articulation secondary to rheumatoid arthritis. A variety of surgical techniques for occipitocervical fusion have been described with variable forms of immobilization, rates of fusion, and successful clinical results (9,20,37,46,66,110). A technique recently described by Wertheim and Bohlman used semirigid fixation and provided successful fusion in all 13 patients in their series (110). Their technique described the passage of wire through burr holes in the external occipital protuberance without going through the inner table of the skull. Additional wires are passed under the arch of the atlas and through the spinous process of C2. A tricortical graft harvested from the posterior iliac crest is then secured (Fig. 26.4). We prefer to use 16- or 18-gauge wire and supplemental external fixation with a halo device for a period of 8–12 weeks.

Possible complications include pseudarthrosis, neuro-logic injury, vertebral artery injury, wound infection, progressive deformity, and/or neurologic deficit in the

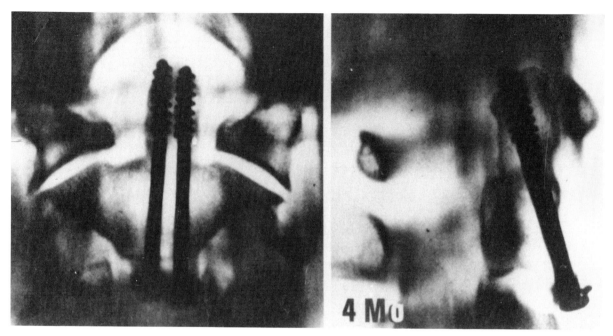

Figure 26.3. AP and lateral tomograms of an initially displaced type II odontoid fracture treated with anterior screw fixation. The fracture appears solidly healed at 4 months, in ideal position. (Reprinted with permission from Bohler J: Anterior stabilization of acute fractures and nonunions of the dens. J Bone Joint Surg 1982;64A:18.)

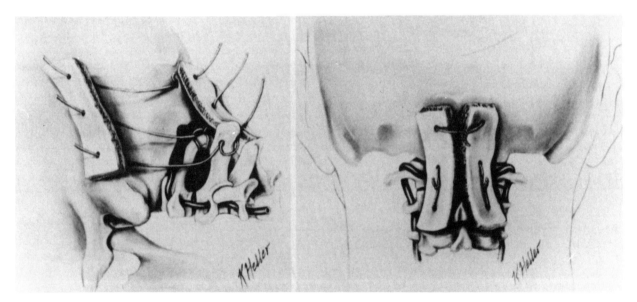

Figure 26.4. Occipitocervical fusion. A burr hole is placed through the external occipital protuberance without penetration of the inner table. A wire is then passed through this burr hole. Additional wires are passed around the posterior arch of C1 and through the spinous process of C2. A tricortical iliac crest bone graft is obtained and secured as shown. (Reprinted with permission from Wertheim SB, Bohlman HH: Occipitocervical fusion: indications, technique and long term results in thirteen patients. J Bone Joint Surg 1987;69A:833.)

presence of solid arthrodesis. Use of intraoperative evoked potentials and attention to detail in passage of wires is imperative in this already compromised patient population.

Additional techniques for occipitocervical stabilization and fusion include plate fixation as described by Roy-Camille (92) and Luque (54) rectangle rod and wire constructs. These methods have not met with general approval. The potential for complications with plate fixation seems great, while limiting the area for placement of graft material. Additionally, there are no biomechanical or clinical studies demonstrating either improved structural stability or successful fusion using either of these techniques.

POSTERIOR C1-C2 ARTHRODESIS

Several techniques of posterior C1-C2 fusion have been described with variable success (13,34,40,79). Based on biomechanical studies, the Brooks fusion appears most sound and has given excellent clinical results (12,43).

Wedges of iliac crest bone are fashioned to fit the C1-C2 interlaminar space, effectively controlling axial rotation, flexion-extension, and lateral bending. These wedges provide a spacer between the posterior arches of C1 and C2, preventing hyperextension of this motion segment with compressive sublaminar wire fixation. This is important, as hyperextension may exacerbate certain pathologic conditions (Fig. 26.5). Another technique of posterior C1-C2 wiring is the modified Gallie method, in which the spinous process of C2 is utilized instead of lamina. This technique is therefore safer than the Brooks fusion and is quite adequate for flexion-type instabilities.

Neurologic complications associated with C1-C2 fusions are most often related to the passage of sublaminar wires. Canal space at C1-C2 is frequently compromised with irreducible subluxation. Nordt and Stauffer reported two cases of quadriplegia with passage of sublaminar wires in the presence of anterior C1 subluxation (86). Pseudarthrosis in posterior C1-C2 arthrodesis has been reported as high as 35%, especially in rheumatoid patient populations. Brooks reported success in 11 of 12 patients;

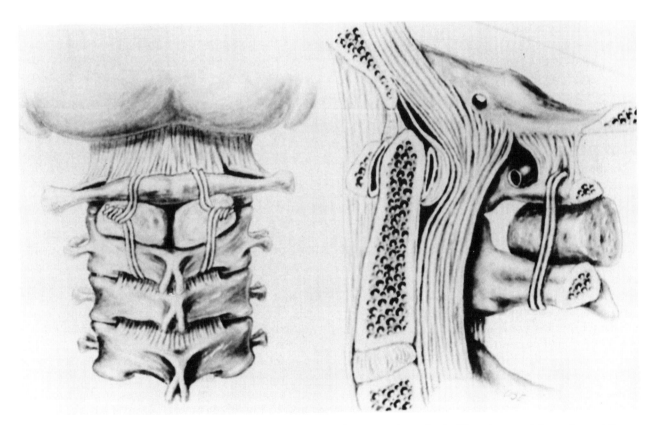

Figure 26.5. Brooks atlantoaxial arthrodesis. Sublaminar wires are passed under the arch of C1 and C2, respectively. Wedges of corticocancellous bone are obtained from the iliac crest. The edges of the graft are bevelled to fit the interval between atlas and axis. The wires are tightened, providing compressive sublaminar fixation. (Reprinted with permission from Brooks AL, Jenkins EG: Atlanto-axial arthrodesis by the wedge compression method. J Bone Joint Surg 1978;60A:279.)

one patient had pseudarthrosis. Adjunctive halo immobilization would appear necessary to optimize results.

The Halifax clamp has recently been introduced and appears to offer rigid C1-C2 fixation without the risk of sublaminar wires. Holness et al. reported on 51 patients treated with the Halifax clamp for C1-C2 and lower cervical spine fusions (52). All patients were immobilized postoperatively in a Philadelphia collar for 3 months. Bone grafting was not performed in this series, yet successful fusion was reported in all those patients followed for a period of at least 4 years. The only reported complication was that of clamp dislodgment in two patients, requiring reoperation to replace the clamp. At the C1-C2 level, insertion of the Halifax clamp and graft may be ineffective in countering the movements of axial rotation, flexion-extension, and lateral bending. Additionally, with the clamp's inherent ability to apply compressive forces across the C1-C2 articulation, there is a tendency to hyperextend the motion segment, which carries a risk of neurologic injury.

The Magerl posterior C1-C2 screw fixation provides a biomechanically strong construct, but it should probably be limited to those cases in which the posterior bony elements are deficient.

LOWER CERVICAL SPINE: ANTERIOR CONSTRUCTS

The majority of anterior cervical fusions do not require internal fixation. Indeed, internal fixation may be associated with significant complication. Anterior plating, however, is receiving more attention. Indications for plate augmentation remain unclear, but may have an advantage in providing immediate postoperative stability. Anterior plating is not advocated for single-level discectomies, but has been used with tumor and multiple-level vertebrectomies for myelopathy.

Biomechanical studies have shown that combined anterior and posterior internal fixation of the cervical spine provides the most rigid construct (105,112). When used alone, dorsal plate and screw fixation is a more stable construct than ventral plate fixation (19). Based on other biomechanical studies, use of anterior devices appears to offer inferior stability against flexion as compared with posterior wiring or plating techniques. However, experience has demonstrated that anterior plate fixation is adequate in the clinical setting (15,16,22,41,50).

Several devices have been designed including those by Roy-Camille, Louis, Caspar, Morscher, and others. Potential complications with these devices include neurologic injury secondary to posterior cortex penetration, loosening, esophageal erosion, or injury to vascular structures during the drilling process (108). There is no re-

ported large series available to estimate the prevalence of such complications.

LOWER CERVICAL SPINE: POSTERIOR CONSTRUCTS

By far, the most common construct used in the cervical spine posteriorly is spinous process wiring. The triple-wire technique described by Bohlman offers rigid fixation and is simple and safe (Fig. 26.6) (8). Recent biomechanical studies in both bovine and human cadaveric specimens have found this technique to provide a rigid construct equal to posterior plating techniques (19,103). Single- and multiple-level fusions can be obtained using this method with minimal associated complications. Indications include traumatic instability secondary to unilateral or bilateral facet dislocation and degenerative cervical spondylolisthesis.

Facet wiring as described by Callahan (14) is a viable alternative for posterior cervical stabilization and fusion, especially in postlaminectomy conditions. With this technique, a small flat elevator is placed into the facet and a burr then used to create a drill hole through the inferior facet. The elevator is positioned to protect the vital anterior structures, namely, the nerve root and the vertebral artery during the drilling process. Eighteen or 20-gauge wire is then passed through the inferior facet pillar and retrieved using a fine-angled clamp. The wire is then advanced and the free end passed through the hole at the next lower facet pillar. Bone graft is harvested and placed under the lateral decorticated surfaces. For multiple-level laminectomies, the wiring technique may be modified, allowing incorporation of a strut-type graft of the surgeon's choice. We prefer a tricortical iliac crest graft (Fig. 26.7).

A commonly encountered postlaminectomy complication is progressive kyphosis, often presenting as a "swan neck" deformity. In this instance, preoperative and intraoperative halo traction may provide some reduction of the swan neck deformity. Postoperatively, we believe halo-vest immobilization is still required for a period of approximately 8–12 weeks.

Biomechanically, the facet wiring construct offers excellent stability against flexion-extension and lateral bending moments, almost equaling that of the intact spine (57). In one study comparing various forms of fixation, facet wiring was found to offer the strongest construct against flexion moments. However, it has been found to provide little stability against either extension or axial rotation (89).

One potential problem with facet wiring relates to the placement of wires through adjacent unfused joints. Accelerated degenerative changes of adjacent joints and as-

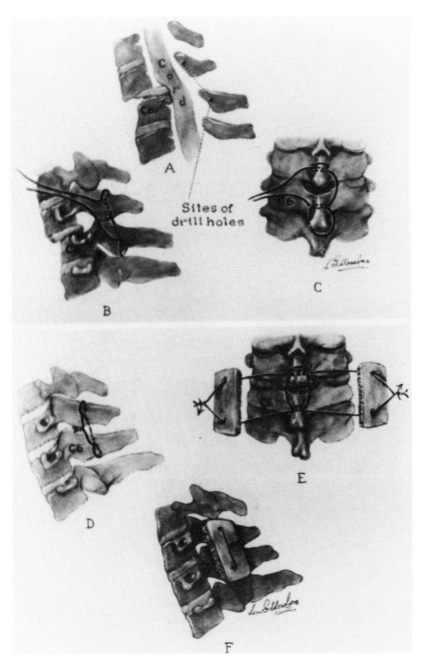

Figure 26.6. Bohlman's triple-wire technique for lower cervical spine stabilization. A hole is placed in the base of the spinous processes (*A*) and a midline tethering wire placed through and around each spinous process (*B*). The facets are most efficiently reduced with Gardner-Wells tong traction (*C*). The wire is tightened, giving initial stability (*D*). Two corticocancellous strips are harvested from the posterior iliac crest and secured with two additional wires (*E* and *F*). (Reprinted with permission from Rifkinson-Mann S, Mormino J, Sachdev VP: Subacute cervical spine instability. Surg Neurol 1986;26:413.)

sociated symptoms are primary concerns, but are not truly appreciated in the literature.

Posterior cervical plating with placement of the screws into the lateral articular mass has been shown to provide rigid structural fixation and may be employed for traumatic and degenerative forms of instability as well as for postlaminectomy arthrodesis (19,21,93,103,105).

The points of screw insertion must be exact to prevent neurovascular injury. Roy-Camille compares the lateral aspect of the posterior cervical spine to a landscape of peaks and valleys. The junctional area where the lamina meets the facet joint represents the valley, while the articular mass is analogous to the peak or hill. The vertebral artery is found directly anterior to the valley, while the nerve roots exit through respective neural foramina at the level of the articular joints. Therefore, to avoid these structures, the plates are placed directly over the articular masses, and screws are implanted into the peak of the articular mass. Drilling for screw placement must be started in the center of the articular mass. The direction

Figure 26.7. Facet wiring technique. *A*, A laminectomy has been completed at C3, C4, and C5 and fusion performed using facet wiring technique. *B*, Wires are placed through the facet joint and around the graft. A second splint of tibial graft is placed and secured, but tends to eliminate normal cervical lordosis. *C*, Rib or iliac crest may be selectively used to maintain lordosis. (Reprinted with permission from Robinson RA and Southwick WO: Surgical approaches to the cervical spine. In: American Academy of Orthopaedic Surgeons: Instruction Course Lectures. St. Louis: CV Mosby, 1960.)

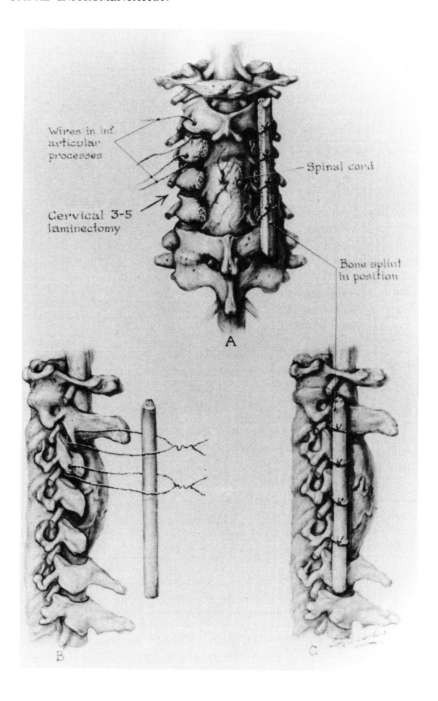

of drilling, however, is variable, depending on the author. Of utmost importance is to direct the bit laterally 10–15°, but never medially, to avoid the vertebral artery and neurologic structures. Based on our own anatomic studies, drilling in the cephalad direction at approximately 10–30° from the perpendicular will avoid nerve root injury as well as facet impingement. The drilling should be more cephalad for the caudad vertebra to avoid the facet joint. Autogenous cancellous bone augmentation

may be performed, but the experience of some has shown that the facets will fuse with plate fixation alone (93).

Severe osteoporosis is the primary contraindication to this technique, as it is for anterior plate fixation. Screw loosening posteriorly does not present the same potential for disaster as anteriorly, since there is no danger to either the esophagus, trachea, or carotid artery. Potential complications include injury to the vertebral artery, cervical nerve roots, failure of fixation, pseudarthrosis, and progressive angulation across the injured segment. In Roy-Camille's series of 221 patients treated posteriorly, he reported no secondary displacement in 85.2% of patients (93). No report of vascular or neurologic injury has been given.

The method of posterior hook-plate fixation was developed by Magerl (76). He reports superior biomechanical fixation for single- or multiple-level injuries. The hook portion of this device is placed under the lamina of the lower vertebrae and secured proximally by screw fixation into the lateral articular mass, as described previously. The hook is placed just medial to the facet joint with a small notch placed in the lamina in order to prevent slippage. Magerl advocates the application of an "H"-shaped interspinous graft to achieve three-point fixation. He reported success in his series of 40 patients using this device and technique with no case of pseudarthrosis (76).

THORACOLUMBAR AND SACRAL SPINE: ANTERIOR CONSTRUCTS

Although not widely used, anterior instrumentation of the thoracolumbar spine has been developed and utilized for deformity, trauma, and tumor conditions. We will briefly discuss the indications for the most commonly used anterior devices and review their respective associated complications.

Due to the early difficulties of surgically dealing with thoracolumbar and lumbar scoliotic curvatures from a posterior approach, anterior forms of correction and stabilization were sought. Dwyer instrumentation was developed in Australia during the 1960s and represented the first anterior system to be widely used in the treatment of flexible thoracolumbar curvatures (30,31). Zielke instrumentation followed, and employs many of the same principles utilizing a solid flexible rod instead of a cable (52,82,117). Dwyer's technique involves insertion of a staple-screw construct placed into the vertebral body from the convex side of the curvature. These screws are then connected by a cable. Correction is obtained with application of compressive forces at each segmental level. Anterior spinal compression produces tensile forces within the cable, creating a corrective bending moment at each of the intervertebral levels. Biomechanically, with a small lever arm, a large tensile force must be created in the cable to effect a corrective force (Fig. 26.8).

Indications for anterior instrumentation are limited, as most deformities can be treated with properly utilized posterior instrumentation. Presently, indications for anterior instrumentation include: (*a*) lumbar scoliosis with deficient posterior elements (e.g., myelomeningocele); (*b*) thoracolumbar curves with extreme lordosis; and (*c*)

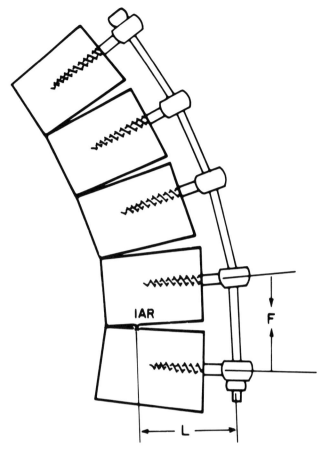

Figure 26.8. This frontal plane diagram demonstrates the biomechanical principle of the Dwyer technique. Compressive force is applied to the convexity of the curve. Force (*F*) is created by applying tension to the wire on the convex side. Correction of the curve is created by the bending moment (*F* × *L*). (Reprinted with permission from White AA, Panjabi MM: Clinical biomechanics of the spine. Philadelphia: JB Lippincott, 1990;152.)

rigid, paralytic thoracolumbar scoliosis requiring a staged anterior and posterior spinal fusion. An absolute contraindication to this anterior procedure is the presence of kyphosis because compressive forces will further induce a kyphotic moment, increasing the sagittal deformity. Advantages of the Zielke instrumentation over the Dwyer technique include its ability to derotate the spinal segments, thus limiting induction of kyphosis. Another advantage is the threaded nuts at each screw site that allow for sequential correction at each intervertebral level.

Complications associated with either the Dwyer or Zielke anterior devices include those common to any major anterior surgical exposure to the spine. These complications include paralytic ileus, pneumothorax, hemothorax, and injury to urologic structures. Neurologic injury may result during the process of discectomy or during insertion of screws into the vertebral body. To avoid neurologic complication, the screws should be placed parallel to the posterior longitudinal ligament and aimed in a posteroanterior direction. The possibility of a vascular insult to the cord also exists. During the exposure, segmental vessels should be ligated near the midportion of the vertebral body. By avoiding the vascular anastomosis at the intervertebral foramina, the risk of vascular compromise is minimal.

Vascular injury is always a concern with an anterior approach to the spine. With Dwyer or Zielke instrumentation, the spine is always approached from the convexity of the curve. The great vessels are found without exception on the concavity. Care must be taken in the process of removing the annulus so as not to damage the aorta, vena cava, or segmental vessels. Placement of a Homan retractor or Chandler elevator anteriorly around the disc is helpful in protecting the vessels. Dwyer (29) and Hall (45) have reported deaths caused by ruptured aortic aneurysm. The incidence of vascular complication is low, but can be minimized by avoiding overpenetration of the screw into the vertebral body and, if possible, obtaining soft tissue coverage over the implant during closure.

Hardware failure with loss of fixation is relatively common and is indicative of potential pseudarthrosis. A pseudarthrosis rate of 50% has been reported in isolated anterior fusions with Dwyer instrumentation for paralytic scoliosis. This finding emphasizes the need for adjunctive posterior stabilization in this particular group. In a recent report by Kohler et al. (60), reviewing 21 cases of idiopathic thoracolumbar or lumbar scoliosis treated with Dwyer instrumentation, evidence of pseudarthrosis was noted in 12% with a 10-year follow-up. Failure may also result from screw pullout, especially in cases of extreme osteoporosis. To minimize pullout, the opposite cortex should be engaged with screw placement, but not overpenetrated, to avoid potential vascular problems. Fracture of the vertebral bodies will result from application of excessive compressive forces, especially in osteoporotic bone. Caution must be used at every level. No more than 30–40 lbs of tension should be applied in the thoracic spine. With more distal curvatures, greater forces may be applied, but should never exceed 100 lbs of pressure.

Several implants have been designed for use in cases of traumatic injury to the thoracolumbar and lumbar spine. Included are screw-rod constructs such as the Kaneda and Kostuik devices (61) and plate and screw systems represented by the Syracuse I-plate and the Armstrong plate.

Anterior decompression is frequently indicated in cases of incomplete neurologic injury following thoracolumbar spine trauma. The indications for anterior implants remain somewhat controversial, but they do appear to have advantages in permitting single-stage decompression, stabilization, and fusion of spinal injuries with short segment fusion. The rod-screw systems additionally permit either compressive or distractive forces to be applied across the injured segment. These rod-screw devices are somewhat bulky, making it difficult to obtain soft tissue coverage of the implant and increasing concerns of vascular injury. The Syracuse I-plate or Armstrong plate is of low profile and allows for nearly as rigid stabilization as the Kaneda system. However, it is unable to employ reduction forces across the injured segment.

Kaneda et al. reported on their series of 27 patients with thoracolumbar burst fractures and neurologic deficit (58). All patients were treated with anterior retroperitoneal surgical approach, decompression, fusion, and instrumentation. The initial 15 patients were treated with the Zielke device, and the remaining 12 with the Kaneda system. Of the 27 patients with an incomplete injury, 26 had some neurologic recovery, 19 improving by at least one Frankel grade. All patients fused. Kostuik, as well, has reported on his experience, and the union rate in his series of 42 patients was 96% (90). Furthermore, 32 patients with partial neurologic deficit improved an average of 1.6 Frankel grades. Yuan et al. have reported successful use of their Syracuse I-plate in 16 patients, with 12–24 months follow-up and minimal complications (115). Use of these devices truly has potential for allowing a single-stage procedure. However, the associated complication inherent in any anterior spinal procedure, as already outlined, must be considered in addition to the loss of position. Loss of fixation is of particular concern in three-column injuries and in the osteoporotic spine.

SURGICAL CONSTRUCTS IN THORACIC, LUMBAR, AND SACRAL SPINE
Posterior Distraction Instrumentation

In contrast to anterior constructs, extensive literature is available reviewing the clinical and biomechanical implications of posterior spinal instrumentation in the thoracolumbar and sacral spine.

Harrington instrumentation was introduced in 1962 for the operative treatment of scoliosis, and employed distraction across the concave side of the curve and compression over the convexity (47). Since that time, its use has been widely expanded to include stabilization of traumatic injuries (23,27,35,114). Occasional use has also been described for both degenerative and tumor conditions. For the purposes of this discussion, the Harrington system will serve as the prototype for posterior distraction instrumentation. Theoretical advantages associated with modifications such as Moe's square-ended rods, Edwards rod-sleeve construct, and others will be reviewed.

The primary use of distraction devices is to obtain correction of deformity secondary to scoliosis and traumatic injuries of the thoracolumbar spine incurred by some axially compressive force. When distraction is applied, tensile forces are developed within the spine that, in turn, create a considerable three-point bending moment (Fig. 26.9). This three-point bending moment is responsible for correction of deformity. The greater the

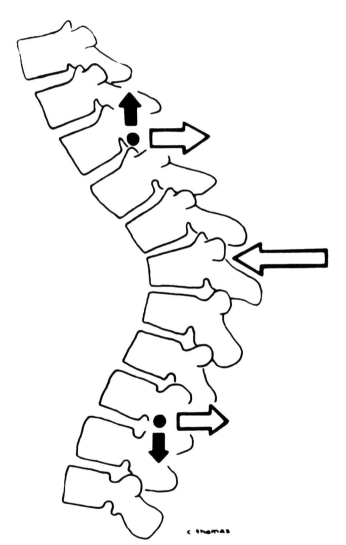

Figure 26.9. Biomechanics of the Harrington distraction rod. The small black arrows represent the distraction forces. The three light arrows represent the forces due to the three-point bending of the spine as the Harrington model is inserted between the two hooks. (Reprinted with permission from White AA, Panjabi MM, Thomas CL: The clinical biomechanics of kyphotic deformities. Clin Orthop 1977;128:8.)

tensile forces created through distraction, the greater the three-point bending moment and potential for correction of deformity. It is additionally noteworthy that the corrective bending moment created by distraction is increased as the deformity is increased. This is in direct contrast to the transverse forces created by segmental forms of fixation, to be discussed later. Hooks are seated proximally and distally under the laminae and fixed by the soft tissue tensile forces created through distraction. In some traumatic cases with severe soft tissue ligamentous destruction, distraction devices may have limited use or even have potential for overdistraction of a motion segment and neurologic injury.

Straight distraction with the Harrington device and the accompanying extension moment provided by three-point bending may lead to a loss of the normal sagittal contours in the thoracolumbar spine. A straight Harrington rod fails to provide the necessary lordosis or rotational control at either the thoracolumbar junction or lordotic lumbar segments (78,80,84,88,101,106). In traumatic injuries, failure to restore these contours may lead to ineffective reduction of the fracture and incomplete decompression of the spinal canal. In traumatic injuries and cases of deformity, distraction without control of lordosis will flatten the normal lordotic contours of the lumbosacral region and may lead to symptomatic flat back syndrome (48,64,81). Such iatrogenic deformity has become increasingly recognized. Distraction across the lumbar spine, especially with fixation to L5 or sacrum, will inevitably lead to a significant loss of lordosis. Compensatory hyperextension of the upper spine and hips is necessary to maintain an upright posture when loss of lordosis is present, and can lead to significant clinical complaints. Many patients will describe a fatiguing muscular ache in the upper spine that may be related to additional stresses placed on the facets in the hyperextended position. Postural and gait abnormalities have also been well documented, especially in patients who lack normal hip extension (48,64).

Lack of rotational control may also lead to distal hook dislodgement, especially when the rods extend below L3. Studies have shown that supplemental use of sublaminar wires or compression rods improve stability of the modified distraction construct in flexion and rotation and limit the possibility of hook disengagement (3,38,49,59,83,88,99). However, these constructs still cannot maintain lordosis and rotational control completely (78).

To circumvent flattening of sagittal contours and to prevent hook dislodgement, Moe developed and recommended a square-ended rod and hook construct (81). However, clinical results have generally failed to show a significant improvement over the straight distraction method of Harrington in preventing either of these complications. Distraction remains the single greatest force of correction. Reported occurrences of hook dislodgement and late kyphotic deformity are similar (1,25,56). These findings are probably related to inherent difficulties in inserting a properly contoured rod into the lower hook and rotational instability that persists as the rod makes contact with only one point.

The Edwards rod-sleeve method was developed in an attempt to address these problems (32). Distraction, extension, and four-point rotational control is offered without the complexities of Cotrel-Dubousset instrumentation or the potential dangers of sublaminar wires. The greatest theoretical advantage of the Edwards system is the constant, elastic lordotic moment provided by the polyethylene sleeve maintaining correction and stability, while minimizing the effects of soft tissue stretch relaxation (Fig. 26.10). Use of pedicle screw fixation in lower lumbar segments with modular systems such as Edwards and Cotrel-Dubousset may be advantageous.

Other complications associated with distraction instrumentation are well documented. Perhaps the greatest fear of spinal surgery is neurologic complication. MacEwen published data based on a survey conducted by the Scoliosis Research Society in 1975 reviewing neural complications (74). A total of 87 patients with acute neurologic deficit were identified with an overall incidence of 0.72% for significant motor deficit. Of this group, approximately 1/3 had no recovery of function; 1/3 had partial recovery; and 1/3 had full return of function. The Scoliosis Research Society reported on 5330 spinal deformity patients treated from 1984–1985, of which 2658 cases involved the use of supplemental sublaminar wires (97). There were seven patients with complete spinal cord injuries in this group, and all seven were treated with removal of instrumentation within hours of

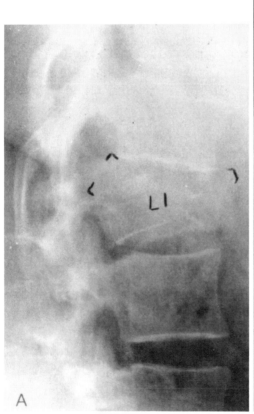
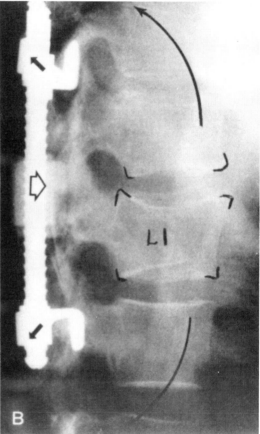

Figure 26.10. Edwards rod-sleeve method. *A,* A flexion-compression burst fracture of L1. *B,* The postoperative radiograph shows the polyethylene sleeve centered over the T12-L1 facet. Anatomic hooks are placed at T11 and L2. Distraction rods coupled with an extension moment created by the sleeves result in full restoration of height and lordosis. (Garfin SR: Complications of spine surgery. Baltimore: Williams & Wilkins, 1989;169.)

the procedure. Four patients had complete recovery, and three had partial recovery. Ten patients had incomplete injuries. Of these, five had a complete recovery and the other five displayed improvement at follow-up. The best results appeared in patients with removal of instrumentation.

Similar rates of neurologic complication have been seen in the treatment of thoracolumbar fractures. Members of the Scoliosis Research Society in 1986 reported only five patients (0.62%) with neurologic worsening in a series of 805 treated operatively (98). Several individual series report an average of 1% incidence of neurologic injury (26,27,32,36,42,87).

Inappropriate laminar hook placement or choice can be a factor in the development of a neurologic injury. Ratcheted rods and hooks have the lowest rate of complication, with a 0.1% incidence, reported by the Scoliosis Research Society (98). Use of Cotrel-Dubousset instrumentation for fracture is reported to have higher rates of neurologic complication with a 1.5% incidence (98). Most of these result from improper hook placement at the L5 or S1 levels. Hooks placed over the normally lordotic L5 lamina often project far into the canal and may cause impingement of a sacral nerve root. Inappropriate use of the tall alar hooks about the lumbar segments may also cause neural impingement (77).

Neural injury may also result from reduction of post-traumatic deformity with distraction-type instrumentation. Failure to first reduce or correct dislocations, translations, or significant kyphotic deformity may induce a significant flexion moment across the injured segment with distraction forces applied. This kyphotic deformity may secondarily lead to neurologic compromise by stretching the neural elements over retropulsed bone. It is therefore imperative that such gross malalignments be corrected prior to application of distraction (77).

Hook dislodgement is the most often reported complication associated with posterior Harrington distraction instrumentation as well as for other posterior rod-hook constructs. Construct failure may result from laminar fracture, laminar resorption, dislodgement of the hook from the lamina, or disengagement at the hook-rod interface, and in large series are reported at 2–17% (23,27,32,36,42,55,87). Proximal hook pullout is the most common form of failure. Flexion and rotation about the upper hook is not well controlled by pure Harrington distraction instrumentation, and hook-lamina contact is reduced, causing forces to be concentrated on the laminar edge and resulting in laminar fracture and/or hook dislodgement. Addition of segmental wire fixation, polyethylene sleeves, multiple-hook construct, and transverse linking devices has been shown to diminish the incidence of single-hook failure by two-thirds (33).

As already indicated, in clinical and laboratory studies, rates of distal hook dislodgement have been shown to increase markedly as one approaches the sacrum (4,62,68,95). Rates of failure at L5 average 10–15%, and increase dramatically to 25–30% with sacral hook fixation. Such hook failures are most likely related to hook design, lack of rotational control, and increased mobility and flexibility of these motion segments. Use of the L-shaped anatomic hooks in the low lumbar segments may increase lamina-hook contact and distribute distraction forces better, minimizing failures. Additionally, consideration of employing pedicular and sacral screw fixation in these lower segments with modular systems such as Edwards or Cotrel-Dubousset may improve fixation and aid in the maintenance of sagittal contours.

Hook-rod disengagement is also a significant problem with the Harrington distraction system. Failure to leave at least 1 cm of rod beyond the proximal hook may lead to disengagement during flexion and subsequent hook dislodgement. Finally, laminar fractures secondary to osteoporosis, excessive laminotomy, failure to obtain bicortical hook purchase, or vigorous distraction may result. Critical attention must be given to hook site preparation and placement to minimize failure. Distraction should be completed gradually to allow for soft tissue stretch, relaxation, and adaptation of the bone-metal interface.

Rates of nonunion are very similar, but generally average 5% in most traumatic and deformity series. Additionally, nonunion rates appear to be higher when fusion and instrumentation approach the lumbosacral junction. This increased incidence of nonunion is probably related to increased mobility and difficulty in obtaining rigid fixation at the lumbosacral junction. Failure of hardware in the form of rod breakage usually follows nonunion. Repetitive loading on implants in the face of nonunion generally results in fatigue fractures. Harrington rod failure invariably occurs at the junction of the shaft and ratchet, where there is an abrupt decrease in rod diameter. This size alteration in the rod creates a significant stress riser. Forces acting across the ratchet-shaft interval may be reduced by using the appropriate-size rod and by minimizing the distance between the proximal hook and shaft-ratchet junction. The Edwards universal rod is larger in diameter for increased strength and is fully ratcheted to eliminate the focal stress risers seen in the Harrington rod. Similarly, the Cotrel-Dubousset rod has a continuously variegated surface and larger diameter designed to limit this potential complication. No large series is available to determine the prevalence of rod failure with the Cotrel-Dubousset system.

POSTERIOR THORACOLUMBAR AND SACRAL SPINE CONSTRUCTS— COMPRESSION INSTRUMENTATION

There are several examples of posterior compression devices. The Harrington compression rod system will serve as the prototype for discussion. Other systems include Edwards compression device, Cotrel-Dubousset system applied in compression, and Gruca-Weiss springs. Compression instrumentation has been applied in cases of scoliosis, kyphosis, and some traumatic conditions.

In the treatment of scoliosis, the corrective compressive device is placed on the convex side of the curve. The rod is placed in tension, applying compressive forces to the spine. The overall ability to correct the coronal deformity is dependent on the bending moments produced at the center of rotation of each vertebra. In cases of scoliosis, the corrective forces created by the Harrington compressive device are quite small or negligible compared to the correction with the distraction component (107). The Harrington distraction rod is 4.7 times as stiff as the compression rod (111). Therefore, the three-point corrected bending moment with the distraction rod is likely to be nearly five times greater than the compression rod. The primary purpose of the compression rod therefore is to provide some immediate clinical stability to the surgical construct through impaction. The second benefit, based on studies by Gaines and Leatherman, is the ability of the compressive rod to preserve or even correct the sagittal plane component of the scoliotic deformity (39).

The causes of thoracic and thoracolumbar kyphosis include congenital and developmental conditions, trauma, tumor, and infection. Scheuermann's disease probably results from an abnormal growth and development pattern of several anterior thoracic vertebral bodies, resulting in kyphosis. Congenital abnormalities such as failure of anterior segmentation and bony bar formation additionally may lead to the development of significant kyphosis. Based on current knowledge and studies, such complex deformities are probably best addressed with combined anterior and posterior procedures (11). Anterior release and fusion are first performed, followed by application of posterior compression instrumentation to correct the deformity. Harrington and Cotrel-Dubousset systems employ multiple-hook constructs, which better distribute corrective forces over several segments and thus lessen the possibility of failure.

Traumatic and posttraumatic development of kyphosis is initiated through injury to both anterior and posterior column structures. With deficits in these two columns, compressive and flexion forces are created and act through the center of gravity, which is anterior to the injured level. Such deforming forces may lead to continued failure of the osseous and ligamentous structures, resulting in progressive deformity. Posterior structures will fail in tension (Fig. 26.11). With large initial kyphotic deformities, a larger flexion bending moment is created, and an increased risk for progressive deformity is likely.

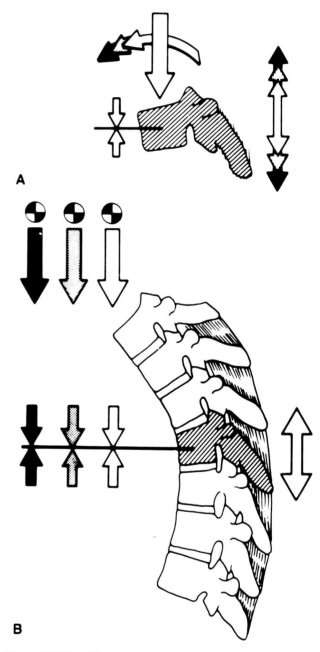

Figure 26.11. The structural and mechanical factors that may contribute to kyphosis are shown. *A,* The anterior elements are in compression and the posterior ones are in tension. *B,* Progressive kyphosis increases the moment arm, which adds more compression and tension. (Reprinted with permission from White AA, Panjabi MM: Clinical biomechanics of the spine. Philadelphia: JB Lippincott, 1990;156.)

Compression rods as treatment for traumatic conditions are ideal for posterior ligamentous disruptions, facet dislocations, and for countering the flexion instability of Chance-type fractures. Compression instrumentation should not be used in any injury with axial instability, i.e., loss of posterior facets and middle column failure. Application of compression rods in such cases may lead to retropulsion of bone in the spinal canal, induction of an iatrogenic scoliosis, or failure to protect against further vertebral collapse. If, however, an anterior decompressive and middle-column reconstruction procedure is performed first, application of compressive instrumentation seems ideal. The major disadvantage of this application is possible overcompression, which may lead to disc space narrowing or herniation.

The Gruca-Weiss springs were first developed by Gruca in 1956 for correction of scoliosis (44). Weiss expanded their use to include thoracolumbar trauma in 1975 (109). This device employs two large springs with hooks on the ends placed under tension on the section of the spine to be corrected. A large tensile force is created in the spring. Because of the curvature of the spine, these springs as well apply a small radially directed force. Use of the spring devices seems to have fallen out of favor within the last decade.

The type of complications associated with compression rod techniques are essentially no different from those described for distraction techniques. Isolated use of dual Harrington compressive instrumentation, however, has a higher rate of rod failure compared with Edwards or Cotrel-Dubousset devices because of the small rod diameter. But, the use of multiple-hook constructs can distribute the load more easily at the hook-rod or bone-implant interface, lessening the risk of failure of the bone or the implant. Other potential complications include neurologic injury, pseudarthrosis, loss of correction, iatrogenic deformity, and infection.

THORACOLUMBAR AND SACRAL SPINE— PEDICULAR SCREW CONSTRUCTS

The idea of pedicular screw fixation through a posterior approach is not new, but only recently has it gained popularity. Boucher, in 1959, first described the passing of long screws through the pedicle and into the vertebral body as a means of temporarily stabilizing lumbar and lumbosacral fusions, with very good results (10). Pennal et al., in 1964, followed up the initial work of Boucher, with similar good results (90). Roy-Camille (94) and Louis (67) developed a system of spine plates and pedicle screws for internal stabilization of the lumbar and cervical spine, which has been closely followed by several other alternatives. Included are systems developed by Steffee (102), Wiltse, Luque (72), Cotrel-Dubousset, Magerl

(75), Louis (67), the Vermont spinal fixator (63), the AO fixateur interne, the Puno-Winter-Byrd system, and others. These systems have all been developed in attempt to address problems of fixation in the lumbosacral spine. Ideally, a pedicle system should offer rigid segmental fixation with the ability to produce and maintain correction of deformity, while limiting the number of immobilized segments. Enhanced fusion rates, improved ease of patient postoperative care, and universal application of pedicle devices to a variety of clinical and pathologic conditions are also important. While there aren't many publications evaluating these devices, certain potential benefits and complications associated with these constructs are evident.

All pedicle screw constructs involve insertion of a screw through the pedicle into the vertebral body from a posteroanteromedial direction. These screws are then stabilized by one of several linkages including rods, plates, internal fixators, etc. Some of these linkages may in turn allow for control and application of sagittal plane and rotational forces on the vertebrae, while others are limited and provide primarily static stabilization. Each system has its own inherent advantages and disadvantages. It is crucial for the surgeon to choose a system based on the particular needs and clinical circumstances of each case.

The primary advantages of pedicular systems lie in its universal application, strength of fixation, and ability to limit the number of fused segments and maintain normal sagittal contour. Based on the studies of Roy-Camille and other biomechanical testing, the pedicle is generally considered to offer the site of most rigid vertebral segment fixation (94). This rigidity may negate the need for multilevel stabilization or even preempt the need for anterior fusion and stabilization procedures. The primary disadvantage of the posterior technique is its limited ability to correct deformity. While newer systems are attempting to address this problem, results of clinical application are limited.

Several biomechanically oriented studies have been published concerning pedicular fixation. Krag's study in 1986 not only introduced results in support for development of the Vermont spinal fixator, but also serves as an excellent review of several issues pertinent to pedicle fixation (63). Krag's results confirm that the vertebra contains ample room for safe pedicle fixation and that an increase in depth of screw penetration from 50–80% is accompanied by a significant increase in pullout strength.

Skinner and associates studied the pullout strengths of various pedicular systems (100). They also concluded that an increase in the major diameter of the screw was associated with an increase in pullout strength. Skinner et al. also proposed that insertion of the screw through the pedicle into the vertebral body endplate significantly enhanced pullout strength, while penetration of the anterior vertebral body cortex failed to improve fixation. Zindrick noted that osteoporosis is a significant negative factor in pullout strength (118). Wittenberg's study supports Zindrick's finding that quality of bone density may be more important than screw design (113). Zindrick noted that larger-diameter screw fixation enhanced overall pullout strength in almost all constructs. However, in contrast to Skinner's study, Zindrick noted improved fixation by engaging the anterior vertebral body cortex. For sacral fixation, screws directed laterally into the ala at 45° or medially into the pedicle offer the best fixation, while those directed straight, anteriorly were weaker.

Few reports are available that elucidate the results and indications of pedicle screw instrumentation. Steffee and Luque have anecdotally reported on the use of their instrumentation for a variety of conditions (72,102). However, no study has truly shown the efficacy of these latter devices in a controlled, randomized fashion. In a recent retrospective study by Bernhardt, fusion rates and clinical results were compared in patients undergoing lumbosacral fusion with or without internal fixation with the variable screw plate (VSP) system (6). The rate of pseudarthrosis was nearly the same as 22% of the VSP group, and 25% of the control group failed to obtain solid fusion. Likewise, clinical results were nearly identical, with 67% of the VSP group and 70% of the control group obtaining good or excellent results. Clearly, data from this study raise questions and concerns about the need and indications for internal fixation.

Several potential complications exist that have been reported in patients undergoing internal fixation with pedicular screw constructs. Possibilities of neural injury, hardware failure, pseudarthrosis, vascular injury, facet joint compromise, loss of correction, and infection exist.

Injury to the nerve root may occur directly by a drill, curette, awl, or screw, or may occur sometime during the postoperative period due to pedicle erosion with subsequent cutout and neural impingement. Rates of reported neural injury, however, have been low. Louis, in his large series of 401 patients, noted only six patients with a postoperative monoradiculopathy (67). All of his complications reportedly improved with removal of the screw. With the application of distractive or compressive forces through the pedicle screw, there is concern for increased risk of pedicle erosion or fracture, which may subsequently lead to development of neurologic injury.

Injury to the aorta, common iliac artery, their branches, or their venous counterparts must also be avoided (Fig. 26.12). Perforation of the anterior cortex at L4 or above may injure the aorta. As indicated earlier, engagement of the anterior cortex with the screw offers questionable improvement of fixation and therefore cannot be strongly advocated. Based on Krag's study, 80% depth of penetration appears to provide adequate strength of fixation for most constructs. At L5, the common iliac artery lies more lateral and is not likely to be injured. Great concern lies in the placement of screws into the sacrum. The common iliac artery bifurcates into the internal and external

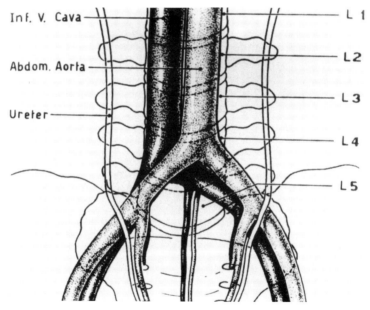

Figure 26.12. Transabdominal view of the abdominal aorta and inferior vena cava. The vertebral column is posterior to the vessels. The aorta lie to the left of the vena cava. (Montorsi W, Ghiringhelli C: Genesis: diagnosis and treatment of vascular complications after intervertebral disc surgery. Int Surg 1973;58:233.)

iliac vessels at this level and are found in the region of the sacral ala, which is considered by some to be the area of optimal fixation. Controversy again exists as to whether penetration of the anterior cortex is needed. Certainly, more than 1–2 mm of anterior penetration must be avoided. Anteromedial screw direction through the S1 pedicle seems to be a safe technique with reasonable biomechanical pullout strength.

A primary reason to use pedicular fixation is to enhance fusion of the lumbosacral segments. Louis reported a 97.4% rate of fusion in his series (67), while Steffee indicated only five failures in 120 patients (102). These findings are in contrast to the study by Bernhardt, who found a 22% incidence of pseudarthrosis in a small series of 18 patients with the VSP system, and a 26% rate of pseudarthrosis in a noninstrumented control group of patients (6). Further clinical data are needed in the form of a randomized prospective study to define the true efficacy of pedicular fixation in promoting fusion and improving clinical results.

Hardware failure has also been a relatively common problem with pedicular screw systems. Roy-Camille reported a 25% failure rate of distal screws in a series of 84 acute lumbar fractures (94). Louis, in his series of 401 posterior pedicle screw-plate cases, noted eight patients with broken pedicle screws and an additional six screws, which had apparently loosened from the sacrum (67). Steffee, reporting on 128 patients, noted hardware problems in eight patients including loosening, migration, or breakage (102). Zucherman reported a higher rate of complications using the VSP system, noting that 18 of 77 patients had one or more broken screws (119). However, similar to Steffee's report, these problems improved with redesigned screws.

A significant problem in pedicular screw fixation appears to be at the site of linkage between the screw and rod or plate. An extremely rigid connection may lead to increased stress at this junction with subsequent risk for breakage. Use of large-diameter screws, improved linkage design, and use of biomaterials more compatible with bone may improve upon these problems and improve fusion rates.

Impingement of the facet joint proximal to the level of instrumentation is a potential problem. Due to the location of the pedicle in relation to the facet joint in the lumbar spine, a portion of the facet capsule and the inferior edge of the facet joint may require removal. Partial arthrectomy may lead to mechanical compromise of the joint and, on a long-term-basis, may accelerate arthritic changes. Arthritic compromise may be limited by angling the uppermost screw in a cephalad and medial direction. The particular design of the screw, plate, or rod also has a direct effect on the mechanical compromise of this joint.

At the level of the sacrum, care must be taken not to direct the screw too laterally. Deep penetration of the sacroiliac joint may be a cause of chronic postoperative pain.

Other potential complications with these pedicle systems include loss of correction or overcorrection of deformity. Higher rates of infection also appear to be a problem with such instrumentation because of increased operative time, larger dissection, and insertion of hardware. When infection has occurred, immediate opening and debridement of the wound are strongly urged, leaving the hardware in place, if at all possible. The wound should be left open initially, and dressing changes completed daily. Depending on the subsequent status of the wound, it may be secondarily closed or allow for secondary intention healing.

Prominence of the hardware is also a potential problem, especially in the very thin patient. These devices generally tend to be bulky and may be bothersome, especially with fusions extending down to the sacrum. In some patients in this latter category, such prominence may necessitate removal of the hardware after the fusion mass has matured.

THORACOLUMBAR AND SACRAL CONSTRUCTS—POSTERIOR SEGMENTAL FIXATION

Luque introduced his segmental form of spinal instrumentation in 1970s as a method of surgically correcting scoliosis (69,71). It involves the use of segmental sublaminar wire fixation to contoured smooth rods. Luque instrumentation has also been employed in the surgical treatment of specific traumatic injuries of the thoracolumbar spine (73).

As indicated earlier, the correctional ability of the Harrington distraction system increases with the severity of the deformity. However, as the deformity is corrected, the system's ability to further obtain correction is diminished. The opposite is true for systems such as the Luque or Drummonds spinous wiring technique, which employs pure transverse loading as the corrective mechanism. The corrected moment for the lateral force decreases as the deformity increases (Fig. 26.13). By the same token, as correction is obtained, the same incremental correction of the deformity can be obtained with less force. Most current biomechanical studies indicate that the use of both axial and transverse corrective forces is superior in obtaining correction. Clearly, segmental forms of instrumentation require little force to support a straight spine, making it an excellent neutralization technique for minimally deformed and nondeformed spinal segments. Additionally, multiple-level fixation sites are

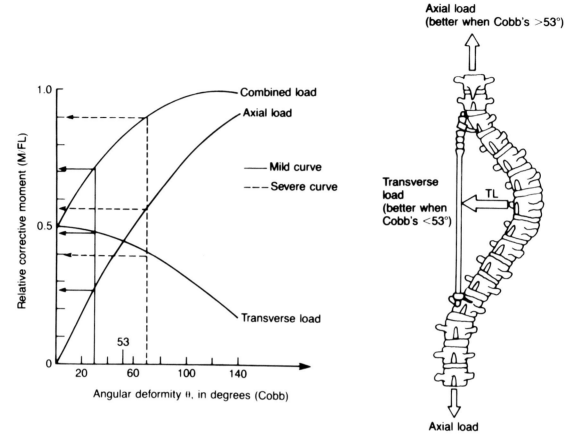

Figure 24.13. A graphic representation of relative corrective moment as a function of spine deformity. According to this model, a combination of axial and transvere loads is the most efficient for any degree of deformity. Axial load efficiency increases with angular deformity while the transverse load efficiency decreases with angular deformity. The deformity angle of 53° is a break-even point for the axial and transverse loads. Examples of two theoretical patients with mild (30°) and severe (70°) curves are shown. (Reprinted with permission from White AA, Panjabi MM: Clinical biomechanics of the spine. Philadelphia: JB Lippincott, 1990;142.)

advantageous in dispersing loads at each vertebra and in diminishing the possibility of hardware or bony failure.

Given the armamentarium of spinal instrumentation now available, the use of Luque segmental wire fixation in traumatic conditions is limited. Purely translational injuries without an axially compressive element may be the primary indication to consider such instrumentation. However, the possibility of neurologic injury to already compromised, edematous tissues may outweigh the potential benefits of this construct.

Luque instrumentation probably remains the technique of choice in dealing with neuromuscular spinal deformities in which soft bone does not allow for use of other techniques. It is able to maintain sagittal contours more effectively, while providing the most secure pelvic fixation currently available.

The greatest fear of employing Luque segmental fixation is neurologic compromise. Recent studies employing this technique in idiopathic scoliosis show only a slight increase in serious neurologic complications compared with the Harrington device (28). However, there appears to be a marked increase in patient complaints of dysesthesia (10%). This neurologic response is most likely related to the trauma associated with passage of sublaminar wires and the fixed, rigid nature of the construct itself. The Luque construct may lead to compromise of blood flow to the cord and may initiate ischemic changes. Use of somatosensory evoked potentials or employment of the Stagnara wake-up test intraoperatively may limit these complications. As indicated earlier, in cases of postoperative paraplegia, the patient should be immediately returned to surgery and hardware removed to optimize outcome. Most cases of dysesthesia resolve over a period of 6–10 weeks without intervention.

Other complications include increased operative time, greater blood loss, hardware failure (wire breakage), and pseudarthrosis. If the implant has to be removed, great care must be taken in removal of cut sublaminar wires. The possibility of cord injury or creating a dural leak exists when wires are extracted. In the region of thoracic cord or conus medullaris, many advocate leaving the wires in place. If wire removal is thought to be necessary, careful and controlled extraction is necessary. Wrapping the wire around the tip of needle-nose pliers during the extraction process may be the most effective and safe method. Drummonds' spinous wiring technique provides a surgical construct that biomechanically is nearly equal in strength to that of the Luque technique and avoids the passage of sublaminar wires. Without sublaminar wires, the incidence of neurologic injury is markedly diminished. Likewise, removal of the device is simpler and should not be associated with the same potential of neural compromise.

THORACOLUMBAR AND SACRAL CONSTRUCTS—UNIVERSAL OR MODULAR INSTRUMENTATION

The Cotrel-Dubousset, TSRH, Edwards, and Isola spinal implants represent systems with universal or modular application. Pedicle screws can be used in conjunction with the various hooks to provide rigid segmental fixation, while also allowing for multidirectional control and correction of deformity. Stability and rigidity of the implants are further enhanced by various cross-linking devices, creating a quadrangular construct. These devices are currently used for deformity, trauma, and degenerative conditions.

The Cotrel-Dubousset system represents the first of such systems. Devised originally for surgical treatment of scoliosis, its use has now greatly expanded to include stabilization of virtually all conditions. The Cotrel-Dubousset system is able to employ distraction, compression, and transverse loading, as well as the ability to contour the rods in obtaining correction. This segmental form of fixation using a hook construct seems ideal in the treatment of deformity. Cotrel reported on 250 patients with scoliosis, kyphosis, and lordosis with the Cotrel-Dubousset instrumentation. Overall correction averaged 66% without utilization of postoperative external support (24). Significant improvement in the sagittal plane of the deformity was also reported through derotation. A mean correction of 77% was seen in paralytic curves.

The universal application of these devices is appealing and probably represents the wave of the future. Those developments add significantly to the complexity of an already vast armamentarium available to the spinal surgeon. It is cautioned, however, that use of such instrumentation by the occasional spine surgeon may be fraught with technical difficulty and complication. Until long-term results are available, the spine surgeon should exercise caution with these instrumentations.

REFERENCES

1. Akbarnia BA, Fogarty JP, Tayob AA: Contoured Harrington instrumentation in the treatment of unstable spinal fractures: effect of supplemental sublaminar wires. Clin Orthop 1984;189:186.
2. Albee FH: Transplantation of a portion of tibia into the spine for Pott's disease. JAMA 1911;57:885.
3. Ashman RB, Birch JG, Bone LB, et al: Mechanical testing of spinal instrumentation. Clin Orthop 1988;227:113.
4. Balderston RA, Winter RB, Moe JH, et al: Fusion to the sacrum for non-paralytic scoliosis in the adult. Spine 1986;11:824.
5. Barbour JR. Screw fixation in fracture of the odontoid process. S Aust Clin 1971;5:20.
6. Bernhardt M, Swartz DE, Clothiaux PL, Crowell RR, White AA III: Posterior lumbar and lumbosacral fusion with and without pedicle screw internal fixation (Abstract). Presented at the Internat Soc Study Lumbar Spine Boston, 1990.
7. Bohler J: Anterior stabilization of acute fractures and nonunions of the dens. J Bone Joint Surg 1982;64A:18.
8. Bohlman HH: Cervical spine and cord: Trauma. Operative Techniques. In: Orthopaedic Knowledge Update 2, AAOS. 1987;275–276.
9. Bosworth D, Cobb J, Ettenson M: Occipitocervical fusion for tuberculosis of cervical spine. Quart Bull Sea View Hosp 1953;14:143–161.
10. Boucher HH: A method of spinal fusion. J Bone Joint Surg 1959;41B:248.
11. Bradford DS, Ahmed KB, Moe JH, Winter RB, Lonstein JE: The surgical management of patients with Scheuermann's disease: a review of twenty-four cases managed by combined anterior and posterior spine fusion. J Bone Joint Surg 1980;62A:705.
12. Brooks AL, Jenkins EG: Atlanto-axial arthrodesis by the wedge compression method. J Bone Joint Surg 1978;60A:279.
13. Burwell RG: The fate of bone grafts. In: Apley AG, ed. Recent advances in orthopaedics. London: Churchill, Livingstone 1969;115.
14. Callahan RA, Johnson RM, Margolis RN, et al: Cervical facet fusion for control of instability following laminectomy. J Bone Joint Surg 1977;59A:991–1002.
15. Caspar W: Anterior cervical fusion and interbody stabilization with the trapezial osteosynthetic plate technique. Aesculap Wissenschaftl. Informationen Aesculp-Werke AG, D-7200, Tuttlingen, West Germany, 1986.
16. Caspar W: Anterior stabilization with trapezial osteosynthetic plate technique in cervical spine injuries. In: Kehr P, Weidner A, eds. Cervical spine I. Wein-New York: Springer-Verlag, 1987;198.
17. Clark CR, White AA: Fracture of the dens. A multicenter study. J Bone Joint Surg 1985;67A:1340.
18. Cloward R: Gas-sterilized cadaver bone grafts for spinal fusion operations. A simplified bone bank. Spine 1980;5:4.
19. Coe JD, Warden KE, Sutterlin CE III, McAfee P: Biomechanical

19. evaluation of cervical spine stabilization methods in a human cadaveric model. Spine 1989;14:1122–31.

20. Conaty JP, Mongan ES: Cervical fusion in rheumatoid arthritis. J Bone Joint Surg 1981;63A:1218–1227.

21. Cooper PR, Cohen A, Rosiello A, Koslow M: Posterior stabilization of the cervical spine fractures and subluxations using plates and screws. Neurosurg 1988;23:300.

22. Correia MMA: Anterior cervical fusion—indications and results. In: Kehr P, Weidner A, eds. Cervical spine I. Wein-New York: Springer-Verlag, 1987;205.

23. Cotler JM, Vernace JV, Michalski JA: The use of Harrington rods in thoracolumbar fractures. Orthop Clin North Am 1986;17:87.

24. Cotrel Y, Dubousset J, Guillaumat M: New universal instrumentation in spinal surgery. Clin Orthop 1988;277:10–23.

25. Denis F, Ruiz H, Searls K: Comparison between square-ended distraction rods and standard round-ended distraction rods in the treatment of spinal injuries: a statistical analysis. Clin Orthop 1984;189:162.

26. DeWald RL: Burst fractures of the thoracic and lumbar spine. Clin Orthop 1984;189:150.

27. Dickson JH, Harrington TR, Erwin WD: Results of reduction and stabilization of the severely fractured thoracic and lumbar spine. J Bone Joint Surg 1978;60A:799–805.

28. Dove J: Segmental wiring for spinal deformity. A morbidity report. Spine 1989;14:229–31.

29. Dwyer AP: A fatal complication of paravertebral infection and traumatic aneurysm following Dwyer instrumentation. In: Proc Austral Orthop Assoc. J Bone Joint Surg 1979;61B:239.

30. Dwyer AF, Newton NC, Sherwood AA: An anterior approach to scoliosis. A preliminary report. Clin Orthop 1969;62:192.

31. Dwyer AF, Schafer MF: Anterior approach to scoliosis. Results of treatment in fifty-one cases. J Bone Joint Surg 1974;56B:218.

32. Edwards CC, Levine AM: Early rod-sleeve stabilization of the injured thoracic and lumbar spine. Orthop Clin North Am 1986;17:121.

33. Edwards CC, York JJ, Levine AM, et al: Determinants of spinal hook dislodgement. Orthop Trans 1986;10:8.

34. Fielding JW, Hawkins RJ, Ratzan SA: Spine fusion for atlanto-axial instability. J Bone Joint Surg 1976;58A:400.

35. Flesch JR, Leider LL, Erickson DL, et al: Harrington instrumentation and spine fusion for unstable fracture and fracture-dislocations of the thoracic and lumbar spine. J Bone Joint Surg 1977;59A:143.

36. Flesch JR, Leider LL, Erickson DL, et al: Harrington instrumentation and spine fusions for unstable fractures and fracture-dislocations of the thoracic and lumbar spine. J Bone Joint Surg 1977;59A:143.

37. Foerster O: Die leitungsbahnen des schmerzgefuhls und die chirurgische behandlung der schmerzzustande. Berlin: Urban & Schwarzenberg 1927;226.

38. Gaines RW, Breedlove R, Monson G: Stabilization of thoracic and thoracolumbar fracture-dislocations with Harrington rods and sublaminar wires. Clin Orthop 1984;189–195.

39. Gaines RW, Leatherman KD: Benefits of Harrington compression instrumentation in lumbar and thoracolumbar idiopathic scoliosis in adolescents and adults. Spine 1981;6:483.

40. Gallie WE: Fractures and dislocations of the cervical spine. Am J Surg 1939;46:495.

41. Gassmann J, Seligson D: The anterior cervical plate. Spine 1983;8:700.

42. Gertzbein SD, MacMichael D, Tile M: Harrington instrumentation as a method of fixation in fractures of the spine: a critical analysis of deficiencies. J Bone Joint Surg 1982;64B:526.

43. Griswold DM, et al: Atlanto-axial fusion for instability. J Bone Joint Surg 1978;60A:285.

44. Gruca A: Protocol of the 41st Congress of Indian Orthopaedics and Traumatology. Bologna, 1956.

45. Hall JE: Dwyer instrumentation in anterior fusion of the spine. J Bone Joint Surg 1981;63A:1188.

46. Hamblen DL: Occipito-cervical fusion. Indications, techniques and results. J Bone Joint Surg 1967;49B:33–45.

47. Harrington PR: Treatment of scoliosis. Correction and internal fixation by spine instrumentation. J Bone Joint Surg 1962;44A:491.

48. Hasday CA, Passoff TL, Perry J: Gait abnormalities arising from iatrogenic loss of lumbar lordosis secondary to Harrington instrumentation in lumbar fractures. Spine 1983;8:501.

49. Herring JA, Wenger DR: Segmental spinal instrumentation: a preliminary report of 40 consecutive cases. Spine 1982;7:285.

50. Herrmann HD: Metal plate fixation after anterior fusion of unstable fracture dislocations of the cervical spine. Acta Neurochir 1975;32:101.

51. Hibbs RH: An operation for progressive spinal deformities. NY J Med 1911;93:1013.

52. Holness RO, Huestis WS, Howes WJ, et al: Posterior stabilization with an interlaminar clamp in cervical injuries: technical note and review of the long term experience with the method. Neurosurgery 1984;14:318.

53. Holt RT, Leatherman KD, Zwemer RJ: Zielke instrumentation experience. Orthop Trans 1983;7:31.

54. Itoh T, Tsuji H, Katoh Y, et al: Occipitocervical fusion reinforced by Luque's segmental spinal instrumentation for rheumatoid diseases. Spine 1988;13:1234.

55. Jacobs RR, Asher MA, Snider RK: Thoracolumbar spinal injuries: a comparative study of recumbent and operative treatment in 100 patients. Spine 1980;5:463.

56. Jacobs RR, Casey MP: Surgical management of thoracolumbar spinal injuries: General principles and controversial considerations. Clin Orthop 1984;189:22.

57. Johnson RM, Owen JR, Panjabi MM, et al: Immediate strength of certain fusion techniques. Orthop Trans 1980;4:42.

58. Kaneda K, Kuniyoshi A, Fujiya M: Burst fractures with neurologic deficits of the thoracolumbar-lumbar spine. Results of anterior decompression and stabilization with anterior instrumentation. Spine 1984;9:788.

59. Keene JS, Wackwitz DL, Drummond DS, et al: Compression-distraction instrumentation of unstable thoracolumbar fractures: anatomic results obtained with each type of injury and method of instrumentation. Spine 1986;11:895.

60. Kohler R, Galland O, Mechin H, et al: The Dwyer procedure in the treatment of idiopathic scoliosis. A 10-year follow-up review of 21 patients. Spine 1990;15:75–80.

61. Kostuik JP: Anterior fixation for fractures of the thoracic and lumbar spine with or without neurologic involvement. Clin Orthop 1984;189:103.

62. Kostuik JP, Hall BB: Spinal fusions to the sacrum in adults with scoliosis. Spine 1983;8:489.

63. Krag MH: An internal fixation for posterior application to short segments of the thoracic, lumbar or lumbosacral spine. Clin Orthop 1986;203:75.

64. Lagrone MO, Bradford DS, Moe JH, et al: Treatment of symptomatic flatback after spinal fusion. J Bone Joint Surg 1988;70A:569.

65. Lee CK: Langrana NA: Lumbosacral spinal fusion. A biomechanical study. Spine 1984;9:574.

66. Lipscomb PR: Cervico-occipital fusion for congenital and post-

traumatic anomalies of the atlas and axis. J Bone Joint Surg 1957; 39A:1289–1301.

67. Louis R: Fusion of the lumbar and sacral spine by internal fixation with screw plates. Clin Orthop 1986;203:18.

68. Lowe TG: Zielke pedicular instrumentation and fusion for instability of the lumbosacral spine. Orthop Trans 1988;12:665.

69. Luque ER: Anatomy of scoliosis and its correction. Clin Orthop 1974;105:298.

70. Luque ER: The anatomic basis and development of segmental spinal instrumentation. Spine 1982;7:256.

71. Luque ER: Segmental spinal instrumentation for correction of scoliosis. Clin Orthop 1982;163:192.

72. Luque ER: Interpeduncular segmental fixation. Clin Orthop 1986;203:54.

73. Luque ER, Cassis N, Ramirez-Weilla G: Segmental spinal instrumentation in the treatment of fractures of the thoracolumbar spine. Spine 1982;7:312.

74. MacEwen GD, Bunnell WP, Sriram K: Acute neurological complications in the treatment of scoliosis. J Bone Joint Surg 1975; 57A:404–408.

75. Magerl FP: Stabilization of the lower thoracic lumbar spine with external skeletal fixation. Clin Orthop 1984;189:125.

76. Magerl F, Grob D, Seeman P: Stable dorsal fusion of the cervical spine (C2-T1) using hook plates. In: Kehr P, Weidner A, eds. Cervical spine I. Wein-New York: Springer-Verlag, 1987;217.

77. McAfee PC, Bohlman HH: Complications following Harrington instrumentation for fractures of the thoracolumbar spine. J Bone Joint Surg 1985;67A:672.

78. McAfee PC, Werner FW, Glisson RR: A biomechanical analysis of spinal instrumentation systems in thoracolumbar fractures. Spine 1985;10:204.

79. McGraw RW, Rusch RM: Atlanto-axial arthrodesis. J Bone Joint Surg 1973;55B:482.

80. Mino DE, Stauffer ES, Davis PK, et al: Torsional loading of Harrington distraction rod instrumentation compared to segmental sublaminar and spinous process supplementation. Orthop Trans 1985;9:119.

81. Moe JH, Denis F: The iatrogenic loss of lumbar lordosis. Orthop Trans 1977;1:131.

82. Moe JH, Purcell GA, Bradford DS: Zielke instrumentation (VDS) for the correction of spinal curvature. Clin Orthop 1983; 180:133.

83. Nachemson A, Elfstrom G: Intravital wireless telemetry of axial forces in Harrington distraction rods in patients with idiopathic scoliosis. J Bone Joint Surg 1971;53A:445.

84. Nagel DA, Koogle TA, Piziali RL, et al: Stability of the upper lumbar spine following progressive disruptions and the application of individual internal and external fixation devices. J Bone Joint Surg 1981;63A:62.

85. Nasca RJ, Whelchel JD: Use of cyropreserved bone in spinal surgery. Spine 1987;12:222.

86. Nordt JC, Stauffer ES: Sequelae of atlantoaxial subluxation in two patients with Down syndrome. Spine 1981;6:437.

87. Osebold WR, Weinstein JL, Sprague BL: Thoracolumbar spine fractures: results of treatment. Spine 1981;6:13.

88. Panjabi MM, Abumi K, Duranceau JS: Three-dimensional stability of thoracolumbar fractures stabilized with eight different instrumentations. Trans Orthop Res Soc 1987;12:458.

89. Pelker RR, Duranceau JS, Panjabi MM: Cervical spine stabilization—a three dimensional, biomechanical, evaluation of stability, strength and failure mechanism. (Submitted for publication in Spine).

90. Pennal GF, McDonald GA, Dale GG: A method of spinal fusion using internal fixation. Clin Orthop 1964;35:86.

91. Quinnell RC, Stockdale HR: Some experimental observations of the influence of a simple lumbar floating fusion on the remaining lumbar spine. Spine 1981;6:263.

92. Roy-Camille R, Gagna G, Lazennec JY: L'arthrodese occipito-cervicale. In: Roy-Camille R, ed. Semes journees d'orthopedie de la Pitie. Rachis cervical superieur, Paris: Masson, 1986;49–51.

93. Roy-Camille R, Mazel C, Saillant G: Treatment of cervical spine injuries by a posterior osteosynthesis with plates and screws. In: Kehr P, Weidner A, eds. Cervical spine I. Wein-New York: Springer-Verlag, 1987;163.

94. Roy-Camille R, Saillant G, Mazel C: Internal fixation of the lumbar spine with pedicle screw plating. Clin Orthop 1986;203:7.

95. Schlapfer F, Worsdorfer O, Magerl F, et al: Stabilization of the lower thoracic and lumbar spine: comparative in vitro investigation of an external skeletal and various internal fixation devices. In: Uhthoff HK, ed. Current concepts of external fixation of fractures. New York: Springer-Verlag, 1982;367.

96. Schneider JR, Bright RW: Anterior cervical fusion using preserved bone allografts. Transplant Proc Suppl 1976;1:73.

97. Scoliosis Research Society: Morbidity and mortality committee report. Park Ridge, IL, Scoliosis Research Society, 1985.

98. Scoliosis Research Society: Morbidity and mortality committee report. Park Ridge, IL, 1987.

99. Scoliosis Research Society: Morbidity and mortality committee report. Park Ridge, IL, 1987.

100. Skinner R, Transfeldt EE, Maybee J, et al: Experimental testing and comparison of screw design variables in transpedicular screw fixation: a biomechanical study. Presented at the AAOS Annual Meeting, Atlanta, 1988.

101. Stauffer ES, Neil JL: Biomechanical analysis of structural stability of internal fixation in fractures of the thoracolumbar spine. Clin Orthop 1975;112:159.

102. Steffee AD, Biscup RS, Sitkowski DJ: Segmental spine plates with pedicle screw fixation. Clin Orthop 1986;203:45.

103. Sutterlin CE, McAfee PC, Warden KE, Rey RM Jr, Farey ID: A biomechanical evaluation of cervical spine stabilization methods in a bovine model. Static and cyclic loading. Spine 1988;13:795–802.

104. Tomford WW, Starkweather RJ, Goldman MH: A study of clinical incidence of infection in the use of banked allograft bone. J Bone Joint Surg 1981;63A:244.

105. Ulrich C, Woersdoerfer O, Claes L, et al: Comparative stability of anterior or posterior cervical plate fixation in vitro investigation. In: Kehr P, Weidner A, eds. Cervical spine I. Vienna-New York: Springer-Verlag, 1987;65.

106. Ward JJ, Nasca RJ, Lemons JE, et al: Cyclic torsional testing of Harrington and Luque spinal implants. Orthop Trans 1985;9:118.

107. Waugh T: Intravital measurements during instrument correction of idiopathic scoliosis. Gothenburg, Sweden, Tryckeri, AB Litotup, 1966.

108. Weidner A: Internal fixation with metal plates and screws. In: The cervical spine research society, eds. The cervical spine, 2nd ed. Philadelphia: JB Lippincott, 1989;404–421.

109. Weiss M: Dynamic spine alloplasty (spring loading corrective device) after fracture and spinal cord injury. Clin Orthop 1975; 112:150.

110. Wertheim SB, Bohlman HH: Occipitocervical fusion: Indica-

tions, technique and long term results in thirteen patients. J Bone Joint Surg 1987;69A:833–836.

111. White AA, Panjabi MM, Thomas CL: The clinical biomechanics of kyphotic deformities. Clin Orthop 1977;128:8.

112. White AA and Panjabi MM: Clinical biomechanics of the spine. Philadelphia: JB Lippincott Co., 1978.

113. Wittenberg RH, Lee KS, Coffee MS, et al: The effect of screw design and bone mineral density on transpedicular fixation in human and calf vertebral bodies. Seventh meeting of European Society of Biomechanics. Aarhus, Denmark, 1990.

114. Yosipovitch Z, Robin GC, Makin M: Open reduction of unstable thoracolumbar spinal injuries and fixation using Harrington rods. J Bone Joint Surg 1977;59A:1003.

115. Yuan HA, Mann KA, Found EM, et al: Early clinical experience with the Syracuse I-plate: an anterior spinal fixation device. Spine 1988;13:278.

116. Zhang Zh, Yin H, Yang K, et al: Anterior intervertebral disc excision and bone grafting in cervical spondylotic myelopathy. Spine 1983;8:16.

117. Zielke K, Stunkat R, Beaujean F: Ventrale derotations—spondylodese. Arch Orthop Unfallchir 1976;85:257.

118. Zindrick MR, Wiltse LL, Widell EH, et al: A biomechanical study of intrapeduncular screw fixation in the lumbosacral spine. Clin Orthop 1986;203:99.

119. Zucherman J, Hsu K, White A, et al: Early results of spinal fusion using variable spine plating system. Presented at North Amer Spine Soc annual meeting, Banff, Alberta, Canada, 1987.

INDEX

Page numbers followed by *t* and *f* indicate tables and figures, respectively.

457